Understanding Lens Surfacing

Understanding Lens Surfacing

Clifford W. Brooks, O.D.
Indiana University

Butterworth–Heinemann

Boston   London   Oxford   Singapore   Sydney   Toronto   Wellington

Library of Congress Cataloging-in-Publication Data

Brooks, Clifford W.
    Understanding lens surfacing / Clifford W. Brooks.
        p.   cm.
    Includes bibliographical references and index.
    ISBN 0-7506-9177-8 (casebound)
    1. Ophthalmic lenses.   I. Title.
    [DNLM: 1. Eyeglasses. 2. Optics.   WW 350 B873u]
    RE976.B78   1991
    617.7′522—dc20
    DNLM/DLC
    for Library of Congress   91-10958
                                                          CIP

British Library Cataloguing in Publication Data
Brooks, Clifford W.
    Understanding lens surfacing.
    1. Ophthalmology
    I. Title
    617.752

    ISBN 0-7506-9177-8

Butterworth–Heinemann
80 Montvale Avenue
Stoneham, MA 02180

10 9 8 7 6 5 4 3 2 1

Printed in the United States of America

To my children—Debbie, Cliff, and Abigail—who are a constant delight to me.

Contents

Foreword

Dr. Clifford Brooks' book *Understanding Lens Surfacing* is the finest and most complete publication on ophthalmic lens surfacing I have ever reviewed. Most of the pages of the work contain descriptions of procedures, calculations, and other information concerning lens surfacing that has never been offered in print.

The book is not only for the laboratory optician. It is an excellent background and source for ophthalmic dispensers and for any ophthalmic professional interested in ophthalmic lens processing.

The major strengths of the book are its invaluable charts, and the meticulous methods the author explains in each section. The explanation of correcting vertical imbalance is extremely well written. Throughout the book there are many examples and homework problems that are useful not only for a classroom, but are also helpful for self-study. The book will serve as an ideal textbook for students or apprentices.

Many budding authors have thoughts about writing a book "someday." Dr. Brooks has already written a number of valuable books for the optical industry: *System for Ophthalmic Dispensing* (1979) with Irvin M. Borish, O.D., and *Essentials for Ophthalmic Lens Work* (1983) are among his most important publications. One of the last prominent sourcebooks on surfacing was the *B&L Job Coach* although lens surfacing was covered in only a part of the book and it was published well over 40 years ago when lens generation did not even exist. My congratulations to Dr. Brooks on producing an extremely useful and valuable book for the ophthalmic industry.

BOYD C. HALSTEAD, M.S., F.N.A.O.
Professor
Director Opticianry Program
Ferris State University

Preface

An understanding of lens surfacing is invaluable for anyone who works in the world of ophthalmic lenses and frames. Dispensers use it in making decisions about frames and lenses, prescribers employ it to realize patient-benefitting new possibilities, while those who work directly in surfacing need it in order to serve knowledgeably those who depend on their optical expertise.

This text is designed for both those who are studying in an academic setting and those who are learning on the job. In an academic setting the traditional approach is to begin with Chapter 1 and work through the chapters in sequential order. When learning on the job, however, an individual does not always have the option of starting at an academically convenient point. Instead one may find oneself in immediate need of information in later chapters. Fortunately, most chapters are independently understandable, even when studied out of order. Those learning on the job should simply turn to that area where they are working and begin there.

Through conscientious study of the text, individuals can attain an optical and mechanical understanding of the surfacing process that will both enhance their present abilities and see them through the rapidly changing optical field of the future.

Acknowledgments

It is difficult to know where to begin in extending proper acknowledgment to those whose help made the writing of this book possible. There are so many who were so helpful during each phase of development that it is not possible to give the proper credit to all who assisted in so many different ways. Each of my students who pointed out omissions, made suggestions, found errors in the working manuscript, and even asked questions which, by their nature, pointed out deficiencies in the text, deserves to be listed by name. Without their input, this project would never have been accomplished. My thanks go out to the many individuals within the optical industry who represent ophthalmic manufacturers and suppliers. These individuals are constantly and conscientiously serving optical laboratories, opticians, optometrists, and ophthalmologists. They have been, and continue to be, an invaluable resource to me. In my attempt to find information and solve unanswered questions, these people have been consistent in their willingness to help, without regard for personal or corporate gain. They are truly an outstanding group.

I must once more extend special thanks to Jacque Kubley for his original photography, exacting illustrations, professional counsel, and personal expertise in bringing understanding through the graphic media.

For help in answers to practical questions, obtaining needed materials for photographs and, in some instances, serving as models in these photographs, my thanks go to Robert Ruff, Sharon Hamontre, Jill Mattingly, and Kathy Billman.

For assistance in helping me master the needed additional computer skills necessary for producing lens layout illustrations, my thanks go to Judith Felty.

For typing and retyping the manuscript, and for keeping a careful eye out for unintended errors in spelling, grammar, and illogical or incomplete thoughts, my thanks go to Laura Shipley, Angela Gray, Robert Cowles, Terri Hahn, and Jane Crowe. Special thanks also go to Gloria Cochran for making certain that secretarial help was available in a timely and consistent manner.

Appreciation for ideas, materials, and information pertaining to this text go also to Harry Cook, Bill and Al White, James Dirheimer, and many of the other employees of Diversified Ophthalmic Optical Lab in Cincinnati; Leo Elsky and Pat Steighner of Coburn Optical Industries; Rodney Tahran and Michael Daley of the Varilux Corporation; and Kevin Thompson of Gerber Scientific.

For reviewing the text in a timely and thorough manner, and for offering many valuable suggestions, thanks to Russell Hess and Boyd Halstead of Ferris State College.

Thanks go to the many individuals and companies who supplied special photos or illustrations. These are acknowledged throughout the text.

Special thanks go to my wife Vickie, who encouraged me to press forward in completing the task.

CLIFFORD W. BROOKS

1

Review of Optics

Lens Power

Lens power refers to where the lens brings light to a focus. The closer the focal point is to the lens itself, the more the light rays are affected by the lens. Lens power is expressed as the reciprocal of the distance in meters from the lens plane to the focal point.

$$\frac{1}{f'_v} = D'_v$$

In this equation f'_v is the distance from the back surface of the lens to the focal point and D'_v is the back vertex power of the lens in diopters of lens power. (Some references use the notation F'_v for back vertex power instead of D'_v.)

If the light rays converge as the light leaves the lens, the distance from the lens is expressed as a positive number and the lens is a *positive* or *plus* lens. See Figure 1-1. For example, if the light is brought to a focus 20 cm beyond the lens, the lens has a power of

$$\frac{1}{0.20 \text{ m}} = 5.00 \text{ D}$$

Units of lens power are called *diopters* and are abbreviated as *D* or *dpt.* Therefore a plus lens with

its focal point 20 cm (i.e., 0.20 m) away from the lens has a power of 5.00 D.

If light rays are caused to diverge as they leave the lens, as shown in Figure 1-2, they may be traced backward to a specific point. Although the rays never physically focus at this point, it is still considered the focal point of the lens. Because this point must be reached by measuring backward, its distance from the lens is given a negative value, making the dioptric value of the lens minus as well. If such a lens has a focal point -20 cm from the lens, its power is -5.00 D.

Sphere, Cylinder, and Axis

The three basic components of an ophthalmic prescription are the sphere, cylinder, and axis values. The *sphere* component has been essentially explained in the context of lens power. If a lens prescription has only a sphere component, there is only one point toward which all light rays converge or from which they diverge. Many prescriptions include only a sphere component.

The *sphere* component of a lens corrects vision for farsightedness or nearsightedness. Plus spherical lenses correct for farsightedness (hyperopia),

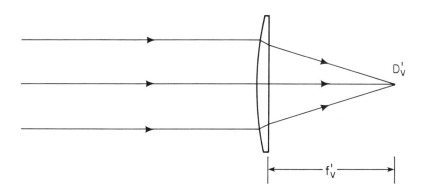

Figure 1-1 A plus lens brings light rays to a single focal point.

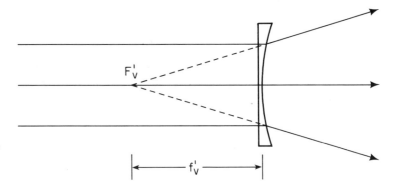

Figure 1-2 A minus lens causes rays to diverge and makes them appear as if they were coming from a single point in space.

whereas minus lenses correct for nearsightedness (myopia).

Cylinder and Axis

Some prescriptions have a zero value for the sphere but do have *cylinder* and *axis* components. If a cylinder value is given, there must also be an axis value so that it is possible to tell which way the cylinder is to be turned.

Just as a plus spherical lens can be visualized as having been cut from one side of a sphere, so can a plus cylinder be visualized as having been cut from a cylinder. However, when parallel light strikes a plus cylinder, the rays converge, not to a single point, but rather to a series of points that form a line focus; see Figure 1-3. The dioptric value of the

cylinder is the inverse of the distance from the lens to its line focus. As with spherical lenses, this focal distance is measured in meters.

Astigmatism results when the front surface of the eye is shaped more like a football than a spherical basketball. The cylinder component of the prescription corrects for this astigmatism.

As shown in Figure 1-4, the midline paralleling the long axis of a cylinder has no power to bend light. The *axis meridian* indicates the orientation of

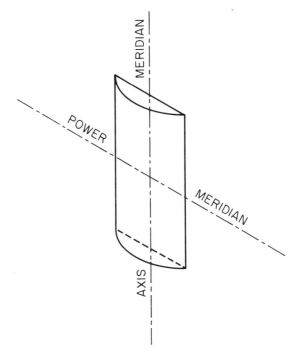

Figure 1-4 The front and back surfaces along the axis meridian are parallel. They have no power to bend light. The front surface of the cylinder along the power meridian is curved differently than the back surface. Therefore the lens bends light in this meridian.

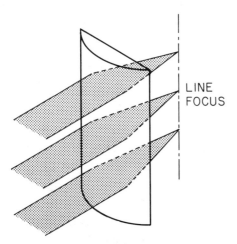

Figure 1-3 A plus cylinder does not converge all rays to a single point focus. Because it refracts light in only one meridian, rays are brought to a line focus.

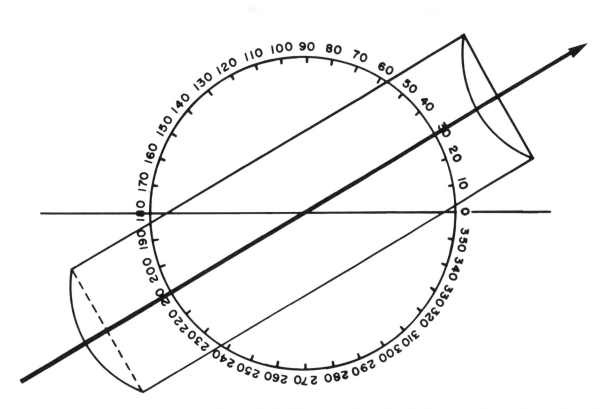

Figure 1-5 The orientation of a cylinder is specified in degrees from 0 to 180. Specifying beyond 180 is unnecessary because values beyond 180 merely duplicate 0 through 180. For example, the axis of the cylinder shown is 30 degrees. (From C.W. Brooks and I.M. Borish, *System for Ophthalmic Dispensing,* Butterworth-Heinemann, Boston, 1979, p. 357.)

the cylinder and may be thought of in terms of the face of a protractor. (The meridian at right angles to the axis has the power to bend light and is referred to as the *power meridian.*) Degree notation begins on the right and goes counterclockwise as viewed from the front of the lens. See Figure 1-5. One need only use degree values from 0 to 180; values from 181 to 360 merely duplicate the 0-to-180 measure. As an example, a cylinder having an axis of 90 degrees would be oriented exactly the same as one having an axis of 270 degrees.

When a cylinder has a minus value, the diverging rays that leave it can be traced backward and appear to emanate from an imaginary line focus. See Figure 1-6.

Combining Spheres and Cylinders

When an individual is either nearsighted or farsighted and also has astigmatism, then both a sphere and a cylinder must be used in combination. Both elements are combined into a single lens. Usually

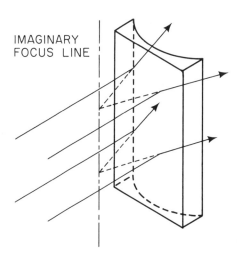

IMAGINARY FOCUS LINE

Figure 1-6 A minus cylinder diverges rays, but because it has no power in its axis meridian, it forms a vertical (imaginary) line focus instead of the point focus of the minus sphere lens.

the back surface incorporates the correction for astigmatism by having two different curves on the same surface. Such a lens is called a *spherocylinder*. It is specified using three numbers in sequence. First the sphere is specified, then the cylinder, then the axis of the cylinder. In the example

$$-2.00 - 1.00 \times 180,$$

the -2.00 (*sphere* value) indicates that the person is nearsighted by 2 diopters; the -1.00 (*cylinder* value) indicates that there is also an astigmatism of 1 diopter; and the *axis* of the cylinder is oriented along the 180-degree meridian.

Transposition of Prescriptions

A prescription as written by the doctor gives a sphere value, a cylinder value, and the axis of the cylinder. The cylinder may be written as either a plus or a minus cylinder, depending on what kinds of lenses the doctor used to find the prescription. If the instrument used by the doctor employs plus cylinder lenses, the prescription will be written in plus cylinder form; if the instrument was equipped with minus cylinder lenses, the prescription will be written in minus cylinder form.

For processing purposes the lab will almost always need to have the prescription in minus cylinder form. This means that if a prescription is written in plus cylinder form, it must be *transposed* to minus cylinder form. The transposition process from plus to minus cylinder form or from minus to plus cylinder form is not difficult. The steps are as follows:

1. Add the sphere and cylinder powers together.
2. Change the sign of the cylinder.
3. Change the axis by 90 degrees.

EXAMPLE 1-1
Change the following prescription from plus to minus cylinder form.

$$+2.00 + 1.25 \times 15$$

SOLUTION
To make the change from plus to minus cylinder form, follow the steps outlined above.

1. Add the sphere and cylinder powers together.

$$(+2.00) + (+1.25) = +3.25$$

The new sphere value is $+3.25$.

2. Change the sign of the cylinder to -1.25.
3. Change the axis by 90 degrees.

$$15 + 90 = 105$$

Putting all of this together results in a minus cylinder form of

$$+3.25 - 1.25 \times 105$$

This prescription has exactly the same refractive power as the plus cylinder form first given.*

EXAMPLE 1-2
A prescription has been written as

$$-2.75 + 1.50 \times 175$$

Write this prescription in minus cylinder form.

SOLUTION
First add the sphere and cylinder. Adding -2.75 and $+1.50$ gives a new sphere value of -1.25. Changing the sign of the cylinder results in a cylinder of -1.50. To change the axis by 90 degrees, subtract 90 from 175, since axis values must be between 0 and 180. Subtracting 90 from 175 gives a new axis value of 85 degrees.† Thus the prescription is written in minus cylinder form as $-1.25 - 1.50 \times 85$.

Prism

Sometimes light is diverted from its path and made to go in a new direction. Light can be redirected by the use of *prism*. A prism is wedge-shaped. The thicker the wedge, the more the rays of light are bent away from their original direction. See Figure 1-7.

An understanding of prism is basic to the optical laboratory. Very little work goes on in the surfacing laboratory without some reference to prism, even for the most elementary of prescriptions.

Prism is measured in terms of how far it bends a

---

*The two prescriptions have the same power because in both prescriptions the power in the 15-degree meridian is $+2.00$ and the power in the 105-degree meridian is $+3.25$. The difference between these two meridians is 1.25, which is the value of the cylinder. For a more complete explanation, see C.W. Brooks and I.M. Borish, *System for Ophthalmic Dispensing*, Butterworth-Heinemann, Boston, 1979, pp. 365–375.

†Remember that axis 85 is really the same as axis 265 on a 360-degree scale. The cylinder line passes through 85 and 265. Adding 90 to 175 would give a value of 265.

ray of light. *Prism diopter* is the unit of measure used for ophthalmic lenses. One diopter of prism is the amount of prismatic effect that causes a ray of light to deviate 1 cm from its original course when

the deviation is measured a distance of 1 m away from the prism. See Figure 1-8.

Prism Caused by Moving a Lens Off-Center

Normally an individual wearing corrective lenses has each lens positioned with its optical center in front of the eye. In this position, when the wearer looks straight ahead there is no displacement of objects from their actual positions. See Figure 1-9.

What happens when the lens is moved so that the center of the lens is no longer in front of the center of the eye? In order to understand what happens, consider the shape of a plus lens. From the side (in cross section), it appears to look much like two prisms placed base to base. See Figure 1-10. A minus lens gives the impression of being a combination of two prisms, but this time placed apex to apex. See Figure 1-11. When the wearer looks right through the center of the lens, the object is not displaced from its actual location. But when a plus or minus lens is moved off-center in relationship to the location of the eye, the object appears displaced as shown in Figures 1-10 and 1-11. This means that a *decentered* lens causes a *prismatic effect*.

Prentice's Rule

There is a relationship between how far the lens is decentered from its original location in front of the eye and how strong the power of the lens is. This relationship can be expressed as a formula known as *Prentice's rule*. *Prentice's rule* states that the prismatic effect is equal to the distance the lens is decentered (in centimeters) multiplied by the power of the lens:

$$\text{Prism diopters} = c \times D$$

or

$$\Delta = cD$$

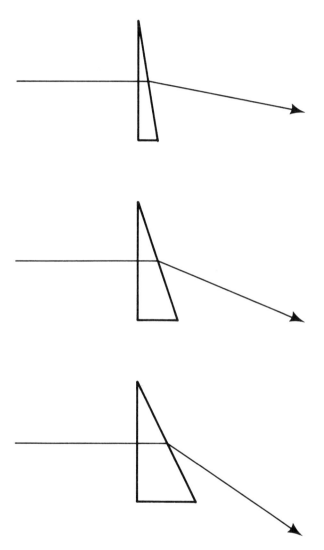

Figure 1-7 The more wedge-shaped a prism is, the greater is its ability to divert light in another direction.

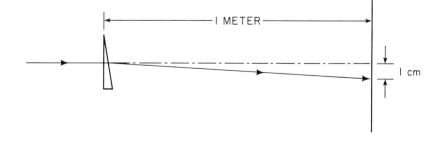

Figure 1-8 One prism diopter is the ability to cause light to deviate 1 cm from its original direction at a distance of 1 m.

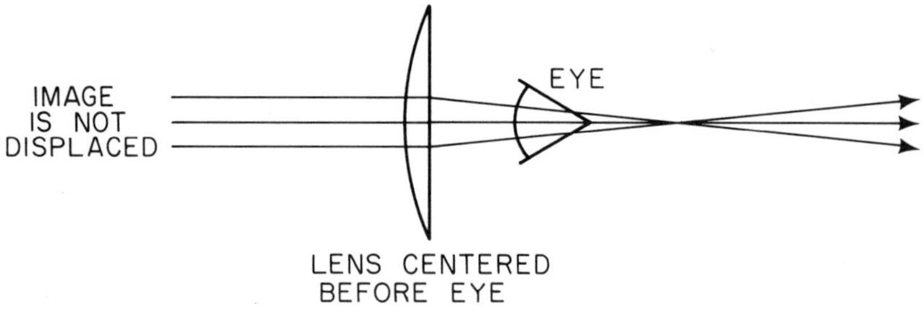

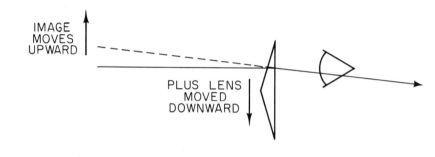

Figure 1-9 When a lens is positioned with its optical center directly in front of the eye, there is no prismatic effect.

Figure 1-10 Moving the optical center of a plus lens downward will produce a base-down prismatic effect.

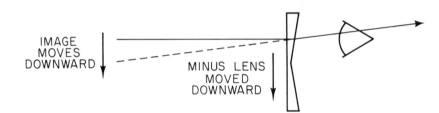

Figure 1-11 Moving the optical center of a minus lens downward will produce a base-up prismatic effect.

where c is the distance the lens is decentered expressed in centimeters and D is the refractive power of the lens expressed in diopters.* The delta symbol (Δ) stands for prism diopters.

EXAMPLE 1-3
If a lens having a power of +3.00 D is decentered 5 mm away from the center of the eye, how much prismatic effect will this cause?

SOLUTION
To find the prismatic effect, simply multiply the distance *in centimeters* that the lens has been displaced by the power of the lens. Since 5 mm equals 0.5 cm,

$$\text{Prism diopters} = 0.5 \times 3.00$$

$$\Delta = 1.5$$

Prism by Decentration

Sometimes a prescription intentionally includes prism in order to relieve a tendency of the eyes to cross or turn outward, upward, or downward in relation to one another. Since prismatic effect can be created by moving the lens away from its optical center, it may be possible to achieve that prismatic effect by *decentering* the lens. If the amount of prism that is needed is greater than what can be created by physically moving the optical center of the lens away from the eye, it can also be created by grinding a prismatic effect onto the whole surface of the lens. If the lens has either plus or minus power, this will displace the location of its optical center. The result will be a prismatic effect at the location of the eye because optical center has been moved to some other point on the lens surface.†

---

*Many sources use F instead of D in this equation to represent lens power.

†If the power of the prism being ground is strong enough, the optical center will be moved all the way off the lens and can no longer be located using a lensmeter.

Specifying Prism Base Direction

As was stated previously, prism causes light to bend, and therefore an object will appear to be displaced from its actual location. Light is bent toward the *base* (thicker end) of the prism, making the object viewed appear to be displaced toward the *apex* (thinnest end or tip) of the prism. The direction of the prism is given in terms of which way the base of the prism is oriented.

How to Specify Prism Base Direction

There is more than one way of specifying prism base direction. Lens prescribers tend to use one method, as it fits in more with how they measure the amount of prism needed. The optical laboratory uses another method, as prism can only be ground in a certain manner.

The Prescriber's Method

The person prescribing prism generally uses the wearer's face to reference the prism direction. The top and bottom of the wearer's face as well as the nose or sides of the head are used to specify base direction. If the prism is "right side up," with the base pointing downward and the apex pointing upward, the prism is said to be a *base-down* prism. If it is "up side down," the prism is said to be *base up*. See Figure 1-12.

If the prism is on its side, so to speak, the base of the prism will be oriented either in the direction of the nose or outward away from the nose. Prism oriented with its base toward the nose is said to be *base in*. See Figure 1-13. Prism turned with its base away from the nose is referred to as being *base out*. See Figure 1-14. This is perfectly adequate for those doing the prescribing, since vertical and horizontal prism elements are considered separately. If both horizontal and vertical prism corrections are required, then two prism elements are prescribed.

Unfortunately, this is somewhat limiting for the optical laboratory. First of all, if base-in or base-out prism is prescribed, it depends on which eye is being referenced as to which direction the base of the prism actually faces. For the right eye, base-in prism means that the base goes to the right, but for the left eye, a base-in prism means that the base goes to the left.

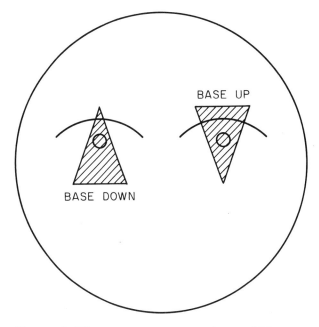

Figure 1-12 It is not necessary to know which eye a prism is on to be certain what "base down" or "base up" means. (However, base down before the right eye has the same effect for the wearer as base up before the left. They are *not* opposite effects!)

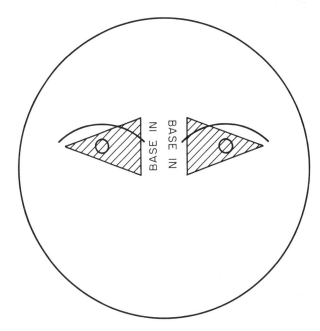

Figure 1-13 When horizontally oriented prism is prescribed for both eyes, it is almost without fail either base in for both eyes or base out for both eyes. Base-in prisms on both right and left eyes do not cancel each other, but rather augment the desired effect.

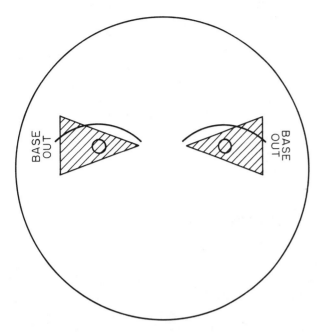

Figure 1-14 Even though the prism bases go in opposite directions, both are classified as "base out." It is not possible to know exactly which way a base-out prism is oriented until a right or left eye is specified.

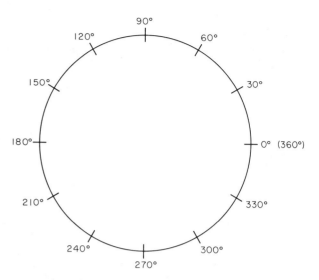

Figure 1-15 The degree system for prism is close to that used for specifying cylinder axis.

A 360-Degree Laboratory Reference System

Although the Prescriber's method of specifying prism is well suited for those examining eyes and those dispensing eyewear, it is not adequate for the optical laboratory. The optical laboratory uses either a *360-degree system* or a *180-degree system* of specifying prism base direction.

The 360-Degree Laboratory Reference System uses the standard method of specifying direction in degrees, as shown in Figure 1-15. When a lens is viewed from the front (convex side facing the observer), the base direction is specified as follows: If the base is pointing to the right, it is specified as Base 0 degrees. If the base is oriented in an upward direction, it is Base 90 degrees. To the left is Base 180 degrees, and straight down is Base 270 degrees.

Converting the Prescriber's Method to the Laboratory System

Suppose a prescription calls for 2 diopters of base-down prism. What is that in the 360-Degree Laboratory Reference System?

Base-down prism is below the 180-degree line. Therefore it must be greater than 180 degrees. Since

there are only four directions in the Prescriber's method, it must be either 0, 90, 180, or 270 degrees. The 270-degree direction is straight down. Therefore 2 diopters of base-down prism corresponds to Base 270.

When there is only one prism element to the prescription lens, there is little difficulty in converting. However, if there are two elements, the conversion may result in any one of the full 360 degrees.

Converting from the Prescriber's Method When Two Prism Elements Are Involved

Sometimes a prescription calls for two amounts of prism in two different directions, both on the same eye. When lenses are ground, it is not possible to work with two prisms. Instead, the two prisms are combined into one new prism. Fortunately, the end result is the same.

Using one prism instead of two is like taking a shortcut across a field. Instead of walking 2 miles east and 2 miles north, it is possible to walk 2.83 miles northeast and arrive at exactly the same location.* Therefore, instead of grinding 2 diopters of base-out prism for the right eye (prism at 180 degrees) and 2 diopters of base-up prism (prism at

---

*Those familiar with geometry will recognize this as simply the sum of two vectors.

base 90 degrees), it is possible to grind 2.83 diopters of prism halfway between (which in this case corresponds to Base 135 degrees).

Although this may seem difficult to visualize initially, anyone who is accustomed to using a lensmeter has already been using this system for some time. The lensmeter uses a system of rings inside the instrument to indicate the amount of prism being measured. If the lensmeter is focused, the lines on the target cross at the location of the optical center of the lens. Normally the lens is moved until the target lines are superimposed on the center of the lensmeter reticle, as in Figure 1-16. If the target lines are not centered, the place on the lens where the lensmeter is measuring creates a prismatic effect. The amount of prism is indicated by the location of the intersection of the target lines.

For example, if the target lines intersect on the reticle ring marked "1," the lens shows 1 diopter of prism. If the target lines are on the "1" reticle ring exactly above the center of the reticle, as shown in Figure 1-17, the prism direction is base up. As would be expected, a base-in or base-out effect will be seen to the left or right, depending on which lens is being measured. See Figure 1-18.

If a lens is placed in the lensmeter and the inter-

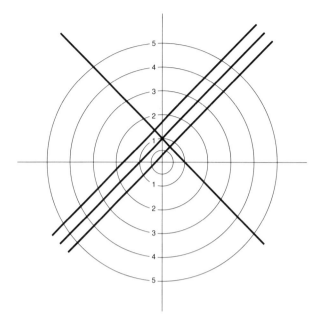

Figure 1-17 If a lens shows this in the lensmeter, there is 1 prism diopter of base-up prism at the point on the lens being looked through. This is true regardless of whether it is a left or a right lens.

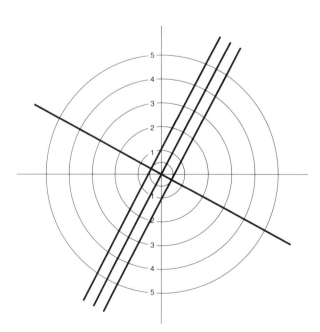

Figure 1-16 When the target is centered in a lensmeter, the optical center of the lens has been located. (From C.W. Brooks, *Essentials for Ophthalmic Lens Work,* Butterworth-Heinemann, Boston, 1983, p. 14.)

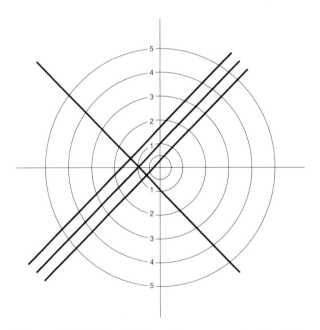

Figure 1-18 For this lens, the amount of prism is 1 prism diopter. However, since we don't know whether the lens is for the left or right eye, we don't know if the prism is base in or base out. If the lens is intended for the right eye, the base direction is base out.

section of the target lines occurs at a location other than on the vertical or horizontal reticle line, then both vertical and horizontal prism are being manifested. The amount of each is found by drawing imaginary lines from the target center to the horizontal and vertical lines of the reticle. In Figure 1-19, if the lens is a right lens, the amount of prism manifested is 2 prism diopters base in and 1 prism diopter base up. However, the location of the center of the target really shows one prism. By looking at the figure it can be seen that the amount of prism is really about 2.25 prism diopters. The base direction is approximately 27 degrees. (Most lensmeters have a degree scale within the reticle that can be used to measure the angle.) We now have a simple system for converting the Prescriber's method to the Laboratory Reference System of recording prism. Since looking into a lensmeter each time is somewhat inconvenient, an alternative is to use a device called a *Resultant Prism Chart*. This chart is shown in Appendix 2-1. Such a chart is used in the same manner but without the lensmeter.

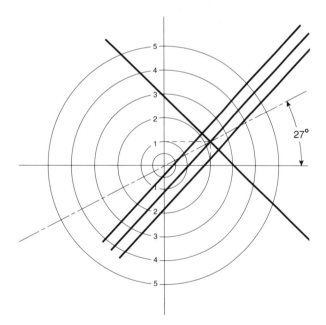

Figure 1-19 Assuming that this lens is for the right eye, the prismatic effect shown is 2△ Base In and 1△ Base Up. The base direction of the resultant prism is 27 degrees. It should be noted that the orientation of the triple and single target lines do *not* tell base direction. Within the eyepiece is a hairline that is turned until it crosses the center of the target. This hairline indicates the correct number of degrees. (The interior degree scale is not shown.)

Some Examples

When a prescription arrives at the optical laboratory, it is necessary to convert the Prescriber's method to the Laboratory method. Following are some typical problems.

EXAMPLE 1-4

If a right lens calls for 1 diopter of base-in prism, what is that in degrees?

SOLUTION

When visualizing prism direction, the lens is always thought of as if the lens (or glasses) has the convex surface facing you (in other words, looking at the glasses as they would appear when being worn by someone else). Therefore, for a right lens the base direction is toward the right. On the Prism Chart this is in the 0-degree direction. Thus the answer is 1 prism diopter, Base 0.

EXAMPLE 1-5

What if the prescription for the left eye in Example 1-4 *also* called for 1 diopter of prism Base In? Expressed in degrees, what would that base direction be?

SOLUTION

When viewing a left lens from the front, the nose will be to the left. Therefore the base direction is to the left. It can be seen from the Prism Chart that the base is now in the 180-degree direction.

The answer is 1 prism diopter Base 180. So now, even though the Prescriber's method indicates base-in prism for both the right and left lenses, the right-eye prism is Base 0, while the left-eye prism is Base 180.

EXAMPLE 1-6

A prescription indicates that the right eye requires 1△BI (1 prism diopter Base In) *and* 2△BU (Base Up). Express this in terms of the Laboratory Reference System.

SOLUTION

Looking at the Prism Chart in Figure 1-20, we find the location of 1△ Base 0. Next we find the location of 2△ Base 90. If we complete a rectangle using these two points as corners, we find the location of the result as 2.25△ Base 64 degrees.

More practice problems are given at the end of the chapter. Answers are provided at the back of the book.

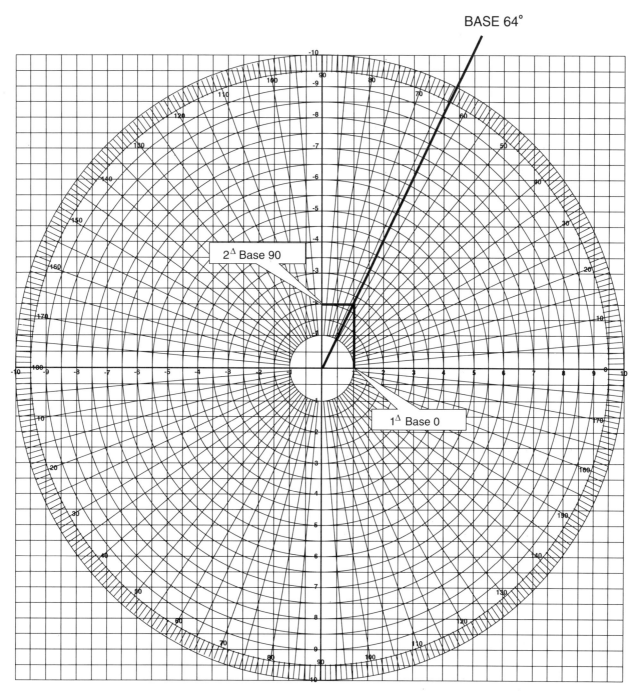

Figure 1-20 Prism Chart for Example 1-6. (Prism Chart redrawn with permission from *Coburn Equipment Catalog*, Coburn Optical Industries, Muskogee, Okla.)

A Modified (180-Degree) Reference System

Since people in the optical industry are familiar with a 180-degree system when specifying cylinder axis, many prefer to use only 0 to 180 degrees when specifying prism base direction. With cylinder axis there is no difference between axis 90 and axis 270: The cylinder axis is one continuous line. This is not the case, however, with prism base direction. With prism, base 270 is exactly opposite base 90. Thus, when using only 0 to 180 degrees, the number must be followed by either "up" or "down." Therefore "Base 90" is "Base 90 Up," and Base 270 is "Base 90 Down."

In practice, if the base direction is between 0 and 180 degrees the word "up" is dropped. But if the base direction corresponds to more than 180 degrees in the 360-degree system, 180 degrees is subtracted from the number and the word "down" is always added. For example, in the 180-degree reference system, Base 270 is 270 − 180 = Base 90 Down (or Base 90 DN, for short).

Prism Tables

Fortunately, in addition to the prism chart, there are several types of aids that have been developed to make the process of converting prism easier. One such aid that is familiar to the laboratory is the *prism table*. Prism tables also allow the values of two prisms to be looked up and the new prism amount and axis to be found.

Unlike the Prism Chart, the prism table requires that the axis indicated on the table be modified depending on the base directions of the two prisms that are being combined. This is shown in Appendix Figure A2-2. The prism table is shown in Appendix 2-2.

EXAMPLE 1-7

A prescription calls for 3 prism diopters Base In and 2 prism diopters Base Up for both right and left eyes. Using the Prism Chart, find the amount of prism required and the correct angle in degrees for each lens.

SOLUTION

On the Prism Chart, the prism amount is listed as 3.6 and the degrees as 34. For the right eye the chart results are used as is. See Figure A2-2. The answer is 3.6 Base 34 Up.

For the left eye the degrees must be modified, as the table shows that for the "up" and "in" combination, the amount shown in the table must be subtracted from 180 degrees (because the degree angle for the left lens will be the symmetrically mirrored angle from that of the right lens). The answer for the left eye is 3.6 Base 146 Up.

There are several different circumstances where it may be necessary to combine two prism amounts into one prism, including the following:

1. when both horizontal and vertical prism are specified in the prescription for the same eye
2. when Rx prism is already specified in the prescription and it is necessary to move the optical center of a lens by grinding in prism
3. when it is necessary to move an optical center in both a horizontal and a vertical direction.

Formulas for Finding Prisms Crossed at Right Angles

The same results as were obtained in the previous section by using tables to find the resultant of two prisms crossed at right angles may be found using formulas instead. The formulas are

$$R^2 = V^2 + H^2$$

or

$$R = \sqrt{V^2 + H^2}$$

where R is the resultant prism, H is the horizontal prism, and V is the vertical prism. The base direction of the prism is found using the trigonometric function

$$\tan \theta = \frac{V}{H}$$

where prism base direction is equal to θ or $180 - \theta$. In other words, after finding θ, it may be necessary to subtract θ from 180 to find the prism axis. This was described in the previous section on prism tables.

EXAMPLE 1-8

What prism results from the following:

Left lens: 2 Base Up
            3 Base In

SOLUTION

$$R = \sqrt{V^2 + H^2}$$
$$= \sqrt{(2)^2 + (3)^2}$$
$$= \sqrt{4 + 9}$$
$$= \sqrt{13}$$
$$= 3.6 \text{ prism diopters}$$

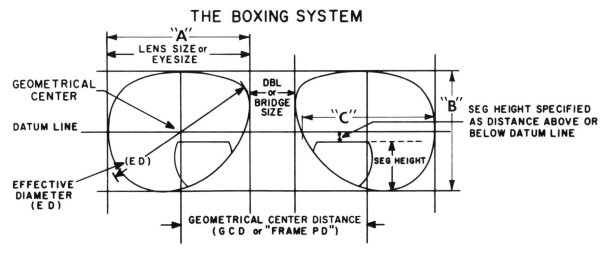

Figure 1-21 The Boxing system. (From C.W. Brooks and I.M. Borish, *System for Ophthalmic Dispensing*, Butterworth-Heinemann, Boston, 1979, p. 20.)

$$\tan \theta = \frac{V}{H}$$

$$= \frac{2}{3}$$

$$= 33.69 \text{ degrees, or about } 34 \text{ degrees}$$

However, since the prism is up and in for the left eye, Figure A2-2 indicates that the prism axis will be 180 − 34 or Base 146. Therefore the resultant prism is 3.6 Base 146 Up.

Frame and Lens Measurement Reviewed

Frames and edged lenses are measured according to the Boxing system. The Boxing system is shown in Figure 1-21 and also appears in the Appendix as Figure A6-1. The frame or edged lens size has several measurements that are especially important.

The first is the *eyesize* or *A* dimension. The eyesize is the horizontal measurement of the lens. However, it is *not* a horizontal measurement of the lens at either the middle* or any other given level of the

*The measure of a lens across the middle is the *C* dimension. The *C* dimension is important if another system, the Datum system, of lens measurement is used. The Datum system is used in Britain, whereas the Boxing system is used in the United States. (The Datum system is shown in the Appendix as Figure A6-2.)

lens. Rather it is a measurement of the horizontal dimension of an imaginary box that encloses the lens, touching that lens on the top, bottom, left- and right-hand sides.

The second measurement is the vertical or *B* dimension of the lens. This is a measurement of the vertical size of the imaginary box that encloses the lens.

A third lens size measurement is the *effective diameter*, ED, of the lens. The effective diameter is twice the distance from the center of the box to the farthest corner of the lens. This measure becomes important when figuring out how large the pre-edged lens must be in order to make the glasses. (The effective diameter will be referred to again in Chapter 2 when minimum blank size is discussed.)

If the lens is a bifocal, the level of the bifocal line can be measured from the bottom of the box up to the top of the segment. A measurement done in this manner is referred to as the *seg height*. (Note that the seg height is measured from the bottom of the box. It is *not* measured from the bottom of the lens at a point directly below the center of the segment unless this is the lowest point on the lens.) The level of the bifocal can also be measured from the center of the box down. If it is measured in this way, it is called the *seg drop*. Dispensers generally specify the vertical position of the segment in terms of seg height. The surfacing lab needs to have this measurement in terms of seg drop and so must convert seg height to seg drop.

The shortest distance between the right and left

lenses as positioned in the frame is called the *distance between lenses,* DBL,* or *bridge size.* This is the distance between the two imaginary boxes; it is not the distance between the lenses at the level of the middle of the lenses.

Questions and Problems

1. A lens has a focal point that is 40 cm behind the lens. What is the power of that lens expressed in diopters?

2. A lens has a focal point that is 10 cm in front of the lens. What is the power of this lens?

3. A cylinder component in a prescription indicates the presence of which condition?
   a. myopia
   b. hyperopia
   c. cataracts
   d. astigmatism

4. If a person looks at an object through a plus lens of spherical power and simultaneously moves the lens, how will the image of that object appear to move?
   a. The image will appear to move in the same direction as the lens moves.
   b. The image will appear to move in the opposite direction from the way the lens moves.
   c. The image will manifest no movement at all.

5. If the optical center of a −7.00 D lens is decentered 4 mm, how much of a prismatic effect is induced at the point where the optical center used to be?

6. How far must a +4.00 D lens be decentered in order to create a prismatic effect equal to 2 prism diopters?

7. If a prism has its base direction to the right (the wearer's left), what base direction is this in reference to the wearer's *right* eye?
   a. base down
   b. base up
   c. base in
   d. base out

   What base direction is this in reference to the wearer's *left* eye?
   a. base down
   b. base up
   c. base in
   d. base out

8. A prescription is received with Rx prism of 2.0

prism diopters Base In for the right eye. How would this be written in the 360-degree Laboratory System?
   a. 2 Base 0
   b. 2 Base 180
   c. 2 Base 90
   d. 2 Base 270

9. A prescription for Rx prism for the left eye reads

   4 Base In
   2 Base Down

   Using the 360-degree Laboratory Reference System, what is the amount of prism and base direction? What would this be when expressed in a 180-degree reference system?

10. What is prism 3.25 Base 287 in the 180-degree reference system?

11. What is prism 1.50 Base 1 DN in the 360-degree reference system?

12. Describe two ways of obtaining Rx prism, first using an uncut lens, and second using a semifinished blank.

13. A prescription calls for prism in the left lens as follows:

    5 Base In
    2 Base Up

    What is this when written as one prism? Give amount and base direction.

14. Suppose a prescription calls for Rx prism in the left lens. The amounts are

    3 Base In
    1.5 Base Up

    What is this when written as one prism? Give amount and base direction.

15. a. What are the two other ways of writing 4 Base 330 for a right lens? (Give the specific base directions and amounts.)

    b. What would the answer be if the lens were a left lens?

In the following instances of prescribed Rx prism, how much prism in what direction would be surfaced onto the lens? (Give the answer in *both* full 360-degree convention as well as the method that employs only 180 degrees of reference. Be able to obtain the answer by any of the methods given in this chapter.)

Two Prism Amounts		Combined Resultant Prism
16. R: 3.00 BO	180	
2.50 BU	360	
L: 3.00 BO	180	
2.50 BU	360	

Two Prism Amounts		*Combined Resultant Prism*
17. R: 1.50 BO	180	
2.00 BD	360	
L: 1.50 BO	180	
2.00 BD	360	
18. R: 6.00 BO	180	
5.00 BU	360	
L: 6.00 BO	180	
5.00 BD	360	
19. R: 3.00 BO	180	
4.00 BU	360	
L: 3.00 BO	180	
4.00 BD	360	
20. R: 4.50 BI	180	
3.00 BD	360	
L: 0.75 BO	180	
4.00 BD	360	
21. R: 5.50 BO	180	
1.00 BD	360	
L: 2.25 BI	180	
4.00 BD	360	
22. R: 3.00 BO	180	
3.00 BD	360	
L: 3.00 BO	180	
3.00 BU	360	
23. R: 0.75 BI	180	
2.50 BD	360	
L: 0.75 BI	180	
2.50 BU	360	
24. R: 2.50 BO	180	
4.25 BD	360	
L: 2.00 BI	180	
4.25 BU	360	

Two Prism Amounts		*Combined Resultant Prism*
25. R: 0.50 BI	180	
1.75 BU	360	
L: 0.50 BI	180	
1.75 BD	360	
26. R: 4.00 BI	180	
0.75 BU	360	
L: 4.25 BI	180	
0.75 BD	360	
27. R: 4.25 BI	180	
2.00 BU	360	
L: 3.75 BI	180	
2.00 BD	360	
28. R: 4.50 BI	180	
2.75 BU	360	
L: 3.50 BI	180	
4.00 BD	360	
29. R: 0.75 BO	180	
1.00 BD	360	
L: 0.25 BO	180	
1.25 BD	360	
30. R: 1.25 BI	180	
0.75 BD	360	
L: 1.00 BI	180	
1.00 BU	360	
31. R: 3.25 BO	180	
0.50 BU	360	
L: 3.00 BO	180	
1.50 BD	360	

2 The Lens Blank

Lens and Lens Blank Terminology and Standards

Introduction

In studying lens surfacing, it is important to understand all aspects of both semifinished and finished lens terminology.

Finished Single-Vision Lenses

Finished single-vision lenses have been finished on both sides at the factory. See Figure 2-1. These lenses have a blank size (lens diameter) and an optical center located exactly at the center of the lens blank.

Semifinished Single-Vision Lenses

Single-vision lenses that have only the front surface finished, as shown in Figure 2-1, really have only a limited number of factors that need be considered. Because there is no second surface, there is no optical center.* Therefore the lens blank has only an overall diameter (blank size) and a base curve. The optical center can be ground to a location anywhere on the lens during processing. (It should be noted that the optical center can be located beyond the edge of the lens in cases where there are large amounts of prism in the prescription.)

Semifinished Multifocal Lenses

As would be expected, when bifocals, trifocals, and other types of multifocal lenses are received in semifinished form, they come with the *segment* on the finished side. The "segment" is the part of the lens through which the wearer looks in order to see clearly when reading. It has extra plus power and makes up for the loss in focusing ability that occurs in the aging process. As with single-vision semifinished lenses, the finished side is almost always the front surface.†

The factors that identify a multifocal lens include the segment style, the size of the segment, and the overall lens blank diameter. The center of the lens blank is called the *blank geometric center.*

On each blank the segment is located at a specific position on the lens. Because most multifocals come as either a left lens or a right lens, the segment is moved over to one side of the lens. The distance the segment is moved away from the blank geometric center of the semifinished lens is called the *blank seg inset.* This inset is measured from the *center* of the segment and not the edge of the segment. See Figure 2-2.

Because the segment will be in the lower portion of the lens when it is being worn, the semifinished blank is made with the segment dropped down somewhat from the center of the lens blank. The distance from the blank geometric center to the top of the segment is called the *blank seg drop.* The blank seg inset and blank seg drop become especially important when calculating how certain lenses are to be ground.

Finished Multifocal Lenses

The semifinished multifocal lens has no optical center. Once finished, however, the lens has an optical center (or, in the case of a lens with prescribed prism, a major reference point). This optical center is usually somewhat above the segment line (3 to 5 mm is average) and 1.5 to 2.5 mm from the midline

---

*Semifinished lenses often come with a back surface that is smooth and polished. Because it has curvature, when examining a lens in the lensmeter it is possible to find an optical center. This, however, has no relationship to any future optical center location and should not be used.

†An exception to this was the older type of Ultex A (large round) bifocal, which was finished on the back surface. In other countries it is not uncommon for multifocals to be finished on the rear surface of the lens.

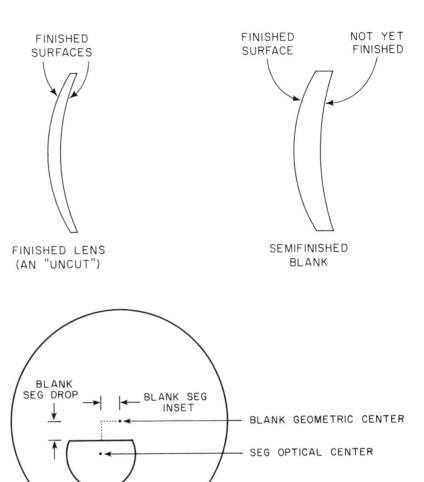

FINISHED
SURFACES

FINISHED
LENS
(AN "UNCUT")

FINISHED
SURFACE

NOT YET
FINISHED

SEMIFINISHED
BLANK

Figure 2-1 The finished lens is ready to edge. The semifinished blank must have one surface (usually the rear surface) ground to the desired curvature, simultaneously removing unwanted lens thickness.

BLANK
SEG DROP

BLANK SEG
INSET

BLANK GEOMETRIC CENTER

SEG OPTICAL CENTER

Figure 2-2 Semifinished multifocal blank dimensions.

of the segment in the direction of the blank geometric center.* See Figure 2-3.

Selecting the Correct Base Curve

It is possible to create the same power using an almost infinite variety of lens forms. A lens with a front curve of $+2.00$ D and a back curve of -6.00 D will produce virtually the same power that a lens with a $+3.00$ D front curve and a -7.00 D back curve will produce. If, then, many lens forms produce the same power, is there a particular front curve that should be chosen for a given lens power?

Although there is a range of possible lens forms that will prove acceptable, there are limits beyond which the overall results will be poor. Spectacle lens wearers can readily demonstrate this to themselves by turning their glasses around and looking through the front surfaces. The quality of vision may be degraded some looking straight ahead, but it will be especially bad when turning the eyes to view an object off to one side. This effect is due to lens aberrations brought about by choosing an incorrect lens form.

Manufacturers' Tables

When requested, lens manufacturers will provide a table to help in the correct selection of lens base

---

*If a lens is plano in power, there will be no specific optical center. If a lens is a plano cylinder, the optical center is not one distinct point, but rather a line corresponding to the axis.

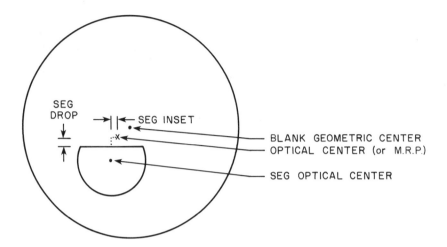

Figure 2-3 Finished multifocal blank dimensions.

curves. Such a table lists the range of powers and tells which lens blank should be used.

American National Standards Institute Guidelines

Previously the American National Standards Institute (ANSI) listed the minimum amount of lens aberration that should be present for lenses of particular powers. (There is a definite correlation between lens base curve and the quality of the image as seen through the periphery of a lens.) These minimum amounts were listed in a series of tables. The American National Standards Institute has discontinued the inclusion of these tables in their Z80.1 Prescriptions Standards, since larger eyesize frames have made it increasingly difficult for the laboratory to adhere to the optimum base curve. (As an example, steeply curved lenses are very difficult to insert into large-size metal frames and make them stay in securely.) However, despite the apparent "loosening" of standards, the optimum base curves should be adhered to as closely as possible. The form of the lens is important to the overall vision of the wearer. Deviation from the manufacturer's recommended guidelines will definitely cause a decrease in vision when looking at objects through the periphery of the lens.

A General Guideline

It will be noted that, as a general rule, plano lens powers have back surfaces with a dioptric power close to −6.00 D. As the dioptric power of the lens increases in the minus direction, the back surface becomes more curved (that is, it becomes more minus in power), while the front surface flattens. For plus lenses, the back surface becomes progressively flatter, while the front base curve becomes steeper.

Base Curve Formulas

One method for finding base curves is to use a simplified formula derived from precalculated base curves. Such a formula is a supplement to, but not a replacement for, manufacturers' recommendations. One commonly used formula is *Vogel's formula*,[1] which states that, for plus lenses, the base curve of the lens equals the spherical equivalent of the lens power, plus 6 diopters. Written as a formula, this is

Base curve = spherical equivalent + 6.00 D

(The *spherical equivalent* of a lens is the sphere power plus half the cylinder power.) For minus lenses, Vogel's formula states that the base curve equals the spherical equivalent divided by 2, plus 6 diopters. Written as a formula, this is

$$\text{Base curve} = \frac{\text{spherical equivalent}}{2} + 6.00 \text{ D}$$

These formulas are summarized in Table 2-1.

EXAMPLE 2-1

Using Vogel's formula, find the base curve for a lens having a power of +2.00 D sphere.

SOLUTION

For spheres there is no need to calculate a spherical equivalent. So for this lens, the base curve is

$$\text{Base curve} = +2.00 \text{ D} + 6.00 \text{ D}$$

$$= +8.00 \text{ D}$$

Table 2-1 Vogel's Formula for Base Curves

Plus lenses:

$$\text{Base curve} = \text{spherical equivalent} + 6.00 \text{ D}$$

Minus lenses:

$$\text{Base curve} = \frac{\text{spherical equivalent}}{2} + 6.00 \text{ D}$$

where

$$\text{Spherical equivalent} = \text{sphere} + \frac{\text{cyl}}{2}$$

EXAMPLE 2-2

Suppose a lens has a prescription of $+5.50 -1.00 \times 70$. Using Vogel's formula, what is the base curve?

SOLUTION

The spherical equivalent of $+5.50 -1.00 \times 70$ is

$$\text{Spherical equivalent} = +5.50 + \frac{(-1.00)}{2}$$

$$= +5.00 \text{ D}$$

The recommended base curve is

$$\text{Base curve} = +5.00 \text{ D} + 6.00 \text{ D}$$

$$= +11.00 \text{ D}$$

EXAMPLE 2-3

A minus lens has a power of $-6.50 -1.50 \times 170$. Using Vogel's formula, what is the base curve?

SOLUTION

The spherical equivalent of $-6.50 -1.50 \times 170$ is

$$\text{Spherical equivalent} = -6.50 + \frac{-1.50}{2}$$

$$= -7.25 \text{ D}$$

The base curve formula for minus lenses is different than that for plus lenses; therefore, the recommended base curve is

$$\text{Base curve} = \frac{-7.25}{2} + 6.00 \text{ D}$$

$$= -3.62 \text{ D} + 6.00 \text{ D}$$

$$= +2.38 \text{ D}$$

Rounded to the nearest ½ D, this is $+2.50$ D. (In practice this would be rounded to the nearest base curve in the series stocked by the laboratory.)

Base Curve Tables

In response to the relaxing of ANSI standards for base curve selection, Glenn A. Fry has urged those engaged in the dispensing process to take a greater role in assuring the optical quality of the lens design.[2] An adaptation of the guidelines he has recommended is found in Table 2-2.

Mancusi[3] lists a sequence of curves that can be used for given powers as a starting point for selecting the correct base curve. Some values based on this idea are given in Table 2-3.

EXAMPLE 2-4

A prescription calls for a crown glass lens having a spherical power of $+3.50$ D. What base curve should be used?

SOLUTION

The solution involves nothing more than looking up the correct curve in a chart corresponding to the appropriate lens material. Most manufacturers make these readily available for every series of lens they produce.

According to Fry's calculations as shown in Table 2-2, the correct base curve for a $+3.50$ D glass lens is a $+8.50$ D front curve. There is a 1.00 D allowance in either a plus or a minus direction permitted.

Using Table 2-3 gives a very similar result, with the base curve of choice being $+8.00$.

EXAMPLE 2-5

What base curve should be chosen for a crown glass lens having a power of $-2.00 -2.00 \times 180$?

SOLUTION

In this case it is necessary to calculate the *spherical equivalent* of the lens before being able to find the base curve using Fry's table. The spherical equivalent is

$$\text{Spherical equivalent} = \text{sphere} + \frac{(\text{cyl})}{2}$$

Table 2-2 Base Curves for Spheres and Minus Cylinder Form Lenses Glass (Index 1.523)

If the spherical equivalent (sphere power + cyl. power/2) is	Then use this base curve (± 1.00 D)
Greater than +7.50	Use an aspheric design
Between +6.37 and +7.50	Use +12.50
Between +4.37 and +6.37	Use +10.50
Between +1.50 and +4.37	Use +8.50
Between −2.12 and +1.50	Use +6.50
Between −5.82 and −2.12	Use +4.50
Between −10.50 and −5.82	Use +2.50
Greater than −10.50	Use +0.50

Source: G.A. Fry, The Optometrist's New Role in the Use of Corrected Curve Lenses, *Journal of the American Optometric Association,* 50(5) : 562 (May 1979).

which in this example turns out to be

$$\text{Spherical equivalent} = -2.00 + \frac{(-2.00)}{2}$$

$$= -2.00 + (-1.00)$$

$$= -3.00$$

Therefore, using Table 2-2, the correct base curve for a −3.00 D spherical equivalent is +4.50 D. (It will be noted that using the sphere power alone would have resulted in choosing a different base curve.)

Using Table 2-3 gives a base curve of +4.00. When using a more complete surfacing chart, all spherocylinder combinations are listed individually, making the calculation of a spherical equivalent unnecessary.

Base Curves and Computers

In spite of the use of computers in lens calculations and the fact that computers can assist in the selection of base curves, many labs choose the lens blank *before* the computer is used. The lens blank can then be individually measured at the time information is fed into the computer, making for a more convenient process. The computer then assists in finding back surface lens curves and desired thickness.

Considering the Right and Left Lenses as a Pair

Up to this point we have only been choosing the base curve on the basis of the power of one indi-

Table 2-3 Base Curve Selection Chart

*Beyond +7.00 D of refractive power, a lens with an aspheric base curve should be used.

This base curve chart shows a great deal of overlap between base curves. It is designed to help in choosing the correct compromise curve when left and right lens powers are unequal. It is not meant as a replacement for manufacturers' recommendations.

vidual lens. This works fine as long as both left and right lenses have exactly the same power. But if the powers are different in the left and right eyes, one lens might call for one base curve, while the other lens requires a different curve. This could be problematic in certain instances.

Consider, for instance, the situation where one

lens in a pair has a power that is only ½ diopter stronger than that of the other. Yet when the correct base curves are looked up on the surfacing chart, the two powers straddle the base curve change. One lens calls for a +6.00 base, while the other calls for a +8.00. If the lenses were chosen with two different base curves, there would be both a visible difference in the appearance of the two lenses and a difference in magnification created between the images seen by the right and left eyes. Therefore a decision needs to be made to modify the base curve(s).

The American National Standards Institute makes the following recommendation:

It is permissible, when supplying corrected curve lenses for a pair in which surfacing charts indicate two different base curves, to supply both lenses in the base curve corresponding to the stronger of the two lenses. If, however, the base curve differential exceeds 2.00 D, the indicated base should be used for each eye. It is also acceptable practice to modify the lens base curvature to be compatible with metal-frame eyewire curvature.[4]

This means that:

1. In instances *where both lenses are plus*, the steeper base curve (higher numerical base curve) of the two should be chosen.
2. *If both lenses are minus*, the flatter base curve of the two should be chosen.
3. *If one lens is plus and one lens is minus*, the base curve for the lens with the highest numerical value should be chosen.

The ANSI quotation indicates that it is advisable to maintain individual lens base curve choices when the difference between the right and left base curves is greater than 2 diopters. A correctly chosen base curve will produce clear vision regardless of whether the wearer is looking through the center or off toward the edges. If the recommended base curve is changed too much, vision in the periphery of the lens will be poor.

Other Factors That Modify Base Curve Choice

Metal and Rimless Frames
It will be noted that the latter part of the ANSI recommendation quoted above states that "it is also

acceptable practice to modify the lens base curvature to be compatible with metal-frame eyewire curvature."[5]

Most metal frames are made so that when a lens with a 6.00 D base curve is edged, it will fit nicely. This is a logical choice, because the majority of lenses are made with base curves close to 6. When a lens has a base curve above 6 diopters, it is often necessary to bend the frame's eyewire so that the lens will fit. The higher (steeper) the base curve, the more the frame must be bent in order to make the lens fit. Flatter base curves require less frame bending and can be fitted into a metal frame more easily. It is also true that lower base lenses, especially for *large* metal frames, are less likely to fall out of the frame.

Therefore plastic frame styles that have a poor lens-retention record may do better with lenses that have flatter base curves.

Large Amounts of Prism
Prescriptions with large amounts of prism end up being thicker. Lens thickness increases lens magnification and makes the eye look larger. This is especially true for plus lenses. Much of this magnification comes from a steep front curve. This means that magnification may be reduced by using a flatter base curve. As an added benefit, large prisms are easier to work with when produced on a somewhat lower base curve.

If finding the correct base curve seems complicated, Table 2-4 should make it easier.

EXAMPLE 2-6
An order calls for a pair of lenses as follows:

R: +2.00 sph 4.50 Base In
L: +2.00 sph 4.50 Base In

The lenses are to be placed in a metal frame. If Fry's tables are used, what base curves should be chosen?

SOLUTION
Fry's tables indicate that for +2.00 spheres, +8.50 D base curves should be used. Yet there are two factors that would argue that the base curves should be flattened. A metal frame can make lenses with high base curves have a bulbous appearance. Some metal frames may not hold high-base-curve lenses as easily. Moreover, there is prism in the prescription, which will thicken the lenses. To counteract the magnification caused by

Table 2-4 Steps in Finding the Correct Base Curves

Part I

---

1. When base curves charts do not consider the cylinder value of a prescription with both a sphere and a cylinder component, calculate the *spherical equivalent* of the lens and use this value, instead of the sphere, to calculate or look up the base curve.

2. Use Vogel's formula or look up the base curve indicated in the chart of choice for each lens individually.

3. Answer the following questions:

   a. Are the base curves of the two lenses the same?
      Yes: Keep these base curves and go to Part II.
      No: Go on to the next question.

   b. Are the two base curves greater than 2 diopters apart?
      Yes: Keep these base curves and go to Part II.
      No: Go on to the next question.

   c. Are both lenses plus?
      Yes: Choose the steeper (higher) base curve and use it for both lenses. Go on to Part II.
      No: Go on to the next question.

   d. Are both lenses minus?
      Yes: Choose the flatter (lower) base curve and use it for both lenses. Go on to Part II.
      No: Go on to the next question.

   e. Is one lens plus and the other lens minus?
      Yes: Choose the base curve of the lens that has the higher numerical power value and use it for both right and left lenses.

Part II

Use the base curves found in Part I unless any of the following apply:

1. Is the frame you are using metal or rimless? If it is and the base curves called for are above 4 D, consider reducing the base curves by 2 D.

2. Does the plastic frame you are using have a reputation for letting the lenses pop out easily? If so and the base curves called for are above 4 D, consider reducing the base curves by 2 D.

3. Does the prescription call for prism over approximately 4 prism diopters per eye? If so and the base curves called for are above 4 D, consider reducing the base curves by 1 or 2 D.

---

the extra lens thickness created by the prism, it may be advisable to flatten the base curve. These factors all point to the advisability of dropping down to a +6.50 base lens.

Certain base curves span a wide range of power. In this instance the +2.00 power is toward the bottom of the +8.50 base curve range. If the lens power had been higher (+4.00 for example), a decrease in base curve might not have been necessary.

EXAMPLE 2-7

A pair of lenses has the following powers:

R: −1.50 −1.00 × 180
L: −4.50 −1.00 × 180

What base curves should be used if the lenses are to be placed in a modestly sized plastic frame? Use Fry's tables to determine base curve.

SOLUTION

Fry's tables are based on spherical equivalents. The spherical equivalent for a spherocylinder lens is found by taking one-half the cylinder power and adding it to the sphere. In the example the spherical equivalent of the right lens is

$$\text{Spherical equivalent} = \text{sph} + \left(\frac{cyl}{2}\right)$$

or

$$-1.50 + \left(\frac{-1.00}{2}\right) = -2.00$$

Fry's tables indicate that for a −2.00 D lens, the base curve is +6.50.

The spherical equivalent for the left lens is

$$-4.50 + \left(\frac{-1.00}{2}\right) = -5.00$$

Looking up a −5.00 spherical equivalent in Fry's tables shows the need for a lens with +4.50 base curve.

Since both lenses are minus in power, the +4.50 base curve should be used for both lenses. According to the tables, we would use a +6.50 base lens for the right eye and a +4.50 base lens for the left. Because these base curves are only 2 D apart, both lenses should be made with the same base. When both lenses are minus, the flatter base should be chosen. In this case a pair of +4.50 D semifinished blanks are used. (Naturally, if the +6.50 lens had been fairly far away from the +4.50 cutoff line, but the +4.50 base lens was only ¼ D away from being a +6.50 base, the logical choice would be to use a +6.50 base anyway.)

Selecting Single-Vision Lens Blank Size

Once the correct base curve has been selected, the next step is to choose a lens that will be big enough to cut out when edged. Although it may seem easiest initially, choosing the largest possible lens blank just to avoid problems is not the answer!

Determining the correct lens blank size for the job is important for the following reasons:

1. The lens should be ground to a minimum thickness. Plus lenses look much better when they are thin.
2. Lens spoilage might result from using a lens blank that was too small.

3. Small blanks are cheaper than large blanks.
4. If a bi- or trifocal lens is too small for the frame, the account needs to know at the earliest possible moment.

Finished Single-Vision Lenses

When using single-vision lenses, the lens blank size should be chosen *as small as possible.* The important things to consider here are

1. the size of the frame's lens opening
2. the distance the lens must be decentered in order to keep the optical center in front of the eye

With *minus lenses*, price is the only reason to use a small blank. The larger the lens blank, the more expensive it will be. Therefore it makes good sense to use the smaller lens.

With *plus lenses*, however, it is important to choose the smaller lens blank not only for economic reasons, but also for optical and cosmetic ones.

With single-vision uncut lenses, the larger the plus lens blank is, the thicker the lens ends up being. A thicker plus lens will be heavier. It will also cause magnification. Everything will look bigger to the wearer, and, to make matters worse, the wearer's eyes will also look bigger to everyone else.

The most economical choice for single-vision lenses is to use a finished lens. This avoids all the costs associated with the surfacing process. But in order to decide if an "uncut" can be used, one needs to know if it is large enough for the frame. This can be done by using either a formula or a scale drawing.

Using a Formula

Years ago, frames were chosen so that the wearer's eyes were positioned at the center of the frame's lens opening. This made the selection of a blank size incredibly easy. When there is no decentration required, the minimum blank size equals the effective diameter of the frame.* Because a slight safety margin is needed to allow for lens chipping, 2 mm is added to the minimum calculated lens blank size. (Increasing the size by 2 mm effectively increases the lens by 1 mm in every direction.) This means

---

*The effective diameter of a frame is twice the longest radius of the frame's lens aperture as measured from the boxing center. See Chapter 1.

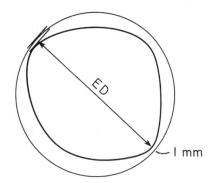

Figure 2-4 If the lens required no decentration, the minimum blank size would equal the ED plus 2 mm as a safety factor.

that if the wearer always looked out the center of the frame's lens opening, the formula for minimum blank size (MBS) would be

$$MBS = ED + 2 \text{ mm}$$

This is shown visually in Figure 2-4.

However, people just don't choose frames this way anymore. Nowadays the optical center of the lens is seldom in the geometric or boxing center of the frame's lens opening. Instead it is in a decentered position. One allows for decentration this way: For every millimeter the lens must be moved inward (or outward), the size of the lens from the center to the edge of the blank must increase by 1 mm. (In other words, the overall lens blank size must increase by 2 mm for every 1 mm of decentration per lens.) This can be visualized by looking at Figure 2-5. Written as a formula, the minimum blank size for uncut single-vision lenses is

$$MBS = ED + 2(\text{decentration per lens}) + 2 \text{ mm}$$

Twice the decentration per lens equals total decentration. Thus, for single-vision lenses the formula for minimum blank size can also be expressed as

$$MBS = ED + \text{total decentration} + 2 \text{ mm}$$

(It should be noted that this formula is no longer valid if there is prism in the lens prescription.)

EXAMPLE 2-8

What would be the minimum blank size for a finished single-vision lens that is to be placed in a frame having the following dimensions?

A = 53 mm
DBL = 17 mm
ED = 59 mm

where A is the horizontal dimension of the Boxing system rectangle. The wearer has an interpupillary distance (PD) of 63 mm.

SOLUTION

The first step is to figure total decentration so that the formula for the MBS may be used. Total decentration is

$$\text{Total decentration} = (A + DBL) - PD$$

In this case,

$$\text{Total decentration} = (53 + 17) - 63$$
$$= 7 \text{ mm}$$

Now that the total decentration is known, the MBS can be found.

$$MBS = ED + \text{total decentration} + 2$$
$$= 59 + 7 + 2$$
$$= 68 \text{ mm}$$

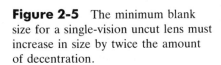

Figure 2-5 The minimum blank size for a single-vision uncut lens must increase in size by twice the amount of decentration.

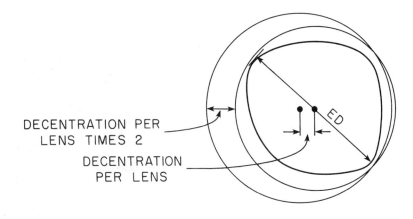

DECENTRATION PER LENS TIMES 2

DECENTRATION PER LENS

Thus, assuming that the prescription has no prescribed prism component, the smallest uncut (finished) lens blank that can be used is one having an overall diameter of 68 mm.

Using a Lens Drawing

One can use scale drawings of lens blanks to determine whether or not it is possible to use a finished single-vision lens. If no lens blanks are large enough, it will be necessary to surface a lens. A scale drawing is shown in Figure 2-6, where it is also explained.

Semifinished Single-Vision Lenses

Semifinished lenses come with only one curve ready for use. This is usually the front curve. When the lens is surfaced, some variables are especially important, particularly the curvature of the second surface and the location of the optical center. The optical center can be placed anywhere on the lens. For especially large frames, the optical center can be moved sideways on the lens so that it will end up in front of the wearer's line of sight. This means that the lens does not have to be physically moved

over. Since no movement of the lens is required, the minimum blank size for a semifinished lens is

$$MBS = ED + 2 \text{ mm}$$

(This is true even if there *is* prescribed prism in the final Rx.)

Selecting Multifocal Lens Blank Size

It is possible to obtain bi- or trifocals already ground to certain spherical prescriptions. These are referred to as "finished bifocals." However, because of the multitude of power combinations possible, multifocals are not usually ordered this way. Most bi- and trifocals go through the surfacing lab.

Because multifocal lenses begin with a semifinished blank and are therefore surfaced, the optical center can be positioned anywhere on the lens. But the location of the multifocal segment on the blank cannot be changed, nor can the location of the segment in the frame. It is also "locked in" vertically by the seg height, and horizontally by the near PD. With the segment positioned as specified on the

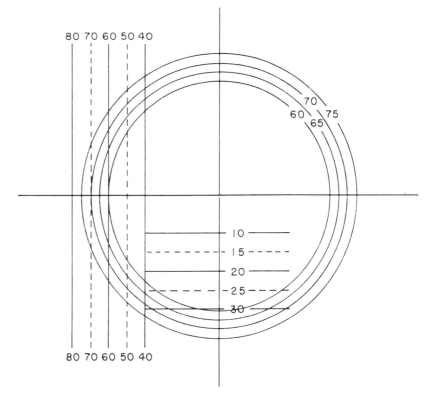

Figure 2-6 Single-vision minimum blank size chart. The blank size chart shown is used as follows: (1) Place the frame front face down on the chart with the right lens opening over the simulated lens circles. (2) Center the frame bridge over the correct binocular distance PD as indicated by the scale on the left. (3) Ensure vertical centration. This is done by positioning the lowest point on the inside groove of the lower eyewire on the lower chart scale. The correct level is one-half the B dimension of the frame. (If a vertical positioning for the optical center of the lens is specified, use this height instead.) (4) Note which diameter lens circle will just enclose the lens opening of the frame including the eyewire groove. This is the minimum blank size required for a non-prismatic, single-vision lens. (From C.W. Brooks, *Essentials for Ophthalmic Lens Work*, Butterworth-Heinemann, Boston, 1983, p. 49.)

order, the lab needs to know if the semifinished blank is large enough to cover the entirety of the frame's lens opening.

Using the Frame to Find Minimum Blank Size

One method for determining if a lens is big enough is to use the frame itself. The lens blank is held in front of the frame. The segment is moved up and down until the correct seg height is obtained, then left or right until it is positioned for the correct near PD. If the frame's lens opening is completely covered by the lens, the lens blank is large enough. If it leaves a gap, a larger lens blank size should be chosen. See Figure 2-7.

The most difficult part of the process is having enough hands to complete the job: One hand is needed to hold the frame, another to hold the lens, and a third to hold the millimeter ruler for measuring seg height and near PD. Despite the awkwardness of the situation, this method is used quite often.

Using Actual-Size Lens Drawings to Find Minimum Blank Size

To help overcome the awkwardness of using the lens blank itself, lens manufacturers have resorted to using actual-size drawings of the lens blank. An exact reproduction of the lens blank is drawn and millimeter markings are added from the top of the seg down to the bottom of the lens. These markings allow the frame to be placed on the drawing and

the correct seg height duplicated without using a ruler. By adding a second millimeter scale extending from the middle of the near segment to a location beyond the nasal edge of the lens blank, the near PD can be found with only a minimal amount of effort. See Figure 2-8.

Each lens blank manufacturer places the bifocal segment at a slightly different location on the lens. Manufacturers also sell lens blanks in a variety of sizes. This means that a separate drawing, or series of drawings, is required for each multifocal style made by a given manufacturer. It is helpful to know how to construct a home-made lens blank size chart. Such charts are not difficult to make. When a new lens series becomes available, such a chart can be quickly constructed and used to figure MBS for new prescription orders. The steps in making such a chart are as follows.

1. Draw a large cross in the middle of a sheet of centimeter graph paper.
2. To the left of the center of the cross draw vertical lines every 5 mm, beginning at 20 mm to the left and ending at 40 mm to the left.
3. Label these lines at twice their measured value. This will allow the middle of the frame bridge to be placed directly on the labeled line. (Although the distance from the center of the frame bridge to the center of the drawn cross is actually half the near PD, doubling the labeled distances will allow the near PD to be read off directly without having to divide by 2 every time.)

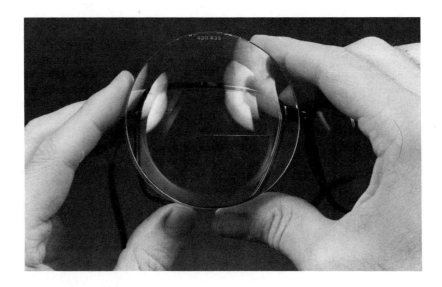

Figure 2-7 Blank size charts do the same thing that can be done by holding the actual lens blank up to the frame. By positioning the bifocal at the ordered location, it is easy to see if the semifinished lens blank will be large enough for the frame. Here the blank will be too small. In order for the lens to cut out, either the seg height must be reduced or the near PD increased.

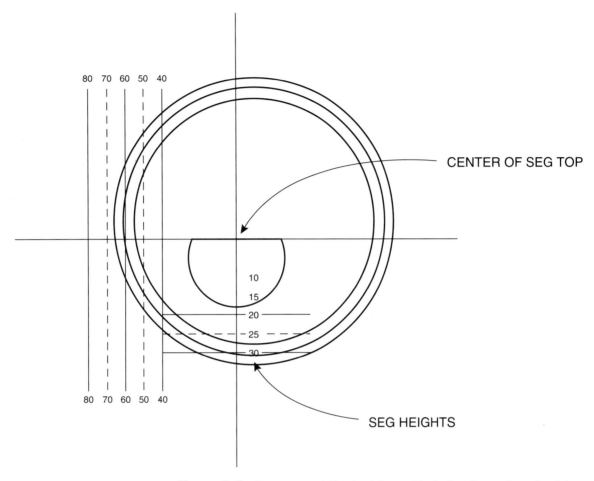

80 70 60 50 40

CENTER OF SEG TOP

10
15
20
25
30

80 70 60 50 40

SEG HEIGHTS

Figure 2-8 To use a multifocal minimum blank size chart, place the right side of the frame face down over the chart. Move the frame left or right until the near PD line corresponding to the ordered near PD is directly in the center of the frame bridge. Move the frame up or down until the correct seg height corresponds to the lowest part of the inside bevel of the lower eyewire. The smallest circle that completely encloses the lens shape is the smallest blank possible for this manufacturer.

4. Now draw horizontal lines below the center of the cross at 5-mm intervals, starting 10 mm below the center of the cross.
5. Label these lines according to their actual distance from the center of the cross. (This will be the multifocal height corresponding to the place where the lowest point of the inside bevel of the lower eyewire of the frame will be placed. See Figure 2-9.)
6. Draw the segment so that the center of its top falls at the center of the originally drawn cross.
7. The blank seg inset and blank seg drop of the lens must be known. Starting from the center of the cross, measure up and over. Measure up the number of millimeters equal to the blank seg drop. Then measure over to the right the number of millimeters equal to the blank seg inset. Mark this spot with a dot.
8. Using a compass, draw circles corresponding to the blank sizes that are available. The center of each circle is the spot found in step 7.

It should be apparent that because each manufacturer may have different blank seg insets and drops, one chart will not work for every brand of

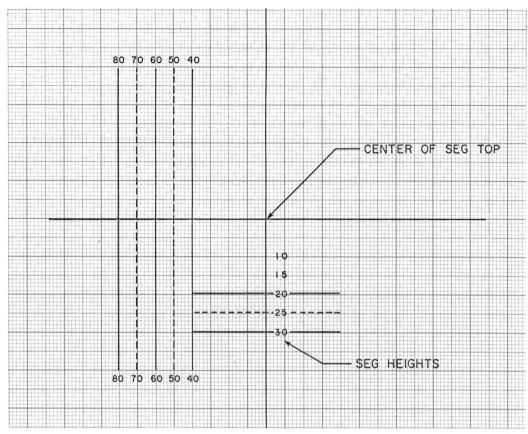

Figure 2-9 The basic drawing for a multifocal lens blank size chart. Any lens or lens series can be superimposed on this drawing by placing the center of the seg at the origin of the cross.

flat-top bifocal, even if the segment sizes are all the same.

Using the Drawn Lens Chart

To use a scale-drawing lens diagram, place the frame front face down on the drawing. Next slide the frame up or down until the lowest part of the inside bevel of the lower eyewire is exactly on the correct seg height line. (The seg height is given on the original order form.) Care must be taken to always keep the frame straight so that the frame front parallels the horizontal. Do not tilt the frame.

After the correct seg height is attained, the frame front must be positioned so that the seg will be at the correct near PD. Remember that the scale from the center of the seg to beyond the nasal edge of the lens drawing is in millimeters, but for ease of reference the measurements are marked as twice

the actual distance. Because of this the center of the frame bridge can be placed over the marking that corresponds to the wearer's near PD.

Now the bifocal segment occupies the position where it will be located after the lens has been cut and edged. If there are any areas within the frame's lens opening that are not covered by the drawn lens, the blank is too small for the frame. This explanation is summarized in Table 2-5.

Helping the Dispenser Correct a Blank Size Error

If a lens blank is too small to process the order, larger blanks are generally available and the order can be completed as specified. Unfortunately, this is not always the case. Sometimes, if the seg height and near PD that has been ordered is to be adhered to, there will be no available lens blank that can be

Table 2-5 How to Use Scale Lens Drawings to Determine MBS

1. Place the frame face down on the drawing.
2. Move the frame up or down until the inside bevel of the lower eyewire is over the line corresponding to the correct seg height.
3. Move the frame left or right until the center of the bridge is over the line corresponding to the near PD.
4. Note whether the lens blank completely encircles the frame's lens opening.
5. If encirclement is complete, the blank is large enough. If it is not, the blank is too small.

used. In this case the account must be contacted and informed. At this point it is most helpful if alternatives can be suggested instead of simply saying that the frame is too big for the blank size and the job can't be done.

The limiting factor in most cases is not that the diameter of the blank is physically smaller than the needed lens size. Rather it is because of the required segment location. The segment height or inset causes the blank to be shifted too far upward, downward, or inward.

For example, if the near PD is exceptionally small, the outermost edge of the lens may not quite cover the frame's lens opening. In this case the suggestion could be made that increasing the near PD by a given amount would solve the problem. The practitioner can then decide if this is permissible. If it is, the same frame can be used and the inconvenience of having the wearer select a different one can be avoided.

The same problem can be encountered with segment height. When the segment is too high for the blank size, there will be a gap between the lower eyewire and the lower edge of the lens drawing. If the segment is only a millimeter or so too high, the practitioner may prefer to lower the seg by a slight amount than completely change frames or multifocal styles. The lab should be able to tell the account *exactly* how much lower the segment must be placed. This amount equals the distance the frame must be moved in an upward direction in order to remove the gap between the lens edge and the frame eyewire.

In short, move the frame away from the direction of the "air hole" or space until it disappears. Read the new seg height and/or near PD from the scale drawing. It is not unusual to find that combining a

slight increase in near PD with an increase or decrease of the seg height will be just what is needed in order to make the lens blank diameter and frame eyesize compatible.

Having the Laboratory Layout Computer Warn of Blank Size Problems

Most laboratory lens layout computers are programmed to indicate the approximate minimum blank size required for a prescription. Even though most people associate the function of this computer with finding the required lens center thickness, the needed lap tool curvatures, and the amount of prism required for decentration, it will also give the minimum blank size required to assure that the lens will cut out.*

The minimum blank size that has been calculated by the computer should be compared to the blank that is to be used. This will assure that the lens does not go all the way through surfacing and into edging before it is discovered that the blank is not large enough.

Knowing How Lenses Are Categorized and Organized

After establishing which lens should be used for a given job, the lens must be pulled from stock. A variety of methods may be used for keeping the many lenses needed in a lab in a logical order so that they may be located when needed.

Sorting Finished Single-Vision Lenses

Some labs put all the spheres together in one area and all the spherocylinders in another. Other labs keep the spheres together with the spherocyls.

When spheres are combined with spherocyls, the lenses are sorted first according to their spherical component, then by their minus cylinder power. Lenses are arranged from lowest to highest sphere powers. Lenses with a cylinder are further arranged

---

*Most computers give an estimated minimum blank size since they do not normally ask for the angle of the effective diameter, though they may ask for a generalized shape.

from the lowest to the highest cyl. For single-vision finished lenses, the sorting order would be

1. by lens material
2. by plus or minus sphere power
3. by sphere power
4. by cyl power (within the context of sphere power)

For example:

+0.25 sph
+0.25 −0.25
+0.25 −0.50
+0.25 −0.75
+0.25 −1.00
etc.
+0.50 sph
+0.50 −0.25
+0.50 −0.50
+0.50 −0.75
+0.50 −1.00
etc.

5. by blank size, if desired

Sorting Semifinished Lenses

Semifinished lenses can be categorized in the following order:

1. by lens material
2. by seg style, such as flat top, round, etc.
3. by seg size, such as FT-25, FT-28, etc.
4. by base curve
5. by add power
6. by lens size, if desired

Questions and Problems

1. What minimum blank size is required for the following single-vision lens if
   a. the lens is ground with no prism for decentration
   b. the lens is ground with prism to give the correct decentration

   Rx +6.00 −1.00 × 180
   A = 54 mm
   B = 49 mm
   ED = 57 mm
   DBL = 18 mm
   PD = 64 mm

2. If the lens in Problem 1 is being surfaced from a 71-mm blank, which method would be fastest and least likely to produce errors?

   a. grinding the lens without prism for decentration
   b. grinding the lens with prism for decentration

3. How large must a finished single-vision lens blank be in order to allow the following Rx to be placed in the frame described?

   Right lens
   −5.00 D sphere
   PD = 62 mm
   A = 46 mm
   B = 40 mm
   DBL = 20 mm
   ED = 48 mm

4. How large should a semifinished lens be for the Rx specified in Problem 3?

5. How large must a finished single-vision lens blank be in order to allow the following Rx to be placed in the frame described?

   Left lens
   Rx power −4.00 −2.00 × 90
   PD = 62 mm
   A = 48 mm
   B = 42 mm
   DBL = 20 mm
   ED = 52 mm

6. How large should a semifinished lens be for the Rx specified in Problem 5?

7. Of the following base curves, which is the best choice in order to create a −10.00 D sphere?
   a. +6.00 D
   b. plano
   c. +8.00 D
   d. +4.00 D

8. When lens base curves are properly selected, the farther from plano the lens power goes in the plus direction, the _____ the back curve of the lens becomes.
   a. steeper (more concave)
   b. flatter (less concave)

9. If you normally choose a 6.00 D base curve for a −2.00 D lens power, what base curve might be chosen for a large rimless or metal frame?
   a. a plano base
   b. a 2.00 D base
   c. a 4.00 D base
   d. the same base (6.00 D)
   e. an 8.00 D base

For each of the following lens powers, use Vogel's formula to find the needed base curve. (Do not round off your answers.)

10. +3.00 D sph

11. +4.50 − 1.50 × 25

12. $+2.00 - 0.50 \times 175$
13. -4.00 D sph
14. $-1.00 - 1.00 \times 90$
15. $-2.75 - 0.75 \times 75$
16. $-2.75 - 2.75 \times 160$
17. $-5.25 - 1.50 \times 15$
18. Using Fry's tables, what base curve would be chosen for a lens having a power of $+1.75 - 1.00 \times 180$?

Using Fry's tables and American National Standards Institute recommendations, what base curves should be used for the following lens pairs?

19. $+2.50 - 1.00 \times 30$ R base curve_____
    $-2.00 - 0.75 \times 150$ L base curve_____
20. $+5.25 - 1.00 \times 30$ R base curve_____
    $+4.25 - 0.75 \times 150$ L base curve_____
21. $-6.00 - 1.00 \times 30$ R base curve_____
    $-5.00 - 0.75 \times 150$ L base curve_____
22. $+2.50 - 1.00 \times 30$ 5 BO   R base curve_____
    $+3.50 - 0.75 \times 150$ 5 BO   L base curve_____

23. What would the minimum blank size be for the following lens/frame combination if the lens were to be edged from a finished uncut?

    Single-vision lens
    A = 54 mm
    B = 45 mm
    DBL = 17 mm
    ED = 61 mm
    Distance PD = 62 mm

24. What would the minimum blank size be for the lens/frame combination in Problem 23 if the lens were to be ground from a semifinished blank?

25. **a.** What is the minimum blank size necessary when using a single-vision *finished* lens if the lens is to be placed in the following frame?

    A = 55 mm
    DBL = 20 mm
    ED = 59 mm
    PD = 64 mm

    b. What is the minimum blank size necessary when using a single-vision *semifinished* lens if the lens is to be placed in the same frame?

26. From the following information, draw and label a flat-top bifocal lens blank with the dimensions requested below.

    Blank seg inset = 6 mm
    Blank seg drop = 7 mm
    A = 50 mm

    B = 47 mm
    DBL = 18 mm
    Wearer's PD = 62/59
    Seg height = 18 mm

    These are the dimensions to be drawn and labeled (when appropriate, include the actual measure of the dimension):

    blank seg inset
    blank seg drop
    seg inset
    seg drop
    blank geometric center
    MRP

27. You are checking blank size with a chart and find that in spite of using the largest blank available, there is still a slight gap in the upper temporal corner between the lens and the inner frame eyewire. What could you do so that you could still use the blank with the same frame? The lens is a flat-top bifocal lens. (You should consult with the account before doing this.)

28. A frame with a moderately large ED has been chosen and sent to you for fabrication. The lenses are high minus. It can be fabricated from stock (uncut) lenses using either a 65-mm lens blank or a 72-mm lens blank. Will the 65-mm lens blank yield better cosmetic results than the 72-mm lens blank?

29. Assume that single-vision uncuts are available up to 71 mm. Will an uncut work for the following Rx?

    $+1.00 - 3.00 \times 90$
    2.0 Prism Base Up
    A = 54 mm
    DBL = 18 mm
    ED = 59 mm
    PD = 63 mm

References

1. Borover, W.A. *Opticianry: The Practice and the Art, Vol. II—The Science of Opticianry.* Gracie Enterprises, Chula Vista, Calif., 1982, pp. 195, 203, 205.
2. Fry, G.A. The Optometrist's New Role in the Use of Corrected Curve Lenses. *Journal of the American Optometric Association,* 50(5):561–562.
3. Mancusi, R.J. *Ophthalmic Surfacing for Plastic and Glass Lenses.* Butterworth-Heinemann, Boston, 1982, p. 7.
4. American National Standards Institute. ANSI Z80.1-1987, American National Standard for Prescription Ophthalmic Lenses—Recommendations. American National Standards Institute, New York, 1987, p. 22.
5. Ibid.

3

Layout for Single-Vision Lens Surfacing

Introduction

The most important part of lens surfacing is lens layout. If the lens is inaccurately marked, no matter how exact all of the following steps are, the lens will not be usable. The lens must be marked with absolute accuracy. To be able to do lens surfacing, one must know how to mark the lens accurately.

There are two principal methods for marking a lens. One is termed *off-center blocking*. This is the older, more traditional method. In many cases it is still the method of choice. The other method is termed *on-center blocking*. With the advent of the lens computer, this method is now the most frequently used method.

Why Surface a Single-Vision Lens?

It makes sense to use a finished lens instead of surfacing a semifinished lens whenever possible. Yet there are times when surfacing a single-vision lens is either preferable or necessary. Here are a few.

1. Either the sphere or the cylinder power of the needed lens may be greater than is normally stocked in uncut lenses.
2. The lens may be glass and require a special tint that is not often used.
3. The lens may be ordered in a material (such as a high-index material) that is rarely needed. Keeping a stock of seldom-used finished lenses is not a wise investment.
4. Using a semifinished lens may allow a small-sized plus lens to be ground thinner than would normally be possible with a finished lens blank. (This is an advantage especially

for young children, who might otherwise have to wear unnecessarily thick lenses.)
5. The lens may be intended for an especially large frame. A normal finished lens blank would be too small.
6. The wearer's PD may be small in comparison to the frame size. The large amount of decentration required could make normal uncuts too small.

Traditional Blocking Practice: Off-Center Blocking

Before a curve can be ground onto the surface of a lens, it must be attached to a block. The block holds the lens in place. When the generator grinds the lens, it places the optical center on the lens at the center of the block (unless prism is ground on the lens). See Figure 3-1. If the block is moved to one side of the lens, the optical center moves with it.

Because this traditional blocking method moves the location of the lens optical center by moving the lens block toward one side of the lens or the other, it is referred to as *off-center blocking*. It retains this name even though, at times, the block may be positioned *on* the geometric center of the lens.

Blocking on the Geometric Center

Sometimes the only reason for surfacing a single-vision lens is because there was no finished lens in stock. A normal-sized lens would be perfectly acceptable. If the semifinished lens blank is large enough, the block may simply be mounted on the

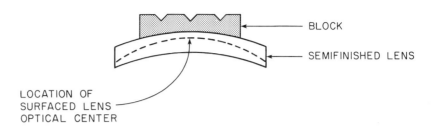

Figure 3-1 When a lens is ground using a conventional block, the location of the lens optical center will coincide with the center of the block unless steps are taken to induce prism.

– – – – (INDICATES LOCATION OF LENS SURFACE AFTER GENERATION)

geometric center of the lens blank. Once ground, the lens optical center will be located at the geometric center of the lens blank. This is just like a factory-finished (uncut) lens. If a semifinished lens blank of sufficiently large size is used, there is no reason for blocking anywhere but on the blank geometric center.

A lens that is spherical and is to be blocked on the geometric center of the lens is the easiest type of lens to mark. Actually, the only reason this lens needs to be marked at all is so that the person blocking the lens can find the geometric center of the lens blank.

How to Find the Blank Geometric Center

The easiest way to find the center of a single-vision semifinished lens blank is to estimate where it is and dot it with a marking pen. This is not always the most accurate way, though.

For many years, laboratory personnel took the blank and positioned it on a lens protractor. The lens blank was centered on or around a larger lens circle found on the protractor. Next a long horizontal line was traced across the center of the lens. A short vertical line was drawn across the center of it. Then, by tracing the major lines at the center of the protractor, the exact center of the lens was located. For spheres this is all the marking that is required.

In order to reduce production time, many laboratories prefer to use a *lens center locator*. This device centers the lens using three inverted, cone-like holders. See Figure 3-2. Once the lens is positioned, it is inked by touching an ink-dotted pin to the lens surface. Theoretically, this dot is all that is be required in order to block the lens. However,

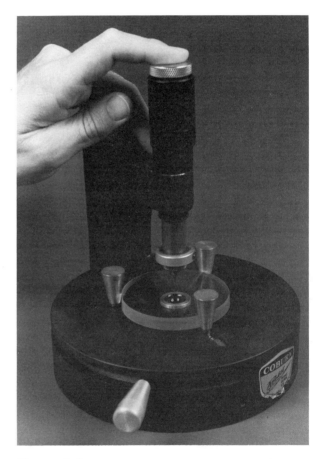

Figure 3-2 The lens center locator cuts time from the lens marking process. However, because some semifinished plastic lenses are molded slightly askew, the lens center found in this manner may not always be 100% accurate. With single-vision lenses this is relatively unimportant. With multifocals, a small error in the PD may result.

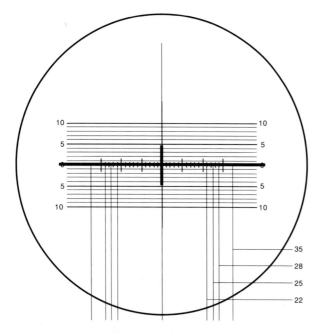

Figure 3-3 A sphere which does not require decentration is centered in the lens layout marker and marked. The marked cross shown here is oriented at 180 degrees. However, the cross is only used to help in finding the center of the blank quickly when blocking the lens.

because such a small dot is hard to see and is easily wiped off, the lens is subsequently placed in a lens marking device and a conventional marking cross (————|————) is applied over the dot. See Figure 3-3.

Now many lens marking devices come with circles corresponding to standard blank sizes. The blank is centered in the circle, then marked.

Off-Center Blocking

So far it has been assumed that the semifinished lens blank is large enough that it can be used in the same manner as a finished lens. If, however, the blank is *not* large enough, the lens can be blocked "off center." It will be recalled that when a lens is surfaced, the optical center will follow the location of the block center. This means that the optical center is moved away from its customary location at the center of the lens. See Figure 3-4. Thus the optical center can be moved to its desired location without having to use a big lens. By moving the optical center a bit off center, a much smaller lens can be used. Figure 3-5 shows how much of a difference this can make in required lens size.

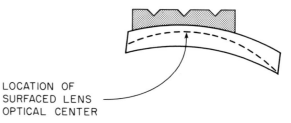

LOCATION OF
SURFACED LENS
OPTICAL CENTER

Figure 3-4 If a block is moved sideways on a semifinished lens blank, the lens optical center will correspond with the block center.

How Far Off Center Should the Block Be Moved?

To move the optical center of a single-vision lens, the block must be moved over by an amount equal to the distance decentration per lens.* This is how to do it.

1. *Find the "frame PD."* The frame PD† is the distance between the boxing centers of the frame's lens openings.

$$\text{Frame PD} = A + DBL$$

2. *Subtract the wearer's PD from the frame PD and divide by 2.*

$$\text{Decentration per lens} = \frac{(A + DBL) - PD}{2}$$

The distance decentration per lens equals the needed block decentration. The steps in marking a single-vision lens for off-center blocking are listed in Table 3-1.

Marking for Off-Center Blocking of Spherical Lenses

Example 3-1 shows how to mark a spherical lens for off-center blocking. It uses the steps given in Table 3-1.

EXAMPLE **3-1**

Mark a lens for the following:

A = 55mm
DBL = 19 mm
PD = 64 mm

The lens is a right lens.

---

*The exception would be instances where single-vision reading glasses are required. For reading glasses, decentration is calculated using the near PD.

†The correct term for "frame PD" is *geometric center distance*.

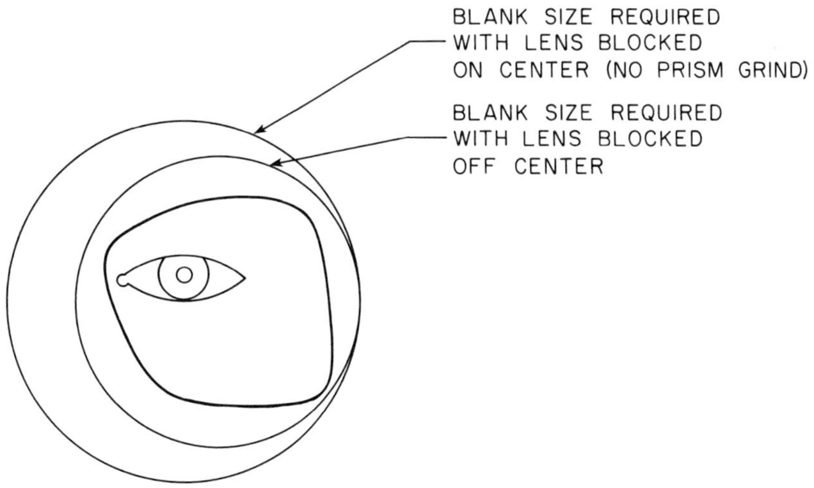

BLANK SIZE REQUIRED
WITH LENS BLOCKED
ON CENTER (NO PRISM GRIND)

BLANK SIZE REQUIRED
WITH LENS BLOCKED
OFF CENTER

Figure 3-5 If a lens is ground with the optical center exactly in the middle of the lens blank, the semifinished blank used must be considerably larger than it would have to be if the optical center were decentered during surfacing. If a lens blank with the optical center exactly in the middle is not sufficiently large, the frame's lens opening will not be fully covered.

Table 3-1 Marking Single-Vision Semifinished Lenses for Off-Center Blocking

1. Figure the block decentration required.

$$\text{Block decentration} = \frac{(A + DBL) - PD}{2}$$

2. Dot the center of the semifinished lens.

3. Place the lens on the lens marking device and move the dot outward (temporally)* by an amount equal to the block decentration.

4. For spheres, mark the lens with a cross (—+—). For spherocylinders, turn the lens marker to the correct axis, lock it securely in place, and mark the lens.

5. Print an "R" or an "L" and the job tray number on each lens. These should be placed on the front surface of the lens using reverse or "mirror" writing, so that it can be read through the back surface once the lens has been blocked. The "R" or "L" is written in the upper half and the tray number in the lower half of the lens.

*Those familiar with the edging process will note that this is opposite to the direction of decentration for edging. With decentration for edging, the position of the block does not correspond to the position of the optical center.

SOLUTION

1. Find the block decentration.

$$\text{Block decentration} = \frac{(55 + 19) - 64}{2} = 5 \text{ mm}$$

The movable vertical line in the lens marking device is moved 5 mm temporally. Since the lens is a right lens and will be placed on the marker with the front side up, the line is moved to the left.

2. Dot the geometric center of the lens.

3. The lens is placed front side up on the lens marking device. The center dot is placed on the horizontal midline of the marking grid at the location of the movable vertical line. See Figure 3-6.

4. The lens is marked as shown in Figure 3-7. (Note that the mark is at the center of the background grid—not at the decentered point where the movable line crosses.)

5. Mark a reverse "R" on the front of the lens in the upper half and the tray number in the lower half. See Figure 3-8.

Initially it may be difficult to write backwards. However, it is necessary to mark the lenses this way in order to keep accurate track of the lenses during processing.

Marking Spherocylinder Lenses

Spherocylinders That Require No Block Decentration
Blocking a spherocylinder lens on its geometric center produces an "uncut" lens. Once it has been surfaced, this lens is just like a finished (uncut) lens. During edging the cylinder axis can be turned in any direction needed. Because the cylinder axis can be turned later, the lens is marked for blocking exactly as the sphere lens was. The location of the axis doesn't matter.

Marking Spherocylinders for Off-Center Blocking
When a lens is blocked off center, it is no longer symmetrical. The optical center has been decentered in a specific direction for the purpose of getting more usable area out of the available lens diameter. Once the lens has been surfaced, it can no longer be rotated. This means that the axis of

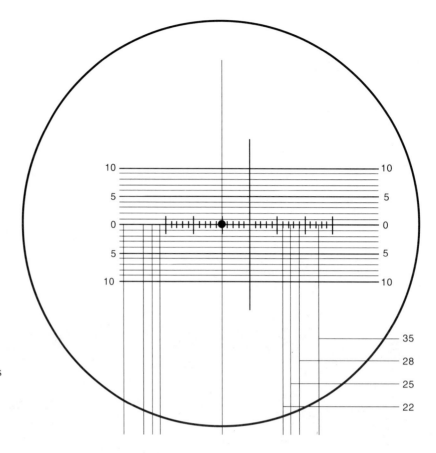

Figure 3-6 The long vertical line is first moved to the correct block decentration. It then helps as a "place holder" to make positioning of the dotted blank geometric center easier.

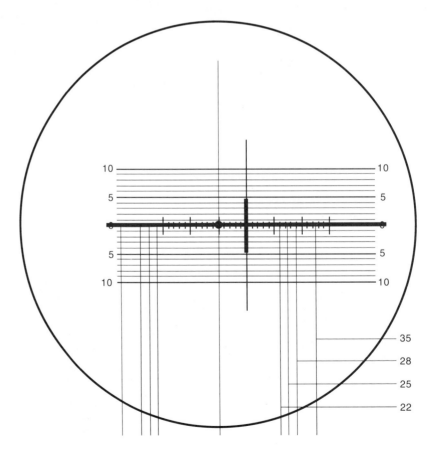

Figure 3-7 Every time the cross is stamped on the lens, it will be centered on the stationary background grid. The short vertical line does not move, nor does the center of the stamp.

36

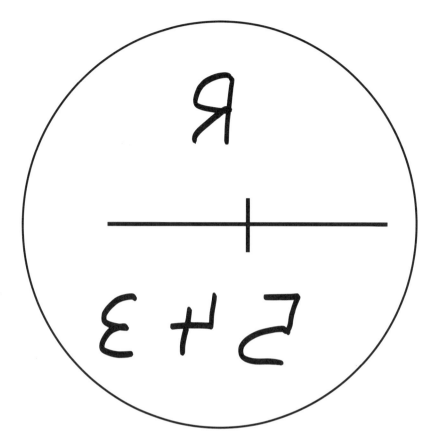

Figure 3-8 Once the lens has been stamped, the job number and an "R" or an "L" needs to be written on the lens. The "R" is written on the front surface in the upper half of the lens in reverse writing. This way the top is always distinguishable from the bottom. The job number is also written in reverse lettering. When the lens has been taped and blocked, and the back surface of the lens ground away, these numbers will still be readable through the back surface of the lens. When viewed from the back, the writing is not reversed.

the cylinder needs to be clearly indicated on the semifinished lens blank during the layout process.

When marking a lens for the correct cylinder axis, it is important to note whether the convex surface (front side) or the concave surface (back side) is facing the operator. This is especially important since there are two degree scales used on lens protractors and marking devices. One scale runs counterclockwise, from the right to the left. This scale is used when the lens is placed convex or front side up. When the lens is placed front side down, the "backward" scale, which runs from left to right in a clockwise direction, is used. Lenses may be marked on either the front or the back side. Hence both scales are important. However, most laboratories mark the front side of the lens.

The steps in marking a spherocylinder lens for off-center blocking are listed in Table 3-1.

EXAMPLE 3-2

Using a lens layout marker, mark a right lens for surfacing using off-center blocking. The frame and lens are to have these specifications:

Lens power required is $-2.00\ -3.25 \times 30$.
Frame A is 54 mm.
Frame DBL is 20 mm.
Wearer's PD is 62 mm.

SOLUTION

1. Block decentration is figured as

$$\frac{(54 + 20) - 62}{2} = 6\ mm$$

2. The geometric center of the lens blank is dotted as required.
3. The lens is positioned front side up for marking. Since the lens is a right lens, temporal is to the left. The lens is moved 6 mm to the left.
4. Because the lens is front side up, the regular degree scale on the marking device or protractor is used. Mark the lens at axis 30 degrees. See Figure 3-9.
5. Print a backwards "R" and the job tray number on the front surface of the lens.

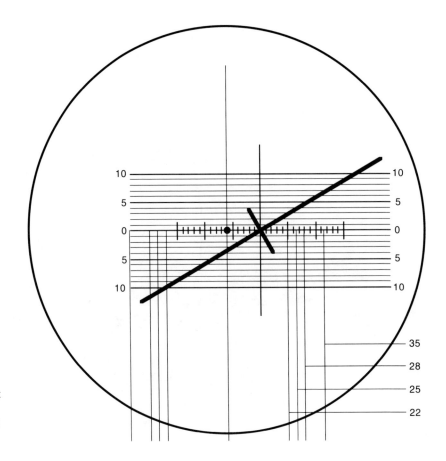

Figure 3-9 This right lens is front side up. The cylinder axis is marked for 30 degrees. The blocking method used is off-center blocking.

Marking for Rx Prism with Off-Center Blocking

Rx prism is prism that is prescribed by the practitioner. This is not the only type of prism referred to in the laboratory, however. Often prism is used in the optical laboratory to cause the optical center to move to a desired location. In order to distinguish between the two uses for prism, the term "Rx prism" is used to make clear that this prism is to be a part of the final prescription.

If there is to be prism ground into the lens, the direction of the prism must be indicated. Prism direction is indicated by an arrow. This arrow may be drawn on the lens when using a lens protractor. With a lens marking device, the so-called *prism axis* is stamped on by turning the marking cross to the correct degree meridian. After the prism axis is stamped, this prism axis line is lengthened with a marking pen so that it extends out to the edges of the lens. An arrowhead is drawn as either ─┼─> or <─┼─. The arrowhead should be drawn on the front of the lens. If it is drawn on the back, the marks disappear as the lens is generated. If the lens must be removed from the generator to be checked,

there will be no way to tell how to orient the prism ring on the lens again.

Unfortunately, there is no general agreement among laboratories as to whether the arrowhead indicates the apex or the base of the prism. Some say the arrowhead should point toward the apex of the prism, as the prism itself seems to point. Others say the arrow should indicate the base direction.* Therefore, when changing laboratories, it is important to find out which system is being used. In this book we will use the system with the arrow pointing in the apex direction, but either system is valid. Often layout computers will dictate which system must be used.

When a prescription calls for both cylinder and prism, there will be two lines on the lens. Let's consider an example.

---

*Although most sets of prism rings used in the generating process are marked at both the apex and the base, some sets are marked only at the apex, whereas others are marked only at the base. If prism ring sets are marked on only one side, then the direction of the arrow must conform to the marking on the prism ring.

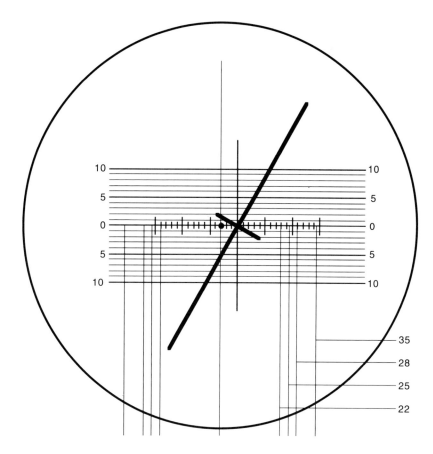

Figure 3-10 The axis of this right lens is marked for 60 degrees and is front side up. The major reference point of the lens is decentered 3 mm. Whenever a lens has Rx prism, the optical center and major reference point are no longer at the same spot on the lens.

EXAMPLE 3-3

A prescription calls for

R: +2.00 −2.25 × 60 with 2 prism diopters Base In
L: +2.00 −2.50 × 120 with 2 prism diopters Base In

The lenses are to be placed in a frame with dimensions of

A = 48
DBL = 18
Wearer's PD = 60 mm

Mark the lenses for off-center blocking using a lens layout marker.

SOLUTION

1. The block decentration is

$$\frac{(48 + 18) - 60}{2} = 3 \text{ mm}$$

2. The right lens is dotted at its geometric center.
3. The lens is positioned front side up on the layout marker and moved 3 mm to the left.

4. Because the lens is front side up, the right lens cylinder axis is marked at 60 using the regular (right-to-left) scale. (Remember that the same scale as was used to mark the cylinder axis is also used for marking the prism axis.) The lens is marked for axis as shown in Figure 3-10.

    For production purposes, Rx prism base direction must be converted from an "in-or-out" system to a degree system.* Base in always indicates that the base is turned toward the nose. For the right lens, this is in the 0-degree direction. To mark a 0-degree base direction, the marker axis is turned and a prism line is marked along the 0–180 line. See Figure 3-11. The arrowhead is hand-drawn so that it points the same way the prism apex points. The apex points *away* from the 0 and *toward* the 180. This indicates that the prism base is at 0 degrees. See Figure 3-12.

5. An "R" is marked at the top of the lens and a job number at the bottom.

---

*For a review on how this is done, see the section on prism base direction in Chapter 1.

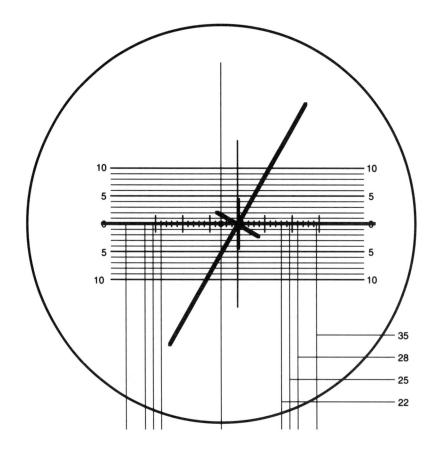

Figure 3-11 This right lens has an axis of 60 degrees and has been marked for horizontal prism. Without an arrowhead on the 180-degree-marked cross, there is no way to tell if the prism is base in or base out.

For the left lens, the blank is moved 3 mm to the right. The cylinder axis is marked at 120. Before marking the prism, remember that for the left lens, Base In is not in the 0-degree direction, but in the 180-degree direction. After prism for the left eye has been marked, compared to the right lens, the left lens arrow will point in the opposite direction. See Figure 3-13.

Marking for Two Prism Components on the Same Lens

Suppose we wish to mark for off-center blocking a lens that has two Rx prism components prescribed for the same lens. Since we can only grind prism in one base direction, the two components must be combined into a single prism component. That new component is marked on the lens.

EXAMPLE 3-4

A prescription calls for

R: −2.75 −1.00 × 25 with 3 prism diopters Base In and 1 prism diopter Base Up

L: −2.50 −1.25 × 160 with 3 prism diopters Base In and 1 prism diopter Base Down
Frame A = 50
Frame DBL = 18
Wearer's PD = 60 mm

How should the prism components be marked? What will the lenses look like after they have been marked?

SOLUTION

The block decentration is

$$\frac{(50+18) - 60}{2} = 4 \text{ mm}$$

The prism components are combined using one of the methods given in Chapter 1. Methods include a Prism Chart or a Prism Table. Using one of these methods, we can calculate the resulting prism for the right eye. For the right eye, 3 BI and 1 BU result in 3.2 prism diopters, Base 18 degrees.

For the left eye we also have 3.2 prism diopters, but this time the base direction is Base 198 (or Base 18 DN).

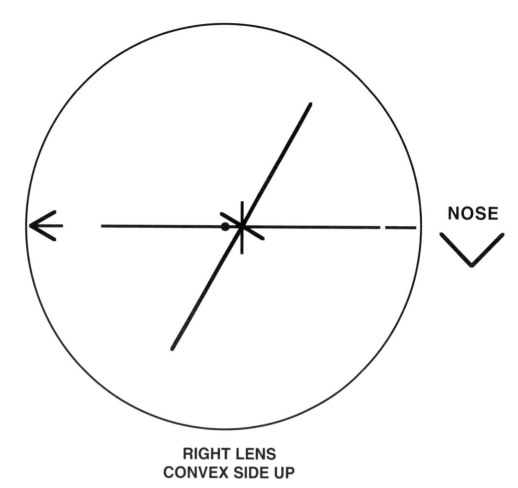

**RIGHT LENS
CONVEX SIDE UP**

Figure 3-12 With the lens turned with the front facing forward, the 60-degree axis is readily apparent. The arrows point toward the apex of the prism and away from the base. The arrow heads are marked on the *front* surface of the lens and indicate a 0-degree prism base direction. (Remember, many laboratories will want the arrowhead pointing to the base of the prism. It does not matter which system is used, as long as there is consistency.)

The correctly marked lenses are shown in Figure 3-14, with the convex (front) side of the lenses facing up.

On-Center Blocking

Sometimes the optical center needs to be moved too far over on the lens for off-center blocking. If off-center blocking were used, part of the block would start to go over the edge of the lens. When this happens, off-center blocking is no longer practical.

With plastic lenses, it is not advantageous to block off center. This is because the part of the lens that extends farthest out from the block tends to flex somewhat when the lens is fined and polished. The extended part of the lens is called *overhang*. See Figure 3-15. This uneven pressure due to lens flexure can result in either unwanted prism in the lens, or a waviness of the surface, or both.

When the semifinished lens blank is small, grinding the optical center in the middle produces a lens that is not big enough for the frame. If lens size is not checked ahead of time, the problem will not show up until edging. Then it results in a space between the edge of the lens and the frame eyewire. Because the traditional method of off-center block-

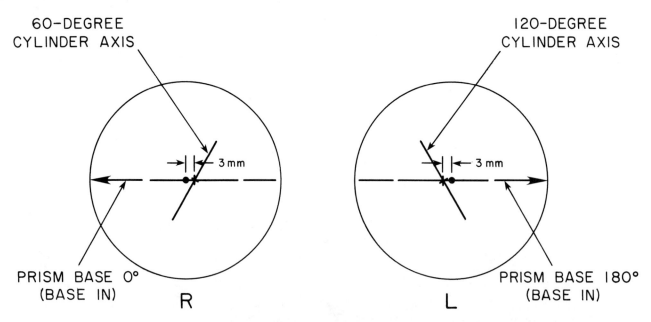

Figure 3-13 Normally, in a pair of lenses with prism the arrows will point in opposite directions. If this is not the case, prism calculations should be immediately rechecked. Here the lenses are convex side up and are viewed from the front.

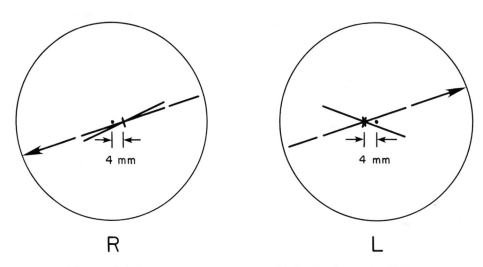

Figure 3-14 When marking lenses with both prism and cylinder, care must be taken to assure that the two marks are not accidentally switched.

Figure 3-15 Off-center blocking poses more of a problem with plastic than with glass lenses. A plastic lens needs as much support from the block as possible in order to keep the lens from bending.

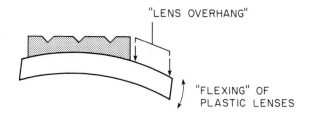

Table 3-2 Marking for On-Center Blocking Using a Layout Computer

1. Dot the blank geometric center.
2. Center the layout marker so that the movable vertical line has no decentration, place the lens on the marker, and center the dotted blank geometric center on the grid.
3. Mark the cylinder axis.
4. Mark the prism axis.
5. Remove the lens from the layout marker and draw an arrow on the front surface to indicate the direction of the prism *apex*.
6. Mark an "L" or an "R" in the upper half of the lens and a tray number in the lower half.

ing may be undesirable in certain circumstances, an alternative is necessary. That alternative is to block the lens on center and then grind prism into the lens. This is called *on-center blocking*. If the correct amount of prism is chosen, the optical center is moved exactly to the desired location.

On-centering blocking is almost always done in conjunction with a lens layout computer. Once the prescription information has been fed into the computer, the computer tells the amount of prism needed to move the optical center to its correct position. The steps for marking the lens from computer-given information are listed in Table 3-2.

Calculating Prism for On-Center Blocking Using Prentice's Rule

The amount of prism needed to move the optical center may be calculated using Prentice's rule. As discussed in Chapter 1, Prentice's rule states that the amount of prismatic effect created is equal to the distance in centimeters from the optical center of the lens to the referenced point on the lens times the power of the lens. Or, as a formula,

$$\Delta = cD$$

Here Δ equals prism diopters, c equals the decentration desired, and D is the power of the lens in the meridian of decentration. In this case the meridian of decentration is the 180-degree meridian.

EXAMPLE 3-5
Suppose it is necessary to block a lens on center, but the blank chosen is not large enough to use with its op-

tical center in the middle of the lens. Let's assume the following:

The lens in question is a left lens.
Its power (D) equals +5.00 D.
The frame has an A dimension of 50 mm and a DBL of 17 mm.
The wearer's PD is 62 mm.

How much prism must be ground and in what base direction in order to move the optical center nasally by an amount equal to the needed decentration? How would this lens be marked for surfacing?

SOLUTION
The following steps may be used as a general guideline for on-center blocking of single-vision spherical lenses:

1. Calculate the distance decentration per lens.

$$\frac{(A + DBL) - PD}{2} = \text{distance decentration per lens}$$

$$\frac{(50 + 17) - 62}{2} = 2.5 \text{ mm}$$

2. Using Prentice's rule, calculate the prism needed to move the optical center the desired amount.

$$\Delta = cD$$

$$\text{Prism needed} = (0.25 \text{ cm}) \times (5.00 \text{ D})$$

$$= 1.25$$

3. Determine the base direction of the prism.
   To help in determining which base direction is necessary, imagine what the lens will look like with the block still in place after surfacing. The center of the block is not at the optical center. The point on the lens where the block center will rest after the lens has been generated has either base-in or base-out prism, depending on whether the lens is plus or minus. To help visualize base direction, Figure 3-16 shows a simplified drawing.
   To determine the base direction, remember that the lens is plus. Decentration of the optical center is nasal, or inward. Since the optical center of a plus sphere lens is the thickest part of the lens, base direction is toward the optical center. The optical center is positioned nasally, so the base direction is base in. This is a left lens. For a left lens, Base In is Base 180.

The lens is marked as follows.

1. The blank geometric center is found and dotted.
2. The lens is placed on the layout marker with the

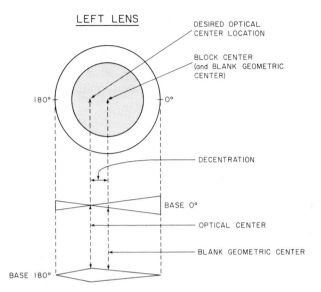

LEFT LENS

DESIRED OPTICAL
CENTER LOCATION

BLOCK CENTER
(and BLANK GEOMETRIC
CENTER)

180°

0°

DECENTRATION

BASE 0°

OPTICAL CENTER

BLANK GEOMETRIC CENTER

BASE 180°

Figure 3-16 How a lens looks on the block after having been surfaced. (Center blocking and prism for decentration were used.)

dotted blank geometric center in the middle of the grid. There should be no decentration of the movable vertical line, nor should the lens be decentered. See Figure 3-17.

3. Ordinarily, the next step is to mark the lens for cylinder axis. However, since this lens is a sphere, it does not have a cylinder axis. Because the lens will have prism ground, it will be marked for prism only.

4. Mark the lens for prism axis. Because the prism base direction is Base 180, mark the lens along the 180-degree meridian. See Figure 3-18.

5. Draw an arrowhead to show the direction of the prism's apex. (Because the base direction is 180 degrees, the arrowhead points toward 0 degrees.) See Figure 3-19. The arrowhead is drawn on the *front* of the lens so that it is not ground away during surfacing.

6. Mark a reverse "L" in the upper half of the lens on the front surface. The job number is marked in reverse writing in the lower half.

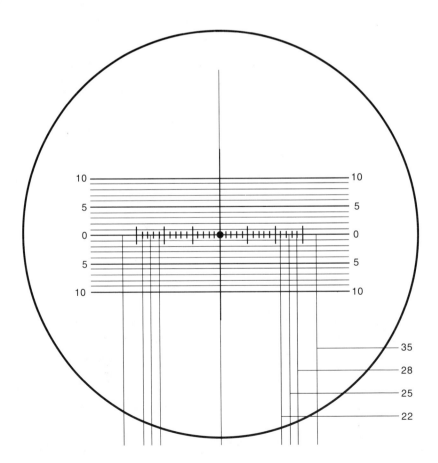

Figure 3-17 Standard positioning of a single-vision lens that is to be marked for on-center blocking.

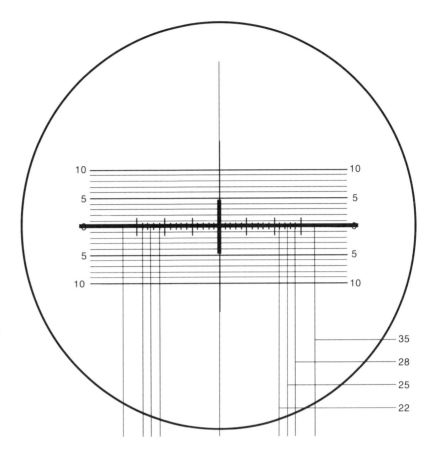

Figure 3-18 How all sphere lenses will look when marked for on-center blocking when prism for decentration is to be ground. The figure does not yet show the direction of prism for decentration. Plus lenses will require base-in prism, whereas minus lenses will require base-out prism.

Determining Prism Using a Prism Power Decentration Chart

Rather than using Prentice's rule, it is possible to refer to a Prism Power Decentration Chart to calculate prism for decentration. This chart is shown as Appendix 2-3. To use the chart, look up decentration. This is found at the top of the chart. Next locate the power of the lens at the 180-degree meridian. Lens power is listed on the left. Find the intersection of the correct column and row. This is the prism power needed to move the optical center over to where it should be.

Example 3-6

How much prism must be ground in what base direction for on-center blocking using the following lens and frame?

The lens is a left lens.
Power = +3.50 D
Frame A = 53 mm
DBL = 19 mm
Wearer's PD = 64 mm

Solution

1. The decentration required is

$$\frac{(53 + 19) - 64}{2} = 4 \text{ mm}$$

2. Using the Prism Power Decentration Chart, look up 3.50 D in the left column of the chart and 4.0 mm in the top row of the chart. Follow row and column, over and down, until they meet. The chart tells us that we need 1.4 prism diopters to move the optical center 4 mm.

3. Because the lens is a plus lens, the thick center of the lens should end up being nasal. Therefore the prism direction is nasal, or base in. Since the lens is a left lens, base in is the same as 180 degrees.

Determining Decentration Prism for Spherocylinders

With glass lenses there is no overriding advantage for blocking on center, even when decentration of the major reference point (MRP) is required. Sim-

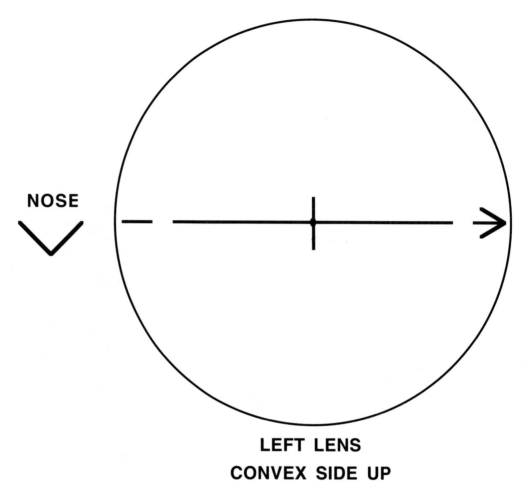

NOSE

LEFT LENS
CONVEX SIDE UP

Figure 3-19 Can you tell if this on-center blocked lens is a plus or a minus lens just by the prism base direction?

ply blocking at the desired MRP location will usually work well and requires no calculation for prism. With plastic lenses, though, the tendency of the lens blank to flex during fining results in unwanted prism and waviness. This makes blocking on center with as large a block as possible the most desirable method.

When a lens has a cylinder component to the prescription, the amount of prism needed for on-center blocking must take the cylinder power and axis into consideration. When the cylinder is oriented with its axis on the 90- or 180-degree meridian, calculation is easier. Not so when the cylinder is oriented obliquely (at other than 90 or 180 degrees)! An extra step is required.

In the next section we discuss what to do when the cylinder axis is at either 90 or 180 degrees. Then a workable method for determining layout and

marking spherocylinder lenses whose axes are oblique is given.

On-Center Blocking of Spherocylinders with Axes at 90 or 180 Degrees
For spherical lenses the required prism for decentration was found by multiplying the sphere power times the decentration in centimeters. With spherocylinder lenses whose axes are at 90 or 180 degrees, the power in the meridian of decentration can be found using a *power cross*.* [The meridian of decentration will be the horizontal (0–180) meridian.]

---

*If the reader is unfamiliar with the workings of the power cross, it may be advisable to review the concept. See, for example, C.W. Brooks and I.M. Borish, *System for Ophthalmic Dispensing,* Butterworth-Heinemann, Boston, 1979.

EXAMPLE 3-7

A prescription reads as follows:

R: −3.00 −2.00 × 90
L: −3.00 −2.00 × 90

The lens is to be placed in a rather large frame, which requires the maximum use of the full lens blank diameter.

Frame A = 56 mm
DBL = 18 mm
Wearer's PD = 64 mm

How much prism in what base direction must be ground for on-center blocking?

SOLUTION

Place the prescription on a power cross to find the power in the meridian of decentration (the 180-degree meridian). See Figure 3-20. From the power cross we see that the power in the 180-degree meridian is −5.00 D.

Next the amount of decentration is calculated.

$$\text{Decentration per lens} = \frac{(A + DBL) - PD}{2}$$

$$= \frac{(56 + 18) - 64}{2}$$

$$= 5 \text{ mm or } 0.5 \text{ cm}$$

Using the Prism Power Decentration Chart in Appendix 2-3 and finding the intersection of 5 mm and 5.00 D, the needed prism for decentration is 2.5 prism diopters.

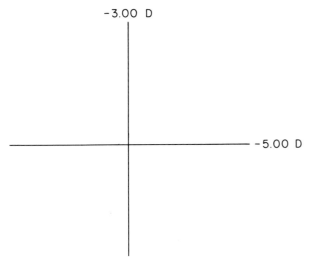

Figure 3-20 To place a prescription on a power cross, think of placing the sphere power (−3.00) in both meridians. Then add the power of the cylinder (−2.00) to the meridian 90 degrees away from the cylinder axis.

Some operators find it just as quick to use Prentice's rule. The answer may be found by mental calculations or by using a hand-held calculator. To find the answer directly using Prentice's rule (Δ = cD), the needed prism for decentration is

$$\Delta = (0.5 \text{ cm}) \times (5 \text{ D})$$

$$\Delta = 2.5$$

Because the lens is minus in power, the prism will be base out. For the right lens this is prism Base 180; for the left lens, it is prism Base 0 degrees.

On-Center Blocking of Spherocylinder Lenses with Oblique Axes

When all surfacing calculations were done by hand, it was necessary to utilize the most straightforward methods possible. In arriving at a workable method for calculating decentration prism for lenses having oblique axes, certain simplifications and assumptions were made.

A plano cylinder has zero dioptric power in the meridian of its axis and full dioptric value in the meridian 90 degrees away from its axis. Based on the fact that cylinder power is zero in the axis meridian and of full value in the power meridian, the assumption was made that the power of the cylinder must increase gradually, degree by degree, from the axis to the power meridian. On this basis, a method for finding this power in a given meridian was developed using the formula

$$D = D_{cyl} \sin^2 \theta$$

In the formula

D = the power of the cylinder in the 180-degree (horizontal) meridian
D_{cyl} = the power of the cylinder
θ = the axis of the cylinder

For cylinders with oblique axes (at neither 90 nor 180 degrees), this allowed the "power" of a cylinder along the horizontal meridian to be found. Once the cylinder "power" in the horizontal meridian was found, it was assumed that Prentice's rule for calculating prism by decentration could be applied in order to move the optical center in surfacing.

Unfortunately, the assumption that a cylinder gradually increases in power from the axis to the power meridian is false. When the principle is applied using sin² θ, the results are not always as expected. Yet surprisingly enough, with a large percentage of lenses this method is helpful in achieving a workable result. It has been used with some success in optical laboratories for quite a number of years. This *sine-squared formula* is especially helpful when used with single-vision lenses.

The main *disadvantage* to the $\sin^2 \theta$ method is that when horizontal prism for decentration is ground, the optical center drifts slightly up or down as it is being moved over. The *farther* from 90 or 180 degrees the axis of the cylinder is, the greater the vertical drift will be. In the same way, the *stronger* the power of the oblique cylinder, the more the optical center will have a tendency to drift up or down.

With single-vision lenses this may not be a serious problem. Vertical optical center drift may be compensated for in the edging process. However, when vertical drift occurs for multifocals in only one lens of a pair, or when the optical centers drift by differing amounts for right and left lenses, unwanted vertical prism results. With multifocals the safest bet is to make use of a good layout computer. (*Caution:* Some of the earlier computer programs mistakenly utilized the $\sin^2 \theta$ calculations instead of the more accurate methods currently available.)

The sine-squared calculation applies to the cylinder only—not to the sphere. Once the result is found, it is added to the sphere power. This new total value is used with Prentice's rule or the Prism Power Decentration Chart. The steps are shown in Table 3-3.

Table 3-3 Decentration Prism for Spherocylinders

1. Calculate the needed decentration.
2. Find the "power" of the cylinder in the 180-degree meridian. To do this, either
   a. use the formula $D = D_{cyl} \sin^2\theta$, or
   b. look up the result in a set of sine-squared tables. (These are shown in Appendix 3-1.)
3. Add this reduced cylinder value to the sphere power to find the total power in the 180-degree meridian.
4. Use the total power in the 180-degree meridian to find the prism needed to move the optical center. This can be done
   a. using Prentice's rule and calculating, or
   b. by looking up the value in the Prism Power Decentration Chart.
5. Find the base direction of the prism.

EXAMPLE 3-8

Find the amount and direction of prism needed to decenter the optical center for each of the single-vision lenses in this pair. Mark the right lens for on-center blocking.

R: $-3.00 -2.00 \times 15$
L: $-2.50 -1.75 \times 155$
Frame A = 50 mm
Frame DBL = 18 mm
Frame ED = 53 mm
PD = 58 mm

SOLUTION

The steps for the right lens are as follows.

1. Calculate needed decentration.

$$\frac{(50 + 18) - 58}{2} = 5 \text{ mm}$$

2. To find the power of the cylinder in the 180-degree meridian, either the formula or sine-squared tables may be used. Sine-squared tables are shown in Appendix 3-1. If tables are chosen, look up the intersection of the cylinder axis and power.

   For a right lens with 2 diopters of cylinder at axis 15 degrees, the "power" of the cylinder in the 180-degree meridian is found to be -0.13 D.

3. To find the power in the 180-degree meridian, the cylinder power in the 180-degree meridian is added to the sphere value:

$$-3.00 + -0.13 = -3.13$$

4. The prism needed to push the optical center over by 5 mm is therefore

$$(0.5 \text{ cm}) \times (3.13 \text{ D}) = 1.565 \text{ prism diopters}$$

5. Because the power in the 180-degree meridian is minus and the decentration desired is inward, the prism direction is base out. Since this is a right lens, the base direction expressed in degrees is Base 180.

To mark the right lens for on-center blocking:

1. Dot the blank geometric center.
2. Center the layout marker so that the movable vertical line has no decentration. Place the lens on the marker and center the dotted blank geometric center on the grid. (These steps are always done when marking a lens for on-center blocking.)

3. Next mark the cylinder axis for 15 degrees.
4. Mark the prism axis for 180 degrees. See Figure 3-21.
5. Remove the lens from the layout marker and draw an arrow on the front surface of the lens to indicate prism direction. See Figure 3-22.
6. Mark an "R" in reverse lettering on the upper half of the front surface of the lens and the job number in reverse lettering on the lower half.

The steps for the left lens are as follows.

1. The needed decentration is the same for the left lens as it was for the right—5 mm.
2. Using the sine-squared table in Appendix 3-1 for the left lens, the "power" of the −1.75 D cylinder in the horizontal meridian is found to be −0.31 D.
3. Therefore the total power used to calculate prism by decentration is

$$-2.50 + (-0.31) = -2.81$$

4. The prism needed to push the optical center over the needed 5 mm for the left lens can be found using Prentice's rule or the Prism Power Decentration Chart in Appendix 2-3. This time, instead of calculating, we will use the chart. Using the chart, the prism needed falls between 1.38 and 1.44 prism diopters (using 2.75 D and 2.875 D for the lens powers, respectively). To the nearest tenth, this is 1.4 prism diopters.
5. Since the power in the horizontal meridian is minus and the decentration desired is inward, the prism base direction must be base out. However, since this lens is a left lens, the base direction in degrees is Base 0.

All the steps needed to calculate prism and mark a single-vision lens for on-center blocking are summarized in Table 3-4.

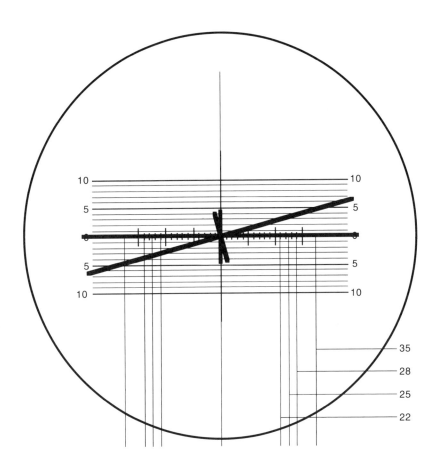

Figure 3-21 This lens is front side up and is marked for a 15-degree cylinder axis and horizontal prism for decentration. The prism arrowheads will be drawn on the prism axis when the lens is removed from the layout marker. It is easy to lose track of which line is the prism axis when taking the lens out of the marker; care should be taken at this point in the process.

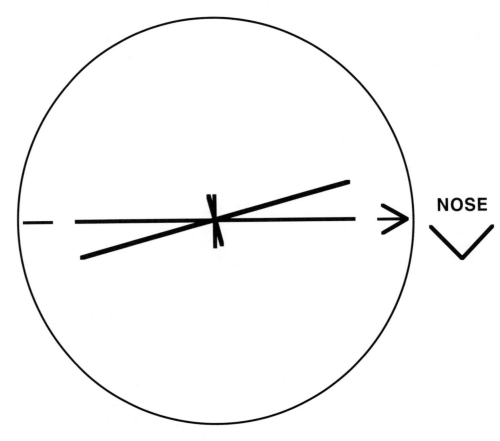

**RIGHT LENS
CONVEX SIDE UP**

Figure 3-22 Is the axis of this lens (a) 0, (b) 180, (c) 15, or (d) 165? Is this lens (a) plus in power in the 180, or (b) minus in power in the 180? If you answered (c) for the first question and (b) for the second, you are correct.

Questions and Problems

General Questions

1. Why might it be necessary to grind prism if a lens is blocked off center?

2. If the Rx listed is to be surfaced on center, how much prism must be ground and in what direction? (Give your base direction in degrees.)

>   Right lens
>   −5.00 D sphere
>   PD = 62 mm
>   A = 46 mm
>   B = 40 mm
>   DBL = 20 mm
>   ED = 48 mm

3. If the following Rx listed is to be surfaced on center using the minimum blank size, how much prism must be ground and in what base direction (in degrees)?

>   Left lens −4.00 −2.00 × 90
>   PD = 62 mm
>   A = 48 mm
>   B = 42 mm
>   DBL = 20 mm
>   ED = 52 mm

4. Use the following information to answer the questions.

>   R: −5.50 −2.00 × 90
>   L: −4.75 −1.75 × 90
>   Frame A = 58

Table 3-4 Steps Used to Calculate Decentration Prism and Mark a Single-Vision Lens for On-Center Blocking

A. Calculating Prism for Decentration

1. Calculate decentration per lens:

$$\frac{(A + DBL) - PD}{2}$$

2. For oblique cylinders, use the sine-squared formula or sine-squared tables to look up the reduced cylinder power in the 180-degree meridian.

3. Find the "power" in the 180-degree meridian ("power" in the 180 = sphere power + reduced cyl power).

4. Use Prentice's rule or the Prism Power Decentration Chart to find the prism amount needed.

5. Determine the prism base direction. (Almost always, plus power will be base in and minus power will be base out.)

B. Marking the Lens

1. Dot the blank geometric center.

2. Set the layout marker for zero decentration and center the lens on it.

3. Mark the cylinder axis.

4. Mark the prism axis.

5. Remove the lens from the marker and draw an arrowhead on the front surface of the lens to indicate prism direction.

6. Mark an "R" or an "L" in reverse lettering on the upper half of the front surface of the lens and the job number on the lower half.

Frame DBL = 15
Frame ED = 65
PD = 61

a. How much prism would be required for each lens and in what base direction in order to grind prism for decentration? (On-center blocking is used.)

b. What would be the smallest semifinished blank size that could be used?

5. Use the following information to answer the questions.

R: + 3.75 −1.25 × 80   2.50 Base Out and
                       1.25 Base Up
L: +3.25 −1.50 × 115   2.25 Base Out and
                       0.75 Base Down

Frame A = 48
Frame DBL = 20
Frame ED = 52
PD = 59

a. If on-center blocking were to be used *without* grinding prism for decentration, how much prism would be required for each lens and in what base direction? (Don't forget your Rx prism.)

b. Using the conditions specified in part a, what would the smallest semifinished blank size be that could be used and still have the lens cut out?

6. Use the following information to answer the question.

R: +2.50 −1.25 × 30
L: +3.25 −1.50 × 165
Frame A = 51
Frame DBL = 19
Frame ED = 59
PD = 60

How much prism (total) would be required for each lens and in what base direction in order to grind prism for decentration when on-center blocking is used?

Off-Center Blocking
Using semifinished single-vision lens blanks or a mock acetate lens, determine where and how each of the following lenses would be marked. Use off-center blocking.

7. Right lens

Power = −2.00 D
A = 50
DBL = 17
Wearer's PD = 62

8. Left lens

Power = −3.00 D
A = 54
DBL = 18
Wearer's PD = 66

9. Right lens

Power = −1.75 D
A = 48
DBL = 20
Wearer's PD = 60

10. Left lens

Power = −1.00 D
A = 53
DBL = 16
Wearer's PD = 62

11. Right lens

> Power = +2.00 D
> A = 44
> DBL = 15
> Wearer's PD = 62

12. Left lens

> Power = +1.00 D
> A = 51
> DBL = 17
> Wearer's PD = 61

13. Right lens

> Power = +0.50 D
> A = 44
> DBL = 15
> Wearer's PD = 55

14. Left lens

> Power = +1.50 D
> A = 59
> DBL = 14
> Wearer's PD = 62

On-Center Blocking

For each of the following lens pairs, determine how much prism must be ground into the lens in order to move the optical center over by the amount required for distance decentration.

Lay out and mark the lenses for on-center blocking, indicating prism direction and amount.

15. Both lenses

> Power = −2.50 D
> A = 50
> DBL = 17
> Wearer's PD = 62
> Prism amount _____
> Prism base direction
> R: _____
> L: _____

16. Both lenses

> Power = +1.50D
> A = 54
> DBL = 18
> Wearer's PD = 66
> Prism amount _____
> Prism base direction
> R: _____
> L: _____

17. Both lenses

> Power = −0.75 D
> A = 48
> DBL = 20
> Wearer's PD = 60

> Prism amount _____
> Prism base direction
> R: _____
> L: _____

18. Both lenses

> Power = +2.00 D
> A = 53
> DBL = 16
> Wearer's PD = 62
> Prism amount _____
> Prism base direction
> R: _____
> L: _____

19. Both lenses

> Power = +2.25 D
> A = 44
> DBL = 15
> Wearer's PD = 62
> Prism amount _____
> Prism base direction
> R: _____
> L: _____

20. Both lenses

> Power = −1.50 D
> A = 51
> DBL = 17
> Wearer's PD = 61
> Prism amount _____
> Prism base direction
> R: _____
> L: _____

21. Both lenses

> Power = +2.50 D
> A = 44
> DBL = 15
> Wearer's PD = 55
> Prism amount _____
> Prism base direction
> R: _____
> L: _____

22. Both lenses

> Power = −0.25 D
> A = 59
> DBL = 14
> Wearer's PD = 62
> Prism amount _____
> Prism base direction
> R: _____
> L: _____

On-Center Blocking, Rx Prism, and Minimum Blank Size

Use a set of dummy semifinished single-vision lenses for

the following. (Plano uncut single-vision lenses or mock acetate lenses will work.)

Mark the "semifinished single-vision lens blanks" for surfacing using on-center blocking. Use a felt-tip, water-soluble marking pen. Answer these questions for each set of example lenses.

a. How far would the optical center (or major reference point, when Rx prism is present) be from the geometric center of the lens?

b. What amount of prism must be ground? (Remember to combine prism for decentration with Rx prism, if necessary.)

c. What is the minimum blank size for this blank if it is ground for decentration?

d. What would the minimum blank size for this blank have to be if the lens were ground with no prism for decentration and the block on the blank geometric center?

23. R: $+3.00 -2.00 \times 180$
    L: $+2.50 -1.75 \times 180$
    Frame A $= 50$
    Frame DBL $= 18$
    Frame ED $= 53$
    PD $= 60$

24. R: $+4.00 -2.00 \times 90$
    L: $+3.50 -1.75 \times 90$
    Frame A $= 51$
    Frame DBL $= 19$
    Frame ED $= 55$
    PD $= 60$

25. R: $+5.00 -2.50 \times 20$
    L: $+4.50 -1.75 \times 170$
    Frame A $= 52$
    Frame DBL $= 18$
    Frame ED $= 53$
    PD $= 62$

26. R: $-1.50 -2.00 \times 80$
    L: $-2.50 -1.75 \times 120$

Frame A $= 58$
Frame DBL $= 15$
Frame ED $= 65$
PD $= 60$

27. R: $+0.25 -3.50 \times 97$
    L: $+0.50 -3.25 \times 75$
    Frame A $= 55$
    Frame DBL $= 17$
    Frame ED $= 59$
    PD $= 61$

28. R: $+5.50 -2.50 \times 90$ 2 Base In
    L: $+4.75 -2.75 \times 90$ 1.5 Base In
    Frame A $= 52$
    Frame DBL $= 16$
    Frame ED $= 53$
    PD $= 59$

29. R: $-2.25 -1.50 \times 90$ 1 Base Up
    L: $-3.25 -1.25 \times 90$ 1 Base Down
    Frame A $= 56$
    Frame DBL $= 16$
    Frame ED $= 60$
    PD $= 62$

30. R: $-3.00 -1.50 \times 90$ 1 Base Up and 2 Base Out
    L: $-3.25 -1.75 \times 90$ 1 Base Down and 2.5 Base Out
    Frame A $= 55$
    Frame DBL $= 15$
    Frame ED $= 59$
    PD $= 61$

31. R: $-2.75 -2.25 \times 85$ 2.00 Base In
    L: $-3.25 -1.50 \times 135$ 2.25 Base In
    Frame A $= 53$
    Frame DBL $= 19$
    Frame ED $= 65$
    PD $= 60$

4 Layout and Marking of Flat-Top and Curved-Top Lenses

Layout and Marking of Flat- and Curved-Top Multifocal Lenses Using Off-Center Blocking

Historically, surface blocking of multifocal lenses was done by using the method called "off-center" blocking. Off-center blocking places the lens block where the optical center or major reference point of the lens should be located. In many laboratories off-center blocking is still used for glass lenses. The steps used to lay out flat-top bi- or trifocal lenses for off-center blocking are as follows:

1. *Preset the layout marker for seg inset.* Position the movable vertical line in the layout marker for the correct seg inset. When the lens is placed in the layout marker front side up, the direction of inset will be to the right for a right lens and to the left for a left lens.
2. *Position the lens for seg inset.* Place the lens in the marker front side up. Center the seg between the appropriate guidelines in the layout marker. The lens is now centered for the correct seg inset.
3. *Position the lens for seg drop.* Move the lens up or down until the top of the seg is at the level of the correct seg drop or raise.
4. *Mark the cylinder axis.* Set the layout marker for the prescribed cylinder axis and mark the lens.
5. *Mark the prism axis.* If Rx prism is present, set the prism for the correct prism axis and

Table 4-1 Layout of Flat- or Curved-Top Lenses for Off-Center Blocking

1. Preset the layout marker for seg inset.
2. Position the lens for seg inset.
3. Position the lens for seg drop.
4. Mark the cylinder axis.
5. Mark the prism axis.
6. Mark the base direction.
7. Mark "R" or "L" and job number.

mark the lens again. Because very few prescriptions have prescribed prism, this step is usually unnecessary.
6. *Mark the base direction.* Remove the lens from the lens marking device and draw arrowheads on the prism line to indicate base direction.
7. *Mark "R" or "L" and job number.* These steps are summarized in Table 4-1.

EXAMPLE 4-1

Consider the following prescription, which is to be made up in a flat-top 25 bifocal.

Left lens power = +2.00 −1.25 × 30
Frame B = 50 mm
Wearer's PD = 64/60
Seg height = 20 mm

How would the lens be marked for off-center blocking?

54

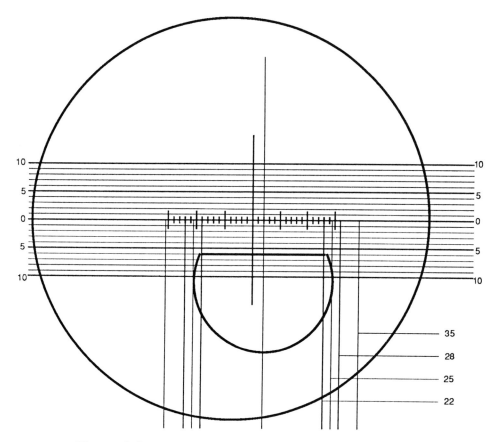

Figure 4-1 This lens is a left lens placed front side up in a lens marking device. The movable vertical line (which is the longer of the two vertical lines) is moved 2 mm to equal the seg inset. The segment is centered between the guidelines.

SOLUTION

To see how the lens is marked, we can go through the steps listed on page 54.

Steps 1 and 2. In order to position the movable line for the correct seg inset, we need to know the amount of seg inset needed. In the example, the PD is 64/60. This means that the seg inset will be

$$\text{Seg inset} = \frac{\text{distance PD} - \text{near PD}}{2}$$

$$= \frac{64 - 60}{2}$$

$$= 2 \text{ mm}$$

The lens is a left lens, so the movable vertical line is positioned 2 mm to the left. The lens is placed on the marker front side up and the segment is centered between the guidelines. See Figure 4-1.

Steps 3 and 4. To set the lens at the correct seg drop,

we must first know what that drop is. Seg drop is figured as

$$\text{Seg drop} = \text{seg height} - \frac{B}{2}$$

$$= 20 - \frac{50}{2}$$

$$= -5 \text{ mm}$$

Because the seg drop is known to be -5 mm,* move the lens seg top to the fifth millimeter line below the horizontal midline of the background grid. When the lens is properly positioned, turn the layout marker to the correct

---

*Technically, seg drop is a negative number, because it is below the midline of the lens, and seg raise is a positive number. In practice, most think in terms of B/2 − seg height, since most lenses have seg drop, not seg raise.

cylinder axis and stamp the lens. See Figure 4-2. Because there is no Rx prism, steps 5 and 6 are unnecessary.

EXAMPLE 4-2

Now consider a lens that has prescribed prism. For the following order, lay out and mark the lens using off-center blocking.

Right lens power is −2.00 −0.75 × 135.
This lens calls for 2 diopters of base-out prism for the right eye.
Frame B = 48 mm
Seg height = 21 mm
Wearer's PD = 62/59

SOLUTION

Layout for this lens is begun in exactly the same manner as was done for the previous example. The main difference is that this lens calls for Rx prism.

Steps 1 and 2. The seg inset for this lens is

$$\text{Seg inset} = \frac{62 - 59}{2}$$

$$= 1.5 \text{ mm}$$

Since this is a right lens, the movable line can be preset 1.5 mm to the right of center.

Steps 3 and 4. The seg drop for this lens is

$$\text{Seg drop} = 21 - \frac{48}{2}$$

$$= 21 - 24$$

$$= -3 \text{ mm}$$

The lens is placed front side up on the layout marker and the seg is centered horizontally between the segment reference grid lines. Next the segment is centered vertically for a −3 mm drop. Once centered, the lens may then be marked for a 135-degree axis as shown in Figure 4-3.

Step 5. Because the Rx prism is horizontal, the axis marker on the instrument is turned to the 180-degree

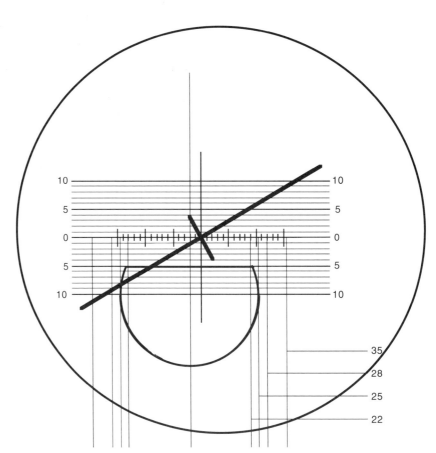

Figure 4-2 This left lens has been marked for off-center blocking. Since there is no prism after surfacing is completed, the optical center will be at the location of the marked cross. Seg inset is 2 mm and seg drop is 5 mm. Distance decentration is not used when surfacing bifocals.

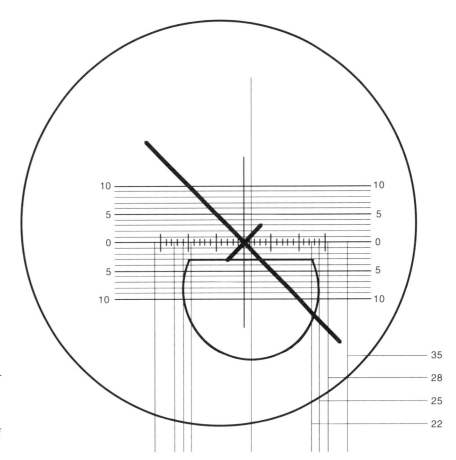

Figure 4-3 For layout of flat-top bifocals using off-center blocking, the seg drop (3 mm) and seg inset (1.5 mm) are positioned before marking. Here the lens has been marked for a cylinder axis of 135.

meridian. The lens is now marked a second time as shown in Figure 4-4.

Step 6. For a right lens, base-out prism is the same as Base 180. When the lens is removed from the marker, it is marked for Base 180 as shown in Figure 4-5.

EXAMPLE 4-3

Occasionally a lens will be prescribed with both horizontal and vertical prism. When this happens, the horizontal and vertical components are combined into one prism at an oblique axis. The procedure for combining horizontal and vertical prism was explained in Chapter 1. What would the following curved-top lens look like when marked for off-center blocking?

Left lens: +6.00 −2.00 × 155
Rx prism: 3△ Base Out
          1△ Base Up
Frame B = 46 mm
Seg height = 19 mm
Wearer's PD = 64/61

SOLUTION

It is likely that this prescription is for someone who has a tendency for crossed eyes. Curved-top lenses are marked and blocked in a manner that is practially identical to that for flat-top lenses. There are only a few differences. To lay out the lens, we go through the steps as used previously.

Steps 1 and 2. The seg inset is found to be 1.5 mm and the layout marker line is moved 1.5 mm to the left. The lens segment is positioned horizontally.

Steps 3 and 4. The seg drop (or raise) is

$$\text{Seg drop (or raise)} = 19 - \frac{46}{2}$$

$$= -4 \text{ mm}$$

Because the seg height is less than half the frame B dimension, the segment is dropped.

As with all multifocals having visible segments, seg height is measured to the highest portion of the segment top. In flat-top lenses the top of the segment is the same all the way across. In a curved-top lens, however, the

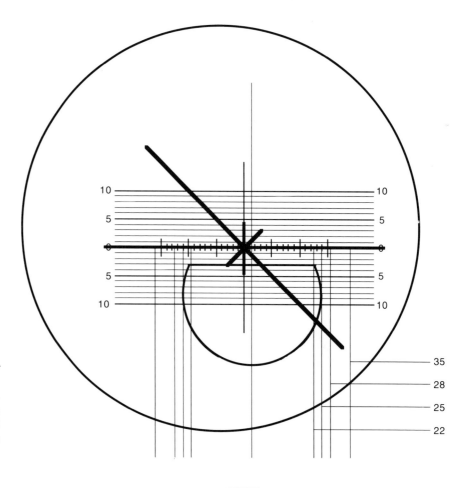

Figure 4-4 A lens that is blocked using an off-center blocking technique will be marked for prism only when there is prism in the prescription (Rx prism). Here the prism is base out for the right eye. The layout marker is used to stamp for horizontal prism.

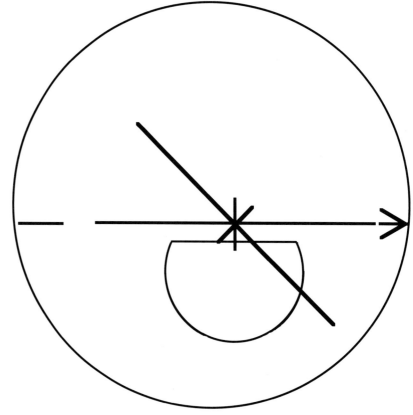

Figure 4-5 Once a prism axis has been stamped, the direction of the prism is applied with an arrowhead. Here the arrowhead goes in the direction opposite the base. Base out for this right lens means that the prism apex will point to the right. (Remember that many laboratories mark the *base* of the prism with an arrowhead, not the apex.)

gradual curve of the upper segment edge means that only the uppermost arch of the curve determines segment height. Fortunately, this presents no problem.

It is important that the segment portion of the lens not be tilted once it is in the frame. With the flat-top segment it was easy to tell if the segment was tipped. With the curved-top segment lens, the two outer corners are used to assure that the lens segment is straight. Both corners must be at an equal height as viewed on the lens marking device or protractor. Once the seg has been properly positioned, the cylinder axis is marked for 155 degrees. See Figure 4-6.

Step 5. Before the prism axis can be marked, we need to know the prism axis direction. Using a Prism Graph or Prism Table (Appendix 2-2) for a left lens having 3 diopters base-out prism and 1 diopter of base-up prism, we find the prism axis to be 18 degrees. The lens is now marked as shown in Figure 4-7.

Step 6. For prism Base 18, the arrowheads are shown as being drawn away from the base and toward the apex as seen in Figure 4-8. (Some laboratories do the opposite.) The arrowheads are always drawn on the front of the lens so that they are not ground off during the generating process.

Step 7. Mark a reverse "L" on the lens, along with the job number.

Layout and Marking of Flat- and Curved-Top Multifocal Lenses Using On-Center Blocking

Theory

Whenever a lens is blocked and then generated, the optical center (OC) of that lens will end up at the center of the block. In off-center blocking, the desired OC location is determined and the block center is placed at that point. However, if the lens is ground for prism, the OC will be pushed away from the center of the block.

On-center blocking places the block at the geometric center of the lens for optical stability, but must use prism to move the OC to its desired location.

When a flat-top lens is marked for surfacing using on-center blocking, prism must be ground in order

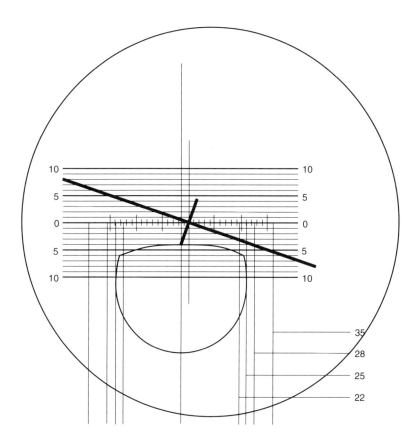

Figure 4-6 When marking curved-top lenses, the top of the curve is placed on the line for the near seg drop. Here the seg drop is 4 mm. The two points on the left and right of the seg curve must be on the same horizontal line so that the lens segment will not be tipped when the lens is placed in the frame.

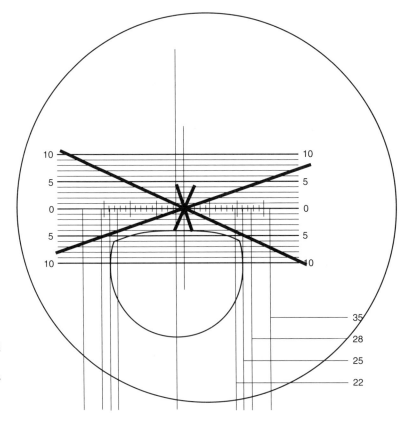

Figure 4-7 Sometimes a prism axis and cylinder axis end up close to being mirror images of one another. When this happens it is easy to confuse the two and mark the arrowheads on the wrong axis.

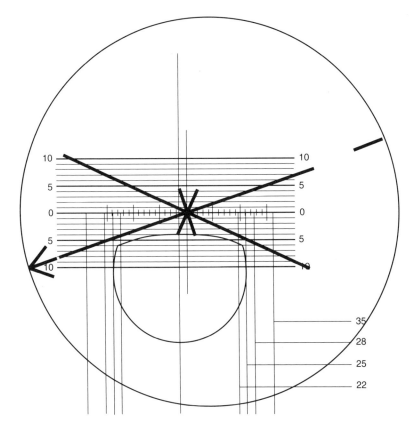

Figure 4-8 One of the most confusing aspects of lens marking is the axis direction. This is especially true for prism. Here the cylinder axis is 155 and the prism axis is 18. (Remember, in this figure, the arrow points *away* from the prism base direction. Some laboratories point the arrow *toward* the base direction.)

to move the optical center from the center of the block (and lens) to where it should be in relationship to the segment. With single-vision lenses this was a purely horizontal movement. If multifocal lenses are truly blocked on the blank geometric center, the optical center must be moved both horizontally and vertically.

EXAMPLE 4-4

A lens that is to be ground has dimensions as follows:

Power = −5.00 D sphere
A = 50 mm
B = 46 mm
DBL = 18 mm
Seg height = 20 mm
PD = 64/60

The semifinished lens that is to be used has a blank seg inset of 6 mm and a blank seg drop of 7 mm. What prism must be ground when on-center blocking is used in order for the optical center to come out in correct relation to the segment location?

SOLUTION

(Before solving this example, it should be understood that these calculations are practical for production purposes only when using a layout computer. However, going through an example calculation manually provides a much better understanding of on-center blocking.)

To find the answer to this question, visualize where the geometric center of the lens blank is in reference to the needed optical center location. This is best demon-

strated by means of a diagram, which can be sketched after the seg inset and seg drop are known.

The seg inset is

$$\text{Seg inset} = \frac{\text{far PD} - \text{near PD}}{2}$$

$$\frac{64 - 60}{2} = 2 \text{ mm}$$

The seg drop is

$$\text{Seg drop} = \text{seg height} - \frac{B}{2}$$

$$20 - \frac{46}{2} = -3 \text{ mm}$$

With this information, we can construct Figure 4-9. First the future position of the optical center is located using seg inset and seg drop. It is 3 mm above and 2 mm to the right of the center of the seg line. Next we must determine where the blank geometric center falls in reference to the distance optical center. This is shown in Figure 4-10. It is 4 mm above and 4 mm to the right of the distance optical center.

The amount of prism required to move the optical center to where it should be is the same as the amount that will be found at the geometric center of the lens blank once the lens is surfaced. This may be easier to visualize by thinking of what it would be like to look through a lensmeter at the blank geometric center of the lens after it has been surfaced. The prismatic effect seen in the lensmeter will be the amount that is used for off-center blocking.

To help understand this better, in Figure 4-10 a set of

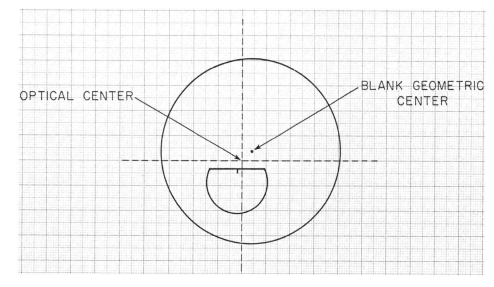

Figure 4-9 With the lens block in the middle of the lens and no prism grind, the optical center and blank geometric center are at the same point. The object of on-center blocking is to move the optical center to the desired location by using a prism grind.

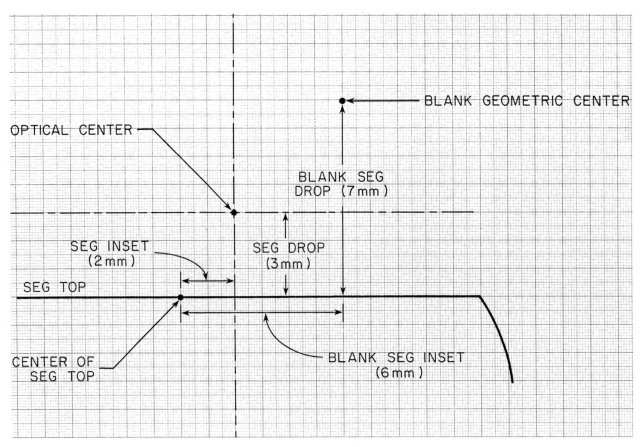

Figure 4-10 Here the relationship between the semifinished lens blank dimensions (blank seg inset, blank seg drop) and the finished lens dimensions (seg inset, seg drop) can be visualized.

coordinate axes is drawn through the desired optical center location. This shows the blank geometric center to be 4 mm up and 4 mm out from the distance optical center. By geometry it can be determined that the blank geometric center is 5.66 mm away from the optical center and is at an angle of 45 degrees to it. Using Prentice's rule, the prismatic effect at the blank geometric center will be

$$(0.566 \text{ cm}) \times (5.00 \text{ D}) = 2.83 \text{ prism diopters}$$

once the lens has been surfaced. Since the lens is minus in power, the prism base direction is Base 45.

Practice

It can be seen that, although it is possible to calculate prism using on-center blocking, even "easier" calculations like the one in Example 4-4 are cumbersome. The problem becomes considerably more

difficult in the presence of a cylinder. In practice, therefore, such calculations are done with the aid of a surface layout computer.

Centering the Lenses for On-Center Blocking

There are three ways to find the center of a multifocal lens for on-center blocking. The first uses a lens center locator to find the geometric center of the lens blank. The second uses the circles found on some layout markers to center the lens. The third finds the lens center by using the seg as a reference point. Methods of on-center layout are outlined in Table 4-2.

Using the Lens Center Locator
The lens center locating device presses on the edge of the lens from three locations and thereby dots

Table 4-2 Layout of Flat- or Curved-Top Lenses for On-Center Blocking

A. Using a Lens Center Locator
   1. Dot the blank geometric center of the lens.
   2. Place the center dot on the center of the layout marker grid.
   3. If necessary, rotate the lens so that the top of the segment is perfectly horizontal.
   4. Mark the lens cylinder axis.
   5. Mark the lens prism axis.
   6. Mark the prism base direction.
   7. Mark "R" or "L" and job number.
B. Using Layout Marker Circles
   1. Position the lens on the layout marker so that it is centered in the circle(s) on the layout marker screen.
   2. Follow steps 3 through 7 in part A above.
C. Using Blank Seg Inset and Drop for Reference
   1. Preset the layout marker for blank seg inset.
   2. Position the lens on the layout marker for blank seg inset.
   3. Position the lens for blank seg drop.
   4. Mark the lens cylinder axis.
   5. Mark the lens prism axis.
   6. Mark the prism base direction.
   7. Mark "R" or "L" and job number.

the center of the semifinished lens blank. This center spot is used as the reference point, and after the lens blank has been rotated so that the seg will be straight, the lens is marked on the dotted center for surfacing. The primary advantage to this method is speed. The only pitfall is the assumption it makes that all lens blanks are consistently made to a high degree of accuracy.

If lenses are made consistently, the distance from the center of the seg top to the blank's geometric center will always correspond to the manufacturer's listed blank seg inset and blank seg drop. However, depending on the quality consistency of the individual manufacturer, blank seg inset and drop may vary. This can happen if the gasket that holds the front and back surface molds together was skewed during casting of a plastic lens. Should this happen, the lens center locator will be unable to locate the center of the front surface accurately. Therefore, all persons must decide for themselves if the lens blanks

they are using will deliver reliable results when using a lens center locator.

Using the Segment for Reference in Centering

A method that yields a higher degree of accuracy uses the lens segment for reference. To find the blank center using this method, the lens is placed on the layout marker and the seg moved down and in by amounts corresponding to the blank seg drop and blank seg inset. The lens is marked and blocked using these measurements. This is the "theoretical" geometric center of the lens blank. Using such a method assures that the computed results will correspond to the actual distances for which they were intended. This method works even when there is a variation in the location of the blank geometric center due to slightly out-of-tolerance semifinished blanks.

EXAMPLE 4-5

A lens is to be marked for on-center blocking. It has the following dimensions:

   Blank seg inset = 6 mm
   Blank seg drop = 6 mm

The right lens power is to be $-3.75 -1.25 \times 180$.

After inputting all other frame and prescription specifications such as frame B dimension, seg height, and PDs, the lens layout computer indicates that the prism needed to move the optical center to its proper location is Base 21. How should the lens be marked for blocking? (Use the steps in Table 4-2, which use blank seg inset and drop to mark the lens.)

SOLUTION

Step 1. In order to preset the layout marker for blank seg inset, the direction of that inset must be known. If a right lens is positioned front side up, the movable line is inset to the right. In this case the amount of inset is 6 mm.

Steps 2 and 3. Next the lens is placed in the layout marker. The segment is positioned horizontally between the segment reference grid lines. Next it is moved up or down until a drop of 6 mm is achieved.

Steps 4 and 5. The cylinder axis is marked for 180 degrees, and then the lens marking device is turned to 21 degrees and the lens is marked for prism. See Figure 4-11.

Steps 6 and 7. Lastly, the lens is removed from the layout marker and the prism axis is marked with arrow-

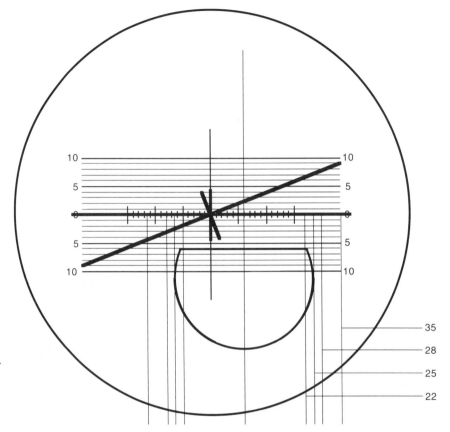

Figure 4-11 For on-center blocking, the lens is marked at the location of the blank geometric center. For layout purposes, however, the segment can still be used for reference. Simply set the movable vertical line for the *blank* seg inset. Center the seg between the seg reference lines and move the seg top to the *blank* seg drop.

heads to indicate base direction. Mark a reverse "R" on the lens, along with the job number.

Multifocal lenses which are blocked off center may surface easier if they are cribbed ahead of time. *Cribbing* is the process of removing some of the lens blank that will only be ground off later when the lenses are edged to fit the frame. Cribbing will be covered in Chapter 9.

A Simplified "On-Center" Bifocal Blocking Method—No Computer Required

When using on-center blocking for single-vision lenses, it is possible to determine the needed prism for decentration using either simple calculations or a decentration chart. Unfortunately, with bifocals the distance optical center not only moves sideways, it also must be moved up or down. Yet there is a way to use the same on-center blocking technique for

bifocals that was used for single-vision lenses. The lens will be on-center horizontally but not quite on-center vertically. Following are the steps in this *simplified on-center blocking* method.

1. *Find the decentration for the distance optical center.* This decentration is the horizontal distance from the blank geometric center to the distance optical center. It may be found by subtracting the seg inset from the blank seg inset.
2. *Find the power in the 180-degree meridian.*
3. *Find the horizontal prism for decentration.* This is done using either Prentice's rule or the Prism Power Decentration Chart.
4. *Position the lens in the layout marker.* Lens layout is accomplished by dropping the segment by an amount equal to the seg drop and insetting the seg by an amount equal to the *blank* seg inset.
5. *Mark the lens.* The lens is marked for cylinder axis and horizontal prism.

EXAMPLE 4-6

A prescription is as follows:

R: −4.50 sph
L: −4.50 sph
A = 56 mm
B = 48 mm
DBL = 20 mm
Seg height = 20 mm
PD = 64/60

The semifinished lens that will be used has a blank seg drop of 7 mm and a blank seg inset of 6 mm. How much prism for decentration is required using the simplified on-center method? Where will the lens block be placed?

SOLUTION

Step 1. We must first find how far horizontally the blank center is from the distance optical center.

Blank seg inset − seg inset = horizontal decentration distance

$$6 - 2 = 4 \text{ mm}$$

Step 2. Since the lens is spherical, the power in the 180-degree meridian is easy to find. It is −4.50 D.

Step 3. The horizontal prism for decentration needed is

$$(0.4)(4.5) = 1.8 \text{ prism diopters}$$

Since the lens is minus, the direction will be base out.

Step 4. The seg drop is calculated as

$$\text{Seg drop} = 20 - \frac{48}{2}$$
$$= 20 - 24$$
$$= -4 \text{ mm}$$

Therefore the segment is dropped 4 mm vertically and moved in by an amount equal to the blank seg inset. The blank seg inset is 6 mm.

Step 5. Lay out the lens for marking by presetting the movable vertical line at the blank seg inset of 6 mm. Center the seg between the seg reference marks and move the top of the seg to the correct seg drop. This was calculated as 4 mm. There is no cylinder axis to mark. The prism axis is along the 0−180 line.

Figure 4-12 shows what the lens looks like when it is marked.

EXAMPLE 4-7

Determine the correct amount of prism for decentration needed for the right lens of the following pair using the simplified on-center blocking technique. Lay out and mark the lens for surfacing.

R: +3.50 −1.00 × 20
L: +3.50 −1.00 × 160
A = 55 mm
B = 46 mm
DBL = 19 mm
Seg height = 20 mm
PD = 66/62

The semifinished lens has a blank seg drop of 7 mm and a blank seg inset of 7 mm.

SOLUTION

Step 1. The horizontal decentration distance is

Horizontal decentration distance = (blank seg inset)
$$- \text{(seg inset)}$$
$$= 7 - 2$$
$$= 5 \text{ mm}$$

Step 2. The power in the 180-degree meridian is a combination of the full sphere power and a portion of the cylinder. The power of the cylinder in the 180-degree meridian is found using the sine-squared table shown as Appendix 3-1. It is −0.12 D. The total power in the 180-degree meridian is

$$\text{Power in } 180 = (+3.50) - (0.12)$$
$$= +3.38$$

Step 3. The horizontal prism for decentration is

$$(0.5)(3.38) = 1.69 \text{ prism diopters}$$

Since the lenses are plus, the prism base direction will be base in.

Step 4. Seg drop is

$$\text{Seg drop} = 20 - \frac{46}{2}$$
$$= 20 - 23$$
$$= -3 \text{ mm}$$

Step 5. For layout, first preset the movable vertical line to equal the blank seg inset. In this case, blank seg inset is 7 mm. Next move the lens up until the seg top is at the 3-mm line below the horizontal. Lastly the lens is marked—first for cylinder axis, then for prism axis.

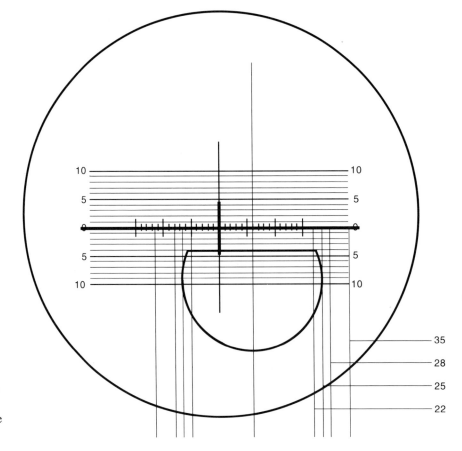

Figure 4-12 When using the simplified on-center blocking method, position the seg horizontally for the *blank* seg inset but vertically for the *seg* drop, not the blank seg drop.

Figure 4-13 shows how the lens will look positioned on the layout marker and stamped for cylinder and prism axes.

Drawbacks of the Simplified On-Center Method for Bifocals

One drawback of the simplified on-center method for bifocals is that the block is not centered vertically. There is more lens at the top than at the bottom. To overcome this drawback, the lens may be "cribbed" down to a round shape again. (See Chapter 9 for more on cribbing.) The extra lens at the top will not be used and may be ground away during the cribbing process. Thus, in spite of a lack of vertical centering, after cribbing the block ends up being fairly well centered anyway.

A second drawback can occur when the lens pair contains an oblique cylinder. To calculate power in the 180 meridian, we use the sine-squared method described earlier for single-vision lenses. However,

when prism for decentration is ground for oblique cylinders, the lens centers will tend to drift up or down, depending on the power of the cylinder and the obliqueness of the cylinder. If the cylinders are equal in power and the cylinder axes are mirror images* of one another, then both will drift up or down the same distance. No unwanted vertical prism will result.

Some individuals have worked in surfacing layout so long that they are able to compensate for the vertical drift in centers. They do this by turning the prism axis away from the horizontal somewhat. (For example, they may stamp the prism at 005 or 175 degrees instead of 180.) This introduces a slight vertical component and keeps the center from moving up or down. This vertical prism helps to counteract the vertical dirft caused by the oblique cylinder.

---

*An example of mirror-imaged cylinder axes would be a right lens of axis 10 and a left lens of axis 170.

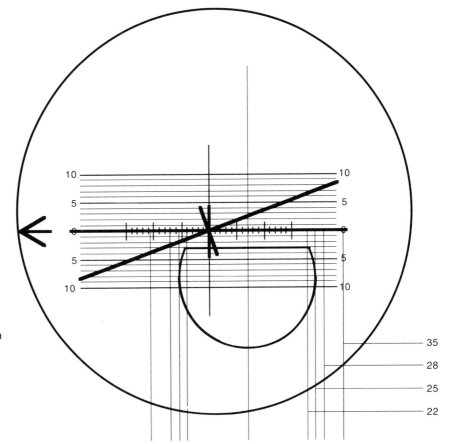

Figure 4-13 This lens has been marked to grind horizontal prism for decentration. Although this method is termed the "simplified" method, it is simple only when compared to calculating on-center blocking without the use of a computer.

Frame Center Blocking

Another method of blocking used by CMSI Prism of Portland, Oregon, is frame center blocking. *Frame center blocking* incorporates parts of both on- and off-center blocking. It is unique because the layout system is identical to that of the edging process. Persons already familiar with edging can make the transition quickly. Frame center blocking is extremely close to what was just described as the simplified on-center method of blocking.

To mark the lens, the segment is moved down by an amount equal to the seg drop, and in by an amount equal to the total seg inset. The *total set inset* is the horizontal distance from the boxing center of the frame's lens opening to the segment center location. Written as a formula, total seg inset is

$$\text{Total seg inset} = \frac{(A + DBL) - \text{near PD}}{2}$$

where *A* equals the frame eyesize, DBL equals the distance between lenses, and the near PD is the wearer's interpupillary distance when measured for reading or other close work.

EXAMPLE 4-8

A lens is to be surfaced using frame center blocking. The lens and frame dimensions are as follows.

Right lens power = −2.00 −1.00 × 25
A = 55 mm
B = 50 mm
DBL = 17 mm
Seg height = 21 mm
PD = 64/60

Explain how the lens would be marked for surfacing.

SOLUTION

In frame center blocking, neither the blank seg inset nor blank seg drop are used directly in the layout process. Instead, the total seg inset and seg drop are needed.

Begin by finding the total seg inset.

$$\text{Total seg inset} = \frac{(A + DBL) - \text{near PD}}{2}$$

$$= \frac{(55 + 17) - 60}{2}$$

$$= \frac{12}{2}$$

$$= 6 \text{ mm}$$

The seg drop is

$$\text{Seg drop} = \text{seg height} - \frac{B}{2}$$

$$= 21 - \frac{50}{2}$$

$$= -4 \text{ mm}$$

Because the lens is a right lens and will be placed front side up, the movable vertical line in the lens marking device is shifted 6 mm to the right. The segment is positioned between the seg reference marks and the top of the segment is moved to the seg drop position 4 mm below the horizontal reference line. The lens is marked for a 25-degree cylinder axis. With frame center blocking the lens must be marked with prism for decentration. When using a computer layout program, prism for decentration has already been calculated.*

After a lens has been marked for frame center blocking, it must be reduced in diameter or "cribbed" to eliminate unneeded areas of the lens. Because the lens is blocked on what will become the center of the edged lens, it is cribbed down to a size equal to the effective diameter (ED) of the frame, plus an extra 4 mm to allow for possible edge chipping during processing. In other words,

Cribbing size for frame center blocking = ED + 4

---

*To figure prism for decentration without a computer, the same procedure as was described in the simplifed method of on-center blocking can be used. However, with on-center blocking, horizontal decentration distance was figured as

$$\text{Horizontal decentration distance} = (\text{blank seg inset}) - (\text{seg inset}).$$

With frame center blocking the calculation is

$$\text{Horizontal decentration distance} = (\text{total seg inset}) - (\text{seg inset}).$$

Once horizontal decentration distance is known, it is multiplied by the power of the lens in the 180-degree meridian to find the required prism.

Cribbing a frame center blocked lens has the advantage of producing minimal surfacing size. This reduces the possibility of surface waviness and may save on fining and polishing times. The cribbing process is described in more detail in Chapter 9.

Questions and Problems

Off-Center Blocking
The following exercises can be done using a lens protractor and semifinished lenses, or mock acetate lenses. A lens-marking pen and flexible ruler will be needed.

Use a semifinished bifocal lens or a mock acetate lens. For each of the prescriptions listed below, layout and mark the lenses for surfacing using off-center blocking.

1. R: $+ 2.25 - 1.75 \times 35$
   A = 52 mm
   B = 38 mm
   ED = 58 mm
   DBL = 22 mm
   PD = 66/62
   Seg height = 18 mm
2. L: $-0.75 - 0.25 \times 65$
   A = 56 mm
   B = 50 mm
   ED = 62.3 mm
   DBL = 19 mm
   PD = 67/63
   Seg height = 22 mm
3. R: $+1.25 - 0.50 \times 110$
   A = 48 mm
   B = 42 mm
   ED = 50 mm
   DBL = 24 mm
   PD = 64/61
   Seg height = 21 mm
4. R: $-1.75 - 3.25 \times 15$
   A = 52 mm
   B = 44 mm
   ED = 55.5 mm
   DBL = 19 mm
   PD = 61/59
   Seg height = 18 mm
5. L: $+4.25 - 1.50 \times 120$
   Rx prism = 1 BO
   A = 53 mm
   B = 51 mm
   ED = 61.5 mm
   DBL = 15 mm
   PD = 62/59
   Seg height = 21 mm

6. R: $-1.75 -3.25 \times 175$
 Rx prism = 2 BD and 1 BI
 A = 51 mm
 B = 48 mm
 ED = 57.5 mm
 DBL = 14 mm
 PD = 54/52
 Seg height = 20 mm

7. R: pl -3.75×167
 Rx prism = 3.25 BI and 1.50 BD
 A = 50 mm
 B = 40 mm
 ED = 54.5 mm
 DBL = 24 mm
 PD = 71/68
 Seg height = 19 mm

8. R: $-5.00 -2.00 \times 17$
 Rx prism = 2 BI
 A = 51 mm
 B = 48 mm
 ED = 54 mm
 DBL = 62/59 mm
 Seg height = 20 mm

9. R: $+2.75 -1.50 \times 75$
 Rx prism = 2 BO and 4 BU
 A = 52 mm
 B = 48 mm
 DBL = 17 mm
 ED = 57 mm
 PD = 64/61
 Seg height = 20 mm

10. R: $+2.75 -1.50 \times 35$
 Rx prism = 4 BU and 2 BU
 A = 54 mm
 B = 49 mm
 DBL = 17 mm
 ED = 57 mm
 PD = 65/61
 Seg height = 20 mm

On-Center Blocking

The prescriptions listed below have already been computed for the prism needed in order to move the optical center (major reference point) to the desired location.

 a. Lay out and mark a semifinished lens or a mock acetate lens as indicated so that it will be correct after surfacing. (Use the blank seg inset and blank seg drop listed, even if the lens blank you are using does not have that same blank seg inset and drop.)

 b. Determine where the major reference point will be on the lens once the lens has been surfaced. Mark this point with a dot using a marking pen. (In order to do this you will have to determine the seg inset and seg drop.)

11. L: $+0.25 -0.50 \times 165$
 A = 51 mm
 B = 47.5 mm
 ED = 57 mm
 DBL = 21 mm
 PD = 68/65
 Seg height = 22 mm
 Blank seg drop = 6 mm
 Blank seg inset = 6 mm
 Prism amount = 0.1
 Prism axis = 116 DN
 Seg drop_____
 Seg inset_____

12. R: $+3.25 -0.75 \times 83$
 A = 56 mm
 B = 47 mm
 ED = 65 mm
 DBL = 15 mm
 PD = 58/55
 Seg height = 23 mm
 Blank seg drop = 7 mm
 Blank seg inset = 6 mm
 Prism amount = 1.7
 Prism axis = 131 DN
 Seg drop_____
 Seg inset_____

13. L: $+ 2.50$
 A = 48 mm
 B = 44 mm
 ED = 56 mm
 DBL = 18 mm
 PD = 57/54
 Seg height = 18 mm
 Blank seg drop = 2 mm
 Blank seg inset = 6 mm
 Prism amount = 1.5
 Prism axis = 163 DN
 Seg drop_____
 Seg inset_____

14. L: $+3.25 -0.75 \times 145$
 A = 55 mm
 B = 49.5 mm
 ED = 60 mm
 DBL = 12 mm
 PD = 57/54
 Seg height = 23 mm
 Blank seg drop = 2 mm
 Blank seg inset = 6 mm
 Prism amount = 1.5
 Prism axis = 163 DN
 Seg drop_____
 Seg inset_____

15. L: $+0.75 -1.75 \times 90$
 A = 57 mm
 B = 48 mm

ED = 65 mm
DBL = 17 mm
PD = 66/61
Seg height = 22 mm
Blank seg drop = 6 mm
Blank seg inset = 7 mm
Prism amount = 0.5
Prism axis = 146 DN
Seg drop_____
Seg inset_____

16. R: +1.00 −2.00 × 90
A = 57 mm
B = 48 mm
ED = 65 mm
DBL = 17 mm
PD = 66/61
Seg height = 22 mm
Blank seg drop = 6 mm
Blank seg inset = 7 mm
Prism amount = 1.5
Prism axis = 37 DN
Seg drop_____
Seg inset_____

17. L: +0.25 −0.25 × 94
A = 57 mm
B = 50.5 mm
ED = 65.5 mm
DBL = 14 mm
PD = 63/59
Seg height = 24 mm
Blank seg drop = 6 mm
Blank seg inset = 7 mm
Prism amount = 0.1
Prism axis = 94 DN
Seg drop_____
Seg inset_____

18. R: +0.25 −0.25 × 85
A = 57 mm
B = 50.5 mm
ED = 65.5 mm
DBL = 14 mm
PD = 63/59
Seg height = 24 mm
Blank seg drop = 6 mm
Blank seg inset = 7 mm
Prism amount = 0.1
Prism axis = 86 DN
Seg drop_____
Seg inset_____

Simplified "On-Center" Blocking
Use an actual semifinished lens blank or a mock acetate lens in conjunction with a protractor or lens marking device. For each of the following prescriptions, calculate the amount of prism required and the base direction needed in order to mark the lenses using the simplified method of on-center blocking. Use the blank seg inset listed in the problem to mark the lens, regardless of the blank seg inset of the actual practice lens blank you are using.

19. R: +3.00 sphere
Rx prism = none
A = 50 mm
B = 46 mm
DBL = 20 mm
PD = 64/60
Seg height = 17 mm
Blank seg drop = 7 mm
Blank seg inset = 7 mm

20. L: +5.00 −1.00 × 90
Rx prism = none
A = 56 mm
B = 50 mm
DBL = 16 mm
PD = 66/62
Seg height = 20 mm
Blank seg drop = 6 mm
Blank seg inset = 6 mm

21. R: +6.00 −1.00 × 60
Rx prism = none
A = 52 mm
B = 48 mm
DBL = 19 mm
PD = 65/61
Seg height = 21 mm
Blank seg drop = 6 mm
Blank seg inset = 6 mm

22. L: −6.00 −1.50 × 30
Rx prism = none
A = 48 mm
B = 42 mm
DBL = 22 mm
PD = 63/60
Seg height = 19 mm
Blank seg drop = 6 mm
Blank seg inset = 7 mm

23. R: −4.75 −1.00 × 90
Rx prism = 2 Base In
A = 49 mm
B = 44 mm
DBL = 20 mm
PD = 64/60
Seg height = 19 mm
Blank seg drop = 6 mm
Blank seg inset = 6 mm

24. L: +0.25 −1.75 × 80
Rx prism = none
A = 55 mm

B = 49 mm
DBL = 19 mm
PD = 63/60
Seg height = 20 mm
Blank seg drop = 7 mm
Blank seg inset = 7 mm

25. R: +2.50 −1.00 × 20
Rx prism = 1 Base Down

A = 53 mm
B = 48 mm
DBL = 17 mm
PD = 65/61
Seg height = 19 mm
Blank seg drop = 6 mm
Blank seg inset = 6 mm

5 Layout and Marking of Round Segment and Blended Bifocal Lenses

Layout and Marking of Round Segment Lenses

Some Preliminary Remarks

Round segment lenses do not come from the manufacturer as a "right" or "left" lens as do flat-top lenses. This is because the lenses may be rotated in order to throw the segment either to the right or to the left. The semifinished round seg lens can serve as either a right *or* a left lens. Because the seg is round, once the lens has been edged, it is impossible to tell that the segment was rotated.

Because the round seg lens does not have any specific blank seg inset, inexperienced individuals can become easily disoriented. With a round seg, who can say where the center of the top of the seg is? In essence, the lens becomes vastly more flexible than a flat-top multifocal. Simultaneously, it is somewhat confusing to work with. Because of its flexibility, there are numerous ways of laying out the lens, all of which may yield perfectly acceptable results. It should be understood that the procedures this text uses to lay out round seg bifocals will not include every workable method. The first methods presented are more traditional and help the learner understand the workings of a round seg lens. However, they do not make full use of the available lens blank as do some of the methods shown later in the chapter.

Layout and Marking of Round Segment Lenses Using Off-Center Blocking Methods

For layout of round seg lenses using off-center blocking, the only information required is

> seg drop
> seg inset
> cylinder axis
> Rx prism base direction

With this information the lens can be marked for surfacing. There is little difference in technique when using a lens layout marker or a lens protractor.

Using a Layout Marker

The traditional method as explained in Table 5-1 is the most straightforward method for marking round segment lenses. However, it does not make the best use of the full lens blank. When using a lens layout marker, follow the steps as outlined in Table 5-1.

EXAMPLE 5-1

A lens has the following dimensions:

Left lens
Power = +2.25 −0.75 × 30
A = 52 mm
B = 46 mm
ED = 58 mm

Table 5-1 Round Seg Off-Center Blocking—
Traditional Method Using a Layout Marker

1. Mark the geometric center of the lens blank.
2. Put the lens in the lens marking device.
3. Place the marked geometric center of the lens blank at the center of the target.
4. Preset the movable vertical line nasally for the correct seg inset and rotate the lens seg inward (nasally) until the seg is centered between the segment guidelines.
5. Move the lens up (or down) until the top of the seg is at the correct seg drop.
6. Recheck to see that both seg inset and drop are correct.
7. Mark the cylinder axis and, if Rx prism is present, the prism axis. (In the absence of cylinder, the lens is marked along the 180-degree meridian.)
8. If the frame is available, hold the lens up to the frame to be sure the lens will cut out.

DBL = 20 mm
PD = 66/62
Seg height = 20 mm

Mark the lens for off-center blocking using a lens marking device and the method outlined in Table 5-1.

SOLUTION
Steps 1, 2, and 3. The geometric center of the lens is spotted. The lens is placed in the marking device, and the spotted lens center is positioned at the center of the background grid. This is shown in Figure 5-1.

Step 4. The inset is

$$\frac{66 - 62}{2} = 2 \text{ mm}$$

The movable vertical line is inset 2 mm and the lens segment is rotated inward until it is bordered by the segment guidelines as shown in Figure 5-2.

Step 5. The seg drop is

$$20 - \frac{46}{2} = -3 \text{ mm}$$

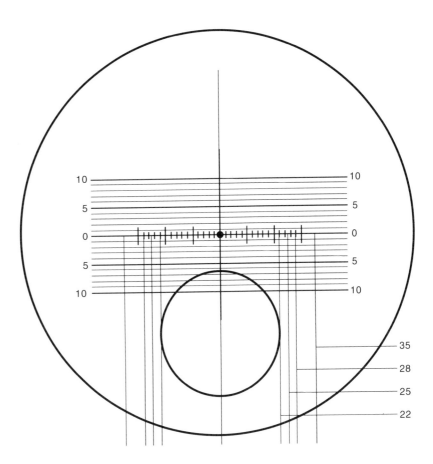

Figure 5-1 The most straightforward method for marking round seg lenses begins by placing the geometric center of the lens blank at the center of the lens marking device target. (Remember that even though this method is the easiest to work with, it will usually require a larger lens blank than some of the methods described later in the chapter.)

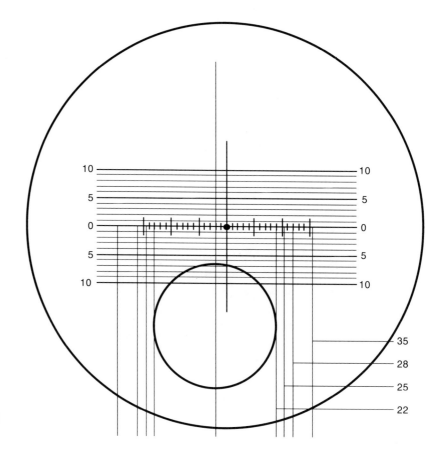

Figure 5-2 Here the left lens is placed front side up on the layout marker. The movable vertical line (longest line) is moved 2 mm nasally. The lens is rotated around its center until the segment is centered between the 22-mm segment guidelines.

The whole lens is moved up until the top of the segment is 3 mm from the horizontal.

Step 6. Drop and inset are rechecked.

Step 7. The lens is marked along the 30-degree cylinder axis. See Figure 5-3.

Step 8. If the frame is with the job, the lens can be held up to the frame to assure that it will cut out.

Using a Lens Protractor

There is little difference between using a lens marking device and a lens protractor. In fact, the lens marking device is simply a mechanized lens protractor.

The steps outlined in Table 5-2 are used to mark a round seg lens using a lens protractor. Notice that after step 4, the remaining steps are identical with those when using a lens marking device.

Table 5-2 Round Seg Off-Center Blocking—Traditional Method Using a Lens Protractor

1. Outline the seg border with dots to help increase segment visibility.

2. Spot the exact center of the seg. (This dot will be used for purposes of finding the seg inset.)

3. Center the lens on the protractor.

4. Rotate the lens seg inward (nasally) until the correct seg inset has been achieved.

5. Move the lens up (or down) until the top of the seg is at the correct seg drop.

6. Recheck to see that both seg inset and drop are correct.

7. Mark the cylinder axis and, if Rx prism is present, the prism axis. (In the absence of cylinder, the lens is marked along the 180-degree meridian.)

8. If the frame is available, hold the lens up to the frame to be sure the lens will cut out.

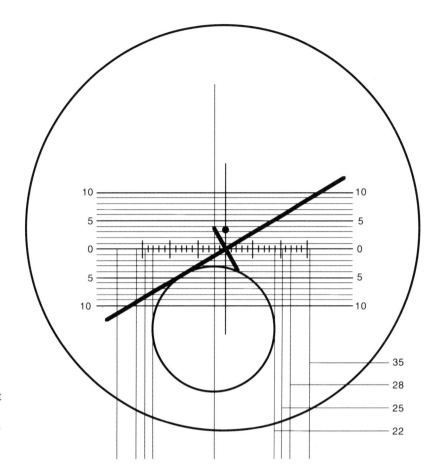

Figure 5-3 Once the segment inset is correct, the entire lens is moved up until the lens is positioned for a 3-mm seg drop. The cylinder axis is set for 30 degrees and the lens is stamped.

Procedures for Round Segment Layout That Maximize Blank Size

At times it is advantageous to know a few tricks in the layout of multifocal lenses to avoid certain limiting factors. Two primary limiting factors are blank size and lens overhang. How can a small round segment lens blank be used most efficiently? How can off-center blocking be modified in order to avoid overhang? The methods shown for off-center blocking are useful for on-center blocking, as will be seen later.

Round Segs: Getting the Most Out of a Small Semifinished Lens

With flat-top lenses, the slightest tilt of the segment causes the lens to be cosmetically unacceptable and optically annoying. Yet because of the very nature of round seg lenses, the symmetry of the segment prevents anyone from knowing if the seg is tilted or straight. Even if the lens is rotated, the segment doesn't look crooked! There is no reference point. Therefore there is no reason for a manufacturer to mark a round seg lens as being a left or a right blank. If the lens is rotated in one direction, it may be used as a left blank. It if is rotated in the other direction, it becomes a right.

Although the conventional method for layout of round seg lenses will prove satisfactory in many cases, there are times when the lens blanks will appear to be too small for the frame. When this occurs it is usually the temporal side of the frame that is not covered by the lens. See Figure 5-4. As a general rule, the most likely cause for this difficulty stems from too little blank seg inset. If the seg were positioned more nasalward in the blank, there would be more blank available temporally to cover

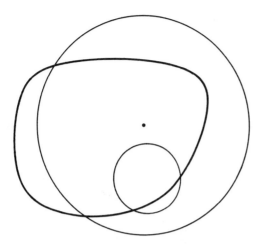

Figure 5-4 If lenses are not referenced to the frame shape before surfacing, what could have been a large enough semifinished blank may end up being too small.

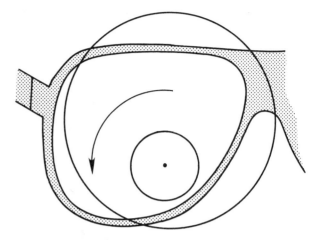

Figure 5-5 While maintaining the necessary seg height and decentration, manually rotate the semifinished lens blank around the correctly positioned seg center until the frame shape is covered.

the open space. When faced with this problem with flat-top lenses, the options are limited. These options are

1. change the near PD,
2. change the seg drop,
3. choose a larger blank,
4. find a blank with a larger blank seg inset.

When we use the conventional procedure for round seg layout, we are artificially creating a blank seg inset. The blank seg inset we create is equal to the seg inset. If flat-top semifinished blanks were made with such small blank seg insets, there would be *many* instances where lenses would not cut out. However, since *we* created the blank seg inset for our round seg initially, there is no reason why we cannot change it to a *bigger* blank seg inset. This can be done by rotating the lens more. In further rotating the lens, we are creating a blank with a larger blank seg inset. Now we are no longer limited to the inset found in our original method.

Determining Blank Seg Inset

Several different approaches can be taken to determine the correct amount of blank seg inset to use for the lens. These include

1. the horizontal midline method,
2. the centering circles method, and
3. an assigned blank seg inset method.

The Horizontal Midline Method

The horizontal midline method may be used when it is evident ahead of time that cutout will be close. It can only be done if the frame is available, or if the laboratory happens to have a pattern that corresponds exactly to the size and shape of the edged lens.

To use this method, hold the lens blank up to the frame with the segment at the correct seg height and near PD. This will show if the lens will cut out. If the lens does not cover the frame's lens opening, it will not cut out. Taking care to keep the seg height and near PD correct, rotate the semifinished lens blank until the blank completely covers the frame's lens opening. See Figure 5-5.

Now draw a dashed horizontal line on the lens. (To avoid a lens with too many marks, it may be helpful to make only two dash marks toward the lens periphery on the 180-degree line.) This dashed line should be along the datum line. The *datum line* is halfway between the lowest and highest points on the inside groove of the frame. See Figure 5-6.

Next place the lens on the lens marking device so that the marked line is horizontal. Move the lens to the left or right until the seg is positioned at the correct inset. See Figure 5-7. Keeping the marked line horizontal, move the lens up or down until the seg top arrives at the correct seg drop. See Figure 5-8. (If a person is skilled, the segment will already be close to its desired location and will require very

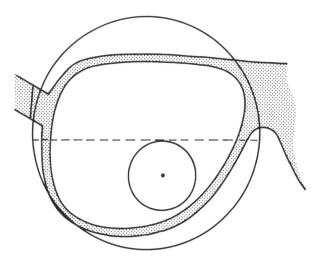

Figure 5-6 Mark the 180-degree line for reference. This will assure that the lens is not inadvertently turned later on.

little extra movement.) The lens may now be marked for cylinder and prism. This method is summarized in Table 5-3.

The Centering Circles Method

Some layout markers have circles on the screen of the instrument. Although they are used primarily for finding the blank geometric center, these circles can also alert the surfacing technician to a problem with semifinished blank size. In order to use the circles effectively, however, it is necessary to simulate edging layout.

EXAMPLE **5-2**

A lens is to be surfaced for a frame with the following dimensions:

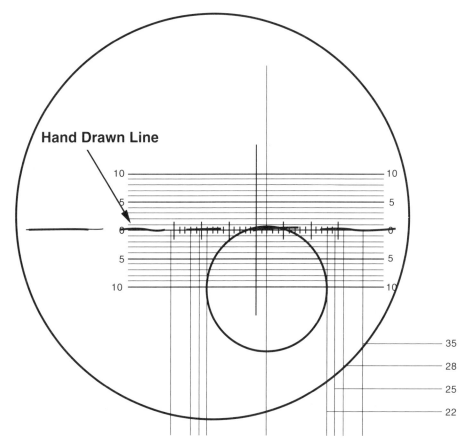

Figure 5-7 The purpose of the hand-drawn line is to keep the lens in the position that will cover the frame's entire lens area. The drawn line should be parallel to the 180-degree line and the segment should be decentered for seg inset. In this case, seg inset is 2 mm. At this point, seg drop has not been considered. Seg drop is shown in Figure 5-8.

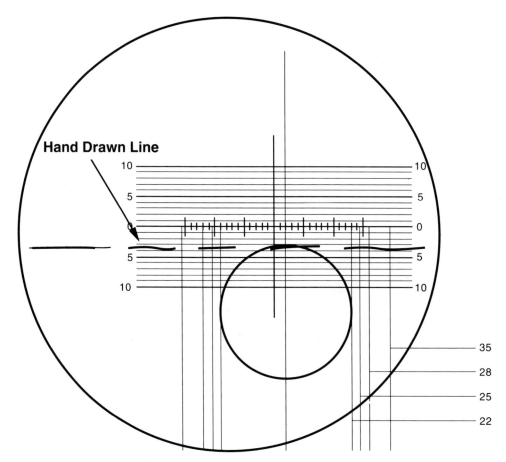

Figure 5-8 Once the segment is inset correctly, the entire lens is moved up or down to achieve the drop called for. Here the drop is 3 mm. Care should be taken to assure that the hand-drawn line still parallels the 180-degree line.

A = 56 mm
B = 50 mm
DBL = 20 mm
ED = 58 mm

The wearer's PD = 66/62, and the seg height is 20 mm.

SOLUTION

Inset the movable vertical line for *total* seg inset, rather than just seg inset. Total seg inset is

$$\frac{A + DBL - near\ PD}{2}$$

Place the lens on the layout marker with the seg between the segment bordering lines. The total seg inset per lens will be

$$\frac{56 + 20 - 62}{2} = 7\ mm$$

When the lens is edged, the seg will be inset 7 mm. Therefore, to check for cutout, the movable line is inset 7 mm and the seg positioned between the segment bordering lines. The seg drop is placed at 5 mm.

At this point the lens should be checked to make sure that it completely encloses the circle in the layout marker that corresponds to the ED of the frame. See Figure 5-9. (If there is no circle corresponding to the frame ED, a reasonable estimation of ED circle size can be made using those circles that are present.) If the circle is *not* enclosed, *do not move the segment.* Keep it exactly where it is on the marking device (that is, at the correct total seg inset and seg drop). Next, rotate the lens around the *seg center* until the lens blank completely encloses the circle on the screen of the marking device corresponding to the frame ED. (It should be noted that a lens may still cut out even if the complete ED circle is not

Table 5-3 Horizontal Midline Method for Round Seg Layout and Marking

1. Hold the lens blank up to the frame with the seg at the correct seg inset and drop. If the lens does not cover the frame's lens opening, proceed to step 2.
2. Without changing the segment location, rotate the lens blank until the frame's lens opening is completely enclosed.
3. Mark the lens along the frame's horizontal midline.
4. Place the lens on the layout marker with the marked line oriented horizontally.
5. After presetting the marker for seg inset, move the lens left or right until the correct seg inset is achieved.
6. Keeping the marked line parallel to the horizontal, move the lens up or down until the seg is at its correct drop.
7. Mark the lens for cylinder and prism axes.

enclosed, especially if it is not enclosed nasally, or at the top or bottom of the circle. Since the ED encircles the outermost part of the frame shape, this will in most cases be the lower temporal corner or sometimes both the lower temporal and upper nasal corners.) See Figure 5-10. When the circle is enclosed, the lens should not be rotated. Move the movable vertical line back to the seg inset (2 mm). Slide the lens over until the seg is once more bordered. Mark the lens for surfacing. For a summary of steps in this method, see Table 5-4.

An Assigned Blank Seg Inset Method

Perhaps the easiest method is simply to assign the round seg lens blank a reasonable blank seg inset and proceed. Most flat-top semifinished lenses have a blank seg inset of 6 or 7 mm. Table 5-5 gives the correct procedure for using the assigned blank seg inset method. See also Figure 5-11.

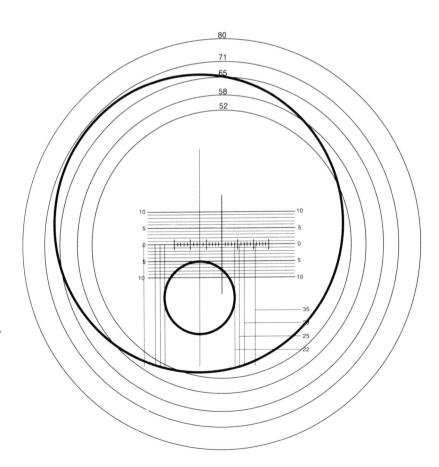

Figure 5-9 The frame for this prescription has an ED of 58 mm. The round seg is positioned correctly, but the lens does not cover the 58-mm ED circle very well. (The lens is represented by the dark circle.) This means that, unless the lens blank is rotated, the surfaced lens will not cut out during edging.

Table 5-4 Centering Circles Method of Assuring Round Seg Lens Cutout

1. Lay out the semifinished round seg lens as if for edging.
2. Find the circle corresponding to the ED of the frame and see if the lens covers all of this circle.
3. If the circle is not covered, rotate the lens (without moving the seg) until at least the temporal portion of the circle is enclosed.
4. Reposition the layout marker for surfacing. Slide the lens over for correct seg inset and drop.
5. Mark the lens for cylinder and prism axis in the customary manner.

Table 5-5 Assigned Blank Seg Inset Method for Round Seg Layout and Marking

1. Dot the blank geometric center of the lens.
2. Preset the marker for the chosen blank seg inset (6 or 7 mm).
3. Place the lens center dot at the center of the marking device.
4. Rotate the seg to the blank seg inset. See Figure 5-11a.
5. Move the lens up (or down) until the top of the seg is at the correct seg drop. See Figure 5-11b.
6. Reset the marking device for the seg inset and move the lens horizontally to the left or right until the segment arrives at the seg inset. See Figure 5-11c.
7. Mark the cylinder axis and, if Rx prism is present, mark the prism axis.

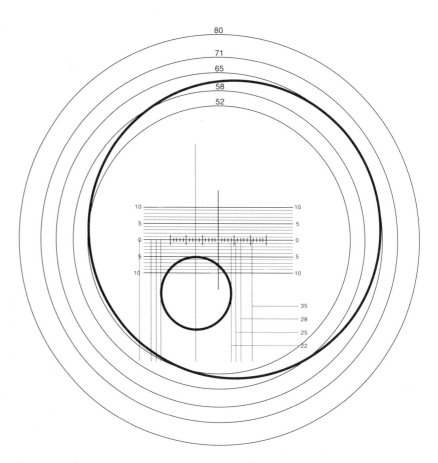

Figure 5-10 Keeping the segment stationary, the lens blank is rotated around the segment until it encloses the 58-mm ED circle at the critical areas. The most critical area is usually temporal and somewhat inferior. Now we know that the surfaced lens will cut out when edged.

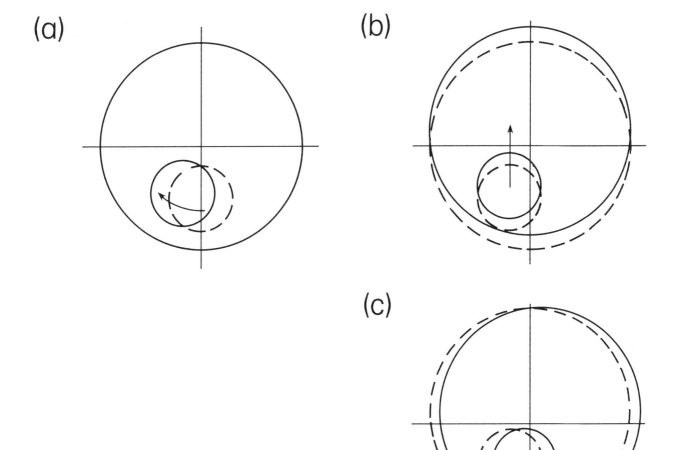

Figure 5-11 The sequence for round segment lens layout using a large blank seg inset is (a) rotate the lens to the blank seg inset that has been determined as being advantageous, (b) move the entire lens up until the seg arrives at the correct seg drop, and (c) move the lens back horizontally until the seg inset is correct.

Layout and Marking of Round Segment Lenses Using On-Center Blocking Methods

When grinding multifocal lenses using on-center blocking, prism for decentration is almost always required. A round segment lens is no exception. Because there is no blank seg inset for a round seg lens, it is not readily apparent how on-center blocking is achieved. Three methods can be used: no-inset on-center marking, computer-assigned blank seg inset and drop, and round seg on-center blocking using a method that simulates flat-top layout.

No-Inset On-Center Marking

Because round seg semifinished lens blanks are not right–left specific, manufacturers list only a blank seg drop. They do not give a blank seg inset. Therefore, some layout computers are programmed so that the lens is marked with no inset. The lens is positioned with the center of the seg on the vertical line directly below the geometric center of the lens blank (as pictured in Figure 5-1). When all necessary information is given to the layout computer, the computer calls for a different cylinder axis than the one given in the prescription! In the end, however, the axis will be as indicated in the prescription. By altering the cylinder axis, the computer rotates the lens for seg inset.

EXAMPLE 5-3

A prescription calls for a 170-degree axis. Using on-center blocking, how should the lens be marked?

SOLUTION

After giving all lens and frame information to the layout computer, the computer calls for a 165-degree cylinder axis. The lens is marked for cylinder axis as shown in Figure 5-12. Figure 5-13 shows how turning the lens to the prescribed axis causes the seg to rotate to the proper inset. In addition, the lens is also marked for the decentration prism called for by the computer so that the optical center will come out right.

Computer-Assigned Blank Seg Inset and Drop

A good computer program can calculate the optimum blank seg inset and drop for semifinished round seg lenses. It needs to know both the blank size and the blank seg drop. The computer then does mathematically the same thing that was described in the horizontal midline method. A new blank seg inset and drop is calculated. The operator rotates the lens to the new inset and drop, then marks the cylinder axis and the prism axis as specified by the computer.

Round Seg On-Center Blocking Using a Simulated Flat-Top Layout Method

Some earlier computers may not have the capability of mathematically creating a new blank seg inset and drop. If this is the case, it is possible to use on-center blocking after having created a new blank seg inset and drop for round seg lens blanks manually. This is done by telling the computer the lens is a flat top instead of a round seg lens and is very close to the method described earlier for on-center blocking.

When the computer asks for seg type, a response of "flat top" should be given, even though a round seg is being used. (Caution: If your computer keeps an inventory of lenses used, this will create inaccuracies in monthly reports.) Later the computer

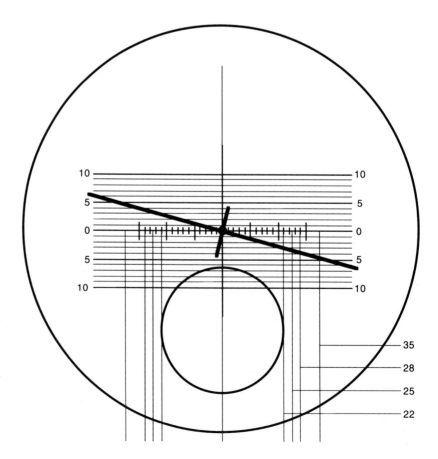

Figure 5-12 Some computers require that round seg lenses be positioned with a zero inset. The computer program recalculates the cylinder axis to allow for inset. In this case, the prescription indicates a 170-degree axis, but the computer calls for 165 degrees. When the lens is laid out for edging at 170 degrees, the segment will swing inward the required 2-mm inset.

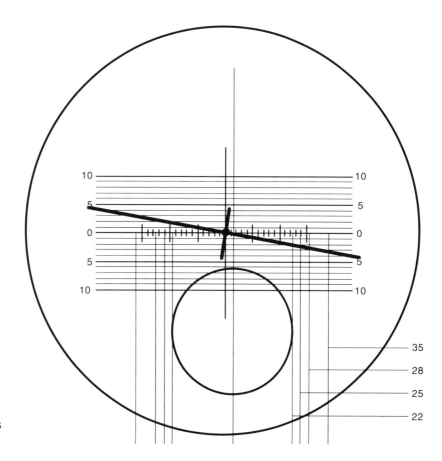

Figure 5-13 Turning the lens shown in Figure 5-12 5 degrees results in a 2-mm segment inset.

will prompt for a blank seg inset. The blank seg inset that was obtained by rotating the lens an extra amount should be entered. This may have been obtained by using the horizontal midline, centering circles, or assigned blank seg inset method. In Figure 5-14, the blank seg inset is 9.5 mm.

When the computer asks for the blank seg drop, use the blank seg drop that results when the geometric center of the blank is in the middle of the lens-marking-device grid and the blank seg inset is positioned correctly. In Figure 5-14 this would correspond to a blank seg drop of 3 mm.

When it is finished, the computer will give a prism axis and amount. This amount and direction will move the major reference point to its correct location.

The lens is properly marked by placing the blank geometric center in the middle of the lens marking device and rotating the lens around the blank geometric center until the seg corresponds to the blank seg inset and drop that was input into the computer. Cylinder and prism axes are marked on the blank

geometric center as is customary for on-center blocking. This procedure is summarized in Table 5-6.

Blended Bifocals

Blended bifocal lenses are treated in a manner that is practically identical to round segment bifocals. This is because the blended bifocal is functionally the same as a one-piece (nonfused) round segment lens. The only difference is that in the blended lens the junction between the segment portion and the rest of the lens is smoothed out so that it is no longer visible upon casual observation.

Blended bifocals are not to be confused with progressive addition lenses, although both have invisible near portions. The progressive addition lens starts to change power at the distance optical center. Plus power for near viewing gradually increases until full add power is reached at the near reading area. The progressive addition lens can be thought of as

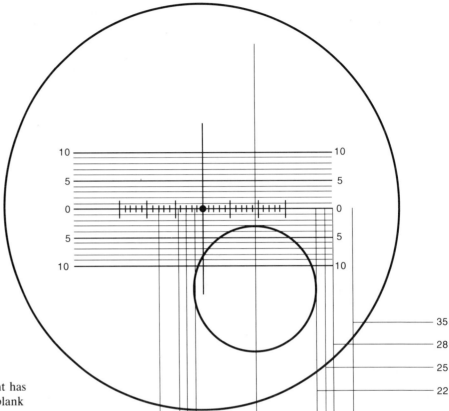

Figure 5-14 Here the segment has been rotated nasally to create a blank seg inset of 9.5 mm.

Table 5-6 Maximizing Round Seg Blank Size Using On-Center Blocking

1. If your computer does not assign round seg lenses a blank seg inset and drop, tell the computer that the lens is a flat top.

2. Spot the blank geometric center of the lens.

3. If the computer does not assign blank seg inset or drop values, assign the lens a blank seg inset according to one of the previously recommended methods. Preset the layout marker for that blank seg inset.

4. Center the lens in the marking device and rotate the seg nasally for the blank seg inset. See Figure 5-14.

5. Note the vertical height of the seg. This is the blank seg drop.

6. Feed the assigned blank seg inset and the newly found blank seg drop into the computer along with all other information.

7. Mark the lens according to the cylinder axis and the prism axis indicated by the computer.

a super trifocal. For more on progressive addition lenses, see Chapter 15.

Thus, the blended bifocal is really a round seg lens with the bifocal line blurred out. The blurred portion of a blended bifocal is approximately 5 mm across, although the exact width may vary with the manufacturer or the power of the near addition.

When a surfacing laboratory receives the semifinished lens blank from the manufacturer, the outermost portion of the blurred area is marked with a circle of dots. See Figure 5-15. During lens layout, the circle of dots is used in the same way one would use the visible segment line.

If these bordering marks have been removed before layout, they can be re-marked by either

finding hidden marks on the lens when such marks have been placed there by the manufacturer, or
looking through the lens at a mottled background and marking the outermost border of the blurred area.

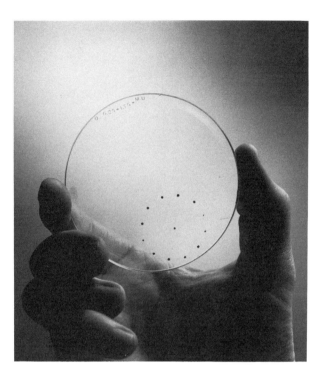

Figure 5-15 Blended bifocal lenses come with the segment borders marked with a circle of dots. These dots should be left in place. They also serve for reference in the edging laboratory.

Remarking Blended Bifocals Using Hidden Engraving

Some blended bifocals have hidden engraving. These hidden engravings are intentional flaws on the surface of a lens, which were created for the purpose of either identifying a specific location on the lens or providing brand-name identification. Such marking may be seen by holding the lens at an angle and looking at a light reflected off the lens surface. It is helpful to have a plain background behind the lens— preferably black. Markings can also be seen by viewing the lens with a mottled surface behind the lens. The Younger Seamless lens has a hidden circle in the center of the segment. Thus if the dotted circle is removed, Younger recommends the following procedure:

> *Locate* the segment by holding the lens away from you at arms length and look at a contrasting surface or at a Younger Seamless Seg Locating Chart. The surface or the chart must be at least 10 feet away from the lens.
>
> Once the seg is located, the "hidden circle"

can be found exactly in the center of the seg. *Mark* the circle with a felt pen, then *measure 15 mm out* from that point in at least 3 directions and the seg "line" has been re-established.[1]

Questions and Problems

General Questions

1. Semifinished round segment lens blanks are made specifically to be used for either a right or a left lens.
   True or False

2. How can a large "blank seg inset" be created for a round segment lens?
   a. by rotating the blank around the segment optical center
   b. by rotating the blank around the distance optical center
   c. by rotating the blank around the major reference point
   d. by rotating the blank around the blank geometric center
   e. The blank seg inset of a round segment lens cannot be increased.

3. Which is the correct order for round segment lens layout for surfacing?
   1. Dot the center of the lens.
   2. Rotate the lens around the blank geometric center until the desired blank seg inset is obtained.
   3. Slide the lens up or down until the seg is at the correct seg height.
   a. 1, 2, 3
   b. 3, 2, 1
   c. 1, 3, 2
   d. 2, 1, 3

4. One method of round seg layout for surfacing begins as follows: Holding the lens over the frame, the blank is rotated until the seg is at the indicated position and the frame's entire lens opening is covered by the blank. Next a horizontal line is drawn across the blank. This line is used for what purpose?
   a. The lens will be marked exactly on this line.
   b. The line serves to help in keeping the lens from rotating during layout. It might be marked somewhat above or below the line.
   c. The line is used to position the lens on the protractor or layout marker. Afterward the line is angled as the lens is rotated for blank seg inset.

5. When a lens-surfacing layout marker has concentric circles on the layout grid, the circle that corresponds to which measure must be covered by the

semifinished lens in order to be sure that the lens will cut out?
   a. ED + (A + DBL −PD)
   b. ED + (A + DBL −PD)/2
   c. chord size
   d. ED
   e. none of the above

6. On-center blocking can be used with round seg bi-focals even if the lens is rotated for a large blank seg inset.
   True or False

7. A blended bifocal
   a. has an invisible near segment. The near portion starts at the MRP and gradually increases in power until the full add power is reached 12 to 14 mm below the MRP.
   b. has an invisible near segment that is essentially round with the segment edge blurred out.
   c. has an invisible near segment that is basically shaped like a flat-top bifocal. The upper line and outer edges are smoothed.

Traditional Off-Center Blocking
For each of the following lenses, use a round seg semi-finished lens or mock acetate lens to lay out and mark the prescription using the traditional method for off-center blocking.

8. Left lens
   F = +0.25 −0.50 × 165
   A = 55 mm
   B = 46 mm
   ED = 62 mm
   DBL = 15 mm
   PD = 64/61
   Seg height = 19 mm
   Seg drop_____
   Seg inset_____

9. Left lens
   F = +3.25 −0.75 × 83
   A = 54 mm
   B = 50 mm
   ED = 59 mm
   DBL = 14 mm
   PD = 63/59
   Seg height = 24 mm
   Seg drop_____
   Seg inset_____

10. Right lens
    F = +6.25 −1.50 × 144
    A = 52 mm
    B = 44 mm
    ED = 59 mm
    DBL = 18 mm
    PD = 66/63
    Seg height = 22 mm
    Seg drop_____
    Seg inset_____

11. Left lens
    F = +2.00 −0.75 × 99
    A = 51 mm
    B = 49 mm
    ED = 65.4 mm
    DBL = 16 mm
    PD = 59/56
    Seg height = 18 mm
    Seg drop_____
    Seg inset_____

12. Right lens
    F = −3.25 −0.25 × 115
    A = 50 mm
    B = 43 mm
    ED = 59.5 mm
    DBL = 16 mm
    PD = 58/54
    Seg height = 21 mm
    Seg drop_____
    Seg inset_____

13. Right lens
    F = −1.25 sph
    A = 51 mm
    B = 42 mm
    ED = 59 mm
    DBL = 17 mm
    PD = 63/60
    Seg height = 18 mm
    Seg drop_____
    Seg inset_____

14. Left lens
    F = +4.75 sph
    A = 50 mm
    B = 43 mm
    ED = 51 mm
    DBL = 19 mm
    PD = 63/60
    Seg height = 18 mm
    Seg drop_____
    Seg inset_____

15. Right lens
    F = pl −3.75 × 17
    A = 51 mm
    B = 47 mm
    ED = 56 mm
    DBL = 18 mm
    PD = 62/59
    Seg height = 19 mm
    Seg drop_____
    Seg inset_____

On-Center Blocking Using Simulated Flat-Top Layout
Each of the following prescriptions has been given a blank

seg inset and a new blank seg drop. This information was given to the computer and a prism axis and amount generated.

Using a semifinished lens blank or a mock acetate lens, lay out and mark the lenses according to the specifications given. (Since the size of the lens you are using will probably not correspond to the size lens for which the calculations were made, you will not be able to block exactly in the center of the lens. However, your grind will still give you the desired optics if you make certain that the segment is positioned at the blank seg inset and drop for which the prism was calculated.)

Once the lens has been marked, determine where the major reference point will be on the lens after surfacing. Spot the MRP with a lens marking pen.

16. Left lens
    $F = +0.25 -0.50 \times 165$
    A = 51 mm
    B = 47.5 mm
    ED = 57 mm
    DBL = 21 mm
    PD = 68/65
    Seg height = 22 mm
    Blank seg drop = 6 mm
    Blank seg inset = 6 mm
    Prism amount = 0.1
    Prism axis = 116 DN
    Seg drop_____
    Seg inset_____

17. Right lens
    $F = +3.25 -0.75 \times 83$
    A = 56 mm
    B = 47 mm
    ED = 65 mm
    DBL = 15 mm
    PD = 58/55
    Seg height = 23 mm
    Blank seg drop = 7 mm
    Blank seg inset = 6 mm
    Prism amount = 1.7
    Prism axis = 131 DN
    Seg drop_____
    Seg inset_____

18. Left lens
    $F = +2.50$
    A = 48 mm
    B = 44 mm
    ED = 56 mm
    DBL = 18 mm
    PD = 57/54
    Seg height = 18 mm
    Blank seg drop = 2 mm
    Blank seg inset = 6 mm
    Prism amount = 1.5
    Prism axis = 163 DN
    Seg drop_____
    Seg inset_____

19. Left lens
    $F = +3.25 -0.75 \times 145$
    A = 55 mm
    B = 49.5 mm
    ED = 60 mm
    DBL = 12 mm
    PD = 57/54
    Seg height = 23 mm
    Blank seg drop = 2 mm
    Blank seg inset = 6 mm
    Prism amount = 1.5
    Prism axis = 163 DN
    Seg drop_____
    Seg inset_____

20. Left lens
    $F = +0.75 -1.75 \times 90$
    A = 57 mm
    B = 48 mm
    ED = 65 mm
    DBL = 17 mm
    PD = 66/61
    Seg height = 22 mm
    Blank seg drop = 6 mm
    Blank seg inset = 7 mm
    Prism amount = 0.5
    Prism axis = 146 DN
    Seg drop_____
    Seg inset_____

21. Right lens
    $F = +1.00 -2.00 \times 90$
    A = 57 mm
    B = 48 mm
    ED = 65 mm
    PD = 66/61
    Seg height = 22 mm
    Blank seg drop = 6 mm
    Blank seg inset = 7 mm
    Prism amount = 1.5
    Prism axis = 37 DN
    Seg drop_____
    Seg inset_____

22. Left lens
    $F = +0.25 -0.25 \times 94$
    A = 57 mm
    B = 50.5 mm
    ED = 65. 5 mm
    DBL = 14 mm
    PD = 63/59
    Seg height = 24 mm
    Blank seg drop = 6 mm
    Blank seg inset = 7 mm
    Prism amount = 0.1
    Prism axis = 94 DN

Seg drop_____

Seg inset_____

23. Right lens

F = +0.25 −0.25 × 85

A = 57 mm

B = 50.5 mm

ED = 65.5 mm

DBL = 14 mm

PD = 63/59

Seg height = 24 mm

Blank seg drop = 6 mm

Blank seg inset = 7 mm

Prism amount = 0.1

Prism axis = 86 DN

Seg drop_____

Seg inset_____

Reference

1. Younger Optics. *Seamless Plus Layout for Surfacing*, Publication 104TF. Younger Optics, Los Angeles, Calif., undated.

6

Layout and Marking of Franklin-Style Lenses

Introduction

The lens referred to in this chapter as the "Franklin-style" multifocal lens is better known by the name Executive. Executive is a trade name of the American Optical Company.

The Franklin-style lens is a full segment lens, with the entire lower half of the lens blank being occupied by the segment. The appearance of the lens makes it difficult to tell how the lens is constructed optically. Without understanding the optics, layout and marking of the lens become difficult. As a result, errors that would never be tolerated with other common lens styles sometimes pass through unnoticed with the Franklin-style lens.

Lens Construction

The Franklin-style lens gets its name from its visual similarity to the first known pair of bifocals. Benjamin Franklin had an optician friend make the first known pair of bifocals for him by fitting the upper half of a pair of lenses used for distance vision and the lower half of a pair of reading glasses into the same frame. Both pairs of lenses were, in all likelihood, cut through their optical centers.

Present-day Franklin-style lenses resemble the originals only slightly. To help in visualizing the optics of today's Franklin-style lenses, imagine a semifinished flat-top 35 lens blank with the segment centered horizontally on the lens; see Figure 6-1. (Note in Figure 6-1 that the optical center of the

segment is on the seg line.) Now consider what the lens would be like if the flat-top segment were increased in size from 35 mm to 68 mm in width. Such a size would completely fill the lower half of a 68-mm lens blank. From an optical standpoint, this is precisely what happens in a Franklin-style lens. From Figure 6-2, it is evident that the segment has an optical center with a specifically localized position on the lens.

Finding the Segment Optical Center of a Franklin-Style Lens

With other multifocal lenses the seg optical center is easily located. For round segs it is at the center of the seg. For small flat-top segs it is directly below the midpoint of the seg line—usually 5 mm below, to be exact. In the past the seg optical center for Franklin-style semifinished lenses was always found at the midpoint of the seg line. In other words, it was on the seg line and right in the middle of the semifinished lens.

Although many semifinished lenses are still constructed in this manner, some lenses are made differently. An alternative method of construction is to make the semifinished lens blank with a small blank seg inset. In contrast to traditional construction, these lens blanks are made as either a right or a left lens.

Even if we know the optics of the semifinished lens blank, how can the center of the seg be found after the lens has been edged? For round and flat-top segs, the job is easy. The same seg center-

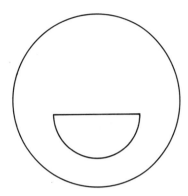

Figure 6-1 The optics of some flat-top 35 bifocals and all flat-top 40 bifocals are very similar to that of Franklin-style bifocals. The seg center is on the seg line. Normally flat-top 35 lens blanks have the segment decentered left or right. This drawing has the segment centered to help illustrate Franklin-style multifocal lens optics.

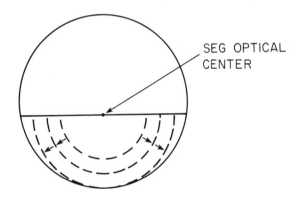

SEG OPTICAL CENTER

Figure 6-2 To understand the optics of a Franklin-style lens, imagine a flat-top 40-mm bifocal segment that has expanded and now fills the entire lower half of the lens.

locating methods that were previously described may still be used. Unfortunately, the task is not as straightforward with Franklin-style lenses.

The Segment Optical Center May Not Be Found Using a Lensmeter

Sometimes people try to find the seg center with a lensmeter. This works only when the distance portion of the lens is plano. Because the distance portion of the lens has no power, all that remains to be seen through the near portion are the optics of the segment. Attempts to use a lensmeter with lenses having any refractive power in the distance prove futile, because the distance lens will exhibit a pris-

matic effect everywhere except at its distance optical center. When attempting to find the optical center of the segment, the prismatic effects from the distance lens interfere and prevent the segment optical center from being located. (It should be noted that this is not just an artifact of the Franklin-style lens. The same phenomenon may be observed through any multifocal segment.)

Finding the Segment Optical Center by Using Reflected Images

It is possible to find the segment optical center of a Franklin-style lens by using reflected images. The easiest way is to look at an image of a fluorescent tube reflected from the front surface of the lens. Hold the lens like a hand mirror until the fluorescent tube is seen at right angles to the seg line. The image is split in two by the seg line, as shown in Figure 6-3. By tilting the lens back and forth, the image can be seen to split apart on the periphery of the lens and reunite in the center. The position on the lens where the tube is seen as continuous (not split apart) is the center of the segment. See Figure 6-4.

The Segment Optical Center Is Found Where the Segment Ledge Is Thinnest

The most direct, though perhaps not the most accurate, method for finding the segment optical cen-

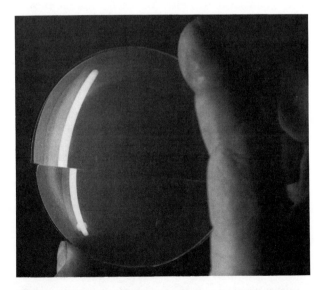

Figure 6-3 The segment optical center of a Franklin-style lens can be found by viewing the reflected image of a fluorescent light tube. When the lens is tilted, the image splits.

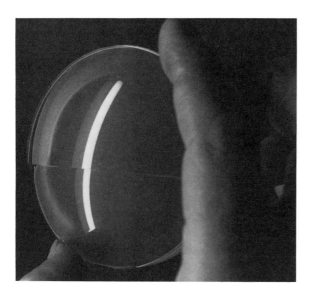

Figure 6-4 When the image of the fluorescent tube is continuous, the segment optical center has been located.

ter is to look for the thinnest point on the segment line. The higher the power of the near addition, the easier it is to find this point.

Five Methods of Grinding Franklin-Style Bifocal Lenses

There are five techniques that have been or are currently being used for grinding Franklin-style lenses:

1. the monocentric method
2. the zero-inset method
3. the preferred (flat-top-style) inset method
4. the optically poor method
5. the near prism reduction method

The first four of these methods will be discussed in the remainder of this chapter. The fifth will be covered in Chapter 16.

Method 1: The Monocentric Method

In the *monocentric method,* the lens is ground with no seg inset and no seg drop. The near optical center of a Franklin-style lens is found on the seg line. This is in contrast to, for example, a round seg bifocal. The optical center of a round seg bifocal will be in the middle of the segment. The closest optical example that visually demonstrates the sit-

uation of a Franklin-style segment is a large segment flat-top lens (such as a flat-top 40). Such a segment looks like the lower half of a circle. This places the center of the circle right on the line.

To understand the monocentric bifocal, consider a pair of bifocal lenses ground with a zero seg drop. With zero seg drop, the segment line is on the datum line. If the normal rules for vertical placement of the distance optical center are followed, the lens would end up with the distance optical center exactly on the seg line. Now consider what would happen if the lens segment were not inset during layout. The distance optical center will fall at exactly the same place on the lens as the segment optical center. The lens then has only one center. It is said to be *monocentric.*

Grinding a Franklin-style lens according to the *monocentric method* means that the distance optical center will always be placed on the seg line at the location of the seg optical center, as seen in Figure 6-5. Thus, during the edging process, both distance and near PDs are placed at the distance PD. This method was used extensively in the past but is currently out of use. Yet many still refer to the Franklin-style lens as a monocentric bifocal and falsely assume that its optics are still monocentric. For a summary of the monocentric method, see Table 6-1.

EXAMPLE 6-1

Suppose the following prescription is ordered for the right lens:

R: +3.00 −1.00 × 95
A = 52 mm
B = 48 mm
DBL = 18 mm
PD = 64/60
Seg height = 22 mm

Table 6-1 Monocentric Method for Grinding Franklin-Style Lenses

1. Use a lens blank having a centered seg optical center.
2. Spot the center of the seg line (the seg optical center).
3. Place the spotted seg line center at the center of the marking grid in the lens marker.
4. Do not move the lens. Simply mark the cylinder axis (and prism axis, if appropriate) through the spotted center.

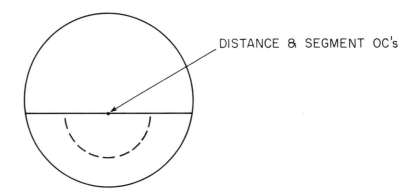

Figure 6-5 With the monocentric method of bifocal grinding, the distance and segment optical centers fall at the same place on the seg line.

If the monocentric method is used, how should the lens be positioned and marked in the layout marker? Use off-center blocking.

SOLUTION

The center of the seg line is spotted and the spot centered as shown in Figure 6-6. Note that the seg is not dropped. Next the lens is marked for blocking as shown in Figure 6-7. The distance optical center will be right on the segment line and at the location of the segment optical center.

Method 2: The Zero Inset Method

In the *zero inset method*, the lens is ground with no seg inset, but with the customary seg drop. The zero inset method and the monocentric method have

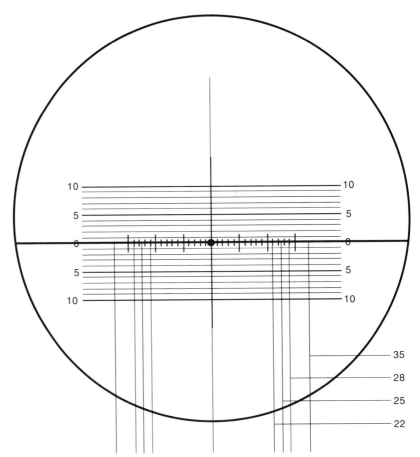

Figure 6-6 If a Franklin-style lens is ground monocentrically, lens centration for surfacing is always the same. The seg optical center (in this case, the center of the seg line) is placed at the middle of the lens marking grid. There is no inset.

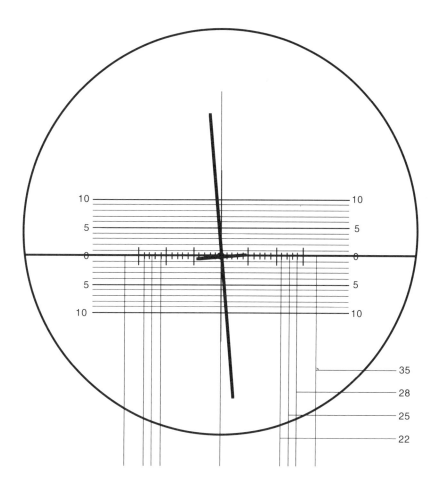

Figure 6-7 Once the segment is centered, with no drop, the monocentrically positioned Franklin lens is marked for cylinder axis. This monocentric method is no longer used when surfacing Franklin-style lenses.

much in common. In fact, there is only one major difference: The zero inset method takes the seg drop into consideration when surfacing. However, there is still no seg inset. The near PD is ignored, and both distance and near PDs are placed at the location of the distance PD. Because there is a seg drop, the distance optical center is exactly above the seg optical center, as shown in Figure 6-8.

Laboratories that use this method most often purchase the more traditional lens blanks, since in these blanks the seg optical center is centered horizontally. These blanks are not right/left specific. (It is possible to use this method with lens blanks that have decentered near optics in order to grind lenses for larger frame sizes.) The zero inset method is summarized in Table 6-2.

To see how lens layout is done, we will use the prescription of Example 6-1 but lay the lens out using the zero inset method instead of the monocentric method.

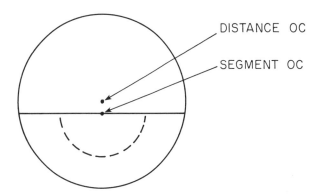

Figure 6-8 The zero inset method yields a distance OC that is directly above the segment OC.

EXAMPLE 6-2

Using the zero inset method, how would lens layout be done for the lens order shown in Example 6-1? Use off-center blocking methods.

Table 6-2 Zero Inset Method for Grinding Franklin-Style Lenses

1. When using a lens blank with no blank seg inset, spot the geometric center of the blank.
2. Place the geometric center on the centered vertical line of the lens marking device.
3. Move the lens up or down until the seg line is at the correct seg drop.
4. Check to be sure the spotted geometric center is still on the vertical line.
5. Mark the lens for cylinder axis (and prism axis when Rx prism is present).

SOLUTION

First the blank geometric center (instead of the center of the seg line) is spotted. Then the lens is placed with this spot on the vertical line in the layout marker. (The movable line is centered.) This is shown in Figure 6-9.

Next the lens must be moved to the correct seg drop. The seg drop is

$$22 - \frac{48}{2} = -2 \text{ mm}$$

or a 2-mm drop. Leaving the center dot on the vertical line, the seg is moved up to the correct drop. See Figure 6-10. At the correct drop, the lens is stamped. See Figure 6-11.

Method 3: The Preferred (Flat-Top-Style) Inset Method

In the *preferred inset method,* the lens is ground with both seg inset and seg drop. Franklin-style lens optics are identical to the optics of flat-top 40 bifocals, but because the Franklin-style semifinished lens is often manufactured with a centered seg optical center, insetting the segment is not always feasible. Attempts to inset the lens will quite often prevent it from cutting out. Insetting the seg effectively renders the blank too small. However, when a small blank is usable, Table 6-3 shows how to do the job.

From an optical point of view, not insetting the seg of a Franklin-style lens is no more justifiable than not insetting a flat-top lens. If optics demand that a flat-top lens be inset, they also demand that

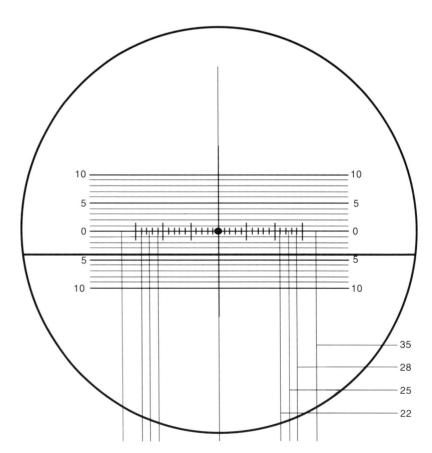

Figure 6-9 To begin the centration for surfacing using the zero inset method, the blank geometric center of the lens is placed on the center of the marking grid.

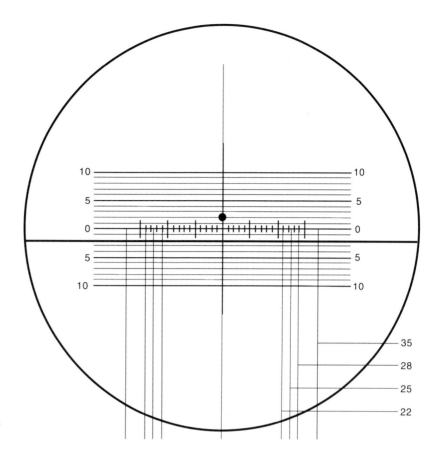

Figure 6-10 Once the lens has been centered horizontally as in Figure 6-9, the seg is moved to the correct drop or raise. In this case a 2-mm drop is called for.

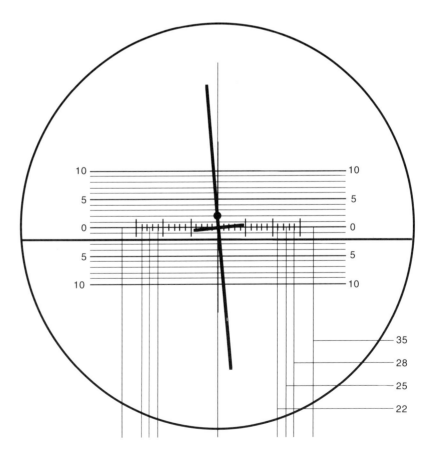

Figure 6-11 For the zero inset method the lens has no segment inset and is stamped for cylinder axis when the correct drop has been achieved. The lens shown is front side up and is stamped for Axis 95.

Table 6-3 Preferred Inset Method for Grinding Franklin-Style Lenses Using a Semifinished Lens Having No Blank Seg Inset*

1. Spot the blank geometric center of the lens. (It will be assumed that the seg optical center is immediately below the blank geometric center.)
2. Decenter the spotted blank geometrical center inward by an amount equal to the seg inset called for in the prescription. (Seg inset is half the difference between the distance and near PDs.)
3. Move the lens up or down until the seg line falls at the correct seg drop.
4. Stamp the lens for cylinder axis and, when appropriate, for prism axis.

*Note that the preferred inset method is not recommended when using a semifinished lens having no blank seg inset. Blank size limitations greatly reduce the probability of success.

Table 6-4 Preferred Inset Method for Grinding Franklin-Style Lenses

1. Look up the amount of blank seg inset for the blank being used.
2. Spot the blank geometric center of the lens.
3. Place the spotted blank geometric center on the center of the lens marking device. (The seg center is now automatically inset by an amount equal to its blank seg inset.)
4. If the amount of seg inset called for in the prescription is less than the blank seg inset, move the spotted geometric center of the lens outward until the correct inset is achieved. (For example, if the blank seg inset is 3 mm and the seg inset required is 2 mm, the spotted geometric center of the lens is outset by 1 mm.)
5. Move the lens up or down until the seg line falls at the correct seg drop.
6. Stamp the lens for cylinder axis and, when appropriate, for prism axis.

Franklin-style lenses be inset. As a result, some manufacturers offer a Franklin-style lens with blank seg inset. Generally the amount of blank seg inset is slightly more than the value for seg inset calculated from the prescription. (For example, blank seg inset may be 3 mm per lens. The average calculated seg inset per lens would be expected to vary from 1.5 to 2.5.) By using a lens with a blank seg inset, the laboratory will be able to cut lenses for larger eye size frames from a lens with a smaller overall diameter. The procedure for using the preferred inset method with a blank having seg inset is summarized in Table 6-4.

Why Not Use a Large Blank Seg Inset for Franklin-Style Lenses?

Franklin-style lens blanks are made with a smaller blank seg inset than flat tops for at least two reasons.

1. Using Franklin-style lenses in extremely large frames will result in a thick lens. The ledge between distance and near portions increases in direct proportion to both the power of the add and the distance from the seg optical center. As a result, the larger the seg ledge becomes, the thicker the lens must be.
2. Manufacturers reason that if the laboratory ignores seg inset and simply lays out the lens using the zero inset method, no serious problems will result. Blanks could be made with a larger blank seg inset (6 mm, for example). However, grinding such a lens in the manner customary for Franklin-style lenses

(the zero inset method) would result in unwanted base-in prism induced through the seg.

Those who desire to use the preferred (flat-top style) inset method for Franklin-style lenses must first establish which type of lens blank is being used. If the semifinished lens blank has no blank seg inset, then the steps given in Table 6-3 are followed. Those who desire to use the preferred inset method for Franklin-style lenses when the semifinished lens blank has a blank seg inset must follow the steps given in Table 6-4.

EXAMPLE 6-3

Using the preferred inset method, lay out a Franklin-style lens for the same prescription as was ordered for Example 6-1. Assume that the semifinished lens is glass and has no blank seg inset. Use off-center blocking methods.

SOLUTION

Dot the center of the lens blank (or the center of the seg line). Prepare the layout marker by setting the movable vertical line for the correct seg inset. In this case, since the lens is a right lens, the movable vertical line is offset to the right by 2 mm. The lens is positioned so that the center dot is on the movable vertical line. See Figure 6-12. Next the seg line is moved upward to the correct 2-mm drop, as in Figure 6-13. The lens is then marked for surfacing as seen in Figure 6-14.

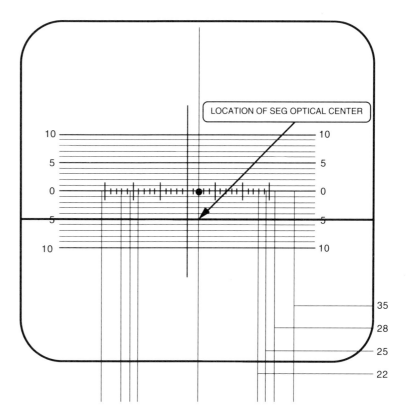

Figure 6-12 When a Franklin-style lens has no blank seg inset, the seg optical center will be directly below the blank geometric center. To use the preferred inset method, the dotted blank geometric center becomes the visible reference point and is inset 2 mm.

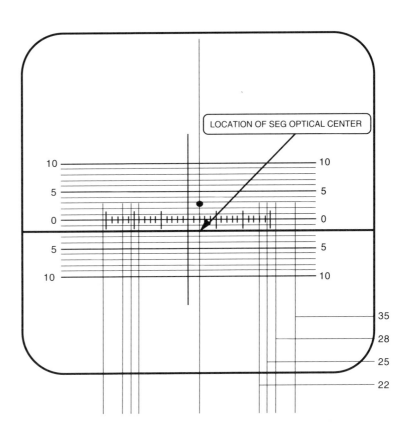

Figure 6-13 Keeping the blank geometric center on the movable vertical line, the segment is moved upward to the calculated 2-mm drop.

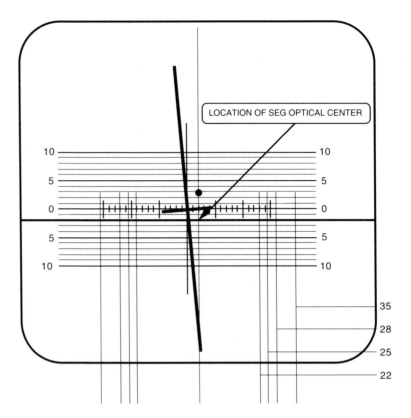

LOCATION OF SEG OPTICAL CENTER

Figure 6-14 Using the preferred inset method with a traditionally centered Franklin-style lens segment means that most of the lens blank ends up on the nasal side. Since more blank is needed temporally than nasally, this centration method is really feasible only for lens blanks that have a blank seg inset, or for frames with a very small eyesize.

EXAMPLE 6-4

Most often the preferred inset method is used only when the lens blanks are manufactured with blank seg inset. To see how this works, use the preferred inset method and a plastic lens with a 3-mm blank seg inset and a 4-mm blank seg drop. Mark the lens for the same prescription as in the previous examples.

SOLUTION

Dot the center of the lens blank. This can be done using a lens center locator, if available. (Alternately, the center of the seg line could be marked.)

Subtract the blank seg inset from the seg inset. In this case,

$$\text{Marker setting} = \text{seg inset} - \text{blank seg inset}$$

$$= 2 - 3$$

$$= -1$$

Because the lens has a greater blank seg inset than the wearer's seg inset, the spotted center of the lens must be outset 1 mm. Move the movable vertical line in the layout marker outward 1 mm and position the spotted lens center on this line. See Figure 6-15. Move the lens upward until the segment line is positioned for a 2-mm

drop as shown in Figure 6-16. The lens is marked for surfacing as shown in Figure 6-17.

An Often-Used Alternative Procedure

Quite often, when a Franklin-style lens having a blank seg inset is used, the laboratory ignores the blank seg inset and lays out the lens using the zero inset method. When this is done, the seg inset always equals the blank set inset. Since few dispensers verify near PDs for Franklin-style lenses, an objection is seldom raised. In fact, the near PD in the glasses is no farther off than when the monocentric method is used for lenses that have a zero blank seg inset. This is not to say, however, that this custom is a recommended procedure.

Method 4: The Optically Poor Method

In the *optically poor method*, the lens is ground with a seg drop, but the grinding for decentration ignores the location of the seg optical center.

One of the biggest problems experienced by those working with the Franklin-style lens is an inability to make a lens that will be large enough for some

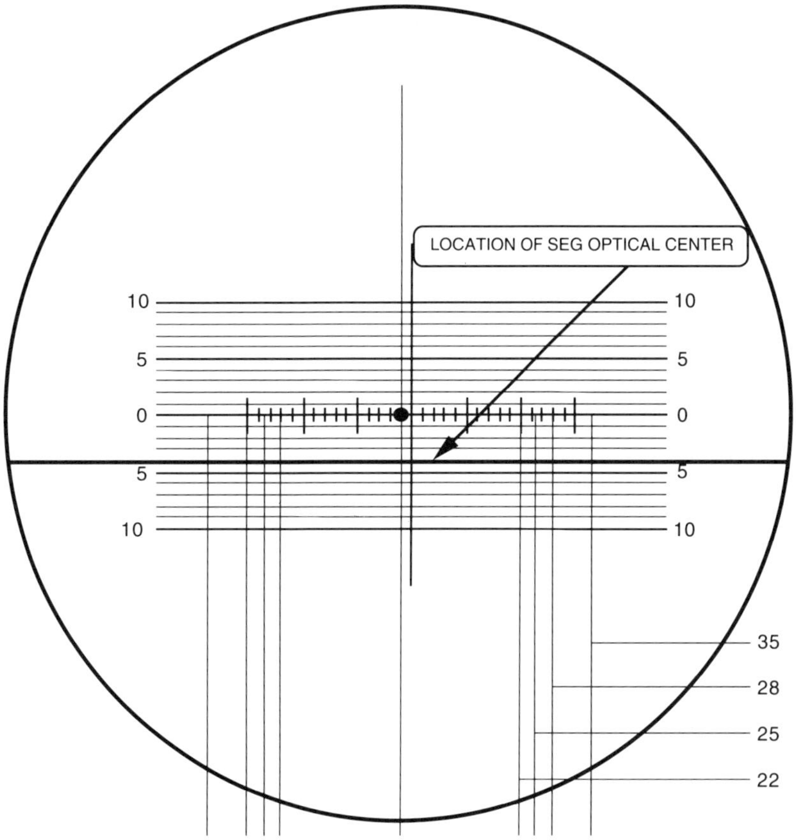

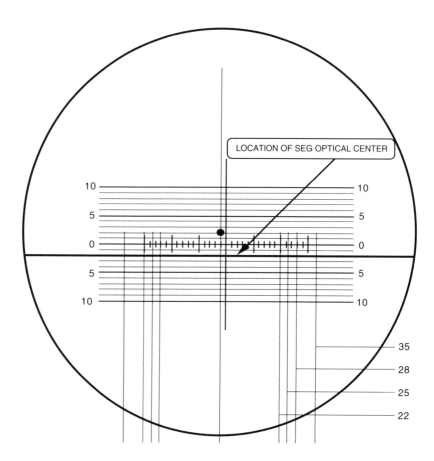

Figure 6-15 Because the seg optical center is not visible or easily located on Franklin-style lenses, the easiest reference point becomes the blank geometric center. This lens is known to have a blank seg inset of 3 mm. To achieve a seg inset of 2 mm, the blank geometric center is outset 1 mm.

Figure 6-16 Keeping the blank geometric center on the movable vertical line, the lens is raised until the indicated 2 mm seg drop is achieved.

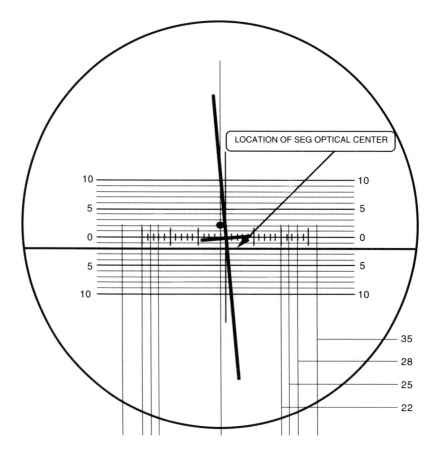

Figure 6-17 The marked cross shows the location of the distance optical center. It can be seen that using the preferred inset method on a right/left-specific lens blank yields good segment decentration and still allows for sufficient lens material temporally, where it is needed most. This is the method of choice for Franklin-style lenses that are right/left specific.

of the larger frames. Because the lenses have either a limited blank seg inset or none at all, the use of the Franklin-style lens with some frames is difficult. Perhaps manufacturers are experienced enough to know that an exceptionally large Franklin-style lens is not advisable. Such a lens would be so thick and heavy that many prescriptions would nonetheless have to be remade in a different lens style.

There is a way to get around this limitation of blank size, even though at times it can yield extremely poor results optically. This method treats the Franklin-style bifocal as if it were a single-vision lens. In order to achieve the desired distance PD, the distance optical center is pushed nasally to the appropriate point while completely ignoring the position of the seg optical center. This would mean, for example, that if the PD were 59/55, the distance PD would be ground for 59 mm, but the near PD could end up being 70 mm instead of 55 mm. With any other bifocal, the error would be immediately obvious. See Figure 6-18. Unfortunately, because the seg location cannot be easily measured on the

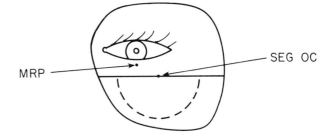

Figure 6-18 The optically poor method of surfacing Franklin-style lenses may result in a near PD that is vastly larger than the wearer's distance PD. If the lens were a flat-top bifocal, it would actually be *out*set, as shown by the dashed line in the figure.

Franklin-style lens, many accounts never know the difference. Table 6-5 explains how to use this method with off-center blocking. Table 6-6 presents an on-center option.

The best solution is not to use this method. If an account becomes belligerent about not getting the

Table 6-5 Optically Poor Method for Grinding Franklin-Style Lenses Using Off-Center Blocking

1. Spot the geometric center of the lens.
2. Move the lens up or down on the marking device until the correct seg height is achieved.
3. Calculate the distance decentration required and decenter the lens for surfacing exactly as if it were a single-vision lens.
4. Mark the lens.

Table 6-6 Optically Poor Method for Grinding Franklin-Style Lenses Using Modified On-Center Blocking

1. Find and spot the geometric center of the lens blank.
2. Calculate the distance decentration required per lens.
3. Calculate how much prism in what base direction would be required to move the optical center laterally for the distance decentration.*
4. Place the lens on the protractor and center the spotted geometric center of the lens blank.
5. Move the lens blank up or down to achieve the correct seg drop.
6. Mark the lens for cylinder axis.
7. Using the base direction calculated above in step 3, mark the prism axis. (If there is Rx prism in the prescription, it will be necessary to combine the Rx prism and the prism for decentration.)

*For more information on how this is done, review the section titled "A Simplified 'On-Center' Bifocal Blocking Method" in Chapter 4.

lenses as desired, one may choose to make the lenses anyway, with results being the account's responsibility.

Incidentally, the plus lens wearer will end up with a worse optical situation than the minus lens wearer. Do you know why? (The answer to this question is found in Chapter 16.)

Marking E/D and F/D Trifocals

Some lenses are constructed like a Franklin-style lens but with a flat-top segment located below the Franklin-style line. For an E/D trifocal the flat-top segment is 8 mm below the line, and for an F/D lens it is 13 mm below the line. These lenses have an intermediate add power below the full-width Franklin-style line, except for the area occupied by the flat-top segment. The flat-top segment area contains the full add power.

With off-center blocking, layout of these trifocal lenses is done by positioning the uppermost Franklin-style line for the calculated seg drop. The flat-top segment is used to position the lens for seg inset horizontally. (Since these lenses are plastic lenses, off-center blocking is not generally recommended.)

To block an E/D or F/D lens on-center, the best method is to use the flat-top segment for reference in centering the lens. This is done according to the manufacturer's listed blank seg inset and blank seg drop.

EXAMPLE 6-5

Lay out the following E/D lens for surfacing, using off-center blocking techniques:

Left lens power is $+1.50 -0.75 \times 15$.
A = 55 mm
B = 48 mm
DBL = 16 mm
Seg height = 26 mm
PD = 66/62
Blank seg inset = 6 mm
Blank seg drop to top of Franklin line = 0 mm

SOLUTION

The procedure needed to lay out this lens using off-center blocking is so much like the flat-top lens that the steps listed in Table 4-1 can be used.

Steps 1 and 2. The seg inset is figured as (66 − 62)/2 = 2 mm, and the flat-top segment is positioned for this amount.

Step 3. The seg drop is 26 − 48/2 = +2 mm up. The Franklin line is set for a seg raise of 2 mm. Figure 6-19 shows the lens positioned correctly for marking.

Step 4. The lens is marked for axis 15.

Steps 5 and 6. There is no Rx prism, so no prism axis needs to be stamped and no base direction needs to be marked.

Step 7. The lens is marked with an "L" on the front upper half and the job number is written on the lower half, both in mirror writing.

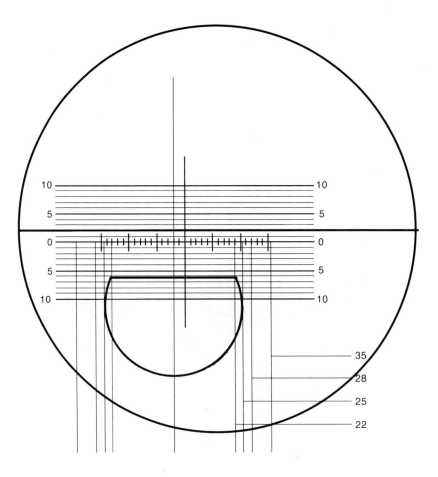

Figure 6-19 With E/D or F/D trifocals, the seg inset uses the flat-top segment for reference; the seg drop, however, uses the Franklin seg line for reference. This lens is positioned for off-center blocking. (Some laboratories may desire to place the OC 2–3 mm above the upper seg line. If so, they would drop the upper seg line by 2–3 mm. The seg height would still be positioned correctly during edging, but the optical center would fall above the line in the distance portion, instead of 2 mm below the line, in the intermediate position. Placing the optical center above the uppermost trifocal line has distinct advantages and should be considered.)

EXAMPLE 6-6

Lay out the E/D trifocal in Example 6-5, this time using on-center blocking techniques.

SOLUTION

The procedure needed to lay out an E/D lens using on-center blocking is the same as that found in Table 4-2. Using the steps listed in Part C, we can proceed as follows.

Steps 1 and 2. The flat-top portion of the lens is positioned with an inset (blank seg inset) of 8 mm.

Step 3. The Franklin line is placed right on the 180 line in the layout marker with no drop. There is no drop because the blank seg drop is 0 mm. Figure 6-20 shows the lens positioned correctly for marking.

Step 4. The lens is marked for axis 15.

Steps 5 and 6. The computer indicates the correct prism axis and base direction.

Step 7. The lens is marked with an "L" on the front upper half and the job number is written on the lower half, both in mirror writing.

Questions and Problems

General Questions

1. The optics of a Franklin-style lens are most similar to those of
   a. a round segment bifocal
   b. a flat-top 28 bifocal
   c. a flat-top 40 bifocal
   d. None of the above is anything like the optics of a Franklin-style lens.

2. Regardless of lens power, the near PD can be verified with a lensmeter for
   a. single-vision lenses in reading glasses
   b. Franklin-style bifocals
   c. flat-top bifocals
   d. a, b, and c are correct.
   e. a and c are correct.
   f. None of the above is correct.

3. Which of the following methods for grinding Franklin-style lenses is/are not in use today?
   a. monocentric method
   b. zero inset method
   c. preferred (flat-top style) inset method

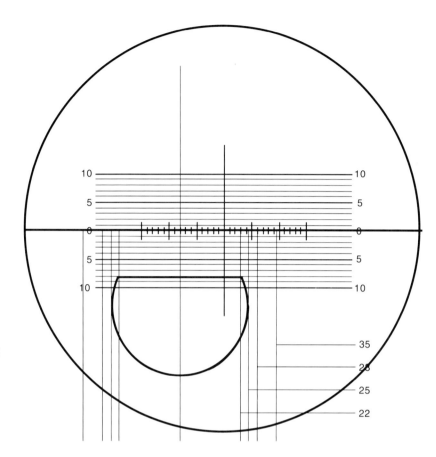

Figure 6-20 For on-center blocking an E/D or F/D lens, the blank seg inset references the flat-top seg, while the blank seg drop references the Franklin seg. This lens has a blank seg inset of 8 mm and a zero blank seg drop. It is positioned for on-center blocking.

    d. optically poor method
    e. near prism reduction method

4. Which method for grinding Franklin-style lenses treats the lens as if it were a single-vision lens?
   a. monocentric method
   b. zero inset method
   c. preferred (flat-top-style) inset method
   d. optically poor method
   e. near prism reduction method

5. For which method or methods would you expect to find the near PD equal to the distance PD after the lens has been ground?
   a. monocentric method
   b. zero inset method
   c. preferred (flat-top-style) inset method
   d. optically poor method
   e. near prism reduction method

6. For which method or methods would it be no surprise to end up with a near PD in the glasses that is significantly different than the wearer's near PD?
   a. monocentric method
   b. zero inset method
   c. preferred (flat-top-style) inset method
   d. optically poor method
   e. near prism reduction method

7. Which of the following allow the smallest possible lens blank to be used?
   a. monocentric method
   b. zero inset method
   c. preferred (flat-top-style) inset method
   d. optically poor method
   e. near prism reduction method

8. Suppose that the optically poor method is used to grind Franklin-style bifocals. If the lenses have a great deal of calculated distance decentration, in which situation does the near horizontal prismatic effect end up being less for the wearer?
   a. when the distance power is moderate to high minus
   b. when the distance power is moderate to high plus
   c. It doesn't really matter.

9. Franklin-style lenses are not made with blank seg inset, only blank seg drop.
   True or False

10. Which method of grinding Franklin-style lenses completely ignores the location of the segment optical center?
   a. monocentric method
   b. zero inset method

c. preferred (flat-top-style) inset method
d. optically poor method
e. near prism reduction method
f. None of the above methods ignores the location of the seg optical center.

11. In which method(s) of grinding Franklin-style lenses will the distance PD and the near PD be equal?
    a. monocentric method
    b. zero inset method
    c. preferred (flat-top-style) inset method
    d. optically poor method
    e. near prism reduction method
    f. none of the above

12. In which method(s) of grinding Franklin-style lenses would you expect the near PD to be greater than the distance PD in a vast majority of cases?
    a. monocentric method
    b. zero inset method
    c. preferred (flat-top-style) inset method
    d. optically poor method
    e. near prism reduction method
    f. none of the above

13. Why should one locate the geometric center of a Franklin-style lens blank during the layout process, even if the lens is to be blocked off center?

14. How can the seg optical centers be physically located and dotted on a pair of cut, edged, and inserted Franklin-style bifocals?

15. Draw and label a Franklin-style lens for each of the listed philosophies of surfacing, including the locations of the distance and seg optical centers. Also include how far apart the centers are from one another in both the horizontal and vertical directions. The lens has the following dimensions:

    A = 48 mm
    B = 44 mm
    ED = 53 mm
    DBL = 20 mm
    PD = 64/60
    Seg height = 18 mm

    a. monocentric philosophy
    b. the more common variation on the monocentric philosophy whereby distance and near PDs are always equal
    c. the method of considering the Franklin-style lens in the same manner as a flat-top lens

16. What optically questionable method is sometimes used in order to get a Franklin-style lens to cut out for a large frame?

Layout Exercises
Using Franklin-style semifinished lens blanks or mock acetate lenses, lay out and mark each lens for the layout method specified according to the prescription information given.

Monocentric method: Using the information given for the following lens pair, mark the lenses provided according to the monocentric method. (Do not be confused by the presence of extra information.)

17. R: $-3.00 -1.00 \times 18$
    L: $-2.75 -1.25 \times 157$
    A = 50 mm
    B = 40 mm
    ED = 54.5 mm
    DBL = 24 mm
    PD = 71/68
    Seg height = 19 mm

Zero-inset method: For the lens pairs listed below, use the zero inset method and mark the Franklin-style lens blanks provided.

18. R: $+2.00 -1.00 \times 110$
    L: $+2.00 -1.00 \times 70$
    A = 50 mm
    B = 43 mm
    ED = 51 mm
    DBL = 19 mm
    PD = 64/62
    Seg height = 15 mm

19. R: $-3.00 -1.75 \times 35$
    L: $-3.00 -1.75 \times 145$
    A = 52 mm
    B = 49 mm
    ED = 55 mm
    DBL = 17 mm
    PD = 62/59
    Seg height = 19 mm

20. R: $+0.25 -0.50 \times 20$ 2 prism diopters Base In
    L: $+0.25 -0.50 \times 135$ 2 prism diopters Base In
    A = 50 mm
    B = 43 mm
    ED = 51 mm
    DBL = 19 mm
    PD = 64/62
    Seg height = 15 mm

21. R: $-0.75 -0.75 \times 135$ 2 prism diopters BI and
                                              1.25 BU
    L: $-0.75 -0.75 \times 45$ 1.50 prism diopters BI
                                              and 1.25 BD
    A = 52 mm
    B = 49 mm
    ED = 55 mm
    DBL = 17 mm
    PD = 62/59
    Seg height = 19 mm

Preferred (flat-top-style) method: For the lens pairs listed below, use the preferred (flat-top-style) method and mark the Franklin-style lens blanks provided. Assume that the lens blanks will have a 3-mm blank seg inset.

22. R: +2.00 sph
    L: +2.00 −1.00 × 110
    A = 50 mm
    B = 40 mm
    ED = 55 mm
    DBL = 20 mm
    PD = 66/64
    Seg height = 15 mm

23. R: −3.00 −1.75 × 88
    L: −3.00 −1.75 × 39
    A = 52 mm
    B = 47 mm
    ED = 59 mm
    DBL = 16 mm
    PD = 60/57
    Seg height = 25 mm

24. R: +0.25 −0.50 × 10   5 prism diopters BI and 2 BD
    L: +0.25 −0.50 × 175   5.5 prism diopters BI and 1.75 BU
    A = 56 mm
    B = 48 mm
    ED = 64 mm
    DBL = 26 mm
    PD = 70/65
    Seg height = 21 mm

25. R: −0.75 −0.75 × 107   2.75 prism diopters BI and 1.25 BU
    L: −0.75 −0.75 × 72   2.50 prism diopters BI and 1.00 BD
    A = 54 mm
    B = 51 mm
    ED = 63 mm
    DBL = 14 mm
    PD = 68/64
    Seg height = 17 mm

Optically poor method: For the following lens pairs, mark the lenses using simplified on-center blocking.

   a. Indicate the amount and direction of prism required to move the major reference point over to the decentration required for the distance PD. (You can move your block up or down on the lens, but not left or right. Grind horizontal prism instead of moving the block left or right.)

   b. Clearly mark where on your lens the major reference point will fall.

   c. Also mark the location of the seg optical center.

   d. What would the near PD end up being if you actually ground the lenses this way?

26. R: +2.00 −1.00 × 180
    L: +2.00 −1.50 × 180
    A = 58 mm
    B = 46 mm
    ED = 66 mm
    DBL = 19 mm
    PD = 64/62
    Seg height = 20 mm
    Prism amount   R: _____
                   L: _____
    Prism base direction   R: _____
                           L: _____
    Resulting near PD _____

27. R: −3.00 −1.75 × 90
    L: −3.00 −2.25 × 90
    A = 57 mm
    B = 49 mm
    ED = 63 mm
    DBL = 17 mm
    PD = 61/59
    Seg height = 27 mm
    Prism amount   R: _____
                   L: _____
    Prism base direction   R: _____
                           L: _____
    Resulting near PD _____

28. R: +0.25 −0.50 × 90   1 prism diopter BI
    L: +0.25 −0.75 × 90   2 prism diopter BI
    A = 56 mm
    B = 46 mm
    ED = 62 mm
    DBL = 19 mm
    PD = 61/57
    Seg height = 20 mm
    Prism amount   R: _____
                   L: _____
    Prism base direction   R: _____
                           L: _____
    Resulting near PD _____

29. R: −5.00 sph   1.00 BU
    L: −5.50 sph   0.75 BD
    A = 58 mm
    B = 50 mm
    ED = 65 mm
    DBL = 17 mm
    PD = 62/59
    Seg height = 21 mm
    Prism amount   R: _____
                   L: _____
    Prism base direction   R: _____
                           L: _____
    Resulting near PD _____

7

Tool Curves and Lens Thickness: Basic Concepts

Introduction

There are three ways of determining thickness and back curves for lenses:

1. by means of calculations and selected tables
2. by using *surfacing charts* as supplied by the manufacturer (Manufacturer-supplied surfacing charts are meant to be used only for their specific brand of lens.)
3. by using a layout computer

The layout computer is a vast improvement over the first two methods when the lens parameters are especially complicated. It should be understood, however, that the quality of any layout computer results depends on the quality of the program.

Lens Curve Terminology

Several different lens curve values may be used to describe the same lens surface. These front-curve lens values are

nominal base curve (NBC)
true base curve (TBC) or "true power"
refractive power

Nominal Base Curve

The *nominal base curve* (NBC) is a reference number established for the convenience of laboratory personnel. The NBC of the front surface plus the back curve should equal the desired back vertex power.* The NBC is meant to decrease the number

---

*The *back vertex power* is the power measured with the lensmeter. It is the desired power for the lens prescription.

106

and difficulty of calculations required to find the back-surface tool curve.

When a lens increases in thickness, the back vertex power will change even if there is no change in other lens parameters. This is most evident for plus lenses. With a plus lens, the back vertex power will continue to increase in power the thicker the lens gets. This increase is more noticeable with steeper base curves. The steeper the base curve becomes, the more the back vertex power will increase with increased lens thickness.

Manufacturers try to keep things as simple as possible. So that the needed back curve can be found more easily, the manufacturer adjusts the physical curve of the front of the lens somewhat. The nominal value of the front curve is the same, but the actual curve of the front of the lens is flatter.

Vertex Power Allowance

A formula can be used to determine how much the front surface (D_1) must be decreased in curvature (made flatter) in order for the equation to come out correctly.

$$D_2 = D_v' - D_1$$

where

D_1 = the curvature of the front surface in diopters
D_2 = the curvature of the back surface in diopters
D_v' = the prescribed back vertex power of the lens in diopters

This formula allows the tool needed to grind the back surface curve to be found by subtracting the front surface curve from the prescribed power. In this equation D_1 would equal the nominal base curve if the lens had a 1.53 refractive index. This amount of decrease is known as the *vertex power allowance* (VPA).[1] The formula for determining the vertex power allowance is

$$\text{VPA} = \frac{t(\text{NBC})^2}{1000n + t(\text{NBC})}$$

where

VPA = vertex power allowance
t = lens center thickness in millimeters
NBC = nominal base curve desired
n = refractive index of the lens

Once the vertex power allowance has been found, its value is subtracted from the nominal base curve. The lens is then produced according to these new specifications. Now it is possible to find the correct tool curve simply by subtracting the NBC from the back vertex power. Thus

$$D_2 = D_v' - D_1$$

can be thought of as

Tool curve = prescribed power − NBC.

Is This Power Compensation Procedure Exact for Every Lens?

Unfortunately, in order to produce exact results every time, a vast number of base curves would be necessary. The correction factor chosen ends up being one that will give the best possible results for a given grouping of lenses, all having the same base curve. The choice of which compensation to use and how to group the lenses is up to the manufacturer. This explains why surfacing charts supplied by one manufacturer may not work for other brands of lenses.

True Base Curve or "True Power"

Once the curvature of the base curve (front surface) has been modified, the manufacturer refers to the modified curvature as the *"true power"* of the lens. Others may refer to true power as *"actual power."* In this sense, "true" and "actual" are synonymous. Also known as *true base curve* (TBC), true power is expressed in diopters of curvature referenced to an index of refraction of 1.53.* (This is the value

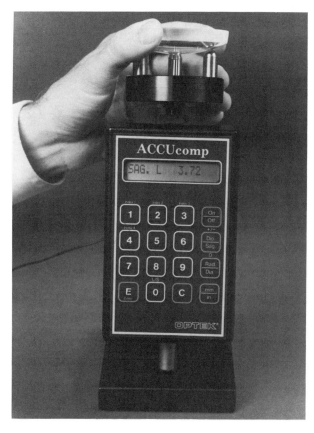

Figure 7-1 Each plastic lens should be checked for its true base curve using a sag gauge so that back curves will be accurately calculated. Reading can be recorded in diopters or as sagittal depth, as shown.

that will be found when using a lens clock.†) One can quickly see that the "true power" is not the refractive power of the surface. Instead, it is a value that is *referenced* to the standard index of 1.53. This standard index is used for lap tools and other optical laboratory measuring devices.

The relationship between nominal and true base curves is not as predictable with plastic lenses. Each lens should be measured for true base curve individually using a sag gauge such as the one shown in Figure 7-1. The value obtained is used by the layout computer in calculating needed tool curves.

---

*Although the glass used today has a refractive index of 1.523, historically lens glass had a refractive index of 1.53. Tools and laboratory measuring devices in use today will employ the previous standard.

†A lens clock or lens measure is a hand-held instrument which resembles a pocket watch with three prongs. When the prongs are pressed against the surface of the lens, the center prong moves and changes the position of a hand on the dial of the "clock." The position of the hand indicates the dioptric power of the lens surface.

Refractive Power

Refractive power is the real value that accounts for what happens to light at the surface of the lens. It can be calculated, but it is not of any *practical* use when surfacing a lens. However, refractive power is the anchor point for all values.

If true power is known, the radius of curvature of the surface can be found using the *lensmaker's formula,*

$$D = \frac{n' - n}{r}$$

or, expressed in terms of r,

$$r = \frac{n' - n}{D}$$

Because the surface is in air, the formula is usually written as

$$r = \frac{n - 1}{D}$$

since air has a refractive index of 1. Because the power of the surface was given in terms of the true base curve, the refractive index is 1.53. This is true *regardless* of what the lens material is, since TBC is always 1.53 referenced to an index of 1.53. Therefore

$$r = \frac{1.53 - 1}{D_{1.53}}$$

From this radius, the refractive power of the surface can be determined once the index of the lens material is known. For example, with crown glass,

$$r = \frac{1.523 - 1}{D_{1.523}}$$

Because both equations refer to the same radius, these two equalities can be combined to yield

$$\frac{1.53 - 1}{D_{1.53}} = \frac{1.523 - 1}{D_{1.523}}$$

which transposes to

$$D_{1.523} = \left(\frac{0.523}{0.53}\right) D_{1.53}$$

and further reduces to

$$D_{1.523} = 0.987 D_{1.53}$$

$D_{1.523}$ is the refractive power and $D_{1.53}$ is the "true power." Thus, for crown glass, the refractive power

will be numerically smaller than either the nominal *or* the "true power."

EXAMPLE 7-1

Suppose a crown glass lens surface has a nominal base curve of +10.25 and a true base curve of +10.09 D. What is the refractive power of the surface?

SOLUTION

Crown glass has an index of refraction of 1.523. Using the equation previously found,

$$D_{1.523} = \left(\frac{0.523}{0.53}\right) 10.09$$

$$= (0.987) 10.09$$

$$= +9.96 \text{ D}$$

Therefore the refractive power of the surface is really +9.96 D. Yet, as previously mentioned, in calculating tool curves and lens thicknesses, refractive power is not used directly.

Tool Curves for Crown Glass Lenses

The nominal base curve is intended to allow the laboratory technician to find the needed tool by simple subtraction. This works well for crown glass lenses and holds true unless the back vertex powers are especially high, or the lens is ground considerably thicker than would be anticipated.

Tool Curves for Spherical Crown Glass Lenses

Back-surface lap tools for crown glass lenses may be found using the formula

Tool curve = back vertex power
− nominal base curve

or

$$D_2 = D_v' - \text{NBC}$$

EXAMPLE 7-2

A crown glass lens has a nominal base curve of +6.25 D. The power called for in the prescription is +1.50 D. (This is the back vertex power.) What tool curve is needed?

SOLUTION

The solution is straightforward:

$$D_2 \text{ (tool curve)} = (+1.50) - (+6.25)$$
$$= -4.75 \text{ D}$$

EXAMPLE 7-3

A semifinished crown glass lens has a nominal base curve of $+4.25$. The prescription calls for a back vertex power of -3.00. What tool curve is need to finish the lens?

SOLUTION

Again, using the formula $D_2 = D'_v - NBC$,

$$D_2 = -3.00 - (+4.25)$$
$$= -7.25 \text{ D}$$

The back tool curve needed is a -7.25 D sphere.

The process of finding the correct tool curve is not quite so direct in cases of high-powered crown glass lenses, or for lenses of a different refractive index such as high-index lenses or plastic lenses. Techniques for finding tool curves for non-crown glass lenses will be explained later in the chapter.

Lens Thickness

Sagittal Depth

The formula that is the basis for determining lens thickness is the *sag formula,* where *sag* is short for *sagittal depth.* Sag is the depth of the lens surface curve and is shown in Figure 7-2. A chord is a

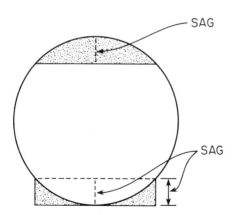

Figure 7-2 A knife-edged plus lens has the same center thickness that the edge of an infinitely thin minus lens would have when both diameters and curvatures are the same.

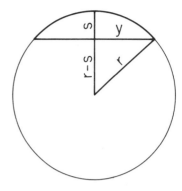

Figure 7-3 The geometry of the figure shows how the sag formula is derived from the Pythagorean theorem. Here $y^2 + (r - s)^2 = r^2$.

straight line joining two points on a curve. In Figure 7-2 the two points on the curve are at the top edges of the lens, and the length of the chord equals the diameter of the lens.

To find the sagittal depth it is necessary to know the length of the chord and the radius of curvature of the lens surface. Figure 7-3 shows the radius (r) as the hypotenuse of a right triangle. The other two sides are y, which is one-half the chord (or ½ the lens diameter), and ($r - s$), which is the radius less the sag. Because this triangle is a right triangle, the Pythagorean theorem* can be used to find the sag:

$$y^2 + (r - s)^2 = r^2$$

By transposition,

$$(r - s)^2 = r^2 - y^2$$

and

$$r - s = \sqrt{(r^2 - y^2)}$$

which simplifies to

$$-s = -r + \sqrt{(r^2 - y^2)}$$

and results in

$$s = r - \sqrt{(r^2 - y^2)}$$

This last equation is called the *accurate sag formula.*†

---

*The Pythagorean theorem states that $a^2 + b^2 = c^2$, where c is the hypotenuse or long side of the triangle while a and b are the short sides.

†Before the advent of hand calculators, simplified formulas yielding an approximate result were used to find the sag of a curved surface. To distinguish the original from these approximations, the formula which did not yield an approximate result was termed the *accurate* sag formula.

EXAMPLE 7-4

A certain lens surface has a radius of curvature of 83.7 mm. The lens has a diameter of 50 mm. What is the sag of the front surface of the lens?

SOLUTION

Using the accurate sag formula,

$$s = r - \sqrt{(r^2 - y^2)}$$

The value for r has been given as 83.7 mm. The *value of y* is half the lens diameter. Since the lens has a diameter of 50 mm, y is 25 mm. Therefore,

$$s = 83.7 - \sqrt{(83.7)^2 - (25)^2}$$

$$= 83.7 - 79.9$$

$$= 3.8 \text{ mm}$$

The s, r, and y can be expressed in meters or millimeters, as long as all are in the same units. In this case all three are expressed in millimeters. The sag of this surface is 3.8 mm.

EXAMPLE 7-5

Suppose a lens has a TBC of +7.19 D. If the diameter of the lens is 52 mm, what is the sag of the front surface at the full 52-mm diameter?

SOLUTION

To find the sag of the surface, we need to know r and y. The y value is easy to find, since it is half the 52-mm diameter. In other words, $y = 26$ mm. However, to find the radius, we must use the *lensmaker's formula*,

$$r = \frac{n - 1}{D}$$

with $n = 1.53$, or

$$\frac{1.53 - 1}{D}$$

To find r for a +7.19 D TBC surface, we use

$$r = \frac{1.53 - 1}{+7.19}$$

$$= \frac{0.53}{+7.19}$$

$$= 0.0737 \text{ m}$$

The sag formula requires that all the terms in the equation be expressed in the same units. Converting 0.0737

to millimeters makes $r = 73.7$ mm. Now we can use the sag formula:

$$s = 73.7 - \sqrt{(73.7)^2 - (26)^2}$$

$$= 73.7 - \sqrt{5431.7 - 676}$$

$$= 73.7 - \sqrt{4755.7}$$

$$= 73.7 - 69.0$$

$$= 4.7 \text{ mm}$$

The sag of a +7.19 D TBC surface on a 52-mm lens is 4.7 mm.

EXAMPLE 7-6

A lens has a TBC of +7.19, a diameter of 52 mm, a plano back surface, and an edge thickness of 1.6 mm. What is the center thickness (CT) of the lens?

SOLUTION

We have already calculated the sag of the front surface of this lens in Example 7-5. To visualize what this plano convex lens looks like, see Figure 7-4a. From the figure we can see that the CT of the lens will be equal to the sag of the front surface (s_1), plus the edge thickness (ET). Therefore the CT of this lens is

$$CT = s_1 + ET$$
$$CT = 4.7 \text{ mm} + 1.6 \text{ mm}$$
$$= 6.3 \text{ mm}$$

(In Figure 7-4 the edge thickness has been drawn exceptionally thick in order to keep front and back surface sagittal depth labels (s_1 and s_2) from overlapping. If drawn to scale, the edge would be much thinner and would correspond more accurately to the example.)

Thickness of Meniscus Lenses

Although some ophthalmic lenses worn today are plano-concave or plano-convex, most lenses have a convex front surface and a concave back surface. These lenses are referred to as *meniscus lenses*. To determine the thickness of a meniscus lens, calculations must be made for both the front and back surfaces.

To better understand the construction of such a lens and how calculations are carried out, think of the meniscus lens as being two lenses glued to-

(A)

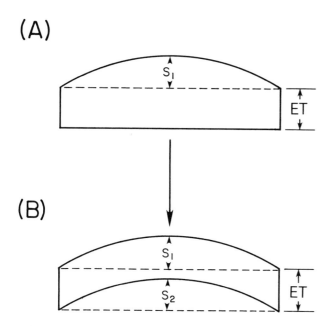

(B)

Figure 7-4 (A) For a plus lens with a convex front surface and a plano (flat) back surface, lens center thickness is equal to the edge thickness plus the sagittal depth of the front surface (S_1). (B) A meniscus lens has a convex front surface and a concave back surface. The center thickness of a meniscus lens is equal to the edge thickness plus the sagittal depth of the front surface (S_1) minus the sagittal depth of the second surface (S_2).

gether. A meniscus lens can first be thought of as a plano-convex lens, as shown in Figure 7-4a. For a plano-convex lens, center thickness is equal to the sagittal depth of the first surface (s_1) plus the edge thickness, or

$$CT = s_1 + ET$$

After center thickness calculations have been carried out for a plano-convex lens, imagine grinding a minus curve on the back of the lens, as shown in Figure 7-4b. This reduces the CT by the sag of this freshly ground concave surface. The CT then becomes

$$CT = s_1 + ET - s_2$$
$$= s_1 - s_2 + ET$$

where s_2 is the sag of the second surface.

Sagittal depths are found using the accurate sag formula

$$s = r - \sqrt{r^2 - y^2}$$

as previously described, or by using sag tables—and sag tables are easier. Sag tables are given in

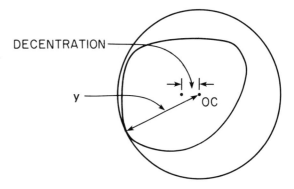

Figure 7-5 The diameter used in calculating lens thickness is basically the same as that used for minimum blank size. The only difference is that the 2- to 4-mm chipping factor is ignored.

Appendix 4-1 and eliminate the necessity of working through the accurate sag formula.

Both the sag tables and the formula require that the lens diameter used to find the sagittal depth be known.

Determining Lens Diameter and Sag Value

The lens diameter needed to find the correct sag value depends on both the frame size and optical center decentration. To visualize the situation, mark the point on an edged lens where the optical center will fall. Next draw a line from the optical center (OC) to the point on the lens edge that is farthest from the OC. See Figure 7-5. The resulting line is the y value we are interested in. Twice y is very close to the *minimum blank size* (MBS). In fact, when considering single-vision uncut lenses, the diameter we are interested in is equal to the minimum blank size, but it does not include the 2- to 4-mm safety factor for lens chipping that is included in the MBS formula.* The formula for this diameter, which we will call the *chord diameter,* is

Chord diameter = ED + (A + DBL − Far PD)

where

    ED = the effective diameter of a lens
    A = the boxing eye size

---

*The MBS formula for single-vision lenses is

    MBS = ED + (A + DBL − PD) + 2
          = ED + (decentration per lens) × 2 + 2

DBL = the distance between lenses

Far PD = the wearer's interpupillary distance for distance viewing

This formula may be used for both single-vision and multifocal lenses.*

Because there is little difference between the sag of the nominal base curve and the sag of the true base curve, in most cases either will work when calculating the sag of the front surface. However, the preferred value for use in determining the sag of the front surface is the sag of the true base curve. The TBC will give a smaller sag value than the NBC and will yield a thinner lens.

To find the sag of the back surface, use the tool curve value as previously determined from the equation

$$D_2 = D'_v - \text{NBC}$$

where, as before, D_2 is the back surface tool curve, D'_v is the back vertex power, and NBC is the nominal base curve.

Center Thickness and Back-Surface Tool Curves for Spherical Lenses

Let us consider some examples of how center thicknesses and back-surface tool curves are found for spherical lenses. The following examples are for plus lenses, as minus lens centers are of standard thicknesses and need not be calculated. Steps in finding tool curves and center thicknesses for sphere lenses are summarized in Table 7-1.

EXAMPLE 7-7

A +3.00 D lens is to be surfaced for a frame having the following dimensions:

A = 54 mm
DBL = 18 mm
ED = 56 mm

The wearer's PD is 64 mm, and the lens chosen has an index of refraction of 1.523, a nominal base curve of +8.25 D, and a true base curve of +8.17 D. If the edge is to be 1.9 mm thick, what back tool curve and center thickness should be used?

---

*A somewhat more accurate formula often used for high-plus lenses is

Chord diameter = $(0.75 \times \text{ED}) + (A + \text{DBL} - \text{far PD})$

This and other ways of further thinning a high-plus lens will be discussed in Chapter 14.

Table 7-1 Finding Lens Thickness and Tool Curves

1. Find the tool curve using

$$D_2 = D'_v - \text{NBC}$$

where D_2 is the tool curve, D'_v is the prescribed lens power, and NBC is the nominal base curve.

2. Find the chord diameter using

Chord diameter = ED + (A + DBL − far PD)

3. Find the sags of the front and back surfaces using sag tables.

4. Find the center thickness using

$$\text{CT} = s_1 - s_2 + \text{ET}$$

SOLUTION

Step 1. To find the back tool curve we use

$$\begin{aligned} D_2 &= D'_v - \text{NBC} \\ &= +3.00 - (+8.25) \\ &= -5.25 \text{ D} \end{aligned}$$

Step 2. The center thickness requires consulting sag tables to find the sags of the front and back surfaces. To find the sags we must know the chord diameter. (Most sag tables call for the chord diameter by simply stating "diameter" on the chart. It should be assumed that "diameter" means chord diameter.) To find chord diameter we use

$$\begin{aligned} \text{Chord diameter} &= \text{ED} + (A + \text{DBL} - \text{far PD}) \\ &= 56 + (54 + 18 - 64) \\ &= 64 \text{ mm} \end{aligned}$$

Step 3. Once the chord diameter is known, it is possible to look up the sagittal depth (sag) of the first and second surfaces. The first surface (D_1) has a true base curve of +8.17 D. Using Appendix 4.1, we see that the sag of an 8.00 D curve having a 64-mm chord diameter is 8.2 mm, and the sag for an 8.25 D curve is 8.5 mm. By estimating from these two values given in the table, we find the closest sag value for 8.17 D as 8.4 mm.

The second surface (D_2) has a curve of −5.25 D. The sag of a 5.25 D curve for a 64-mm chord diameter is 5.2 mm.

Step 4. To find the needed center thickness, we use

$$\begin{aligned} \text{CT} &= s_1 - s_2 + \text{ET} \\ &= 8.4 - 5.2 + 2.0 \\ &= 5.2 \text{ mm} \end{aligned}$$

Thus the center thickness of this lens should be 5.2 mm.

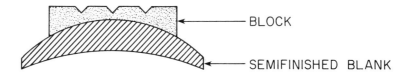

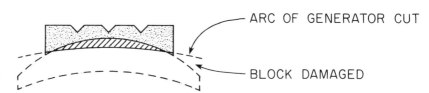

Figure 7-6 When calculating thicknesses for small, plus lenses, the limiting factor may not be the desired size of the lens. The size of the block may prevent the lens from being ground thinner. If the size of the block is not considered and the lens is ground too thin, the lens, the block, and even the generator wheel may be ruined.

EXAMPLE 7-8

A prescription is to be surfaced for a rather small frame. The lens power is plus, and the thinnest edge is to be 2 mm thick. The lenses are to be made up in crown glass with lens power and frame dimensions as follows:

R: +3.25 sph
L: +3.25 sph
Frame A = 38 mm
DBL = 14 mm
ED = 40 mm
Wearer's PD = 50 mm

The laboratory chooses a lens with a nominal base curve of +8.25 D. The true (1.53) base curve is 8.17 D. What tool curve and center thickness should be used?

SOLUTION

Step 1. The back tool curve is

$$D_2 = D_v' - NBC$$
$$= (+3.25) - (+8.25)$$
$$= -5.00 \text{ D}$$

Step 2. To find the thickness, we first need to know the chord diameter.

$$\text{Chord diameter} = ED + (A + DBL - far PD)$$
$$= 40 + (38 + 14 - 50)$$
$$= 42 \text{ mm}$$

Step 3. Using the sag tables, the sag of the true curve of 8.17 D for a 42-mm chord diameter is 3.45 mm, and the sag of the back tool curve of 5.00 D is 2.1 mm. (Note how much smaller the sag value is for this prescription

than it was for the one in Example 7-7, even though the base curves are the same.)

Step 4. The center thickness is thus

$$CT = s_1 - s_2 + ET$$
$$= 3.45 - 2.1 + 2.0$$
$$= 3.35 \text{ mm}$$

(Also notice how much thinner this smaller-sized lens is than the lens in Example 7-7, even though their powers are nearly the same.)

Special Cautions for Small Lenses

During processing, lens blocks are attached to the front surface of the lens to hold the lens in place. Because the back surface of a plus lens is curved less than the front surface, grinding the lens too thin will cause part of the lens block or generator ring* to be ground away. See Figure 7-6. This will both ruin the lens block and dull the cutting wheel of the lens generator. This means that a lens can only be ground so thin, regardless of computations! The minimum thickness a lens may be ground will depend on the sizes of the lens block and generator ring. Most lens blocks used for glass lenses are 43 mm in diameter and use a 50-mm-diameter generator ring. (Blocks used for plastic lenses are usually larger.) Thus, for a plus lens to be ground thinner

---

*When glass lenses are generated, a 50-mm-diameter ring fits around a 43-mm lens block to steady the lens.

than the thickness dictated by the block size, it would be necessary to use a smaller lens block—otherwise the lens block may be destroyed.

EXAMPLE 7-9

Is it possible to grind the lenses in Example 7-8 without destroying the block or ring?

SOLUTION

To see if a lens can be made without destroying the block or ring, calculate what thickness a lens of that same power would have for a 50-mm-diameter chord size if it were to be ground with knife edges.* Using the data from Example 7-8, s_1 for a +8.17 D curve is 5.0 mm, while s_2 for a 5.00 D curve is 3.0 mm. For a knife-edged lens,

$$
\begin{aligned}
CT &= s_1 - s_2 + ET \\
&= 5.0 - 3.0 + 0 \\
&= 2.0 \text{ mm}
\end{aligned}
$$

Therefore, if a +3.25 lens is ground thinner than 2.0 mm, the ring and possibly also the block will be ruined. (Naturally, the prudent person will allow somewhat extra thickness for safety.) Because the thickness called for in Example 7-8 is 3.35 mm, the lens may be ground without ruining either block or ring.

Tool Curves for Lenses with a Cylinder Component

Most ophthalmic lenses in the United States have the cylinder power on the back of the lens. These lenses are spherocylinders and are known as *minus cylinders*. They are ground using lap tools having two curves. The first and weaker curve gives the sphere power and is called the *back base curve* (or *toric base curve*). The second, more minus curve is called the *cross curve* and includes the added value necessary to create the cylinder. These two values quantify the two-curved, or *toric* surface. The tool value is written as

Back base curve/cross curve

An example might be −6.00/−6.50.

To find the needed toric back-surface curves for crown glass lenses having cylinder power, the back base curve is calculated using the sphere power.

---

*A *knife-edged lens* is one having an edge thickness of zero.

Table 7-2 Finding Tool Curves for Spherocylinders

1. Find the back base curve:

$$D_2 = D_v' - \text{NBC}$$

where D_2 is the back base curve, D_v' is the sphere component in a minus cylinder prescription, and NBC is the nominal base curve.

2. Find the cross curve:

Cross curve = back base curve + cylinder

3. The needed tool is

Back base curve/cross curve

The cross curve is found by adding the cylinder power to the back base curve:

Cross curve = back base curve + cylinder

These steps are summarized in Table 7-2.

EXAMPLE 7-10

A prescription lens power is to be −2.00 −1.00 × 180. A base curve of +6.25 D is chosen. (The nominal base curve is +6.25 D, and the true base curve is +6.20 D.) What tool is needed to grind the lens?

SOLUTION

Step 1. The back base is calculated from the nominal base curve and the back vertex power:

$$
\begin{aligned}
D_2 &= D_v' - \text{NBC} \\
&= -2.00 - (+6.25) \\
&= -8.25 \text{ D}
\end{aligned}
$$

Because the lens is minus in power, the center thickness is chosen rather than calculated. Customarily, minus-powered crown glass lenses are ground 2.2 mm thick. Therefore we do not need to know what the true base curve is.

Step 2. The cross curve is the back base plus the cylinder, or

$$
\begin{aligned}
\text{Cross curve} &= -8.25 + (-1.00) \\
&= -9.25
\end{aligned}
$$

Step 3. Thus the needed tool is

−8.25/−9.25

Compensated Power and Tool Curves for High-Minus Crown Glass Lenses

For very low lens powers, there is no significant difference between the 1.523 crown glass lens power and the 1.53 indexed tool. However, for higher-powered surfaces, compensation for differences in index must be made.

High-minus lenses are ground on very low base curves. These base curves are seldom modified, because it is unlikely that there will be enough center thickness to cause any power variation. The nominal base curve and the true base curve are either exactly the same or only slightly different from one another.

Since the front surface of a lens is given in terms of 1.53 index material and the back surface must be ground using a 1.53-indexed tool, a trick referred to as *compensated power* can be used to give the correct back-surface tool curve for high-powered minus lenses. This "trick" references the back vertex power in terms of 1.53. Compensated power for a crown glass lens may be found as follows:

$$D_{1.53} = \left(\frac{0.53}{0.523}\right)D_{1.523}$$
$$= 1.0134\, D_{1.523}$$

In other words, if the back vertex power is multiplied by the constant 1.0134, the compensated back vertex power can be found. Tables are also available, making direct calculations unnecessary. Compensated powers are given in Appendix 3-3. This "new" (compensated) power can then be used to find the needed tool curve from

$$\text{Tool curve} = \text{compensated power} - \text{true base curve}$$

or

$$D_2 = D_c - D_1$$

where D_c is the compensated power. (It should be noted that since NBC and TBC are so similar, the nominal base curve can as easily be used without seriously compromising the final results.)

EXAMPLE 7-11

A prescription calls for a crown glass lens having a power of −8.00 D. If the lens is to be ground on a semifinished blank having a base curve of +0.50, what 1.53-index tool curve must be used in order to make the power come out right? (The nominal and true base curves are both +0.50 D.)

SOLUTION

The compensated power for −8.00 D can be found in Appendix 3-3, or by multiplying by the constant for crown glass:

$$\text{Compensated power} = (1.0134)(-8.00)$$
$$= -8.11\ D$$

Since

$$\text{Tool curve} = \text{compensated power} - \text{TBC}$$

in this instance,

$$\text{Tool curve} = -8.11 - 0.50$$
$$= -8.61\ D$$

To the nearest ⅛th diopter, the correct tool is −8.62 D.

Additional Power Compensations for High-Plus Crown Glass Lenses

Extra tool power compensation is required for plus lenses only in certain cases. This is because the base curve is already compensated for values up through the expected average lens thickness. When compensation is necessary, the amount is usually ⅛th diopter of extra minus added to the tool curve value. This extra compensation is used only if the lens is ground thicker than would ordinarily be anticipated. Extra thickness will generally be needed with executive bifocals or with plus lenses intended for frames having very large eyesizes.

Such additional back-surface tool compensation usually is not made until the lens becomes thicker than approximately 4.7 mm, regardless of power. As a precautionary measure, lenses to be ground for back vertex (Rx) powers over +4.00 D should be checked to see if they will be above average in thickness. Lenses with base curves over +7.00 D should also be checked more carefully for extra thickness. Generally speaking, the higher the base curve, the more likely it is that the lens will require additional compensation.

A handy chart that may be used is given as Appendix 4-2. When a lens differs from its predicted thickness, this chart may be used to figure power compensation.

EXAMPLE 7-12

A crown glass (1.523-index) lens is ground using a semifinished blank with a +10.00 D nominal base curve. We find that the lens will end up being 1.7 mm thicker than expected. If we assume that normally the lens would have a tool curve of −5.25 D, what new tool curve must be used to compensate for the increased thickness?

SOLUTION

Using Appendix 4.2, we see that for a 1.523-index lens having a +10.00 D base curve, the multiplier to be used is 0.071. We multiply the change in thickness by this value:

$$\text{Tool curve change} = \text{multiplier} \times \text{thickness change}$$
$$= 0.071 \times 1.7$$
$$= 0.12$$

For increased lens thickness, the tool curve must be steepened. This increases the minus power of the rear surface, compensating for plus power induced by the thickness. The new curve is

$$-5.25 - 0.12 = -5.37 \text{ D}$$

Low-Plus Crown Glass Lenses

Because of vertex power allowances made by the manufacturer in calculating the needed true base curves, low-plus-powered lenses seldom need added compensation for thickness. For purposes of finding tool curves, a low-plus lens will be considered as having

    a nominal base curve of less than +7.00 D
    a back vertex power of +4.00 D or less
    a thickness of less than 4.7 mm

Lenses above these parameters should be looked at for greater than average thicknesses and, if necessary, adjusted by either adding ⅛th diopter of extra minus power to the tool curve or by using Appendix 4-2.

Low-Minus Crown Glass Lenses

For calculation purposes, a low-minus lens will be considered as having a back vertex power of less than −4.50 D. Tool compensation is seldom required for low-minus lenses. Tool curves for high-minus crown glass lenses may require compensation using the compensated power concept previously explained.

Other Factors

Other factors can and do affect lens thickness and, consequently, the tool curves to be chosen. Some of these factors will be addressed in the next chapter.

Tool Curves for High- or Low-Index Lenses

The compensated power concept for finding lens back-surface curves can be used for lenses of other indexes as well—especially high-index lenses of minus power. Because all lenses have 1.53-referenced front base curves, the back curves can be found by changing the back vertex power to a "compensated" power.

When the compensated power concept is used with lenses having a cylinder component, each meridian must be figured separately. The sphere power is figured first. This is the power of the first major meridian on the power cross. Next the sum of sphere and cylinder is calculated, for this is the power of the second major meridian. See Table 7-3 for the steps required to find tool curves using compensated power.

EXAMPLE 7-13

A lens pair is ordered with the following parameters:

    R: −7.75 −1.00 × 180
    L: −7.75 −1.00 × 180
    Frame A = 50 mm
    DBL = 20 mm
    ED = 52 mm

Table 7-3 Using Compensated Power to Find Tool Curves for Thin Lenses

---

1. If the lens is a spherocylinder, determine the back vertex power in each of the two major meridians. The power in the first meridian equals the sphere power. The power in the second major meridian equals the sphere plus the cylinder.

2. Look up the compensated power for each power meridian using a compensated power table. If the index of refraction of the material is not found in the chart, calculate the conversion constant (k):

$$k = \frac{1.53 - 1}{\text{index of new material} - 1}$$

Multiply the conversion constant by the back vertex power of each meridian separately to find the compensated meridian powers:

    Compensated power = k(back vertex power)

3. Subtract the true base curve from the compensated power to find the tool curve for each meridian:

    Tool curve = compensated power
                − true base curve

The Rx is to be made from high-index material having an index of refraction of 1.7. The semifinished lens has a nominal base curve of +2.00 D. The nominal and true base curves are equal. What tool curves are needed in order to surface the lens?

SOLUTION

Step 1. The first step is to find the back vertex power in each of the two major meridians. The first meridian has a back vertex power equal to that of the sphere, which is −7.75 D. The second major meridian's back vertex power is

(Sphere) + (cyl) = second major meridian power

or

$$(-7.75) + (-1.00) = -8.75 \text{ D}$$

Step 2. Next we look up these two powers in the compensated power table in Appendix 3-3 under the 1.7 index column. The first meridian is −5.87 D. The second meridian is −6.62 D.

Step 3. Finally, the true base curve is subtracted from the compensated powers to find the needed tool curves:

$$\text{First meridian tool curve} = -5.87 - (+2.00)$$
$$= -7.87 \text{ D}$$

$$\text{Second meridian tool curve} = -6.62 - (+2.00)$$
$$= -8.62 \text{ D}$$

The needed tool is a −7.87/−8.62.

EXAMPLE 7-14

A prescription calls for a back vertex power of −5.50 −1.00 × 180. The lens is to be ground in 1.586-index polycarbonate. The semifinished blank chosen has a nominal base curve of +3.25 D and a true base curve of +3.15 D. What 1.53-indexed tool must be used to surface the lens?

SOLUTION

Step 1. Because the lens is minus in power, lens thickness does not influence the power of the lap tool. Back vertex power is −5.50 D in the first meridian and −6.50 D in the second meridian.

Step 2. Compensated powers for these two meridians are found in Appendix 3-3. They are −4.97 D and −5.88 D, respectively.

Step 3. To find tool curves, use

Tool curve = compensated power − true base curve

For the first meridian,

$$\text{Tool curve} = -4.97 - (+3.15)$$
$$= -8.12 \text{ D}$$

For the second meridian,

$$\text{Tool curve} = -5.88 - (+3.15)$$
$$= -9.03 \text{ D}$$

The theoretical tool curve needed is

$$-8.12/-9.03$$

In practice, the tool chosen would be −8.12/−9.00.

Summary of Essential Formulas

Front surface refractive power:

$$\text{Refractive power} = \left(\frac{n - 1}{1.53 - 1}\right) \text{(true power)}$$

Tool curve for lower-powered crown glass lenses:

$$\text{Tool curve} = D'_v - \text{NBC}$$

Accurate sag formula:

$$s = r - \sqrt{r^2 - y^2}$$

Center thickness using sags:

$$\text{CT} = s_1 - s_2 + \text{ET}$$

Chord diameter:

$$\text{Chord diameter} = \text{ED} + (\text{A} + \text{DBL} - \text{far PD})$$

Compensated power:

$$D_{1.53} = \left(\frac{1.53 - 1}{n - 1}\right)D_{\text{new material}}$$

Tool curve for non-crown glass lenses:

$$\text{Tool curve} = D_{\text{compensated}} - \text{TBC}$$

Questions and Problems

1. The "nominal power" of a lens base curve is listed as being +8.25 D. The "true power" of this same surface is +8.17 D. The lens has a refractive index of 1.523. Answer the following questions about this lens.

   a. What is the *refractive* power of the base curve?

   b. If the lens was to have a back vertex power of +2.25 D, what tool curve would be chosen for the back surface?

c. If you checked the base curve using a lens clock, what would you expect the lens clock to read?

2. A high-index lens of index 1.70 comes in a box stamped "+8.25 D." Before surfacing, it is checked on the sag gauge and reads +8.17 D. What are the nominal, true, and refractive powers for this lens surface?

3. A plastic lens of index 1.498 is marked with a base curve of +6.25 D. It measures +6.18 D with a lens clock. What are the nominal, true, and refractive powers for this lens, expressed in diopters?

4. If a lens has an index of 1.498 and a refractive surface power of +9.56 D, what is the true power of the lens surface? What would you expect the nominal power of the lens surface to be?

5. a. What compensated power would you use to find the back surface curve for a −8.75 D lens from 1.7-index material?

   b. If the lens had a true front surface power of +2.00 D, what back-surface tool curve would you use?

6. a. What compensated power would you use to find the back-surface curve for a −5.75 D lens made from 1.7-index material? (You may use a compensated power chart.)

   b. If the lens had a true front-surface power of +2.00 D, what back surface tool curve would you use?

7. Use the compensated power method to find the correct D_2 tool curve for a high-index lens of index 1.70 having a nominal base curve of +2.00 D and a needed back vertex power of −7.25 D. (Assume that the nominal surface power equals the true surface power.)

8. If no precalculated tables were available, using the compensated power method for figuring D_2 tool curves for plastic lenses of index 1.499 would require multiplying by a constant, K. What is the value of this constant?

9. A lens has a true base curve of +10.25 D and a back tool curve of 6.25 D. The frame has the following dimensions:

   A = 50 mm
   DBL = 20 mm
   ED = 53 mm
   Wearer's PD = 66 mm

   How thick should this lens be ground so that the minimum edge thickness equals 1.3 mm when complete?

10. A lens has a true curve of +8.00 D and the back surface is to be ground with a −5.00 D tool. If the lens is to be ground to a 50-mm diameter with no decentration and an edge thickness of 1.3 mm, how thick will the lens be in the center?

In Problems 11–13, find the center thickness and back-surface tool curves for each lens prescription. Begin by determining the chord diameter.

11. D'_v = +4.25 sph
    NBC = +10.00
    A = 51 mm
    DBL = 18 mm
    ED = 54 mm
    PD = 63 mm
    Minimum edge thickness = 1.5 mm

12. D'_v = +3.50 sph
    NBC = +8.50
    A = 52 mm
    DBL = 19 mm
    ED = 53 mm
    PD = 66 mm
    Minimum edge thickness = 2.3 mm

13. D'_v = +7.50 − 0.50 × 180
    NBC = +12.00
    A = 40 mm
    DBL = 15 mm
    ED = 40 mm
    PD = 54 mm
    Minimum edge thickness = 1.6 mm

14. Without using sag tables, find the sagittal depth for a lens surface that has a 50-mm chord size and a true curve of +4.25 based on an index of refraction of 1.53. Show your work.

15. a. Use the compensated power concept to determine the D_2 tool curves for a lens having a refractive index of 1.60, a nominal base curve of +2.00 D, and a back vertex power of −5.25 D.

    b. Suppose the above lens is to be ground 2.1 mm thick and is for a frame with the following dimensions:

       A = 53 mm
       DBL = 18 mm
       ED = 54 mm
       Wearer's PD = 65 mm

    What would the maximum edge thickness be?

16. Suppose an innovative new lens material comes on the market with an index of refraction of 1.64. If you were using tools of index 1.53, by what constant would you multiply the prescribed lens power in order to find the "compensated power" of a lens?

Appendix: Using Compensated Power for Thick Lenses

When a lens begins to increase in center thickness, the vergence* of light changes as it travels from the first to the second surface. The higher the base curve, the more significant the change becomes. In order to offset this thickness-induced power change, the following formula for the back curve is used:

$$D_2 = D_v' - \frac{D_1}{1 - (t/n)D_1}$$

where

D_2 = the 1.53-indexed tool curve
D_1 = the true base curve
D_v' = the *compensated* back vertex power
t = lens center thickness
n = 1.53

EXAMPLE 7-15

What tool curve would be used for a 1.498-index CR-39 plastic lens that is to have a back vertex power of +5.00 D and will be ground on a semifinished blank with a nominal base curve of +8.25 D and a true base curve of +8.36 D? The lens is to have a center thickness of 6.7 mm.

SOLUTION

First find the compensated power for the +5.00 D lens. Using the compensated power table (Appendix 3-3), we find a compensated power of +5.32 D. The terms in the formula are therefore

D_2 = tool curve needed
D_1 = TBC = +8.36 D

---

*Vergence is the reciprocal of the distance from the focal point of converging or diverging light rays to a reference plane crossing these rays. Vergence, like lens power, is expressed in diopters of refractive power. For a more complete explanation, see Brooks, C. W., and Borish, I. M., *System for Ophthalmic Dispensing*, Butterworth-Heinemann, 1979, pp. 385–389. See especially Figure XVII-3 on page 388.

D_v' = compensated power = +5.32 D
t = center thickness = 6.7 mm = 0.0067 m
n = 1.53

Because the powers are expressed in diopters, which are based on meters instead of millimeters, the lens thickness must be written in meters. Thus the formula becomes

$$D_2 = 5.32 - \frac{8.36}{1 - (.0067/1.53)(8.36)}$$

$$= 5.32 - 8.68$$

$$= -3.35 \text{ D}$$

The theoretical tool needed is 3.35 D. The tool closest to this value would be 3.37 D. This procedure is summarized in Table 7-4.

Tool Curves and Lens Thickness for a Thick Lens

When it is necessary to determine thickness for a non-crown glass lens, the procedures shown in Table 7-5 should be followed.

Table 7-4 Using Compensated Power to Find Tool Curves for Thick Lenses

1. Determine the back vertex power for each major meridian.
2. Look up the compensated power for each power meridian using a compensated power table, or use a calculated constant.
3. Use this formula to find each tool curve:

$$D_2 = D_v' - \frac{D_1}{1 - (t/n)D_1}$$

where

D_2 = 1.53 indexed tool curve
D_1 = true base curve
D_v' = *compensated* back vertex power
t = lens center thickness
n = 1.53

Table 7-5 Finding Tool Curves and Thickness for Thick Lenses

1. Find the chord diameter for the lens.
2. Use the chord diameter and true base curve to find the sag of the front surface (s_1) using sag tables (Appendix 4-1).
3. Find the compensated power for the sphere meridian of the lens using Appendix 3.3.
4. Find an *estimated* D_2 tool curve using

$$D_2 = \text{compensated power} - \text{true base curve}$$

5. Find the sag of the back curve (s_2) using sag tables (Appendix 4-1).
6. Find the lens center thickness

$$CT = s_1 - s_2 + ET$$

7. Now find the final back base tool curve using the formula

$$D_2 = D'_v - \frac{D_1}{1 - (t/n)D_1}$$

where

D_2 = the 1.53-indexed tool curve
D_1 = the true base curve
D'_v = the *compensated* back vertex power
t = lens center thickness
n = 1.53

8. Find the compensated power for the cylinder meridian of the lens. (Add the sphere power and the cylinder power together. Look up the compensated power for the cylinder meridian in Appendix 3-3.)
9. Use the formula in step 7 to find the back-surface cross curve tool power.
10. The values found in steps 7 and 9 give the needed tool curves.

EXAMPLE 7-16
A prescription is as follows:

R: +6.50 −1.00 × 180
L: +6.50 − 1.00 × 180
Frame A = 54 mm
Frame ED = 56 mm
Frame DBL = 18 mm
PD = 66 mm

The lenses are to be ground in 1.586-index polycarbonate material with a minimum edge thickness of 1.2 mm. The nominal and true base curves for the semifinished blank are both +9.75 D. How thick should the lens be ground? What tool should be used?

SOLUTION

Step 1. To arrive at a center thickness, we need to know the chord size.

Chord diameter = ED + (A + DBL − far PD)
= 56 + (54 + 18 − 66)
= 62 mm

Step 2. The sag (s_1) of a +9.75 D surface for a 62-mm chord is found from the sag tables as 9.7 mm.

Step 3. The compensated power for a +6.50 D polycarbonate lens is +5.88 D.

Step 4. To find s_2 we need an estimated D_2 curve. The *estimated* D_2 curve is found using

$$D_2 = \text{compensated power} - \text{true base curve}$$

(This is used only for arriving at lens thickness.) Therefore,

$$D_2 = +5.88 - 9.75$$
$$= -3.87 \text{ D}$$

Step 5. The sag of −3.87 D at a 62-mm chord diameter is 3.6 mm.

Step 6. Therefore, center thickness is

$$CT = s_1 - s_2 + ET$$
$$= 9.7 - 3.6 + 1.2$$
$$= 7.3 \text{ mm}$$

Step 7. Knowing a working center thickness, the tool curve can be found as

$$D_2 = 5.88 - \frac{9.75}{1 - (0.0073/1.53)\,9.75}$$
$$= 5.88 - 10.23$$
$$= -4.35 \text{ D}$$

(At this point, in order to be really accurate, the thickness should be recalculated using the sag of 4.35. This would give a thickness of 6.85 mm. Then the tool curve could be refined even further, giving a value of −4.32 D. However, these values are so close to the value already found that they will not be significant.)

Step 8. To find the compensated power for the cylinder meridian, first add the sphere and cylinder powers. In this case,

$$(+6.50) + (-1.00) = +5.50 \text{ D}$$

The compensated power of + 5.50 D is looked up in compensated power tables and found to be +4.97 D.

Step 9. The cross curve becomes

D_2 = 4.97 − (same factor as previously calculated)

  = 4.97 − 10.23

  = −5.26

Step 10. The theoretical tool chosen will −4.35/−5.26, or more likely −4.37/−5.25 when rounded.

The formula method shows the reason why tool curves must be modified as a result of lens thickness. It becomes the basis for understanding why surfacing charts and lens computers require a change in the tool curve when a change in lens center thickness occurs. For more on thick lenses, see Chapter 14.

Reference

1. Jalie, M. *Tables for Surfacing Instruction; Spectacle Crown Glass and CR-39.* ICP Science and Technology Press, Guildford, England, 1972.

8 Tool Curves and Lens Thickness: Additional Factors

Surfacing Charts

Manufacturers of lens blanks have a vested interest in ensuring that their lenses are properly surfaced for the correct thickness and power. Upon request, manufacturers will supply charts indicating what specifications should be used for each power of lens in order to produce the best results. However, because of the variables that affect lens thickness and therefore lens power, different results can be obtained by different individuals using the same tables. Results will depend on the foresight and care of the individual using the tables. All variables should be considered.

Lens tables can be constructed in a variety of ways. Some manufacturers assume much skill on the part of the optician and include a lot of detailed information. Proper use of all the information will result in the preparation of excellent lenses. Other manufacturers fear that, because of a lack of understanding, detailed information in their charts will not be given proper consideration. Hence they present a more averaged set of less complicated tables.

No matter how they are presented, each set of tables requires some study in order to understand the format and logic being used. Familiarity with the way charts are used will make it easier to utilize different types of tables. Used properly, lens charts make it possible to develop a "feel" for why lenses are ground as they are, a "feel" that cannot be obtained by using computers alone.

Determining Lens Parameters

Finding the Base Curve

It is important to follow the rules for finding the correct base curve, as described in Chapter 2. The fact that a lens power is listed under a given base curve does not mean that this base curve is optimum for the lens power. Surfacing charts may include the same lens power under as many as three or more separate base curves, because the base curve of a given lens may have to be altered to conform to the curve of its partner.* The best base curve should be found first, then the lens power looked for under that base curve section of the table.

Using the Main Chart

Lens surfacing charts may contain an area where base curves, back-surface tool curves, and lens thicknesses for given powers are listed. This part of the chart is often called the *main chart*. See Table 8-1. Other, accompanying tables may show allowances for special factors that need to be taken into consideration. An example is the effect of Rx prism on the thickness of a lens.

Some main charts contain more variables within the chart itself. Table 8-1 is an example of a main chart that includes lens diameter variables. As shown in this table, a chart may list "effective diameter" (ED) of the frame rather than "chord diameter," "diameter," or "minimum blank size." In this case, either an average decentration has been estimated and then added to the value, or the term "effective diameter" is not being used in its true sense.†

---

*Equality of base curves is not just for cosmetic purposes. It is important in order to equalize lens magnification between right and left lenses, making image sizes more equal.

†The effective diameter is twice the longest radius of a frame's lens aperture as measured from the boxing center. The ED measure was shown in Figure 1-22 and again in Figures 2-4 and 2-5. The effective diameter does not take lens decentration into account. To obtain an accurate center thickness for plus lenses, decentration must be considered.

Table 8-1 Sample Surfacing Chart—Vision-Ease "Unilite"—8.25 Base (8.36 True Base Curve) Concave Curves for Plus Powers

Plus Power	Center Thickness (CT) / Minus Curve (MC)	Lens Effective Diameter					
		54	58	62	66	70	74
1.25	CT	3.0	3.1	3.3	3.5	3.7	4.0
	MC	7.16	7.17	7.17	7.18	7.19	7.20
1.50	CT	3.1	3.3	3.5	3.7	4.0	4.3
	MC	6.90	6.91	6.92	6.93	6.94	6.95
1.75	CT	3.3	3.5	3.8	4.0	4.3	4.7
	MC	6.64	6.65	6.66	6.67	6.69	6.70
2.00	CT	3.5	3.7	4.0	4.3	4.7	5.0
	MC	6.38	6.40	6.41	6.42	6.44	6.46
2.25	CT	3.7	3.9	4.3	4.6	5.0	5.4
	MC	6.13	6.14	6.15	6.17	6.19	6.21
2.50	CT	3.8	4.1	4.4	4.8	5.2	5.7
	MC	5.86	5.88	5.90	5.91	5.93	5.95
2.75	CT	3.9	4.3	4.7	5.1	5.6	6.1
	MC	5.61	5.62	5.64	5.66	5.68	5.71
3.00	CT	4.1	4.5	4.9	5.4	5.9	6.4
	MC	5.35	5.37	5.39	5.41	5.43	5.46
3.25	CT	4.3	4.7	5.2	5.7	6.2	6.8
	MC	5.09	5.11	5.13	5.15	5.18	5.21
3.50	CT	4.4	4.8	5.3	5.9	6.4	7.1
	MC	4.83	4.85	4.87	4.90	4.92	4.95
3.75	CT	4.6	5.1	5.6	6.1	6.7	7.4
	MC	4.57	4.59	4.62	4.64	4.67	4.70
4.00	CT	4.8	5.3	5.8	6.4	7.1	7.8
	MC	4.32	4.34	4.36	4.39	4.42	4.45
4.25	CT	5.0	5.5	6.1	6.7	7.4	8.1
	MC	4.06	4.08	4.11	4.14	4.17	4.21
4.50	CT	5.1	5.6	6.2	6.9	7.6	8.4
	MC	3.80	3.82	3.85	3.88	3.91	3.95
4.75	CT	5.2	5.8	6.4	7.1	7.9	8.7
	MC	3.54	3.56	3.59	3.63	3.66	3.70
5.00	CT	5.4	6.0	6.7	7.4	8.2	9.0
	MC	3.28	3.31	3.34	3.37	3.41	3.45

Source: From *Vision-Ease Laboratory Processing Data,* Vision-Ease Corporation, St. Cloud, Minn., revised 5/18/88, p. 50, used by permission.

Once the base curve of the lens is known, the next step is to look up the standard lens thickness and tool curve in the main chart. After these values have been found, any special factors can be considered. If there are no special considerations, the thickness and tool curve values given in the main chart may be used to produce the lens. Main chart values may be used in a majority of cases. This is especially true for minus lenses, because center thicknesses are generally standard. The basic steps

Table 8-2 Basic Steps in Using Lens Surfacing Charts

1. Determine the base curve of the lens.
2. Look up the standard lens thickness and tool curve in the main chart.
3. Allow for any special factors that should be considered.

in using lens surfacing charts are summarized in Table 8-2.

Determining Edge Thickness

At this point it may be helpful to consider whether the semifinished lens blank is thick enough to allow for sufficient edge thickness with high-minus lenses. If no edge thicknesses are given on the charts, the edge thickness may be determined by estimation or by using sags.

Estimating Edge Thickness

It can be very useful to be able to estimate edge thickness quickly. Such estimates are useful not only for determining if a semifinished lens blank will be thick enough to grind the prescription, but also to respond to questions about how thick certain lens prescriptions will be. These estimating methods also work for center thicknesses. Center thicknesses found in this manner, however, should not be used for production purposes. Table 8-3 shows a fairly accurate system for estimating thickness based on lens size. This lens size is what has been referred to previously as the chord diameter. Each lens size has a constant, K, which is multiplied by the power of the lens.

EXAMPLE 8-1

Estimate the edge thickness for the following prescription using Table 8-3 and assuming a center thickness of 2.2 mm.

R: −7.00 sph
L: −7.00 sph
A = 53 mm
DBL = 18 mm
ED = 57 mm
PD = 65 mm

SOLUTION

Steps 1. and 2. The chord diameter of the frame is found by adding the total decentration to the frame ED.

Table 8-3 Tabular Method for Estimating Lens Thickness*

Lens Chord Diameter (ED = A = DBL − PD)	Constant (K)
46	0.5
50	0.6
55	0.7
58	0.8
60	0.9
64	1.0
67	1.1

1. Find the ED of the frame.
2. Determine the chord diameter by adding total decentration (A + DBL − PD) to the frame ED.
3. Look up the constant in the table.
4. Multiply the constant by the power of the lens.
5. For minus lenses, to find the edge thickness add the center thickness to the value found in step 4.
   For plus lenses, to find the center thickness add the edge thickness to the value found in step 4.
6. If there is Rx prism in the prescription, one-half the Rx prism power is added to the thickness.

*Based on a circular entitled "An Easy Method of Determining Edge Thickness of Minus Lenses," E. H. Schmidt and Sons, Optical Laboratories, Indianapolis, Indiana, undated.

$$\text{Total decentration} = A + DBL − PD$$
$$= 53 + 18 − 64$$
$$= 7 \text{ mm}$$

$$\text{Chord diameter} = ED + \text{total decentration}$$
$$= 57 + 7$$
$$= 64 \text{ mm}$$

Step 3. The constant in Table 8-3 for a chord diameter of 64 mm is 1.0.

Step 4. For a lens having a power of −7.00D, the constant (1.0) multiplied by the power (7.00) is 7.0 mm.

Step 5. The center thickness of the lens (2.2 mm) is added to the value found in step 4 to find an estimated edge thickness of

$$2.2 + 7.0 = 9.2\text{mm}.$$

A Rule of Thumb In spite of the simplicity of this method, it is still not possible to estimate thickness without calculating chord diameter and referring to the table. In an effort to make estimations easier, most calculations can be dropped by assuming a total decentration of 6 mm for all cases, and by using the effective diameter (ED) of the frame instead of chord diameter. This means that a lens having an ED of 50 mm will have a constant (K) of 0.7. An ED of 50 mm is considered to be small and the constant used for small lenses is 0.7. Lenses with a 58-mm ED call for a constant of 1.0. A lens with a 58-mm ED is considered large and the constant for large lenses is 1.0. If the numbers (50, 0.7) and (58, 1.0) are memorized, constants other than 0.7 and 1.0 can be estimated, depending upon how close the ED of the frame is to 50 or 58. This simplification is summarized in Table 8-4.

EXAMPLE 8-2

Estimate the edge thickness of a −6.00 D lens that has a center thickness of 2.2 mm and is to be placed in a frame with an ED of 55 mm.

SOLUTION

A 55-mm ED is more than halfway between 50 and 58. This means that the constant chosen will be more than halfway between 0.7 and 1.0. (Halfway is 0.85.) The constant chosen will be 0.9. Edge thickness is

$$\text{Thickness} = K(D) + \text{edge thickness}$$
$$= 0.9\ (6.00) + 2.2$$
$$= 5.4 + 2.2$$
$$= 7.6 \text{ mm}$$

When a lens has prism as part of the prescription, for estimation purposes one-half of the prescribed prism amount is added to lens thickness. (The reason why prism changes the thickness of a lens will be explained more fully later in the chapter.)

Table 8-4 Easy-to-Remember Rule of Thumb for Estimating Lens Thickness

Frame Size	Multiplication Factor (K)
Very small	(less than 0.7)
Small (ED of *50*)	*0.7*
Moderate	(between 0.7 and 1.0)
Large (ED of *58*)	*1.0*
Very large	(greater than 1.0)

Thus, the rule of thumb can be expressed as

$$\text{Thickness} = K(D) + (\text{edge or center thickness})$$
$$+ \frac{P}{2}$$

where

$$K = \text{the constant}$$
$$D = \text{the power of the lens}$$
$$P = \text{the power of the prism}$$

EXAMPLE 8-3

Estimate the edge thickness of the lens in Example 8-2 if it is also to have 3 prism diopters of base-out prism.

SOLUTION

The thickness factor for prism is an estimated 0.5 mm for every diopter of prism. This increases the estimated thickness by 1.5 mm. Therefore the estimated edge thickness is

$$\text{Thickness} = 0.9\ (6.00) + 2.2 + 1.5$$
$$= 9.1 \text{ mm}$$

It should be understood that this method of estimation is intended to provide only a rough estimate and cannot be unerringly depended on.

Edge Thickness Using Sags: A More Accurate Method

Edge thickness may be found very accurately by using sag tables. Sag tables are normally used to find the center thickness for plus lenses. The use of sags for this purpose was described in detail in Chapter 7.

To find edge thickness using sags, the same formula is used for minus lenses as for plus lenses:

$$\text{CT} = s_1 - s_2 + \text{ET}$$

where CT is center thickness, s_1 is the sag of the first surface, s_2 is the sag of the second surface, and ET is the edge thickness. However, the formula may be easier to use if it is transposed so that it reads

$$\text{ET} = \text{CT} - s_1 + s_2$$

A very accurate estimate of edge thickness can also be obtained by looking up the sag of the back vertex power and simply adding the center thickness to it.

Other Center Thickness Corrections

Center thickness can be affected by a number of factors. As mentioned previously,* any change in center thickness can conceivably change the back vertex power of the lens. If the tool curve is not compensated appropriately, the lens will be off power when it is surfaced. In this section, some of the factors that can cause a change in thickness are discussed.

Rx Prism

How much Rx prism will affect the edge or center thickness of a lens depends on

1. the size (chord diameter) of the lens
2. whether the lens is plus or minus
3. the base direction of the prism

Surfacing charts generally include tables with titles such as *Thickness Differences for Sharp-Edged* Prisms. See, for instance, Appendix 4-4 or 4-5. These tables will be different for different lens materials and will list the thickness of the base of a prism for various lens diameters. The "thickness difference" amounts to how much thicker the base of the prism is than the apex. If the apex of the prism is assumed to be *knife-edged,* that is, having an edge thickness of zero at the apex, then the difference between prism base and apex thicknesses will be equal to the thickness of the base.

If the difference in thickness between the apex and base is known, the amount of prism present in a lens can be found using the formula

$$P = \frac{100g(n-1)}{d}$$

where

P = the amount of prism present in the lens
g = the difference in thickness between the apex and the base of the prism
n = the refractive index of the lens material, and
d = the distance between the apex and base of the prism

See Figure 8-1.

---

*See the section in Chapter 7 entitled "Additional Power Compensations for High-Plus Crown Glass Lenses," and also the appendix to Chapter 7.

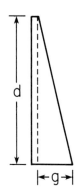

Figure 8-1 The thickness difference, g, is the difference between the thickness of the prism base and that of the prism apex. The formula is $g = \dfrac{dP}{100(n-1)}$.

From this formula we can find the amount of prism in either a plus or minus lens—not just a plano lens.

To find the amount of vertical prism in a lens, we can measure thickness at two points: one point above and one point below the lens center. These two points must be equidistant from the center. If the lens has no prism at the center, both measured points will have the same thickness. If there is a thickness difference, the amount of prism present can be calculated using the formula. See Figure 8-2.

EXAMPLE 8-4
Suppose a plus lens is 50 mm in diameter. We need to know if the lens has vertical prism, and if so, how much. A point at the top of the lens is measured as being 1.8 mm thick. A point at the bottom of the lens is measured

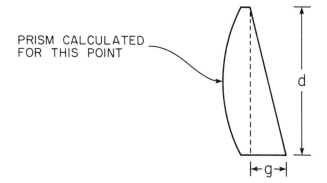

Figure 8-2 When a lens is measured with calipers and the thickness difference is used to compute prism, the amount of prism found is for a point on the lens that is halfway between the two measured thicknesses.

as being 2.8 mm thick. The lens is made from a material with an index of refraction of 1.5. Is there vertical prism present in the lens? If so, how much?

SOLUTION

Because the thickness of the two equidistant points above and below the center of the lens are of unequal thicknesses, there is vertical prism in the lens. The amount of vertical prism is found using the formula

$$P = \frac{100g(n-1)}{d}$$

In this case

g = thickness difference between top and bottom points, or 2.8 − 1.8 = 1.0 mm

n = the index of refraction of this lens, which is 1.5

d = the distance between the top and bottom points, or 50 mm.

$$P = \frac{100\,(1.0)\,(1.5-1)}{50}$$

$$= \frac{100\,(0.5)}{50}$$

$$= \frac{50}{50}$$

$$= 1 \text{ prism diopter}$$

Since the lens is thicker at the bottom, the prism is base down.

This method for finding prism by using thickness differences is often called *calipering for prism*. It gets this name because lens calipers are used to measure lens thickness. This method has been used extensively in the past to check for both wanted and unwanted vertical and horizontal prism during the generating and finishing processes. It is still used upon occasion. If a lens has an index of refraction of 1.5, measuring thickness difference at points 50 mm apart means that a 1-mm thickness difference equals 1 diopter of prism, and a 0.5-mm difference equals 0.5 diopter of prism. The ratio is 1 to 1, making calculations unnecessary. It is not necessary for the lens to be 50 mm in diameter. As the lens being processed is always larger than 50 mm, it is only necessary that each point being measured is 25 mm away from the center. Because crown glass (index 1.523) and CR-39 plastic (index 1.498) are so close to index 1.5, for small amounts of prism this direct measurement without calculation is close

enough. If the lens is blocked for surfacing using a 43-mm glass block, simply caliper the lens at a point 3½ mm away from the edge of the block. If the block is larger than 50 mm, caliper the lens further out from the center using tables or calculations. The caliper is not the only way to measure the amount of prism in a blocked lens. A prism gauge may be used. The prism gauge is discussed in Chapter 10 and is shown as Figure 10-26.

As was seen in Figure 8-2, if prism is present in a lens, the lens center thickness will change. Most of the time it is assumed that a lens will be thicker by ½ g when prism is present, *regardless* of how the prism base direction is oriented. This simplifies the problem, but it is not entirely true. The base direction determines just how much the Rx prism will change the center or edge thickness. How this works is summarized in Table 8-5 and explained in the following.

Plus Lenses

If a plus lens is decentered inward, then after the lens is in the frame the thicker portion of the lens edge will be found nasally and the thinner portion temporally. See Figure 8-3A. This means that if Rx prism is positioned *base inward*, the thickest portion of the lens will become even thicker. See Figure 8-3B. The thinner temporal portion, though, must retain the same minimum thickness. Therefore the center thickness of the lens must be increased by an amount equal to half the value listed in the "thickness differences for sharp-edged prisms" chart.

Table 8-5 Lens Thickness Changes for Rx Prism

Plus Lenses:

Base in: Increase center thickness by one-half of thickness difference.

Base out: Decrease center thickness by up to the full thickness difference, depending upon the amount of decentration present.

Vertical prism with small frame *B:* Do not change center thickness.

Vertical prism with large *B:* Increase center thickness by up to one-half the thickness difference.

Minus Lenses:

Base in: Increase center thickness slightly.

Base out: Increase center thickness slightly. Check to be sure that the semifinished lens blank will be thick enough.

(A)

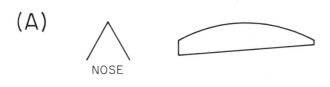

(B)

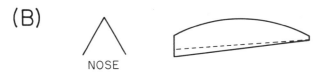

Figure 8-3 (A) Plus lenses that have been decentered inward to correspond to the wearer's PD are thicker nasally. (B) If base-in prism is prescribed for the plus-lens wearer, the lens will be thicker still.

This increase in center thickness is necessary because the middle of the prism will be located at what had been the optical center of the lens. With prescribed prism, this location now becomes the major reference point.

EXAMPLE 8-5

A plus-powered crown glass lens with a chord diameter of 54 mm is calculated to have a center thickness of 3.4 mm without Rx prism being considered. If the prescription also calls for 2.5 prism diopters of base-in prism, what will the center thickness be?

SOLUTION

To figure the thickness induced by the prism, we can either calculate directly using a formula, or we can use the "thickness differences for sharp-edged prisms" tables. The tables are easier to use, but in order to see how they work, we will begin from the formula,

$$P = \frac{100g(n-1)}{d}$$

and transpose it to

$$g = \frac{dP}{100(n-1)}$$

The thickness difference between the thick edge and the thin edge is thus

$$g = \frac{54 \times 2.5}{100(1.523 - 1)}$$

$$= 2.58 \text{ mm}$$

Looking up the thickness difference in the prism tables, we find the value to be 2.6 mm. This is the same answer as before, rounded from 2.58.

The thickness in the center of the prism will be half of this value, or $g/2$. Thus the increase in center thickness should be 1.3 mm.

Base-Out Rx Prism If the Rx prism is *base out*, the thicker portion of the prism is turned outward. This corresponds to the thinnest part of the plus lens. The net effect is a lens that is closer to the same thickness both nasally and temporally. If the lens has sufficient center and nasal edge thickness, it may be *thinned* by an amount up to the full thickness difference g. Therefore a plus lens with base-out Rx prism can be ground thinner than it would be without Rx prism. See Figure 8-4.

Base-Up or Base-Down Rx Prism Small amounts of base-up or base-down Rx prism will not affect the center thickness of the lens if the vertical (B) dimension of the frame is small compared to the A dimension. However, for prescriptions with larger amounts of prism or for frames with larger B dimensions, center thickness will be affected. The amount of center thickness increase may then ap-

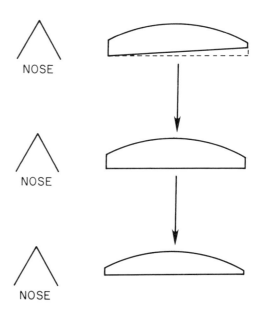

Figure 8-4 When base-out prism is prescribed for a plus-lens wearer, the lens will be thicker temporally. Now, because the thinnest edge is thicker, the whole lens may be thinned.

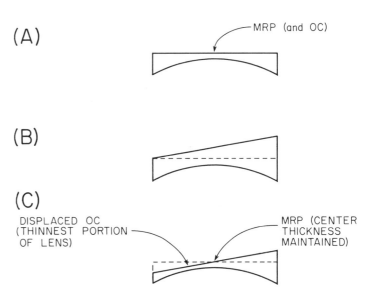

Figure 8-5 (A) A finished but unedged lens with no prism has the major reference point (MRP) and optical center (OC) at the same location. (B) Simply adding extra thickness to a minus lens by an amount equal to one-half the prism's apex–base thickness difference will cause the lens to be unnecessarily thick. (C) Thinning a minus lens with significant prism back to a normal minimum thickness at the MRP can cause the lens to be excessively thin at the now-displaced OC. The displaced OC will be at a location other than the MRP.

proach half the amount listed in the tables (i.e., one-half of *g*).

Minus Lenses

With minus lenses the amount of prism affects edge thickness. *Base-out* prism increases the thickness of the temporal edge by an amount equal to the base thickness of the prism. This is important in terms of how thick the blank must be, but it does not affect the choice of tool curves. Blank thickness will not have to be increased with *base-in* prism unless the amount of prescribed prism is especially large in comparison to the refractive power of the lens.

Center thickness should be increased somewhat when *base-out* or *base-in* Rx prism is ground for minus lenses. If the center thickness is left at the minimum accepted value,* the thinnest portion moves from the major reference point to the location of the displaced optical center, as shown in Figure 8-5. If the center thickness is not increased, the minimum thickness could drop below acceptable

limits. Center thickness must be increased somewhat, but not the full amount of the *g* value.

Lens (Chord) Diameter

If the main chart does not take lens diameter into account, there should be a separate table for plus-lens center thicknesses. This table will give a different center thickness value for each lens diameter. The amount by which this value is greater or less than the standard value listed in the main chart should be noted. This difference will be used later to help in determining how much to modify the tool curve.

Safety Lens Requirements

Prescription lenses to be used for safety eyewear must have a minimum thickness of 3.0 mm, unless they are above +3.00 D. The edge thicknesses of lenses above +3.00 D may be reduced to a minimum of 2.5 mm. This means that the center thicknesses of both plus and minus lenses must be increased. For minus lenses this will not necessitate a change in the back tool curve chosen, but for plus lenses it may, especially when other factors discussed in this section are considered.

Edge Grooving

When lenses must be mounted in a frame that holds them in place by means of a nylon cord, the lens

---

*Minimum accepted values for lens center thicknesses depend upon the material being used and impact resistance standards required by the country. In the United States, current practice places minimum center thickness as follows:

2.2 mm for glass
2.0 to 2.2 mm for CR-39 plastic
1.0 mm for polycarbonate
1.5 mm for most polyurethane lenses
2.4 mm for low-powered and 2.0 for high-minus-powered "Transitions" photochromic plastic lenses

edges must be grooved to accept the cord. If the edges are too thin, there will not be enough room on the edge for grooving.

Although preference may vary slightly from one laboratory to another, an edge thickness of 2.3 mm is usually the minimum size required for grooving. If a chart for an edge thickness other than 2.3 mm was used, the difference must be allowed for. For example, suppose that the main chart gives center thickness values based on a plus lens edge thickness with a value of 1.8 mm. The extra thickness required for edge grooving is

$$2.3 \text{ mm} - 1.8 \text{ mm} = 0.5 \text{ mm}$$

Therefore the lens must be ground 0.5 mm thicker than indicated.

Multifocal Segments

Multifocals can be produced as

1. one-piece multifocals, which means that one piece of lens material is used for both distance and near portions;
2. fused multifocals, which are constructed by fusing a minilens of a higher-index material into the distance carrier lens, or
3. cement segment bifocals, which are made by cementing a small segment lens onto the carrier lens. (Cement segs are seldom used at the present time.)

With most types of one-piece multifocals, the segment sticks out from the front of the lens. Plastic flat-top bifocals are an example of this style of one-piece lens. With these types of lenses no extra thickness allowance is necessary. The edge and center thicknesses of the lens are unaffected.

Franklin-Style Segments

One style of lens achieves its segment power increase by having the lens segment cut *into* the body of the distance carrier lens. The Executive or Franklin-style lens is constructed as if two lenses, a distance and a near, were cut in two and joined together. These "two lenses" have the same center thicknesses and the same back curves. They differ only in their front curves. When the centers of the two front curves are aligned and the upper and lower lens halves "glued" together, the lower lens

recesses farther back than the distance lens because of its steeper front curvature.

Now, for equal-diameter lenses, a higher-powered plus lens will have a greater center thickness than a lower-powered plus lens. Because of this the thickness of the Franklin-style lens must be based on the near (reading) lens power rather than the distance lens power. Therefore, in order to achieve sufficient overall edge thickness, the center thickness of the lens must be increased. The amount of this increase is equal to the difference between what is called for in the chart for the distance lens and what would be used for a lens with a dioptric strength equal to the near power.*

It is fortunate that in many instances separate charts are available specifically for the Franklin-style lens, making these extra steps unnecessary.

There is a technique which will allow plus-powered Franklin-style lenses to be ground noticeably thinner than would otherwise be possible. This technique is called *vertical yoked prism* and is done by using equal amounts of base-down prism on both right and left lenses. Base-down prism will thin a plus-powered Franklin-style lens using the same principle described in the previous section on thinning plus lenses with base-out prism. Vertical yoked prism is used extensively for progressive addition lenses and will be described in more detail in Chapter 15. It is illustrated in Figure 15-8. Yoked prism works well and is to be recommended for producing a thinner, more attractive plus-powered Franklin-style lens.

Fused-Seg Thicknesses

Flat-top glass bifocals are made by fusing a segment into the distance lens. When multifocals are created by fusing a minilens into the distance lens, a bed for this minilens must first be scooped out of the distance-powered lens. After fusing is complete, the front surface is spherical and smooth. The near segment (minilens) is buried in the distance lens. In most cases the "grave" (called the *countersink curve*) created for the segment "burial" is shallow enough to remain undisturbed when the back of the lens is surfaced. It must be remembered, though, that if the lens is ground thin enough, the segment will be cut into from the back. See Figure 8-6.

The depth of the segment's countersink curve is

---

*Near power = distance power + near add.

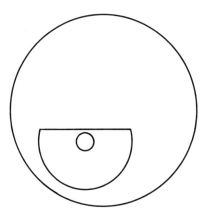

Figure 8-6 Grinding a fused segment lens too thin can mean grinding all the way through to the seg from the back. As the seg is ground away, a circle begins to show up, as shown in the figure.

governed by two factors, the power of the add, and the size of the segment. The segment is a lens in its own right. As with any other lens, the higher the add power, the thicker the seg will be. It should also be evident that a wider fused segment will be a deeper (thicker) segment.

With high-plus lenses, the lens seldom becomes thin enough to cause the seg to be exhumed from the back; but this may be a distinct possibility with low-plus and all minus lenses. Tables listing the seg thicknesses of larger fused-segment lenses such as the flat-top 35 are necessary in order to know how much thickness allowance should be made. Appendix 4-3 gives an example of such a table.

Unless the add power is exceptionally high, the back tool curve will seldom require modification solely on the basis of a fused-segment thickness allowance.

Cover Plates

A specific thickness allowance must be made when surfacing lenses having a cover plate over the front surface of the lens. One example of a lens with a cover plate is a Polaroid lens. A Polaroid lens may require 1.4 mm of extra thickness to be added to the seg thickness to determine minimum center thickness. In most cases special charts are used, or a table is provided that will allow the correct thickness to be chosen. Surfacing the lenses at other than the specified thickness, or failing to allow for in-

creased thickness, may cause the segment or the cover plate to be penetrated during processing.

Summary of Thickness Correction Factors

Once all factors have been taken into consideration, the necessary changes in thickness should be evaluated to see which are additive. For example, two plus-lens thickness increases, such as a large eyesize and a safety Rx, must be added together. If, though, a lens should be increased in thickness because of a large, fused seg and a safety Rx, then adding the two thicknesses is not necessary. It is only necessary to choose the larger of the two increases; the smaller increase is then taken care of automatically.

Tool Curve Compensation

When the final thickness change is known, the back tool curve must be modified so that the correct power will result. This may be done by using a separate chart and finding the amount of compensation. Such a compensation table is shown in Appendix 4-2 and was referred to in Chapter 7. Each listing in the chart is for a lens of a specific refractive index. The given amount of compensation is either added to or subtracted from the tool curve that was originally given in the main chart, depending on whether the lens is to become thicker or thinner.

Other charts, such as the one shown in Table 8-1, list several lens sizes and thicknesses for each lens power in the main chart itself. If this is the case, the final lens thickness may be found for that power. The back tool curve listed with this thickness is used to grind the lens. This is true even if the lens diameter under which the thickness is listed is different than the lens diameter actually being used.

EXAMPLE 8-6

Suppose that a CR-39 plastic lens having a plus power of +5.00 D on an 8.25 base curve is calculated to have a center thickness of 5.4 mm. However, because the lens is to be edge-grooved and string-mounted, the thickness must be increased by 2 mm. If the original tool curve was calculated for −3.28 D, how would the tool curve have to be modified to allow for the increased lens thickness?

SOLUTION

Using Appendix 4-2, we find that the change in center thickness for an 8 Base 1.498 index lens should be multiplied by 0.047. Since the change in thickness is 2 mm,

Base curve change = 0.047 × 2 = 0.094 D

Because the lens is being made thicker, the tool curve must be made more minus to compensate. Therefore,

New tool curve = −3.28 − 0.094 = −3.374

The tool curve must be modified to a −3.37 D to allow for a 2-mm increase in thickness.

Finding the Cross Curve from the Cylinder Value

Some charts give the cross curve in the main body of the chart. Others require that the cross curve be looked up in another table. To find the cross curve when it is not given in the body of the chart, find the chart that gives tool curves for minus cylinders. See, for example, Table 8-6. Table 8-6 gives a value for each minus cylinder and shows the corresponding power that must be added to the base curve to give the cross curve. The cross curve is then added to the base curve. There are different tables for lenses of different refractive indexes.

Crown-glass lens cylinder values need only be compensated for extremely high cylinder powers. However, with CR-39 plastic or high-index lenses, cylinder-power compensation is required most of the time.

EXAMPLE 8-7

Suppose a lens prescription has a power of

+2.75 − 1.75 × 17

The lens material is to be CR-39 plastic (index 1.498). The base curve chosen is +8.25 D, and the diameter to use in calculating the thickness is 58 mm. Using Table 8-1, what tool should be used to grind the lens?

SOLUTION

The spherical portion of the tool, from Table 8-1, is 5.62. Looking up the desired 1.75 D cylinder in Table 8-6, we find that the additional cross curve required is 1.86. The cross curve is thus

Cross curve = 5.62 + 1.86 = 7.48 D

Table 8-6 Tool Curves for Minus Cylinders (1.498 Index CR39)

Desired Cylinder Power	Additional Cross Curve Required
0.12	0.13
0.25	0.26
0.37	0.40
0.50	0.53
0.62	0.66
0.75	0.80
0.87	0.93
1.00	1.07
1.25	1.33
1.50	1.60
1.75	1.86
2.00	2.13
2.25	2.39
2.50	2.66
2.75	2.93
3.00	3.19
3.25	3.46
3.50	3.72
3.75	3.99
4.00	4.25
4.25	4.52
4.50	4.78
4.75	5.05
5.00	5.32
5.25	5.58
5.50	5.85
5.75	6.11
6.00	6.38
6.25	6.65
6.50	6.91
6.75	7.18
7.00	7.44
7.25	7.71
7.50	7.98
7.75	8.24
8.00	8.51

Source: From *Vision-Ease Laboratory Processing Data,* Vision-Ease Corporation, St. Cloud, Minn., revised 5/18/88, p. 50, used by permission.

Rounded to the nearest one-eighth diopter, the cross curve is 7.50 D. The tool that should be used is thus 5.62/7.50.

Rounding the Tool Curves

We can now determine theoretical values for both base and cross curves. However, lap tools come only in certain dioptric increments, so the theoretical values must be rounded to the nearest one-eighth diopter. If the curve is halfway between two dioptric sizes, it is usually rounded to produce a steeper back curve, making the lens somewhat more minus. However, care must be taken in rounding the cross curve so that it is rounded in the same direction as the base curve except when rounding increments less than approximately 0.025 D. If the base and cross curves are rounded in opposing directions, a noticeable cylinder-power error may result.

Questions and Problems

1. **a.** What is the rule of thumb for estimating center thickness for plus lenses (or edge thickness for minus lenses) when no Rx prism is present?

    b. According to this rule of thumb, how much extra thickness must be allowed for when Rx prism is present?

2. How thick might the thickest edge of the following lens be, using the rule of thumb for estimating?

    -6.50 sphere, glass or CR-39 plastic lens
    2.0 Base-Out prism
    Frame ED = 52 mm
    center thickness = 2.2 mm

3. **a.** Use the rule of thumb to estimate the center thickness of a lens with the following characteristics:

    $+5.00$ D sphere
    Frame ED = 58 mm
    Edge thickness = 2.0 mm

    b. Now estimate the center thickness of this same lens, but include 4 prism diopters of base-in Rx prism.

4. A dispenser working in the same establishment has just finished helping someone choose a frame. He is concerned about how thick the lenses are going to be, so he asks you to estimate the thickness. Looking at the prescription form, you see that the Rx is

    R: $+5.00$ -1.00×90 1.00 BI prism
    L: $+5.00$ -1.00×90 1.00 BI prism

    The CR-39 plastic lenses are going into a frame with an ED of 56 mm. Edge thickness will be 1.8 mm. How thick do you estimate the lenses will be?

5. In calipering a crown-glass lens along the 180-degree meridian during surfacing, it is found that the lens is 0.3 mm thicker at a point 30 mm temporal to the center of the block than it is at a point 30 mm nasal to the center of the block. How much prism in what base direction is present at the center of the block? (Give the prism direction in degrees.)

6. A round lens is 5.0 mm thick in the center and 3.0 mm thick on the edges. It has a refractive index of 1.498. If it is 60 mm round and is to be reground with 2 diopters of prism at the center of the lens, how much thicker will the lens edge be toward the base of the prism axis meridian than at the apex?

7. Using a "thickness difference for sharp-edged prisms" chart, tell how much thickness difference there is along the prism axis of a plastic lens of index 1.498 blocked on a block measuring 62 mm in diameter. Assume that the lens was generated using a 3.25 prism ring. Assume also that the lens is calipered as close to the block as possible.

8. A lens is calipered during the surfacing process in order to determine the amount of horizontal prism present. Both points at which measurements are taken on the 1.7 index, -9.00 D lens are 27 mm from the center of the block. (Traditional off-center blocking is used.) If the nasal point on the lens calipers out as 9.7 mm and the temporal point as 8.3 mm, how much prism is present and in what base direction?

9. Use the rule of thumb to estimate the edge thickness expected for a -8 CR-39 plastic lens that is to be placed in a frame with an ED of 50 mm. The center thickness of the lens will be 2.2 mm. Choose your answer from among the following:
    a. 7.8 mm.
    b. 8.2 mm.
    c. 10.3 mm.
    d. 11.7 mm.
    e. None of the above is a reasonable estimate.

10. A prescription is as follows:

    R: -8.00 sphere
    L: -8.00 sphere
    Lens refractive index = 1.498
    A = 48 mm
    DBL = 18 mm
    ED = 48 mm
    PD = 64 mm

Rx prism = 4 BO for the right eye and 4 BO for the left eye

These lenses will change in edge thickness because of the Rx prism. Where will the increased (decreased) thickness be? How much of an increase (or decrease) in edge thickness will occur because of the Rx prism? The formula for sharp-edged prism calculation is

$$P = \frac{100g(n - 1)}{d}$$

11. A prescription is as follows:

> R: +8.00 sphere
> L: +8.00 sphere
> Lens refractive index = 1.498
> A = 48 mm
> DBL = 18 mm
> ED = 48 mm
> PD = 64 mm
> Rx prism = 2 BO for the right eye and 2 BO for the left eye

These lenses will change in thickness because of the Rx prism. Where will the increased (decreased) thickness be? How much of an increase (or decrease) in thickness will occur because of the Rx prism? The formula for sharp-edged prism calculation is

$$P = \frac{100g(n - 1)}{d}$$

12. What is the minimum edge thickness required for high-plus lenses that are to be used for safety eyewear?
    a. 1.8 mm
    b. 2.2 mm
    c. 2.5 mm
    d. 3.0 mm
    e. 3.2 mm

13. A prescription has a power of

> +2.50 sphere
> +2.50 sphere
>   +2.00 add

For Franklin-style bifocals, center thickness is calculated using a power of
    a. +2.00
    b. +2.50
    c. +4.50

14. Which of the following lenses would be thicker?
    a. A plastic minus lens with a flat-top 35 segment in a high-add power.
    b. A plastic minus lens with a high-add flat-top 25 segment.
    c. Both are the same thickness.

15. Which of the following lenses would be thicker?
    a. A glass minus lens with a high-add flat-top 35 segment.
    b. A glass minus lens with a high-add flat-top 25 segment.
    c. Both are the same thickness.

16. Which of the following lenses would be thicker?
    a. A high-plus glass lens with a +2.00-add flat-top 28 segment.
    b. A high-plus glass lens with a +2.00-add flat-top 25 segment.
    c. Both are the same thickness.

17. A lens with a plus front surface is to be ground thicker than is listed in the lens surfacing chart. In order for the power to come out correctly, if a power compensation is necessary the back tool curves must be
    a. steepened compared to the value listed in the chart
    b. flattened compared to the value listed in the chart

18. Assume that your lap tools are calibrated for a reference index of refraction of 1.53. When the refractive index is different than 1.53, compensating the cross curve may be necessary so that the cylinder power will come out correctly. When compensating for a lens of index 1.701, the difference between the base curve and cross curve would be
    a. greater than the prescribed value of the cylinder
    b. less than the prescribed value of the cylinder
    c. the same as the prescribed value of the cylinder

9

Blocking and Cribbing

Lens Blocking

A number of different methods have been used to hold a lens in place during the surfacing process. The method most commonly used at present makes use of a low-melting-temperature alloy. Some older methods that have been used in the past may still be used for specialized purposes.

In blocking using low-melting-point alloys, bismuth, tin, lead, cadmium, indium, and antimony are combined to make an alloy. When they are combined correctly, the alloy melts at a temperature considerably lower than any one of its component elements would melt by itself. Such an alloy can be heated to a temperature that is high enough to cause it to melt, but not so high as to endanger laboratory personnel. The alloy will neither cause a plastic lens to melt nor a glass lens to crack. For example, one alloy that melts at 117 degrees is made from the following combination of metals[1]:

45% bismuth
23% lead
8% tin
5% cadmium
19% indium

Although different alloys are used for glass and plastic lenses, each with its own melting point, mixing a 158-degree low-melting-point alloy that is appropriate for glass lenses with a 117-degree alloy normally used for plastic will not necessarily yield an alloy with a melting point halfway between. The alloys should not be mixed. If there is a possibility of 158- and 117-degree alloys being accidentally mixed, consideration should be given to using 117-degree alloy for both plastic and glass lenses. The 117-degree alloy will work for either plastic or glass lenses, but the 158-degree alloy will only work for glass. The primary advantage to using 158-degree alloy is that it costs less than the 117-degree alloy.

Low-melting-point alloys can be molded onto a lens in the shape of a lens block, or they can be used as part of the "adhesive" between a lens block and the lens.

Precoating or Taping Lenses for Surfacing

Reasons for using tape or a lens coating when surfacing lenses include the following:

1. To keep the lenses from being scratched. During the surfacing process, the front of the lens is already finished to the required curvature and optical polish. If the surface is not shielded in some manner, it will become scratched.
2. To serve as a heat shield. When plastic lenses are blocked, heat from the alloy can cause the lens surface to indent or the lens to warp. This results in an uneven power, or waviness, which is unacceptable.
3. To achieve better alloy adherence. Low-melting-point alloys serve as excellent supports for lenses during surfacing because they conform well to the curve of the lens surface. Unfortunately, these alloys do not adhere directly to the lens. On the other hand, they do stick to the lens coating and blocking tape well, so that the lens holds to the block and does not drop off during processing.

Coating of Lenses

Lens coatings, available in brush-on and spray applications, may be obtained from optical supply houses. The coating is applied to the convex side of the lens. When the coating is brushed on, a plastic dispenser bottle with a brush in the lid is commonly used. See Figure 9-1. This type of dispenser slows evaporation of the coating. Spray coatings are more convenient, but they should be used only in well-ventilated areas.

Any coating should be applied in an area well away from the mist created by lens generators during the grinding process. Drying of lenses can be a problem and is slowed by high humidity. A heat lamp may be used to hasten the drying process.

Coatings are available as either a washable, water-soluble type, or as a peelable form that can be stripped from the lens after the block has been removed. See Figure 9-2. Most laboratories use coatings only on lenses that have large ledges on their front surface. An example is the Franklin-style lens. Lenses with ledges leave air pockets under the surfacing tape and reduce an alloy's holding power. To obtain maximum holding and heat-absorbing power, multiple applications are sometimes used. Brush-on or spray coatings should not be used on polycarbonate lenses.

Surface Taping of Lenses

The cleanest and most common method for protecting lens surfaces and holding the block securely is the use of a surface tape. This tape was first developed by the 3M Company. It is applied by placing the lens in a small chamber (Figure 9-3A), stretching tape over the chamber (Figure 9-3B), and applying a partial vacuum. The lens moves up to the tape and the tape is pulled down over the lens surface (Figure 9-3C). A curved knife blade on a

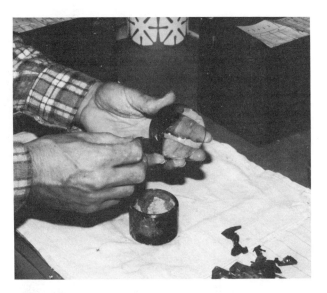

Figure 9-2 Some coatings are peelable and can be stripped off like removed tape after the block has been removed.

handle is used to cut around the lens (Figure 9-3D), removing the excess tape. A hot-tipped instrument,* shown in Figure 9-4, may be used to "cut" the excess tape from the lens, if desired.

Ledges on a lens surface, such as are found on plastic flat-top bifocals, may prevent the tape from sticking to the entire surface of the lens. After the lens has been taped, any such areas should be smoothed out by hand. Failure to get the bubbles out from under the tape is reported to cause optical distortion (waviness) at the position of the bubble. This is assumed to be caused by air superheated in the bubble during alloy blocking. See Figure 9-5. (Note that only the area immediately above the ledge should be pressed against the lens with the thumbnail. Trying to smooth out the whole taped surface with the hand may transfer oil and moisture from the hands to the tape surface and decrease alloy adherence.)

Sometimes it is necessary to resurface an already surfaced lens in order to correct an error. Because the lens is considerably thinner, heat buildup during blocking can become a problem. To help reduce this, it is advisable to use a double layer of surface tape.

Different types of tapes are available, depending on the lens material being used.

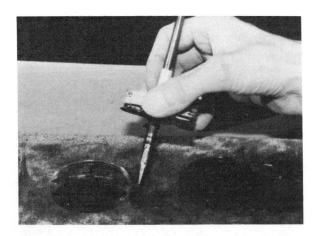

Figure 9-1 Coatings can be applied using a plastic dispenser with a brush in the cap.

---

*The Hot Knife, Practical Systems, Inc., Tarpin Springs, Fla.

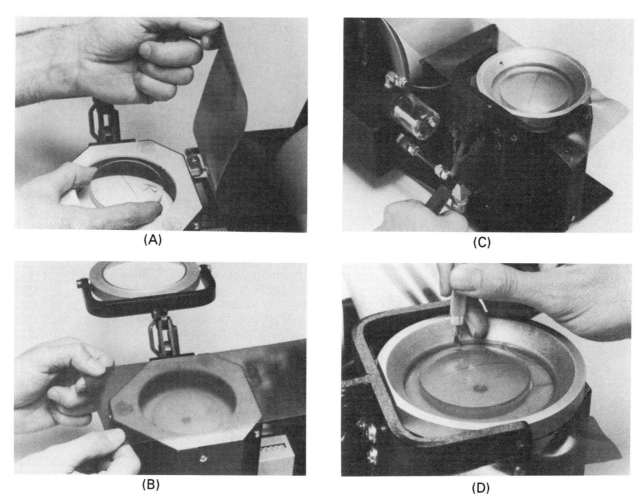

Figure 9-3 Surface taping a lens. (A) The lens is placed in the applicator. (B) Tape is unrolled. (C) Tape is applied to the lens. (D) Trimming and removal. (Photos courtesy of Armorlite, Inc.)

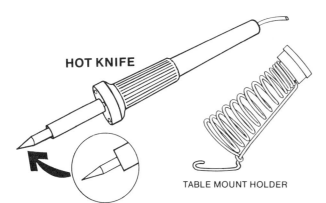

Figure 9-4 The "hot knife" is electrically heated and penetrates the lens tape, "cutting" the tape without snagging. (Courtesy Practical Systems, Inc., Tarpon Springs, Fla.)

Lens Blocks

Glass Lens Blocks

Blocks used for glass lenses ("glass blocks"*) are generally 43 mm in diameter. See Figure 9-6. They do not need to be large, since their purpose is purely to hold the lens during generating.

Plastic Lens Blocks

Blocks used for plastic lenses ("plastic lens blocks") must not only hold the lens in place, they must also

---

*It should be understood that "glass blocks" are really made from steel, not glass. They are normally used for blocking glass lenses. Neither are "plastic lens blocks" made from plastic. Such blocks are normally made from aluminum.

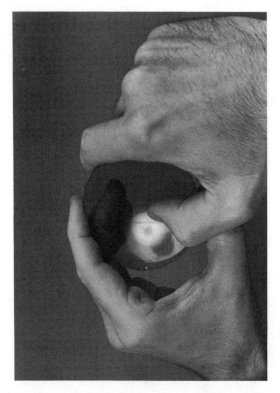

Figure 9-5 For best results on lenses that have ledges on the surface, the tape should be smoothed at the junctures to assure optimum adherence.

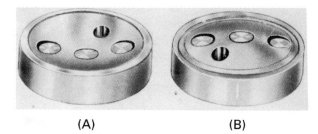

(A)   (B)

Figure 9-6 The standard Coburn block is 43 mm in diameter. The concave (CC) block as shown in (A) is used to hold the front surface of the lens while the back surface is being worked. If the front surface of the lens is to be generated, fined, and polished, a convex (CX) block as shown in (B) is used. Exceptionally strong concave back surfaces will require a thicker convex block when the front surface is worked. A thick block is needed because the normal thin block "disappears" into the steep concave surface and cannot be easily grasped by the generator chuck. (Photo courtesy of Coburn Optical Industries, Muskogee, Okla.)

keep it from flexing (bending) during generating, fining, and polishing. For that reason, plastic lens blocks are considerably larger than glass blocks. See Figure 9-7.

Since blocks for plastic lenses should be made as large as possible for each grinding situation, they are available in a variety of sizes ranging from approximately 55 to 68 mm. Generally, the largest block that can be used on a given semifinished lens blank is chosen. (When a lens must be shock deblocked, the block must be 7 mm smaller than the lens block.) For high-plus lenses, smaller plastic lens blocks must be used. As discussed in Chapter 7, if large blocks were used for a high-plus lens being ground to minimum thickness, the block itself may be in danger of being ground.

Plastic lens blocks are made in different curves so that the contact area of the block will correspond to the front base curve of the plastic lens. Generally, the higher the base curve, the smaller the block will be.

Glass Blocks Used for Plastic Lenses

It is possible to use blocks that are normally used for glass to block lenses made from plastic. Yet it is necessary to use these blocks in conjunction with a *plastic lens blocking ring,* as shown in Figure 9-8, so that a molded support ring of alloy material reinforces the lens. Plastic lens blocking rings come in a variety of sizes and base curves. When using

Figure 9-7 Larger blocks for plastic lenses give support for thin edges and prevent waviness in the optics. Blocks come with a variety of inside curves, which are made to approximate the base curve of the lens. (Photo courtesy of Coburn Optical Industries, Muskogee, Okla.)

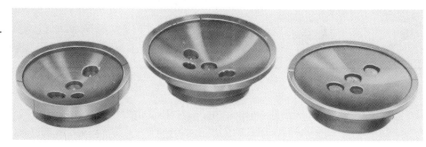

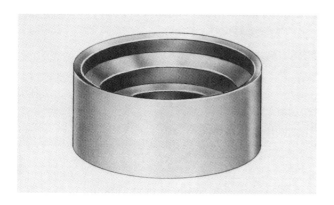

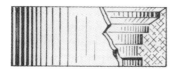

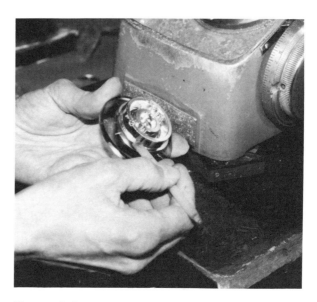

Figure 9-8 A plastic lens blocking ring allows glass blocks to be used with plastic lenses. It molds a lip around the outside of the glass block to give additional support at the periphery of the lens. (Photo courtesy of Coburn Optical Industries, Muskogee, Okla.)

Figure 9-9 A block made entirely from alloy should be free from any small projections of unwanted alloy. Removing these will help avoid unwanted prism in the lens during the generating process.

glass blocks, the molten alloy covers a large area of the lens. Because of the negative effect of heat on a plastic lens, this type of blocking requires close temperature control so that the alloy does not get too hot.

When a plastic lens blocking ring is used in the generating process, it is not necessary to use a generator ring with the block. Ordinarily, when using 43-mm glass blocks, an additional "generator ring" is required while generating the lens.

Blocks Made Entirely from Alloy

Using blocks made completely from alloy solves the problem of both block storage and block chilling. See Figure 9-9. When using blocks made entirely from alloy, the laboratory needs to be especially careful to keep the alloy temperature as close to the melting point as possible in order to avoid lens problems caused by heat from the alloy.

The Blocker

Blockers that use metal alloy either inject molten alloy between the semifinished lens and the block,

or mold a block fully and completely from the alloy material. Both types have a melting pot that is thermostatically regulated, and a feeding tube. The feeding tube is also heated so that the alloy does not "freeze" before getting to the block.

For plastic lenses the idea is to keep the alloy temperature just above its melting point until it fills in the area between the lens and lens block. For example, the 117-degree alloy used for plastic, polycarbonate and polyurethane lenses should be kept at 125 degrees, or even lower if possible.[2] Photochromic plastic lenses require that the alloy temperature be between 120–122 degrees. For glass lenses the alloy temperature may be maintained at 165 to 170 degrees.[3]

Once on the lens, the alloy should be cooled as rapidly as possible so that plastic lenses will not form indentations on the surface of the lens. In addition, time is saved because the block can be removed from the blocker without waiting for the alloy to harden. Furthermore, the lens does not have to cool as long before being generated.

There are two ways to harden the alloy quickly. The first is to circulate cold running water or a coolant through a *water ring*, which fits around the lens block. See Figure 9-10. This causes the lens block and alloy to chill, "freezing" the alloy. The

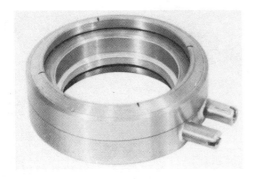

Figure 9-10 A water ring fits on the surface blocker, encircling the block. Small plastic in- and out-flow tubes are attached to the spouts on the water ring. When cooled water passes through the water ring, heat is drawn off from the block, cooling both block and alloy. Different sized rings are available for different sized blocks. An Executive water ring, intended for use with Franklin-style (Executive) lenses, is also available. (Photo courtesy of Coburn Optical Industries, Muskogee, Okla.)

second method is to chill the blocks before they are placed on the blocker.

One of the most straightforward ways to chill lens blocks is to keep them in a refrigerator. The blocks are removed from the refrigerator just before needed, and the lens is blocked before they have a chance to cool. One ingenious laboratory used a restaurant salad bar unit to chill blocks! The blocks could be kept out in the open, yet they remain cool and readily accessible. For quick cooling, blocks can be placed on ice or in ice water. Unfortunately, all of these methods have varying degrees of inconvenience. This inconvenience can be avoided by using a chiller designed especially for chilling blocks and molds to the required temperature—usually 40 degrees. The operator can then select the correct block from any one of several compartments in the chiller.

Blockers that mold the entire block from alloy often have the advantage of being able to block for prism directly. This eliminates the need for prism rings, which must be used in conjunction with the block at the time the lens is generated. To mold prism directly in the block, the correct amount of prism is set. This tips the lens to the correct angle. Next the prism axis is turned into place. Last, the alloy is allowed to flow into the block mold.

It is helpful to place the blocker in a large, shallow cake pan. This helps save on alloy and insulates the blocker for better temperature control.[3]

Blocking the Lenses

Blocking Single-Vision Lenses

When a lens is blocked, there are two points of reference. The first reference point is where the center of the block will be positioned. When marked, the center of the axis cross (——) must be positioned in the center of the block. This is true regardless of whether the lens is to be blocked "on center" or "off center." Second, the cylinder *axis* is positioned horizontally, corresponding to the scored lines on the block. See Figure 9-11. Some blocks use the three replaceable centers to line up the cylinder axis. See Figure 9-12. Care must be taken to be certain that the eye is lined up directly in front of the lens so that a parallax error is not introduced by being off to one side. Some blockers have a sighting ring to help avoid this problem.

With the lens held in place with the lens holding arm or the fingers, the alloy release lever is pulled and the alloy is allowed to flow steadily (not too quickly) into the space between the block and the lens. After the space between the lens and the block is filled with alloy, the lever should be held lightly in place until the alloy just begins to harden. If this is not done, the alloy will have a tendency to flow back out of the hole in the block and harden there.

Note: With plastic lenses, only enough pressure should be applied to the lens to keep the lens in

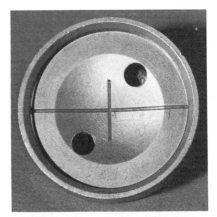

Figure 9-11 The scored lines on this disposable 43-mm glass block are clearly visible. The marked cylinder axis on the lens should overlap the horizontal line when correctly positioned. Disposable blocks do not have replaceable centers. Once the centers become worn, the block is discarded.

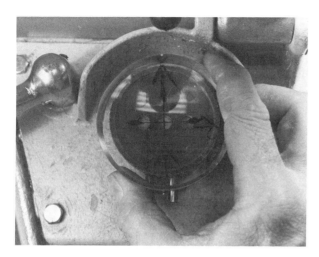

Figure 9-12 When surface blocking a lens, the cylinder axis must always be oriented as marked on the block. This will usually be along the horizontal meridian. When a prism axis is also marked on the lens, care should be taken to avoid blocking on the prism axis.

place. Applying too much pressure will bend the lens blank, causing it to steepen. The alloy will then flow in, harden, and keep the lens in an artificially steepened position. The lens is "bent" while the back curves are being ground. Only when the lens is taken off the block does it reflatten. This causes the lens to be off in power. Just how far it is off varies from lens to lens, but the amounts are significant and unacceptable.

In order to avoid potential problems, many laboratories simply remove the hold-down arm from the blocker. (Not all blockers have hold-down arms.) The lens is then held lightly in place with three fingers.

Blocking Multifocal Lenses

Problems that may occur in blocking multifocal lenses vary, depending on the type of multifocal lens being used. Most problems encountered are caused by a surface ledge or a nonspherical surface.

Fused-Glass Multifocals

Fused-glass multifocals are smooth on the front surface, making them exactly the same as single-vision lenses with regard to how they are blocked. No special considerations are necessary. They are simply blocked along the cylinder axis. It does not matter if the segment ends up at the top, bottom,

left, or right on the blocker, so long as the cylinder has been positioned correctly.

One-Piece Multifocals

One piece bi- or trifocal lenses are made with one kind of lens material only. Because the glass or plastic is of the same index of refraction throughout the lens, the extra power needed in the bifocal portion must be obtained through a change in lens curvature. This means that the bifocal or trifocal portion of the lens is raised and can be felt with the fingers. When the lens is being blocked, this ledge can produce problems.

With plastic lenses, if this bifocal area is positioned so that it rests on the rim of the plastic lens block, the lens will be tilted. This tilting causes unwanted prism to be ground into the lens during processing. Therefore the plastic lens block must be large enough to avoid encountering the segment.

With glass lenses, the lens rests against a *fiber ring,** which fits around the glass block and is used in the generating process. The fiber ring levels the lens, assuring that no unwanted prism will be ground in. Large, round, one-piece "Ultex" segments will touch this ring and tip the lens, inducing prism. Thus, a special *Ultex ring* must be used for this lens. An Ultex ring has a section cut out of the rim where the segment is placed.

Executive (Franklin-Style) Multifocals

Plastic Executives   The Franklin-style bifocal is also a one-piece lens. The difference between this lens and other one-piece bifocals is that the segment is over the entire lower half of the lens and is recessed. See Figure 9-13. If a plastic Franklin-style bifocal is placed on a plastic lens block with its bifocal segment downward, the alloy will simply run out the bottom between the lens and the block. Thus these lenses must be positioned for blocking with their lower segment area up. Furthermore, the operator must keep the lens in place on the blocker by placing fingers on the distance portion of the lens. Only the distance portion of the Franklin-style bifocal is against the block, *not* the segment area. See Figure 9-14. Putting any pressure on the segment area will cause the lens to tilt. As in other cases discussed previously, any tilt at all will result in unwanted prism in the finished lens.

---

*Fiber rings are also referred to as *generator rings.*

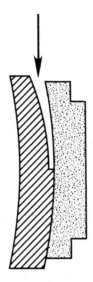

Figure 9-13 The Franklin-style lens has a front surface with two different radii. When a block is attached to the front surface, the block must be positioned solidly against the distance portion of the lens. If a Franklin-style lens is blocked right side up, alloy will flow out the bottom at the location of the arrow. The lens must be turned upside down, as shown in the drawing.

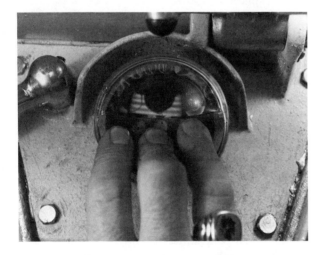

Figure 9-14 For blocking, the Franklin-style lens is turned so that the segment is up. Therefore the operator holds the lens in place by pressing against the distance portion, which is at the bottom.

Alloy should be released slowly and allowed to begin hardening before completely filling the space. This helps to keep it from being too fluid and runny when it reaches the open segment area of the lens and thus it is not as likely to flow out from between

the lens segment and the block, then down onto the blocker and the table.

Glass Executives Because the lower half of the Executive lens is recessed, it is left unsupported in the generating process. The fiber ring that is placed over the lens block and contacts the lens comes into contact only with the upper half of the lens. In order to support the lens fully, alloy must be used to bear up the lens in much the same manner as would be done when using 43-mm blocks on plastic lenses. To this end, an *Executive water ring* is used. Alloy is cast into the form of a fiber ring, which then braces the lens equally in both the upper and lower portions.

Progressive-Addition Lenses

Progressive-addition lenses come in two basic designs. In the first type the upper half of the lens front surface is perfectly spherical, like an Executive lens. The lower half is aspheric (nonspherical) and increases gradually in power. See Figure 9-15A. The second type of progressive-addition lens is somewhat spherical even on the upper portion of the lens. See Figure 9-15B.

Progressive-Addition Lenses with Spherical Upper Halves Progressive-addition lenses with spherical upper halves are blocked in the same manner as Executive lenses. They are positioned on the lens blocker with their segment area up. The lens is held in place by gently pressing the fingers against the distance portion of the lens. (This portion will be turned toward the bottom during blocking.)

Progressive-Addition Lenses with Aspheric Upper Halves The Varilux progressive-addition lens is made with the entire front surface somewhat aspheric. Therefore there is no way that the lens can rest evenly against the outer portion of the lens block without tilting. Tilting of the Varilux lens would result in unwanted prism.

To solve the problem, the manufacturer provides *spacer tabs* or a *spacer shim*. These tabs or shims are of a specific thickness and are applied to the lens surface on the left and right where the aspheric front surface of the lens will come into contact with the outer rim of the plastic lens block. This allows the top of the lens and the two spacer tabs to rest against the ring. These three points of contact form

(A)

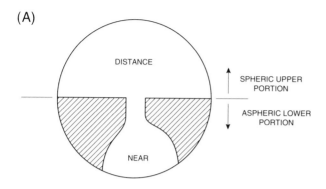

(B)

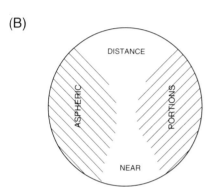

Figure 9-15 (A) In one type of progressive-addition lens, the upper portion of the lens is designed to be spherical. These lenses can be blocked like Franklin-style lenses. (B) The second design uses a front surface that is aspheric in both the upper and lower portions. This type of lens will not fit evenly against a plastic lens block or a glass generator ring. Spacer tabs are therefore required for plastic or a special generator ring for glass lenses.

a triangle and give the lens stability. See Figure 9-16. As with the Executive lens and other progressives, the lens must be blocked upside down.

With glass Varilux lenses, the lens is blocked normally. However, a specially designed fiber ring must be used during generating to lend stability to the lens and prevent prism from being induced.

Blocking in Prism

It is possible to include prism in the lens block (i.e., block in prism) *without* using a special prism blocking unit. In order to do this, *prism blocking rings* are used in conjunction with standard 43-mm glass blocks. These prism blocking rings serve to mold

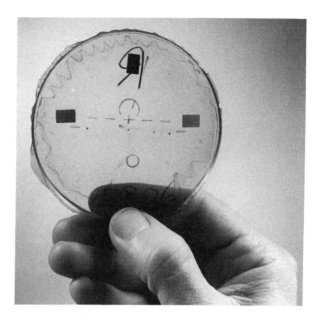

Figure 9-16 Spacer tabs are positioned on a lens so that the unevenly curved surface is allowed to rest evenly on the rim of the lens block. Tabs are of a predetermined thickness and cannot be interchanged with one another.

prism right into the block, eliminating the need for prism rings or prism wedges during generating.

Blocking in Large Amounts of Prism

Some prescriptions require an exceptionally large amount of prism—more prism in fact, than it may be possible to grind using one prism ring. There are several solutions to this problem.

Using Prism Blocking Rings in Combination with Wedges or Rings

As mentioned previously, it is possible to block prism directly into the lens block using either a special lens blocking unit or a regular lens blocker and a specially designed prism blocking ring. One method of grinding more prism into the lens is to block prism into the lens block and then add more prism using a prism ring or wedge. The prism ring or wedge is used in exactly the same manner as if no prism were already contained in the block. For example, suppose a prescription calls for a lens with 10 diopters of base-out prism. If 4 diopters of prism are molded into block and a 6-diopter prism ring or prism wedge is used, then the full 10 diopters of prism are attained.

Using a Combination of On- and Off-Center Blocking

Prism may be ground by combining off-center blocking with a prism grind. By way of review, recall that prism may be achieved in two basic ways: (1) simply grinding prism into the prescription using a prism ring (or blocking it in when a blocker having this capability is used); or (2) producing a prismatic effect by decentering the block. This is "prism by decentration."

For large amounts of prism the methods may be combined. Some of the prism may be produced by decentration and the rest by a prism grind.

Cooling Lenses Before Generating

Once a lens is blocked, it should be allowed to cool before generating. If a lens is generated too soon after blocking, it will not have cooled evenly, producing surface distortion or waviness. A warm lens also causes the heat-producing effects of the generating process to become even more pronounced. The length of time needed for the lens to cool depends upon the lens material. Recommended times are summarized in Appendix 8. These times will be longer if an all-alloy block is used. Polycarbonate lenses which are exceptionally thin (such as 1.0 mm center thickness), should be chilled in a refrigerator or freezer for 5 minutes before generating. If the lenses are to be generated dry, the chilling time should be increased to between 7 and 10 minutes.[4]

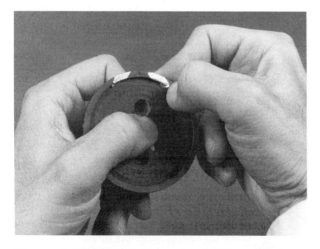

Figure 9-17 Often, excess alloy will come off the block by simply scraping with a fingernail. (The alloy in the photo is a simulation.) If it neither brushes off with a bristle brush nor is easily picked off, it can be scraped off with a hard plastic object or with a knife blade.

Block Maintenance

Before using a lens block, it must be carefully inspected to be sure that there is no old, hardened alloy material sticking to the block. If there is any alloy, burrs, dirt, or other foreign material on the block, the lens may not seat itself fully against the block. If the lens does not rest firmly and evenly against the block, prism is produced during processing because of the lens tilt.

Defects on the *sides* of the block can cause problems in properly *chucking* the lens for generating. Any extra alloy or foreign material should be scraped off. See Figure 9-17.

It is advisable to brush the blocks off with a stiff-bristle brush as they are removed from the alloy reclaim tank (the deblocking unit). Drying glass blocks will help prevent rust.*

Some laboratories add antifreeze to their water-filled alloy-reclaiming deblockers. Although there are powerful rust inhibitors in antifreeze, there are also agents present that may have toxic effects on workers, so this is *not* an acceptable practice. As an alternative, one can add a cup of white vinegar to the reclaim tank.[5] The first time this is done, the vinegar will have plenty of work to do! The water and vinegar will have to be replaced several times in rapid succession. Thereafter, however, water and vinegar will have to be replaced only once a week.

Replacing Block Centers

Each lens block has three replaceable centers, which are used in the fining and polishing process. See Figure 9-18. Pins in the cylinder machines (finers and polishers) fit into these centers during fining and polishing. The holes in these centers are *axis holes*. If they are not kept clean, the axis pins will not hold the blocked lens correctly and the axis will be off. They can be cleaned using a $\frac{3}{16}$-inch drill bit mounted in a tap handle. When the replaceable centers in the blocks become worn, they can cause the axis of the prescription cylinder to be off, or cause waviness on the lens surface. Centers should therefore be replaced as soon as they are worn.

Centers can be replaced by driving them out with a punch and hammer. However, it is easier and safer to use a center replacement punch. A center

---

*Plastic lens blocks are made from aluminum and do not rust, though the replaceable centers may.

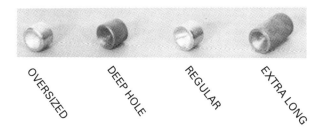

Figure 9-18 Replacement centers come not only in the regular size, but also oversized for blocks that have enlarged holes through wear or mishandling. Extra long centers are sometimes used in the center block hole only. When fining and polishing a spherical lens on a cylinder surfacer, this allows the lens to be held in place by just the center pin. Using the center pin alone permits the lens to rotate freely. Some operators maintain that this rotation produces a sphere that is better optically. (Photo courtesy of Coburn Optical Industries, Muskogee, Okla.)

replacement punch will allow block centers to be removed without damaging the block. See Figure 9-19.

When being replaced, all three centers should be set to the same depth and pressed into place without excessive force so that the block is not "mashed" out of round.[6] Center replacement punches aid in this.

Dual Center Blocker

Semi-Tech, Inc. makes a blocker which molds the block completely from alloy. The unique thing about this blocker is that it allows lenses to be blocked on the optical center of the lens, yet fined and polished on the blank geometric center. The advantages of the *dual center blocker* are

1. Layout can be done using off-center blocking.
2. There is no prism for decentration. Prism rings are only needed during generating when Rx prism is present.
3. When fining and polishing are done on the blank geometric center there is less chance of creating unwanted prism resulting from uneven pressure across the lens surface.

The dual center blocker has two blocking heads. The first is an optical center grid. Here the lens is prealigned on its optical center. The second head is

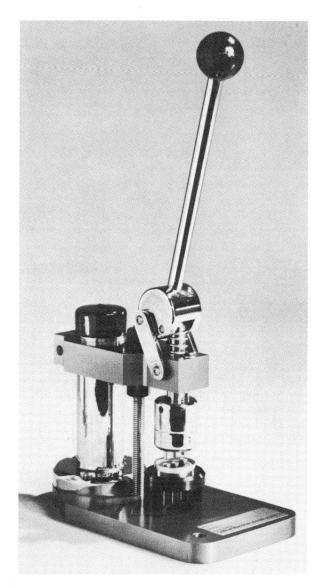

Figure 9-19 A center "knock-out" punch (or replacement press) is used to remove and replace steel block centers without damaging the block. Such presses help in setting all three centers to the same depth. A variety of such presses are available. The one pictured is an OWC-OMI 013 Torres Center Press. (Photo courtesy of Optical Works Corporation, Muskogee, Okla.)

the blocking plate where cylinder axis and blank geometric center are aligned. The alloy block is formed on the second blocking head.

In laying out a lens for dual center blocking, the desired location of the distance optical center must be found and marked with a dot. This is basically the same as off-center blocking, except that a dot is used to mark the O.C. instead of a cross. Then the blank geometric center is located. The lens is marked for cylinder axis at the blank geometric center. (Semi-Tech refers to the blank geometric center as the mechanical center.)

The procedure for dual center blocking is summarized in the following steps:[7]

1. Place the blocking ring on the optical center grid. The blocking ring is a water-cooled mold which will form the block. The dual center blocker creates a block made entirely from alloy.
2. Place the semifinished lens blank on the blocking ring so that the optical center mark is at the center of the grid and the cylinder axis line parallels the horizontal grid lines. See Figure 9-20. Clamp the lens on the blocking ring.
3. Move the blocking ring (with clamped lens) over to the blocking plate. There are three protrusions on the blocking plate. Put the blank geometric center (mechanical center or MC) on the center protrusion. Turn the lens so that the axis line crosses all three protrusions, as shown in Figure 9-21.
4. Hold the lens in place and fill the blocking ring with alloy. As soon as the ring is cool enough, remove the blocked lens.

The lens block created by the dual center block is 5 mm thinner than a conventional lens block. On automatic or semiautomatic generators, this thickness difference requires a 5-mm compensation. If no compensation is made, the lens will be 5 mm too thick. Because of the thickness of the prism ring, a thicker blocking ring and a different thickness compensation is needed when Rx prism is present.

Keeping Alloy Fresh

Lens blocking units have an alloy melting pot that holds the molten alloy in reserve. With time and repeated use, the alloy may oxidize and produce a frothy substance on the top. This substance should be scraped off and discarded. If it is not, this frothy material will clog the feeder lines in the blocker.

The same person who recommends using vinegar in the alloy reclaim tank also recommends it for the blocker alloy pot. Here is his suggestion:

Use white vinegar (¼ cup) in your blocker's alloy pot when you fill up the tank. Stir the alloy around with a rag. When you pull the rag out it will come out with all the loose particles of grit, etc. Also, the rag will pick up the excess old alloy laying on the top of the tank. Shake the rag to remove the particles—clean it and you can use the rag again. Initially, this may have to be done a couple of times to get all the old alloy and excess grit out. Then add the vinegar each time you fill the pot.[5]

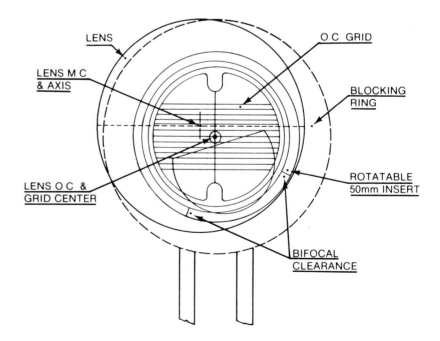

Figure 9-20 When blocking a lens using a dual center blocker, the optical center is placed on the center of the grid and the cylinder axis is made to parallel the horizontal grid lines. The axis does not need to be in the middle of the grid. (Illustration courtesy of Semi-Tech, Inc., Garland, Texas.)

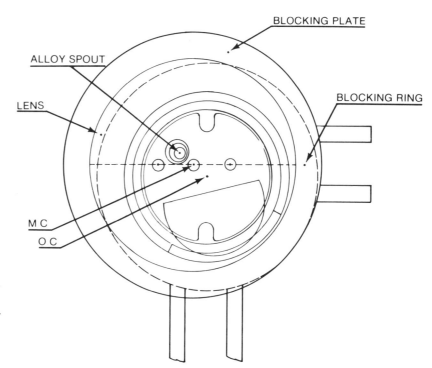

Figure 9-21 The second stage in dual center blocking positions the cylinder axis across the three protrusions and the blank geometric center (sometimes called the mechanical center, or MC) on the center protrusion. (Illustration courtesy of Semi-Tech, Inc., Garland, Texas.)

Over time, the oxidation of the alloy will cause the melting point to change. The balance of metals within the alloy can eventually become upset to the point where the alloy does not perform as it should. If old alloy is constantly replenished because of loss, it may not require complete renewal. However, the alloy needs periodic reprocessing to replace the bismuth content, which oxidizes out of the alloy.[8] These metals are too costly to simply discard. They should instead be exchanged or sent for reprocessing.

Cribbing of Lenses

Semifinished lenses that are large and are blocked off-center have a great deal of "overhang." Overhang is that part of the lens which is off to one side and is not supported by the lens block. Too much overhang can cause difficulty in generating the lens, increased fining and polishing time, waviness, or prism.

When this overhang is larger in certain places than is actually necessary for the size of the frame, the lens can be cut down or "cribbed" to a smaller size.

Previously lenses were cribbed by hand. This procedure was referred to as *hand shanking*. Hand shanking was done with special shanking pliers, and

excess glass was chipped away by a sort of "nibbling" at the lens edge.

Now cribbing is done with a *lens cribber*, which operates in the same manner as an edger and uses a pattern. See Figure 9-22. Patterns may be round, or they may approximate the general shape the lens will eventually have once it has been edged for the frame.

In the absence of an automatic lens cribber, it is possible to take the lens down by hand using a hand edger. For best results, the hand edger should have a coarse-grit wheel, as normal hand-edger smoothing wheels are too slow in removing the amount of lens material required in cribbing. Hand edgers are acceptable alternatives if cribbing is done on an occasional basis only.

Some operators use the roughing wheel in a lens edger with the coolant running to crib lenses by hand. This is *not* a safe procedure and is not recommended.

Determining Cribbing Size

The size to be used when cribbing a lens that is blocked off-center is the same as the calculated minimum blank size. This size should include at least an additional 2 mm to allow for the possibility of chipping the edge of the lens. If no safety factor

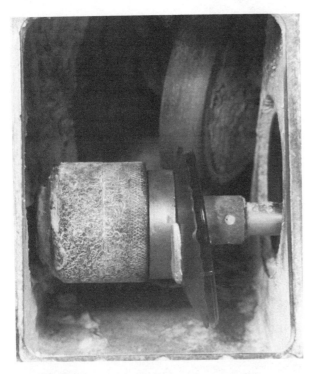

Figure 9-22 A lens cribber works in the same way as a lens edger. One obvious difference is that the cribber accepts surfacing blocks, which the lens edger does not. Because semifinished lens blanks are thick, the cribber must be made with a "heavy-duty" grinding wheel and motor. In the figure an off-center-blocked lens is shown in the grinding chamber of a lens cribber.

is added, the chipped edge will still show after edging, requiring that the job be done over again. The formula for minimum blank size (MBS) is

$$MBS = ED + \text{distance decentration} + 2$$

or

$$MBS = ED + (A + DBL - \text{distance PD}) + 2$$

EXAMPLE 9-1

What size would be used when cribbing a lens for the following prescription?

A = 47 mm
DBL = 18 mm
ED = 49 mm
PD = 61/57 mm

SOLUTION

The needed cribbing size is

$$
\begin{aligned}
MBS &= ED + (A + DBL - PD) + 2 \\
&= 49 + (47 + 18 - 61) + 2 \\
&= 55 \text{ mm}
\end{aligned}
$$

This is shown diagrammatically in Figure 9-23.

A summary of good reasons for cribbing lenses, especially Executive and Ultex lenses, whenever possible is given in Table 9-1.

Figure 9-23 Cribbing a lens removes excess material that will not be within the area of the lens after it has been edged down for the frame.

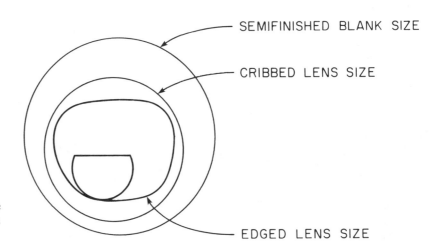

SEMIFINISHED BLANK SIZE

CRIBBED LENS SIZE

EDGED LENS SIZE

Table 9-1 Reasons for Cribbing Lenses

1. Easier generating
2. Less breakage
3. Faster fines and polishes
4. Less tearing of fining and polishing pads
5. Eliminating overhang
6. Reducing unwanted prism

Offsetting the Block

In some cases it is not possible to crib a lens with a great deal of overhang. An example is lenses that are to go into large frames with a great deal of decentration. In order to avoid some of the problems caused by overhang, it may be possible to *offset the block*.

Some blocks have extra sets of small holes into which the pins will fit during fining and polishing. See Figure 9-24. Using one of these sets of offset holes for fining and polishing will cause the pressure to be shifted in the direction of the lens overhang. This helps somewhat in counteracting the unevenness of pressure.

There are also offset block adapters that may be fastened onto the block. See Figure 9-25. These allow the pins to be offset even farther. Offset block adapters are not all of one design, but are available in different styles.

Questions and Problems

Note: Multiple-choice questions may have more than one correct answer.

1. A low-melting-point alloy, such as is used in blocking lenses for surfacing, has a melting point that is the average of the melting points of the metals that make up the alloy.
   True or False

2. Which of the following is not a reason for taping or coating plastic lenses before blocking them for surfacing?
   a. to keep the lenses from being scratched
   b. to keep the lenses from becoming slightly tinted from the generator coolant
   c. to serve as a heat shield
   d. to achieve better alloy adherence

3. On which lens style would you be more likely to use a spray or brush-on coating rather than surface tape?

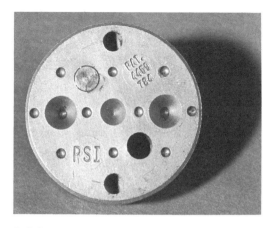

Figure 9-24 Some offsetting can be done using a regular block and placing the pins in the noncentral sets of holes. The holes that should be used are the ones nearest the geometric center of the semifinished lens.

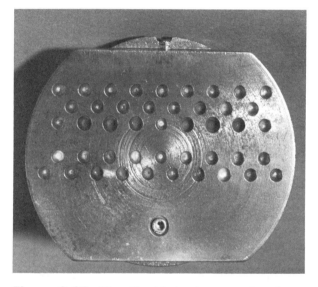

Figure 9-25 The offset block adapter can be adjusted so that the center pin in the cylinder surfacer corresponds to the center of the semifinished lens.

   a. Prescriptions having large amounts of prism.
   b. Progressive-addition lenses.
   c. Franklin-style lenses.
   d. One-piece flat-top-style bifocals.
   e. All of the above are more likely to do better when spray or brush-on coated than when surface taped.

4. Which blocks are generally larger?
   a. plastic lens blocks
   b. glass lens blocks

5. Pick out the true statement(s) concerning plastic lens blocks.
   a. As the plus power of a lens prescription increases, the block diameter will usually become larger.
   b. As the base curve of a plastic lens steepens, the block diameter will usually become smaller.
   c. As the base curve of a plastic lens steepens, the block diameter will usually become larger.

6. Glass blocks can be used to block plastic lenses.
   True or False

7. What is a "water ring" used for?
   a. To quickly cool alloy material when it is molded onto the lens in blocking.
   b. To spray coolant on the lens and grinding wheel during the generating process.
   c. To wash the blocks before reblocking a new lens.
   d. It is a ring-shaped block with water inside which is frozen before using.

8. In a lens block chiller the lenses are cooled to approximately what temperature?
   a. 0 degrees
   b. 30 degrees
   c. 40 degrees
   d. 50 degrees
   e. 60 degrees

9. When blocking a lens of any kind, it is a good idea to apply a fair amount of pressure with the blocker's lens-holding arm so as to avoid the possibility of inducing prism.
   True or False

10. When blocking a lens with cylinder, the lens is always blocked on the cylinder axis, never the prism axis (unless the two axes are the same).
    True or False

11. Choose the plastic lenses from the list below that may cause problems with unwanted prism if blocked with the segment on the edge of the plastic surfacing block.
    a. one-piece flat-top bifocals
    b. progressive-addition lenses with spherical upper halves
    c. Executive (Franklin-style) bifocals
    d. Ultex A bifocals
    e. fused-segment flat-top bifocals

12. Franklin-style bifocals are positioned upside down when being blocked.
    True or False

13. Which type of glass progressive-addition lenses require a special fiber ring for generating?
    a. Progressive-addition lenses with spheric upper front surfaces and aspheric lower front surfaces.

    b. Progressive-addition lenses with their entire front surface aspheric.
    c. Both of the above type of lenses require a special fiber ring for generating.

14. When using plastic lens blocks to block plastic progressive-addition lenses, which type of lens requires no special "spacer tabs" for blocking and is blocked in the same manner as a Franklin-style lens?
    a. Progressive-addition lenses with spheric upper front surfaces and aspheric lower front surfaces.
    b. Progressive-addition lenses with their entire front surface aspheric.
    c. Both of the above type of lenses require special "spacer tabs" for blocking.

15. Which of the following are methods of producing a greater-than-normal amount of prism in a prescription?
    a. Use a prism blocking ring in combination with a prism wedge.
    b. Use a toothpick positioned between the block and the lens in the desired base direction.
    c. Turn the block around and block the lens from the reverse side.
    d. Use off-center blocking combined with a prism ring or wedge.

16. Using antifreeze in the alloy reclaim tank will help reduce block rusting and is recommended practice.
    True or False

17. Failure to replace worn block centers will result in
    a. the refractive power of the prescription being off
    b. the axis of the prescription cylinder being off
    c. waviness on the lens surface

18. Extra long block centers are used for what purpose?

19. A center replacement punch is used to
    a. Remove block centers.
    True or False
    b. Press block centers into the lens block.
    True or False

20. To what size should a lens be cribbed that has the following dimensions?

    A = 50 mm
    DBL = 18 mm
    ED = 52 mm
    PD = 64/60 mm

21. It is impossible to do any offsetting of the block during fining and polishing operations using the standard lens block alone.
    True or False

22. How could the segment of a one-piece multifocal lens cause the lens to be ground with unwanted prism?

23. When might a lens be given a double layer of surface-saver tape? Why would this be done?

24. To what does the term "hand shaking" refer?
    a. Replacing block centers by hand.
    b. Trueing a spherical lap tool by hand.
    c. Generating a lens surface by using a hand pan.
    d. Cribbing a lens by hand.
    e. None of the above is correct.

References

1. Hirschhorn, H. Lens-Blocking Materials. *Optical Index,* 55(3):97 (March 1980).

2. Denison, J. Surfacing Optical Plastic Lenses Made from CR-39ᴿ Monomer—Part 1. *Optical Index,* 55(8):61 (August 1980).

3. *Coburnsystem Program Outline,* Coburn Optical Industries, Muskogee, Okla., p. 1. (Undated)

4. "Surfacing Techniques Update for Liteweights (1.0 mm C.T. Polycarbonate Lenses)," Orcolite, Azusa, California, 4/1/91.

5. Stone, G. Varilux Labs Helpful Hints. *Progressive Addition,* 5(3):11 (August 15, 1985). (Idea contributed by Dale Gluegge, Soderberg, Milwaukee, Wis.).

6. Denison, "Surfacing Optical Plastic Lenses," p. 62.

7. Semi-Tech, Inc., "Layout Procedure for Dual Center Blocker," Garland, Texas, undated.

8. Horne, D. F. *Spectacle Lens Technology.* Adam Helger, Bristol, England, 1978, p. 135.

10 Generating

Introduction

To surface a lens to a specific power, the desired curve must first be ground onto the semifinished lens. The process of putting this curve on the lens is called *generating*. It needs to be done as accurately and rapidly as possible. This chapter describes that process.

Types of Generators

Hand Pans

The oldest and most basic way to generate a lens surface is to use either a *hollow* (or *concave*) or a *mushroom* (or *convex*) *tool*. A large, round *hand pan* with a rotating spindle mounted in the center is used. The tools are mounted on the spindle. See Figure 10-1. An extremely rough abrasive (100 to 400 microns)* in slurry form works the lens blank until it conforms to the sphere power of the tool.[1] See Figure 10-2. This process is called *roughing*. Afterward the surface is worked some more, using a somewhat finer grade of abrasive, to bring it to the exact curve desired. This second step is called *smoothing*. Thereafter a still finer abrasive is used, by which the surface is *fined* in preparation for *polishing*.

Sphere Generators

Sphere generators are no longer used in the surfacing laboratory, because spherical surfaces are just as easily generated with a generator used for toric surfaces. The sphere generator preceded the toric generator in development but is now used only in high-production manufacturing.

---

*A micron is one millionth of a meter or one thousandth of a millimeter.

Toric Generators

A *toric generator* uses a cuplike generator wheel. The lip or rim area of the cup is impregnated with diamond and forms the cutting surface. The cuplike generator wheel can create a variety of curves, de-

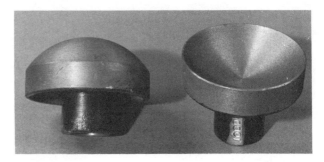

Figure 10-1 A mushroom tool (left) and a rough abrasive were routinely used in the past to create a minus surface on a lens. A hollow tool (right) was used to create a plus surface.

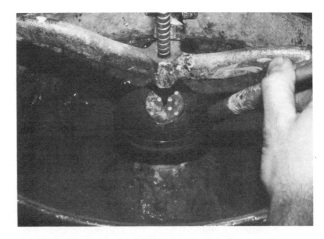

Figure 10-2 Repeatedly brushing an abrasive on the spinning lap tool allows a glass lens to be ground to the correct curvature and thickness. Compared to present-day lens generators, the process is extremely time-consuming. Using the technique today would result in glasses that would be extremely expensive.

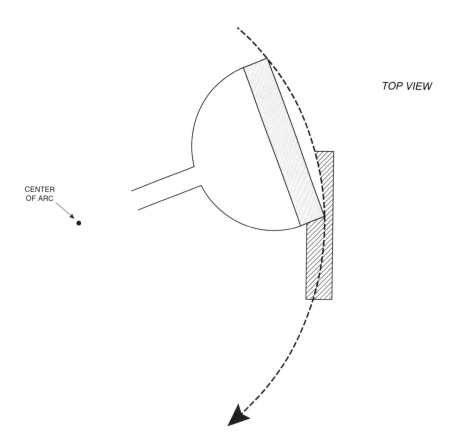

TOP VIEW

CENTER
OF ARC

Figure 10-3 When a spinning, cuplike abrasive tool is swung in an arc across the surface of a lens, a plano minus cylinder is created.

pending on how it is angled with reference to the lens surface.

The generator wheel is mounted so that it can be rotated around a specific point, creating an arc. This arc cuts a curve with a specific radius of curvature. If the cup is held with its surface perpendicular to the radius of the circle as it is swung in an arc, it is possible to create a surface that is close to a plano minus cylinder. As can be seen in Figure 10-3, the power meridian of the cylinder is in the horizontal.

To cut a lens with power in both meridians, the generator wheel is angled. Angling the wheel creates an ellipse. To see how this works, take a teacup and hold it in front of you as shown in Figure 10-4, so that you are looking directly into the cup. The rim of the cup forms a perfect circle. Now turn the cup slightly so that you are no longer looking directly into the cup. See Figure 10-5. Notice that the rim of the cup now forms an ellipse. The side of the ellipse has a longer "radius" than the rim of the cup had when viewed from straight ahead.

If the generator wheel is angled as it rotates in a specific arc, one meridian of the lens will have a radius of curvature equal to the arc of rotation.

(This will be the base curve.) The other meridian will have a "radius" of curvature equal to the side of the ellipse. (This will correspond to the cross curve.) Thus, a spherocylindrical surface is created. This is illustrated in Figures 10-6 and 10-7.

Toric Generators

Manual Toric Generators

A manual toric generator requires that the spinning generator wheel be drawn across the surface of the lens by hand. The operator pulls the grinding assembly in an arc.

Semiautomatic Toric Generators

A semiautomatic generator allows the operator to use the unit as if it were manual. It is also possible to set the base curve, cross curve, and amount of stock removal. The generator then grinds the lens at a speed set by the operator. For certain unusual lens curves or grinds, the manual mode is chosen for greater control.

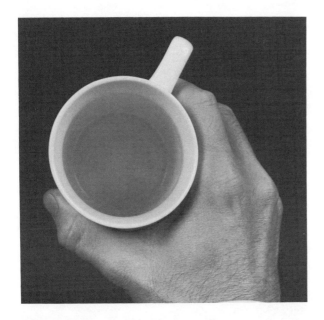

Figure 10-4 Looking directly at the top of a teacup shows the regular, circular appearance of the rim.

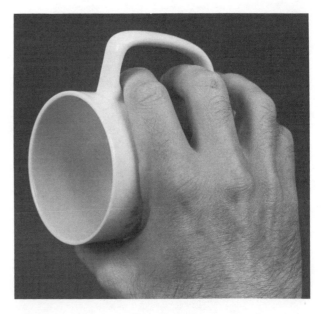

Figure 10-5 Even though the rim of the teacup is perfectly circular, angling the teacup creates an elliptical appearance.

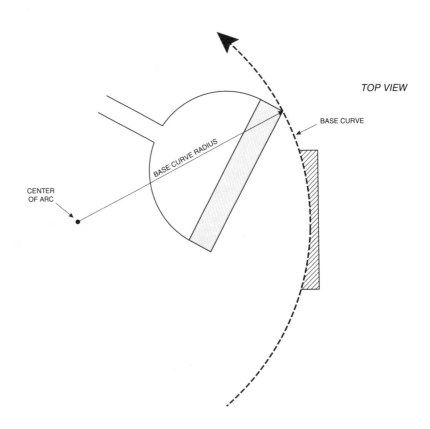

Figure 10-6 The lens base curve depends on how "tight" or short the arc of rotation is.

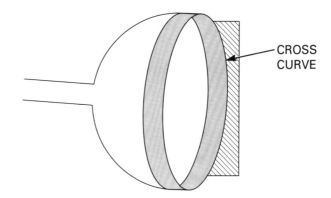

SIDE VIEW

CROSS CURVE

Figure 10-7 Because this meridian of the lens surface is actually created from an elliptical curve, rather than a spherical surface, there is "elliptical error" which must be removed during fining.

Computerized Toric Generators

Computer-controlled toric generators require only a minimum of operator input. By inputting the job number, all needed information is transferred to the machine from the central laboratory computer. Base curve, cross curve, and lens thickness have already been computed. If individual settings are made automatically, setup time per lens is reduced and the next lens can be readied while the previous one is grinding.

Setting the Generator

Calculating Stock Removal

In order to set the generator to grind a lens, the final thickness of the lens must be known. (The procedure for determining finished lens thickness is covered in Chapters 7 and 8.) Some generators are capable of grinding the lens to a desired finished thickness without having to know how much thickness must be removed from the semifinished blank. A great many, however, require this information. To calculate how much lens thickness must be removed from the blank, the following procedure is used.

First, calculate the desired finished lens thickness. Add the amount of lens material that will be removed during fining and polishing to the desired lens thickness. For glass and CR-39 plastic this is 0.3 mm. For other materials, see Table 10-1. Next, measure the center thickness of the semifinished

Table 10-1 Calculating Stock Removal

1. Calculate needed finished lens thickness.
2. Add thickness allowance for fining and polishing.

   For glass add 0.3 mm

   For CR-39 plastic add 0.3 mm

   For polycarbonate add 0.35 mm

   For polyurethane add 0.2 mm for one-step fining, add 0.4 mm for two-step fining.
   (Recommendations may vary with manufacturer.)

3. Measure semifinished blank thickness.
4. Subtract finished lens thickness plus thickness allowance from semifinished lens thickness.

lens. This can be done by using calipers. However, using calipers is unhandy and, due to large blank thicknesses, requires an especially large pair. Center thickness can be measured better by using a center thickness gauge. Center thickness gauges allow the lens to be measured while mounted on the lens block. Finally, subtract the desired lens thickness from the semifinished lens thickness. This is the amount of thickness that must be ground away and is referred to as *take-off* or *stock removal*. See Table 10-1.

To summarize this procedure in equation form,

Stock removal = (semifinished lens thickness)
    − (finished lens center thickness
    + thickness allowance for fining
    and polishing)

EXAMPLE 10-1

Suppose a −5 D crown-glass lens is to be generated. How much stock should be removed in generating?

SOLUTION

To find the amount of stock removal we first need to know the desired center thickness. Because the lens is a "street-wear" minus lens, we want to have a 2.2-mm center thickness when the lens is finished. We know that *after* generating, during the fining and polishing process, 0.3 mm of thickness will be removed. Therefore the lens cannot be less than 2.5 mm thick when it comes off the generator.

Next we must measure the center thickness of the lens blank. We find this to be 11.0 mm thick. So we know that if the lens starts out as an 11-mm semifinished blank and must end up 2.5 mm thick after generating,

$$\text{Stock removal} = 11.0 \text{ mm} - 2.5 \text{ mm}$$
$$= 8.5 \text{ mm}$$

The amount of stock removal needed is 8.5 mm.

Gauging Center Thickness

Center thickness gauges allow the measurement of a semifinished lens blank with the lens mounted on a surfacing block. This is especially handy because it is often desirable to be able to check the thickness of a lens during the surfacing process.

A center thickness gauge is made such that the blocked, semifinished lens is seated in a holder at the base of the instrument. See Figure 10-8. A probe is lowered onto the back surface of the lens. If all lenses had flat front surfaces, the measure would be straightforward with no further adjustment necessary. However, different lenses have differently curved front surfaces. Without compensation, semifinished lenses of different base curves and equal thicknesses will measure differently on the gauge. Therefore the gauge must first be adjusted for the base curve of the lens, as shown in Figure 10-9. When this is done, the probe is lowered onto the back surface of the lens and an accurate measure of center thickness results.

Steps in using a center thickness gauge are as follows:

1. Note the base curve of the lens and set the dial to this measure.
2. Raise the probe.
3. Place the blocked lens on the stand.

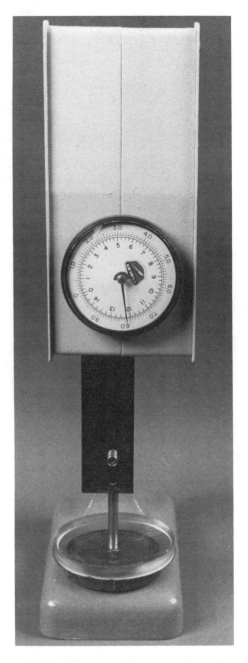

Figure 10-8 A center thickness gauge can be used even when the lens is on the block.

4. Lower the probe.
5. Read the thickness of the lens.

Setting Back Base and Cross Curves

There are two separate scales on the generator. One is for the back base curve and the other for the

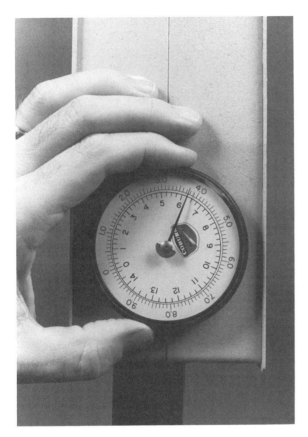

Figure 10-9 If a center thickness gauge is not set for the base curve of the lens, accurate thickness readings are impossible. The dial is turned until the indicator is at the correct base curve.

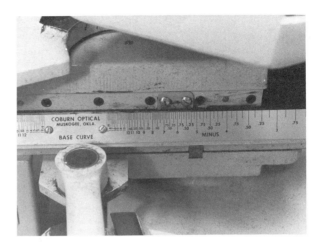

Figure 10-10 Scales that show back base curves vary from generator to generator.

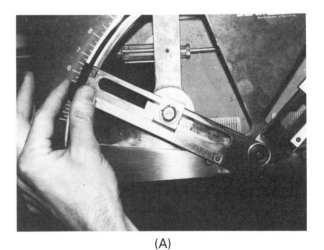

(A)

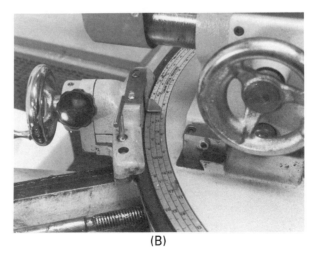

(B)

Figure 10-11 Two of the many types of generator cross curve scales.

cross curve. See Figures 10-10 and 10-11. When setting these curves, remember to approach the setting from the same direction every time. In other words, if the back base is 6.00, always move the pointer or dial into the area that is less than 6.00, and approach from the less-than-6.00 side. If 6.00 is overshot to 6.12, do not just move back to 6.00. Instead move back to 5.75 and approach 6.00 from the low side again.

If the cross curve is 8.00, approach from the less-than-8.00 side. Because of the possibility of some "play" in the system, this procedure will give more consistent results.

Compensating for Elliptical Error
When the cross curve of a toric lens is generated, it is not exactly spherical. It is, rather, an ellipse. This is called *elliptical error*. In order to compensate for elliptical error, cylinder powers may be reduced by approximately 6% when setting the generator

cross curve. Plastic lenses require more compensation than glass lenses. Some guideline starting points are shown in Table 10-2. Each laboratory should adjust compensation based on its own experience, as generators may vary. The larger the lens blank, the more elliptical error will be present. If the lens blank is larger than 75 mm, the cross curve will require a greater reduction than shown in Table 10-2. Compensating for elliptical error will keep fining and polishing pads from tearing, reduce fining time, and keep lenses from "chattering" (making a vibrating noise because of being off-curve) on the cylinder machines.

EXAMPLE 10-2

Suppose a job using glass lenses calls for a back base curve of 4.50 D and a cross curve of 6.50 D. What would the generator settings be when compensated for elliptical error?

SOLUTION

No elliptical error compensation is needed for the back base curve. The difference between the back base and cross curves accounts for 2.00 D of cylinder power. For 2.00 D of cylinder power, the cross curve should be compensated by 0.12 D. The generator cross curve should be set at

$$6.50 - 0.12 = 6.37 \text{ D}$$

It should be noted that some of the newer, more automated generators compensate for elliptical error automatically.

Table 10-2 Elliptical Error Compensation[2]

Prescribed Cylinder Power	Cross Curve Reduction
For Glass Lenses:	
0.00 to 1.75	None
2.00 to 3.75	0.12
4.00 to 5.75	0.25
6.00 to 7.75	0.37
Over 8.00	6% reduction
For Plastic Lenses:	
0.00 to 1.00	None
1.25 to 3.00	0.12
3.25 to 5.00	0.25
5.25 to 7.00	0.37
Over 7.00	6% reduction

Setting the Generator So the Job Fines from the Center Out or the Edges In

Some laboratories advocate setting both the base and cross curves slightly flatter than actually called for. This assures that fining begins at the center of the lens and moves outward toward the edge. Those who use this procedure suggest that curves be flattened by approximately 0.06 D (1/16th diopter). Yet what appears to be just the opposite is recommended by the Varilux Corporation for their 1.6 index polyurethane lenses. They recommend adjusting the generator settings until the lens shows a 30-mm fining hole on the surface after 5 seconds of fining time. This would show that their recommendation is to fine from the edge inward. Although this may appear to be advocating steepening the curves, it is actually a check against having the lens too steep. The fining hole will often have a tendency to be larger than 30 mm after 5 seconds, indicating that the lens was generated steep and requires flattening.

Using Fiber Rings

Lenses blocked with standard 43-mm glass blocks require the use of an additional *fiber ring*, which fits around the block and spaces the lens correctly in the generator. Fiber rings are also referred to as *generator rings*. Plastic lenses blocked with specially designed, large aluminum blocks do not require a fiber ring.

A fiber ring fits between the generator chuck and the lens surface. It keeps the lens steady, preventing unwanted prism and assuring accurate thickness.

The same ring may be used on different base curves. The standard fiber ring is for spherical front surfaces. If a lens with a toric front surface is to be used, the normal fiber ring will allow it to rock. This results in unwanted prism being ground into the lens. A special fiber ring, shaped to conform to the toric surface of the lens, should be used for the occasional front-surface toric lens.

As mentioned in Chapter 9, other specialized types of fiber rings are used for specific lenses. One example is the fiber ring used for Varilux progressive-addition glass lenses.

Chucking the Lens

A blocked lens must be squarely and securely placed in the generator chuck. The suggested method for chucking a lens is to hold the middle of the front surface with the first three fingers. See Figure 10-12. This will aid in keeping the lens from tilting. Tilting of the lens will definitely produce unwanted prism.

Before tightening the chuck, rotate the lens back and forth slightly to assure that the axis pins are fixed securely in the lens block. There should be no rotational movement. Any play in the lens that allows for rotation will result in the axis being incorrect.

Setting the Generator for Stock Removal

After setting the base and cross curves and chucking the lens, some generators require zeroing in. Generators that require calculation of stock removal must be zeroed in. Procedures vary according to machine. For explanation purposes, the Coburn 108 BP generator has been chosen.

To zero in the Coburn 108 BP generator, the chucked lens must be moved up to the generator wheel. This is done by moving the *tailstock ram* of the generator forward. See Figure 10-13. An exact distance between the generator wheel and the center

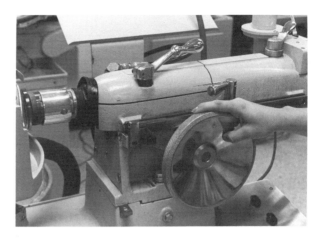

Figure 10-13 Moving the tailstock rim of the generator forward in preparation for grinding.

of the lens must now be set. This is done by using a *zero-in gauge*. Zero-in gauges are usually either *saddle gauges* or *ball gauges*. The zero-in gauge is held in the middle of the lens and the lens is moved forward (by moving the tailstock ram) until the gauge just touches both the center of the lens and the lip of the generator wheel. See Figure 10-14.

Next the *zero-in unit* is set so that this position will be remembered during the grinding phase. The zero-in unit (which contains a hinged bar of equal thickness to the pin of the saddle or ball of the ball gauge) slides down to a stop. With the hinged bar down so that it is between the zero-in unit and the stop, the zero-in unit is locked in place. See Figure 10-15. Now the tailstock ram is moved back. The saddle or ball gauge is removed and the hinged bar is flipped up out of the way. See Figure 10-16.

Next the rotary table is set. The rotary table, shown in Figure 10-17, will cause the diamond wheel to move back and forth across the lens as it rotates. The table is set by rotating it until it is aligned. The clamp on the rotary table slide should be loosened and the cutting head assembly (where the diamond wheel is housed) moved until it clears the edge of the lens. See Figure 10-18. This assures that the sweep of the wheel will go far enough to grind the whole surface of the lens. Finally, the slide is retightened.

Now the tailstock ram can be moved forward so that the lens is in position. When it is in position, the zero-in unit touches the zero-in stop.

Set the gauges or dials for the amount of stock removal per sweep of the wheel. Set the speed of the sweep as well. Now the grinding wheel can be

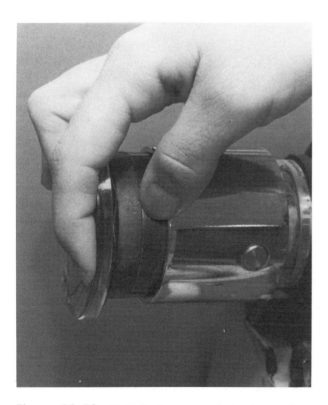

Figure 10-12 Hold the lens squarely in place with three fingers while chucking. It helps to twist the lens back and forth slightly to be certain the block is properly seated and the axis is correct.

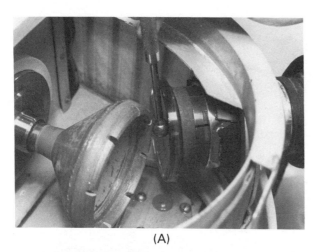

(A)

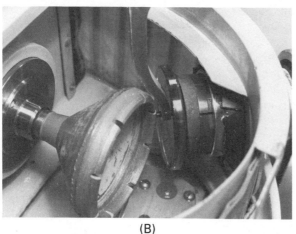

(B)

Figure 10-14 Either a ball gauge (A) or a saddle gauge (B) with a known width is used to bring the lens within a fixed distance from the generator wheel rim.

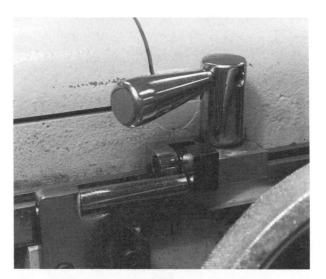

Figure 10-15 With the hinged bar down, the generator is set so that the lens will be the width of the bar away from the lens surface. (The width of the hinged bar equals the diameter of the ball gauge or the length of the saddle gauge pin.)

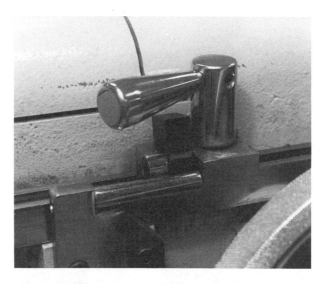

Figure 10-16 Once the hinged bar is swung upward, the back surface of the lens is allowed to travel forward until it just touches the generator wheel.

started. Once the wheel is running, the thickness gauge for the total amount of stock removal can be set. See Figure 10-19.

The lens may now be ground.

Generators Which Grind for Correct Lens Thickness Automatically Many generators do not require figuring the amount of stock removal for the lens. Instead, the base curve and a desired center thickness are set using dials on the generator. Thickness is removed in steps until the final thickness is reached. With plastic lenses, a considerable amount of lens material can be removed with each sweep of the cutting wheel.

Using Prism Rings and Prism Wedges

Generators are designed to grind a lens so that the optical center will end up in the middle of the lens block. As long as the lens is chucked squarely in the generator and is not tilted, no prism will appear

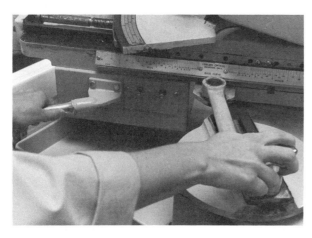

Figure 10-17 The rotary table causes the mechanical turning that moves the diamond wheel across the lens.

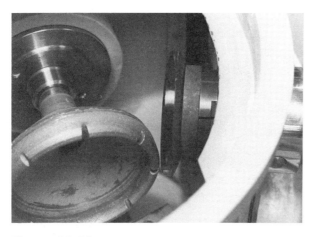

Figure 10-18 The wheel must be positioned so that it will clear the lens at the end of the sweep. Otherwise an unsurfaced lip of lens material will remain.

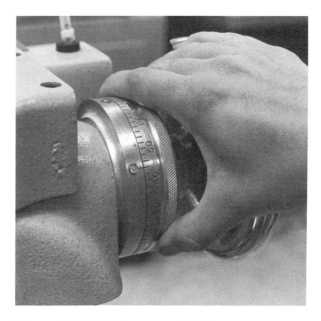

Figure 10-19 The generator's thickness gauge is set for the desired amount of lens take-off (the thickness of the lens that must be removed).

in the lens. However, if it is chucked with a tilt, the tilt of the lens will cause more lens material to be removed on the side of the lens that sticks up. See Figure 10-20.

Fortunately, tilting can be used to advantage when prism is desired. By controlling the degree of tilt of the lens in the chuck, a precise amount of prism can be ground into the lens. Tilt can be controlled by placing a wedge under one side of the block. *Prism wedges* are made in sets. Each wedge has a thickness corresponding to the amount of prism desired. See Figure 10-21. *Prism rings* can also be used. See Figure 10-22. Prism rings are thin on one

side and thick on the other. They fit around the outside of a lens block. The thickest point on a prism ring corresponds to the apex of the prism created. See Figure 10-23. In other words, the location of the prism wedge (or the thickest part of the prism ring) is across the lens from where the base of the prism will be. See Figure 10-24.

A prism ring is placed on the lens right before it is chucked. Lenses that require a prism grind are marked with an arrow. The arrow points to the apex of the prism, showing the generator operator where the prism wedge or the thickest part of the prism ring belongs. See Figure 10-25. The prism ring has a notch at the thickest point for ease in orientation. (Because some laboratories draw the arrow toward the base instead of the apex, there is also a notch at the thinnest edge of the ring.)

Prism Ring and Wedge Calibration

Prism rings are calibrated for a specific index material. Prism rings (and wedges) are marked in prism diopters. Those prism diopter markings are valid only for the lens material for which the set was made. Prism rings made for plastic lenses having an index of 1.498 will not give the same results if they are used for a high-index plastic lens. If index 1.498 rings are used for high-index plastic, more prism

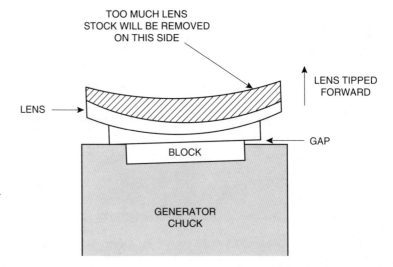

TOO MUCH LENS
STOCK WILL BE REMOVED
ON THIS SIDE

LENS TIPPED
FORWARD

LENS

GAP

BLOCK

GENERATOR
CHUCK

Figure 10-20 If a lens is chucked at an angle, more lens stock will be removed from one side of the lens than from the other, creating prism. The hatched lines on the lens show the part of the lens that will be ground off.

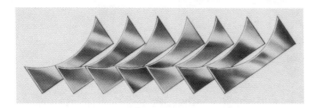

Figure 10-21 A set of prism wedges. When placed under one side of the lens block during the generating process, prism can be ground onto the lens in a predictable manner. (Photo courtesy of Coburn Optical Industries, Muskogee, Okla.)

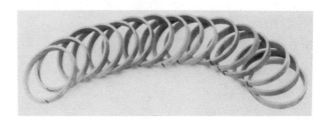

Figure 10-22 A set of prism rings is marked according to the lens material for which they are used. This particular set is for glass. If another index material is to be ground, the prism ring amount must be compensated. (Photo courtesy of Coburn Optical Industries, Muskogee, Okla.)

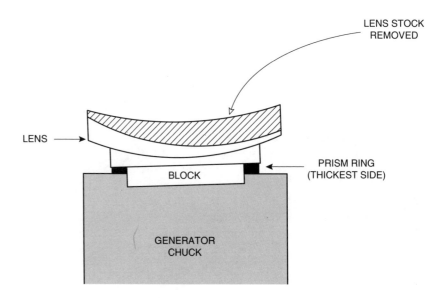

LENS STOCK
REMOVED

LENS

BLOCK

PRISM RING
(THICKEST SIDE)

GENERATOR
CHUCK

Figure 10-23 The angle of tilt in lens chucking can be controlled using a prism ring or a prism wedge. Each angle of tilt will give a different prismatic effect.

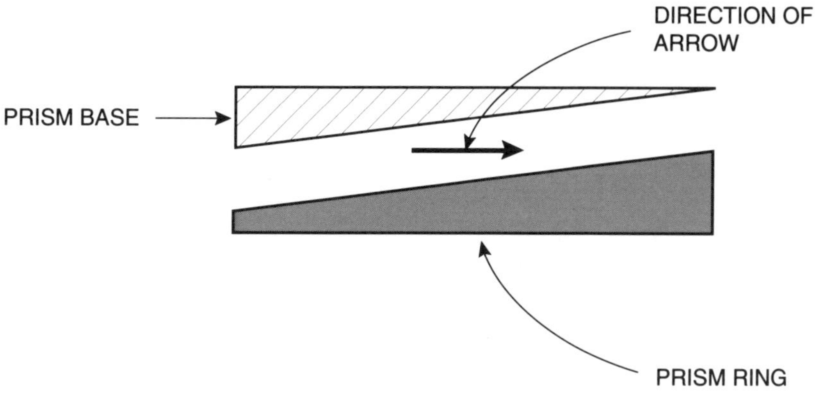

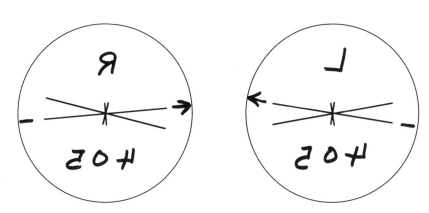

Figure 10-24 The orientation of a prism ring in relation to the desired prism base direction and the layout marking on the lens. (Remember that many laboratories have the arrow pointing the other way, toward the base of the prism instead of toward the apex as shown here.)

Figure 10-25 The arrows show the desired position of the prism *apex*. When paired lenses with prism for decentration are placed side by side, the prism arrows should always point toward each other or away from each other. If both point right or both left, check the prescription for Rx prism. If there is none present and both lenses are plus or both minus, then the lenses are probably mismarked. Marking accuracy should be checked before the lenses are generated.

will result than expected. Ideally a different set of rings should be used for each lens material having a different refractive index. But if the same set of rings is to be used for more than one material, either a conversion table or a computer program will have to be used so that the correct amount of compensation can be made.

Prism Gauges

An instrument that looks a lot like a center thickness gauge can be used to check a blocked lens for prism. The prism gauge replaces the manual procedure of using calipers to check for thickness differences on opposite sides of the lens.* A prism gauge can be used if the generator operator suspects that a lens has unwanted prism, or wants to determine if the correct amount of prism is being ground on a lens. See Figure 10-26.

---

*See Chapter 8, in the section on Rx prism.

The Generating Process

Lenses should be generated as aggressively as possible. This is beneficial for more than one reason. First, more lenses can be produced per day, saving on labor costs. Second, the lens is ground by more of the generator wheel than just the top of the lip, utilizing the full potential of the wheel and the generator. Some generators, when equipped with the correct wheel and properly cooled, are able to generate a lens with one back cut and one forward sweep. Often, though, this will not be possible.

Back Cuts

Whenever a large amount of lens material is removed with one sweep of the generator, there is a tendency for the edge of the lens to break off at the end of the sweep. This is because as the generator wheel reaches the end of its sweep, there is a large chunk of lens material at the edge of the lens. See

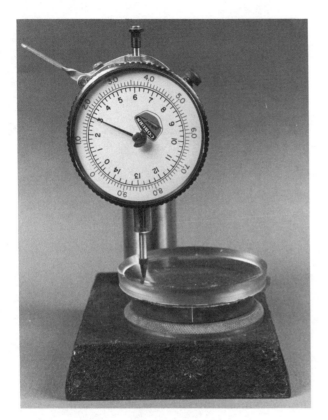

Figure 10-26 The prism gauge replaces hand thickness when measuring prism on a blocked lens.

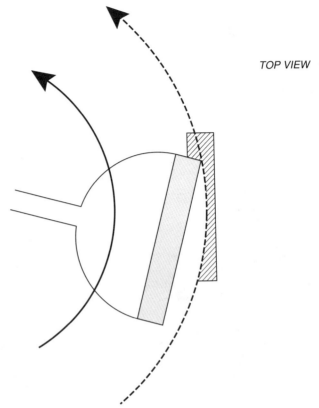

TOP VIEW

Figure 10-27 When there is no back cut, as the wheel reaches the edge of the lens there may be a large chunk of lens.

Figure 10-27. Because of the stress exerted as the wheel presses forward, this chunk of material can tear out a part of the lens edge. See Figure 10-28. This problem can be avoided by making what is called a back cut. A *back cut* is made by beginning with the back edge of the lens first, instead of the front. The back cut makes only a partial sweep of the surface. See Figure 10-29. The wheel is then moved to the front of the lens and the full sweep made. See Figure 10-30. In this manner the lens surface can be swept across without the danger of ripping off part of the edge. Back cutting is essential whenever large amounts of lens material are to be removed in a single pass of the generator wheel.

Many automatic generators can be set to do a back cut routinely. When back cuts are to be done manually, however, the generator should be set from 3 to 5 mm less than the amount of stock removal required. Manual back cuts should be made approximately one-fourth of the way across the lens.

After grinding a manual back cut, the generator is reset and the lens generated in the usual manner.

Generating Glass Lenses

With glass lenses it is not always as easy to remove as much material in one sweep as with plastic lenses. Attempting to remove an inordinately large amount of glass at too great a sweep speed can easily result in lens breakage. There is a relationship between generator sweep speed and the amount of stock removal that can be attempted. Naturally, if the generator is made to sweep rapidly across the lens surface, not as much thickness will be safely removable as during a slower sweep.

Most operators will finish generating a lens with a smaller pass, which removes only 2 or 3 points (0.2 or 0.3 mm). Some maintain that the last 0.4 mm to be removed from the lens should be taken

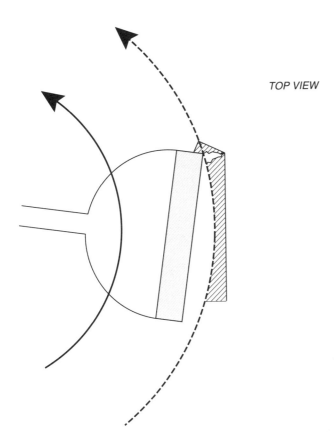

Figure 10-28 Too much force on a thick chunk of lens at the edge can cause the edge to crack off.

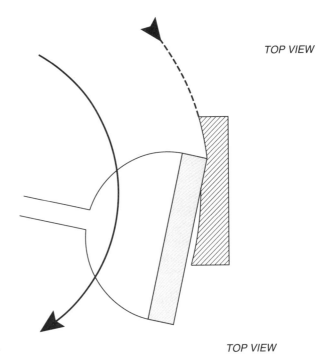

Figure 10-29 The beginning procedure for backcutting a lens. This removes the material that could crack off if no back cut were made.

in two cuts of 0.2 mm each.[3] This is done in order to allow for a smoother surface.

Generating CR-39 and CR-39 Compatible High-Index Plastic Lenses

There are some high-index plastic lenses such as PPG's Hi-Ri 1.56-index plastic which can be processed in the same manner as conventional CR-39 lenses. High-index lenses which are identified as being compatible with CR-39 processing methods should be processed in exactly the same manner as CR-39.

When an electroplated, plastic-only diamond wheel is used with CR-39 plastic lenses, the maximum amount of stock possible should be removed in one pass. A good suggestion is to start with 3 to 4 mm (30 to 40 points) per pass across the lens. This amount will result in less heat buildup and pressure on the lens. Do not take multiple small

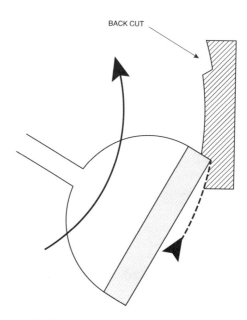

Figure 10-30 A back cut goes only part way. Then the wheel is repositioned and the normal cut is made without the danger of lens breakage.

cuts or be concerned with final surface finish. If final surface finish is of concern, a final cut of 0.2 mm may help.

If a multipurpose wheel for both glass and plastic is used, much smaller cuts are necessary. In this case, normally only 0.3 to 0.8 mm of material is removed per pass. When generator coolant is not refrigerated, stock removal must also be reduced to 0.3 to 0.8 mm per pass. Multipurpose wheels also mean that the final 0.4 mm of material should be removed in two cuts of 0.2 mm each. These final cuts should be made slowly.[4] CR-39 lenses may also be generated using the same methods as are required for polycarbonate, polyurethane, and other high-index plastic lenses. These methods are described in the sections following.

Generating Polycarbonate Lenses

Recommendations vary on generating polycarbonate lenses. Most of these variations are due to using generator wheels of differing grits, styles, or even construction. Although some methods are mentioned here, the laboratory should consult with their generator and wheel manufacturers.

Dry Cutting Polycarbonate

Polycarbonate lenses may be generated dry, with no coolant at all. Cutting can be done using a diamond grit wheel, a fly cutter, or a wheel which combines the characteristics of both. (These wheel types will be explained in more detail later in the chapter.) When using a combination fly cutter/diamond grit wheel, the lens may be generated with three sweeps or less. Opinion varies considerably over the value of small final cuts with dry cutting. Many maintain that polycarbonate responds well to a heavy final cut when a fly cutter is used dry. Some operators dry cut polycarbonate with one sweep only.

If a laboratory is to dry cut lenses, the generator must be equipped with a vacuum system attached to the grinding chamber. See Figure 10-31.

Wet Cutting Polycarbonate

At the time of this writing, the recommended technique for polycarbonate is wet cutting. Generator wheel options for wet cutting are the same as for dry. Some advise limiting the first cuts to between 0.5 and 1.0, with 2 to 3 mm cuts until the last cut. The last cut should be 0.5 mm and take 15 seconds, or as an alternative, two final cuts of 0.5 and 0.2

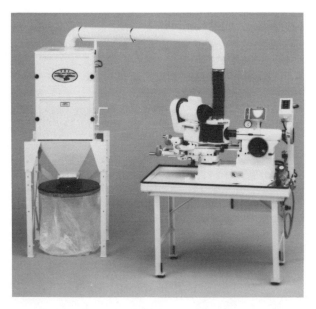

Figure 10-31 A table model FB Lens Generator equipped with a vacuum system for dry-cutting polycarbonate, high-index plastic, and CR-39 lenses. (Photo courtesy FB Optical, St. Cloud, Minn.)

mm each. Using a combination fly cutter/diamond grit wheel yields a surface which will require less fining and polishing than will be obtained when using a regular diamond grit wheel.

Generators used for wet cutting polycarbonate do best with a high-pressure/high-volume coolant pump and a special tank for collecting polycarbonate swarf.*

Generating High-Index Polyurethane Lenses

High-index polyurethane lenses are processed with the same generator wheels as for polycarbonate. They can also be cut wet or dry. Wet cutting with a diamond-plated generator wheel is recommended.[6] The maximum recommended cut is 1 mm at normal speed or 2 mm at slow speed. The final cut is 0.2 mm as slow as possible. If the final cut is done using automatic thickness, a zero final cut is recommended. A zero final cut means that the generator makes another cut across the lens without cutting any deeper. The technique is used to give a smoother surface finish.

If the lens is dry cut with a fly cutter or combi-

---

*Swarf is the ground lens material created by the grinding process.

nation fly cutter/diamond grit wheel, it may be cut aggressively with three sweeps, the final cut being 0.7 mm.

Coolants Used in Generating

Oil-Base Versus Water-Base Coolants

For many years, oil was used exclusively as a coolant in the generating process. Good-quality oils such as Shell Pella were sometimes mixed with a small amount of Stadoil. Unfortunately, when the grinding surface between diamond and lens gets hot enough, it is possible to ignite the mist of oil created by the spinning generator wheel. The mist ignites with a "flash" but usually does not continue burning. It was not uncommon, however, for an optical laboratory to be destroyed by a fire that started at the generator. Gradually, water-based coolants began to increase in quality and popularity.

There are pluses and minuses to both water- and oil-based coolants. Most laboratories now use water-based coolants, but each must decide which is best for them. Here are some of the factors to consider.

Advantages of Oil-Based Coolants
1. Oil-based coolants will not cause rusting, but in fact prevent it.
2. Oil-based coolants do not evaporate.
3. Oil-based coolants can be used for both CR-39 plastic and glass.

Disadvantages of Oil-Based Coolants
1. Oil based coolants are a fire hazard.
2. Oil-based coolants are messy to work with.
3. Oil-based coolants may be more expensive than water-based coolants.
4. Disposal of spent oil is a problem. City, state, and federal laws now prohibit the disposal of oil wastes in sewers and sanitary landfill areas, and require that such refuse be deposited in approved dumping areas.[7]
5. Some inexpensive oils contain wax and animal fats. These are used in order to raise the "flash-point" temperature so that it will not ignite as readily. Oxidation of these fats may allow for bacterial growth.[7]

Advantages of Water-Based Coolants
1. Water-based coolants are less expensive than oil-based coolants.
2. Water-based coolants allow glass particles to settle faster, resulting in a cleaner coolant.

Disadvantages of Water-Based Coolants
1. Water-based coolants evaporate faster than oil-based coolants.
2. Water-based coolants have a tendency to foam.

Mist Collectors

As a generator cuts across the surface of a lens, coolant is sprayed on the wheel at the cutting interface between the wheel and the lens. The rapidly spinning wheel throws off a fine spray of coolant, which is, for the most part, trapped by the confines of the grinding chamber. Some of the spray escapes as a mist around the generator. The mist can be messy as it settles, especially if the coolant being used is oil. Some laboratories have chosen to install *mist collectors* on their generators. Mist collectors vacuum the mist from the grinding chamber area before it can enter the surrounding atmosphere.

Controlling Coolant Cleanliness and Temperature

Keeping the generator coolant clean is more than just a matter of good housekeeping. Clean coolant will increase the life of the generator. Sandpaperlike contaminants are not constantly seeping into the moving areas of the machine, nor do they dry as a thick film on machine surfaces.

If the glass content in the coolant builds up to an amount greater than 2%, the diamond tool will load up, glaze, and may cause breakage.[8] Thus clean means increased generator wheel life and less frequent honing (dressing) of the wheel. Large amounts of lens material in the coolant can also cause dermatitis for the individual whose hands are in constant contact with it.

Several methods are used to keep generator coolant clean.

Settling Tanks
The simplest way to clean generator coolant is just to let the glass or plastic grindings settle to the bottom of the *settling tank* that comes with the generator. The tank is allowed to fill to the point where the sludge builds up. Then it is emptied. The problem with this method is that there is more recirculation of contaminated material as the tank fills with

sludge. Additionally, since less and less of the liquid is actually recirculating, the temperature of the coolant rises more quickly.

Coolant Filtering Systems

By pumping the coolant through an external *filtering system* purchased for this purpose, the coolant remains cleaner and the full volume continues to circulate, less any evaporation that might take place.

Centrifuges

Instead of filtering glass or plastic debris out of the coolant, it is possible to use a large *centrifuge* to spin the debris out. A coolant centrifuge operates in the same manner as a top-loading washer when it is going through its spin cycle. As the tank in a washing machine spins rapidly, the clothes are pressed against the sides of the tank. The tank has a lip at the top so that the clothes do not spin out. A centrifuge unit for an optical laboratory works in the same way. Instead of one tank, though, a coolant centrifuge has a series of tanks nestled in one another. These spin at a rapid rate. Coolant is pumped to the center of the centrifuge and spins outward from one tank to the next. Sludge begins to accumulate against the walls of the tanks. If the walls of the tanks completely fill with sludge before being emptied, the centrifuge will lose its ability to remove any debris. Accumulated glass or plastic should be removed regularly. Because the liquid has been spun off, the remaining sludge is easily disposable. For a summary of the advantages of filtering or centrifuging generator coolant, see Table 10-3.

Table 10-3 Advantages of Filtering or Centrifuging Generator Coolant

1. The life of the generator is extended because less abrasive debris is left on or in the moving parts.
2. The generator wheel can be used longer before it must be dressed and before it must be replaced.
3. The surface quality of the lens is better.
4. There is less breakage and lens rejection.
5. Disposal of wastes is much easier because they are collected as solids.
6. Because the full volume of coolant continues to recirculate, the coolant does not heat up as rapidly.
7. There are fewer problems of dermatitis among generator operators.

In summary, any coolant cleaning system is far superior to attempting to operate an expensive generator with no coolant cleaning device other than a settling tank.

Controlling Coolant Temperature

As the generator wheel grinds across the surface of the lens, a great deal of heat is generated. Coolant should absorb the heat as it is generated. It should keep plastic lenses from warping, melting, or burning and prevent glass lenses from breaking. Unnecessarily high temperature will also decrease diamond generator wheel life.

Throughout the day the constant friction between generator wheel and lens surface raises the temperature of the coolant, reducing its effectiveness. Refrigeration or "chiller" units are available to lower the temperature to the desired level. The desired temperature for glass is about 58 degrees Fahrenheit, and for plastic somewhere between 50 and 60 degrees F. Commonly, such a refrigeration unit will have a reservoir with cooling coils. As coolant flows into and out of the reservoir, the desired temperature is maintained.

Without the use of refrigeration, only small amounts of lens material may be removed with each pass of the generator wheel. This will slow production time and increase the risk of producing an unacceptable lens.

It is not uncommon for either filtering and refrigeration or centrifuge and refrigeration units to be sold as a combination.

Protecting the Operator

Oil and water can both penetrate skin, carrying with them what could be an irritant in solution. If the operator is sensitive to the materials that are in suspension, in solution, or in the coolant itself there are two possible alternatives. One is to use rubber gloves; the second may be the use of a barrier cream applied to the hands. For example, Kerodex 71* is formulated for wet work and protects the skin against water and water-soluble irritants such as cutting oils (coolants), epoxy resins, plating solutions, photographic developers, bleaching compounds, ammonia, detergents, and soaps. A second product,

*Kerodex is available from Ayerst Laboratories, 685 Third Avenue, New York, NY 10017.

Kerodex 51, is recommended for dry or oily work, protecting the skin against irritants that are insoluble in water. Both products can be used together to protect against an even broader range or irritants.

It is sometimes helpful to empty a small bottle of Lysol disinfectant directly into the generator coolant if skin irritation occurs.[9]

Generator Wheels

The choice of a generator wheel depends on several factors. These factors include what type of coolant is being used (oil- or water-based), what lens material is being used, and how aggressively the lens is being cut.

Choosing the Wheel for the Material

There is a great deal of difference in how quickly and effectively a surface can be generated, depending on the suitability of the generator wheel for the lens material.

Glass and "All-Purpose" Wheels
Generator wheels designed for glass lenses can be used for standard CR-39 plastic surfaces, but they will not cut as rapidly. In addition, if the glass "all-purpose" wheel is used for too large a percentage of plastic, it will have a tendency to *load*. *Loading* occurs when plastic material gets between the diamond grit of the wheel, causing a glazing effect and decreased cutting ability. Wheels that will cut glass cannot cut plastic as effectively. The surface of the plastic lens being generated heats up if it is ground too rapidly. This may result in a poor-quality surface. If a regular glass wheel is used to generate plastic lenses, the wheel will have to be honed about once a day to clean the diamond out. Otherwise neither glass nor plastic lenses will cut well.

If photochromic material is ground in quantity, a specially chosen wheel should be selected. Photochromic material grinds hard and is rough on generator wheels.

Wheels for CR-39 Plastic Lenses
Some electroplated diamond generator wheels are used specifically for CR-39 plastic lenses. These wheels use a coarser grit of diamond with a wider spacing between the individual pieces of diamond, preventing the loading effect. This wheel *cannot* be used for glass. Attempting to use an electroplated

wheel designed for plastic on glass will break the glass and severely damage the wheel. Electroplated wheels are never honed. Honing would severely damage the wheel. They may be cleaned using a stiff-bristle brush and kitchen cleanser.

Basically, the same rules that apply to diamond edger wheels also apply to diamond generator wheels. (For a more detailed explanation, see C. W. Brooks, *Essentials for Ophthalmic Lens Work*, Butterworth-Heinemann, Boston, 1983.) Wheels used to cut polycarbonate can also be used for standard CR-39.

Wheels for Lenses Made from Polycarbonate and Other Soft Plastics
Polycarbonate lenses require an extremely coarse diamond wheel* because of the softness of the material. Polycarbonate can be generated wet or dry. "Wet" means that the lens is flushed with coolant during generating. "Dry" means that no coolant is used during generating. When polycarbonate lenses are generated dry, a special vacuum system is needed to remove polycarbonate swarf (the ground lens material created by the grinding process).

Toothed wheels called *fly cutters* or *milling cutters* are sometimes used for cutting polycarbonate lenses. These wheels are more dangerous than diamond wheels and require a safety interlock on the lens grinding chamber lid and an electric braking system on the drive motor, so that if the wheel is running and the chamber lid opens, the wheel stops immediately.

A generator wheel with one to four toothlike protrusions on the wheel edge is an innovative design that creates a very smooth surface on both plastic and polycarbonate lenses. See Figure 10-32. These are a form of a fly cutter wheel. The cutting surface is a "large, full-face polycrystalline (PCD) diamond."[10] It cuts in both directions and can be retrued. The beauty of this wheel is that the plastic surfaces finished by the tool are very smooth. This introduces the possibility of reducing fining and polishing times.

There are combination fly cutter/diamond grit generator wheels which use both diamond grit and diamond cutter blade technology. They are versatile wheels which cut rapidly and smoothly. Combination wheels are available with replaceable, interchangeable diamond grit and cutter blade segments.

---

*The grit for this wheel is approximately a 20 grit.

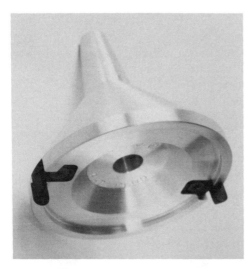

Figure 10-32 The wheel shown is a patented Tiger Tooth™ cutter from CDP Diamond Products, Inc. This wheel is specifically designed for cutting plastic and polycarbonate lenses. It is not recommended for grinding glass. (Photo courtesy of CDP Diamond Products, Inc. of Livonia, Mich.)

With interchangeable segments, grit size can be varied and segments may be retrued, resharpened, or replaced.

Diamond Concentration

With aggressive cutting, the diamond wheels must have a sufficiently high concentration of diamond material. "Aggressive cutting" is where the pass across the surface is fast and/or the cut is deep. If there is not enough diamond material per square inch, the wheel will cut poorly and wear quickly.

Wheel Slotting

Most generator wheels are made with slots along the cutting edge. The purpose of these slots is to allow for a freer exchange of coolant and flushing out of ground lens material.

The Coolant Manifold

The *coolant manifold* distributes coolant over the lens and wheel during cutting. Jets of coolant are sprayed onto the cutting interface through a number of spouts. It is possible for these coolant manifold spouts to become misaligned by being struck by a fragment of lens. Spout alignment should be checked periodically to assure that the coolant is being directed to the intended area. Excessive flashes when using an oil-based coolant, or cracked lenses, could indicate that the spouts are out of alignment. Normally the upper spout sprays coolant around the screw that holds the diamond wheel to the spindle. The other, lower spouts should hit at the outer edge of the diamond wheel, where the wheel grinds the lens.

Wheel Wear

All diamond wheels wear out with time. However, there are certain things that will cause the wheel to wear unevenly, resulting in inaccurate curves and undependable thicknesses.

If the generator operator takes off (grinds away) only a small amount of lens stock at a time, only the outermost portion of the generator wheel rim will be used. This will flatten that particular part of the wheel rim. As much lens material should be removed as possible with each sweep of the generator. This uses the diamond surface more evenly and also saves valuable time.

Another common mistake that causes excess, uneven wheel wear is the practice of separating jobs so that all jobs for one group of base curves are ground on one generator. Grinding only one lens curve (or even only one group of lens curves at a time) will also wear the wheel unevenly. Both of these practices will result in early wheel retrues, inaccurate lens curves, and undependable lens thicknesses.

More expensive, sophisticated, computer-controlled automatic generators have electronic wheel gauging, which measures the wear of the diamond cutting edge. This information is transmitted to the computer so that it can compensate for the wear. This compensation allows lenses to continue to be ground with correct curves and lens thicknesses.

Extending the Range of the Generator

The generator wheel is cup-shaped, and the circular rim of the cup has a given diameter. Half this diameter, or the radius of the circle, is one of the factors that limits the radius of curvature that can be ground on a lens surface. A smaller-diameter wheel will allow steeper curves to be cut on a lens. Yet if the lens blank is large, the smaller-diameter wheel sizes will not be large enough to grind the full surface of the lens. They would only grind the central area. Therefore, for larger lenses a larger wheel is needed. Unfortunately, the wheel may now cover the full surface of the lens but cannot cut the high curves. The lower range of curves is determined by the cutting range of the lens generator.

The larger the wheel size, the smaller the range of curves that can be generated. The curve ranges that correspond to each of the wheel sizes is shown in Table 10-4.

Changing Generator Wheel Size

Once a generator is calibrated for one particular wheel size, a (3½-inch wheel, for example), moving to a smaller wheel will throw the calibration off. Recalibrating the generator takes too long, and would have to be done over again when switching back to the larger wheel anyway. To simplify the process of going from a 3½-inch to, say, a 3-inch wheel, a chart for the smaller wheel can be made so that it will not be necessary to recalibrate. To make such a chart, cut a junk lens with a steep curve and leave it thick. Recut the lens for progressively flatter curves. After each cut, remeasure the curve to see what it actually is, compared to the generator setting. Write down the generator setting and the actual curves in the form of a table. This creates a compensation table that can be used for real lenses.

Remember that if the main 3½-inch wheel wears and the generator is recalibrated, the compensation chart for the 3-inch wheel will no longer be accurate.

One system used to help solve the back-curve range limitation quickly is to have a matched set of generator wheels. These wheels (usually three) have a known relationship to one another. They can be interchanged without having to produce a set of tables experimentally as was discussed earlier. It

should be noted that in order to maintain the correct curve relationship, if one tool is retrued then all three tools must be retrued.

There is an increasing demand to change wheels quickly and accurately. This is spurred not just by the need to extend the curve-power range of the generator. A number of smaller surfacing laboratories are using the same generator for both glass and plastic.

To meet this demand, Coburns' Quick Change Diamond System was developed. This system allows for alignment of the diamond wheels outside the generator, instead of having to adjust the generator itself. It requires replacing the quill in the generator and using a spirally designed stand gauge. Wheel change time, however, is dramatically reduced. This means that whereas it may previously have been necessary to use one diamond wheel for both glass and plastic, the advantages gained by using separate glass and plastic wheels may be possible for the laboratory with only one generator.

Using Coarse Lap Pads or Rough Emery

If the generator has a range from −3.00 D to −11.00 D, it may be possible to create a curve beyond this without changing generator wheels. For plastic lenses this is done by using a coarse fining pad and prefining the lens. With glass lenses a hand pan and rough emery may be used.

For plastic lenses, the pad chosen may be a coarse 400-grit brown pad, for example. Suppose the back curve calls for a −2.00 D surface. To create a −2.00 D surface, begin by generating a −3.00 D curve. Then, using a 2.00 D lap tool and a coarse-grit fining pad, fine the lens down to a −2.00 D curve. When the lens curve must be flattened, as in the just-described situation, the lens does not have to be cut any thicker than normal. See Figure 10-33. The pad grinds the lens from the outside inward, so if the curve is watched closely, no center thickness will be removed.

If, though, the curve must be steepened, then the pad begins grinding from the center outward. In this case, extra center thickness must be allowed. The rule of thumb is to allow 1.0 to 1.2 mm of extra thickness for every diopter that the lens surface must be steepened. See Figure 10-34. The larger the lens size, the greater is the thickness that must be allowed. For especially large lenses, do not hesitate to exceed the 1.2-mm recommendation. Extra lens stock can always be removed by additional fining with the rough-in pad.

Table 10-4 Relationship Between Generator Wheel Size and Curve Range

Wheel Size	Curve Range Upper Limit
2 inch	20.00 D
2½ inch	17.00 D
3 inch	14.00 D
3½ inch	11.00 D
4 inch	9.50 D

Figure 10-33 If a lens surface curve must be flattened, the flattening process begins at the sides and extends inward. Therefore, by the time the center is reached, the lens curve is already down to what it is supposed to be. No extra thickness needs to be allowed.

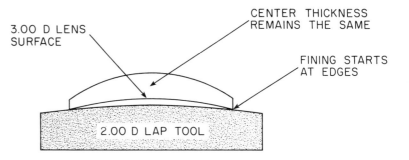

Figure 10-34 If a lens surface curve must be steepened, the steepening process begins at the center. Therefore, extra thickness must be allowed before the lens is generated. If this thickness is not allowed for, the lens will end up without enough thickness on the edge.

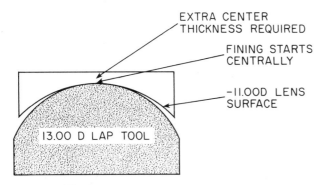

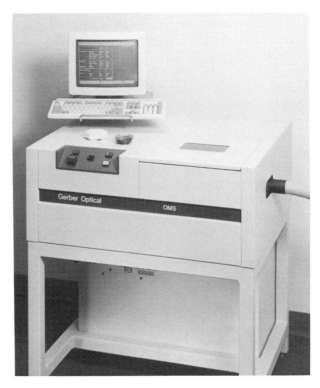

Figure 10-35 The Gerber Optical lens generator takes up little space and does not resemble a conventional generator. (Photo courtesy of Gerber Optical, a division of Gerber Scientific Products, South Windsor, Conn.)

EXAMPLE 10-3

Suppose that a 3½-inch generator wheel will grind up to a −11.00 D, but the back curve called for is a −12.50 D. You wish to surface the lens without changing to a 3-inch diameter wheel. The lens size is moderately large. How much extra center thickness should be included when generating so that the lens will not be too thin after having been changed from a −11.00 D to a −12.50 D curve?

SOLUTION

Since the lens size is moderately large, the full 1.2 mm of extra thickness should be allowed for each diopter the lens is steepened. Therefore, since the lens will be steepened 1.50 D, the extra thickness required will be

$$1.2 \text{ mm} \times 1.5 \text{ D} = 1.8 \text{ mm}$$

The lens must be generated 1.8 mm thicker than would otherwise have been needed with the −11.00 D back curve.

The Gerber Optical SG-8 Surface Generator

The Gerber Optical lens generator, shown in Figure 10-35, uses an entirely different type of surface cutting system. Instead of a generator wheel, a fluted spherical cutter is used. With the Gerber machine, not only does the cutting tool move during surfacing, the lens moves and rotates as well. See Figure

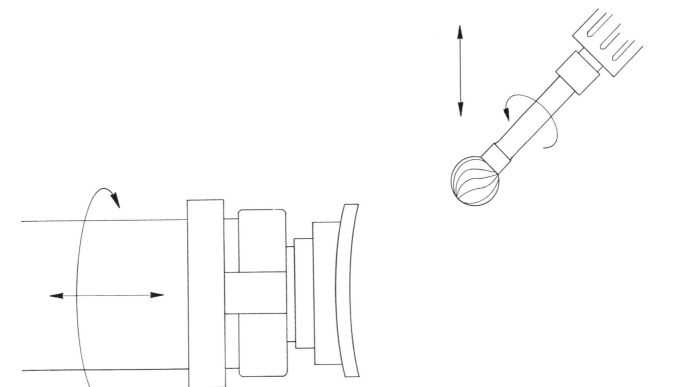

Figure 10-36 With both lens and tool moving, elliptical error does not become a problem with the Gerber Optical system. (Illustration courtesy of Gerber Optical, a division of Gerber Scientific Products, South Windsor, Conn.)

10-36. This innovative design overcomes the problem of elliptical error inherent in cup-shaped wheels.

Another unique feature of the Gerber generator is its ability to cut a disposable tool. See Figure 10-37. This tool, matched precisely to the lens surface, is used to fine and polish the lens. As an added bonus, the generator can retrue aluminum lap tools.

Specific Features of the Gerber Optical SG-8 Surface Generator

The Gerber SG-8 generator will cut from a −30.00 D to a +30.00 D surface, including a plano surface. It can cut up to 15 diopters of prism without prism rings and with no blocked-in prism. See Figure 10-38.

Blank Thinning

At times the edge of a particularly thick semifinished lens blank may interfere mechanically with

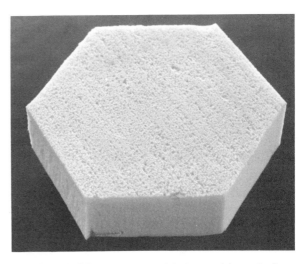

Figure 10-37 The disposable lap tool is made from a strong styrofoam material. (Photo courtesy of Gerber Optical, a division of Gerber Scientific Products, South Windsor, Conn.)

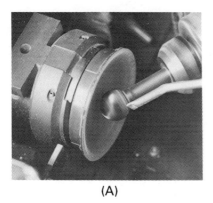

(A)

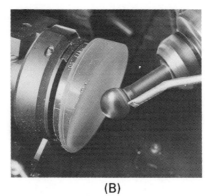

(B)

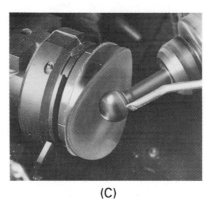

(C)

Figure 10-38 (A) Lenses cut using the fluted cutting wheel are cut cooler. Here a 1.5-mm polycarbonate lens is cut without the problem of thermal stress. (B) Because both the cutting tool and the lens move in all directions, lenses such as this plano-curve 10-diopter prism lens are feasible. (C) Prism is generated without marking the lens for prism or using a prism ring, even with high-toric surfaces as shown here. (Photo courtesy of Gerber Optical, a division of Gerber Scientific Products, South Windsor, Conn.)

the shaft of the cutting tool. From the information given to the SG-8's computer, interference is known in advance. To enable the lens to be surfaced, the machine can make a preliminary cut to thin the blank. If this means that the blank will not surface the curve out to the very edge, the CRT screen first tells the operator what the bowl diameter of the surfaced aperture will end up being. If this diameter is unacceptably small, the procedure can be stopped and the lens removed.

Safety Beveling

Some laboratories routinely safety-bevel the back of all lenses, or at least all plus lenses, to prevent the lens edge from tearing the fining and polishing pads. Gerber generators are capable of putting a safety bevel on the back of each generated lens blank automatically. The width of the bevel can be specified according to laboratory preference.

Cutting CR-39, Polycarbonate, and Other Plastic Lens Materials

The Gerber generator cuts conventional CR-39 lens material with a spherical carbide tool having 12 cutting surfaces. See Figure 10-39. The tool rotates at 22,000 rpm, making 400 cuts per second. Currently the depth of cut for one sweep is 8 mm for

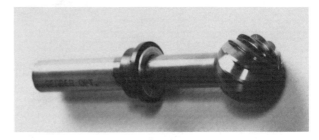

Figure 10-39 The tool used in the Gerber machine for grinding CR-39 lenses is not a cup, but rather a burr. (Photo courtesy of Gerber Optical, a division of Gerber Scientific Products, South Windsor, Conn.)

CR-39, 6 mm for high-index plastic, and 4 mm for polycarbonate. At present, carbide cutting tools last from 1000 to 2000 lens surfaces before they need retruing. A tool can be retrued up to three times.

The ideal tool for cutting polycarbonate is of somewhat different design. The polycarbonate tool has two cutting surfaces, or "flutes," instead of 12. See Figure 10-40. Polycarbonate lenses are cut at low temperature with this tool and, according to the manufacturer, are free from internal stresses. This is not to say that such stress reduction is of major significance when considering the impact resistance of the polycarbonate lens, although testing indicates that low-stress lenses contribute to increased lens coating quality.

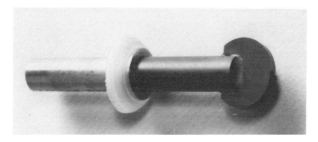

Figure 10-40 Because of the soft nature of polycarbonate, a cutter with fewer cutting surfaces is necessary. Cutting efficiency increases. (Photo courtesy of Gerber Optical, a division of Gerber Scientific Products, South Windsor, Conn.)

Cutting Disposable Laps

A disposable, uncut lap blank is referred to as a *lap master*. See Figure 10-41. Lap master blanks are made from hard styrofoam material.

Laboratories may prefer to use their own existing set of laps on CR-39 through a normal range of curves of 3 D to 8 D. Lap masters can be used outside that range and for all polycarbonate and high-index jobs. Polycarbonate and high-index lenses are typically generated to the hundredth of a diopter on the Gerber SG-8. Incentives for the continued use of disposable laps may be reduced, since existing laps can be trued on the generator to match lens curvature exactly. It should be remembered, however, that the advantage of disposable laps is not with ordinary low-powered CR-39 lens surfaces. Here are four examples of when disposable laps would be especially useful.

1. For special tools used only occasionally. Every lab has tools that are cut for just one job, then are recut and reused for the next special job. Disposable laps are ideal for such occasions.
2. For in-between curves in exacting situations. Existing tools are cut to every one-quarter or one-eighth diopter. If the curve called for is exactly in between, as in polycarbonate and high-index processing, such a tool would be useful.
3. For tools already in use.
4. For new laboratories where space may be a factor. There is then no need for tools, lap racks, or a tool cutter.

A handy use for the disposable tool presents itself when the existing tool is somewhere else, already

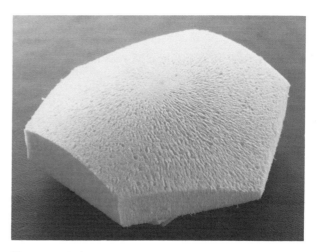

Figure 10-41 The lap master is placed in the generator and ground to match the generated lens exactly. (Photo courtesy of Gerber Optical, a division of Gerber Scientific Products, South Windsor, Conn.)

in use. By making a disposable tool, the job at hand does not have to wait but can be processed immediately.

Layout and Marking

Lens layout for the Gerber generator requires on-center blocking. And because the generator cuts prism at the power and angle specified by the operator, the lens need be marked only for cylinder axis. It does not need to be marked for prism.

Since the generator grinds prism for decentration automatically, it is essential that the lens not be blocked or chucked upside down. For this reason, one should mark the upper end of the axis line with an arrowhead as shown in Figure 10-42. Thereafter this arrowhead can serve as a directional orientation for blocking and chucking.

Blocking

The lens is blocked in the conventional manner, but with one small variation. The arrowhead that was placed on the upper end of the cylinder axis line should be pointing to the left. This is shown in Figure 10-43.

Conventional 43-mm glass-type blocks used in conjunction with 50 × 9 spacer rings work well with the Gerber generator. The generator also accepts large plastic blocks without spacer rings. If larger plastic blocks are used, the base curve of the lens

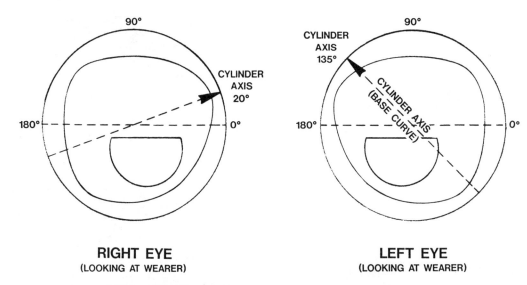

RIGHT EYE
(LOOKING AT WEARER)

LEFT EYE
(LOOKING AT WEARER)

Figure 10-42 Marking lenses for generating with the Gerber generator differs slightly from the procedure for conventional lenses. After marking the cylinder axis, an arrowhead is drawn on the upper end of the cylinder axis line. No prism axis is marked. (Courtesy of Gerber Optical, a division of Gerber Scientific Products, South Windsor, Conn.)

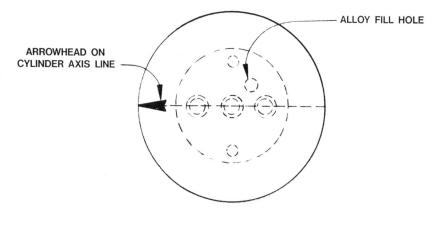

(VIEW FROM LENS SIDE)

Figure 10-43 The position of the arrowhead on the cylinder line becomes important during blocking and chucking. The arrowhead should be pointing left when blocking. It should point toward the operator when generating. (Courtesy of Gerber Optical, a division of Gerber Scientific Products, South Windsor, Conn.)

being generated must not vary from the amount marked on the block by more than 0.50 D. This is because "the height of the support ring at the rim of these blocks is increased from the standard 9 mm to compensate for the front curve of the lens."[11] In practice this means that for every 0.50 difference between block curve and actual lens base curve, finished lens thickness will be thrown off by 0.2 mm. It is possible for the SG-8 to compensate for base curve variations, but all base curve information must be accurately and completely input at the time.

Chucking

For chucking, the lens is oriented with the cylinder axis horizontal and the arrowhead pointing toward the operator, as shown in Figure 10-43. The block base goes into the chuck so that the generator pins slip into the holes in the block. This keeps the lens from slipping off axis.

The same rules as must be observed in chucking lenses for other, more conventional types of generators also apply with the Gerber generator. For example, Franklin-style or progressive lenses may rock if not held firmly. The fingers should press against the top of the lens in the distance portion. Allowing the lens to tip will cause unwanted prism.

The National Optronics Vista I Dry Generator

The Vista I generator is extremely compact, bench mounted, and on first glance could pass for a lens edger. See Figure 10-44. It uses a computer-controlled polycrystalline diamond (PCD) cutting tool capable of 3-axis movement. The Vista I virtually eliminates the problem of elliptical error. The curve range is 0 to -25 diopters with a 60- to 90-second cycle time. Although the National Optronics generator lacks many of the features of the Gerber generator, it cuts any plastic lens currently available, is innovative, versatile, lightweight, compact, and fast. It represents another viable option in the changing technology of lens surfacing.

Questions and Problems

1. When a coarse abrasive (between 100 and 400 microns) is used to create a lens surface with a lap tool and a hand pan, the process is called
   a. grating
   b. trueing
   c. smoothing
   d. roughing
   e. fining

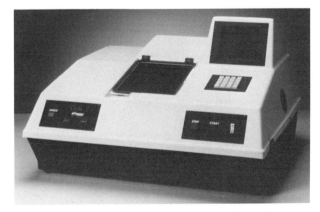

Figure 10-44 The Vista I Dry Generator is bench mounted, weighs 110 lbs and can cut CR-39, polycarbonate, and high-index plastic lenses. It uses a polycrystalline diamond cutter and comes with a vacuum system to keep the cutting chamber free of plastic debris. (Courtesy of National Optronics.)

2. Turning a cup so that the rim is viewed from an angle visually creates the effect of
   a. a parabola
   b. an ellipse
   c. a circle
   d. a sphere
   e. a cylinder

3. A certain CR-39 plastic semifinished lens blank is 12.5 mm thick. The lens that is to be ground should have a finished center thickness of 3.4 mm. How much stock removal is required at the generator?
   a. 3.4 mm
   b. 9.1 mm
   c. 9.4 mm
   d. 8.8 mm
   e. none of the above

4. When using a center thickness gauge to measure the center thickness of a blocked lens, the base curve of the lens
   a. has direct bearing on the final readout of the lens thickness.
   b. has no bearing on the final readout of the lens thickness.
   c. occasionally has a bearing on the final readout of the lens thickness.

5. When setting the back base and the cross curves on a generator, it is advisable always to approach the setting
   a. from the plus direction.
   b. from the minus direction.
   c. from the plus direction for base curve and the minus direction for cross curve.
   d. from either direction as long as both directions are the same and it is done consistently every time.
   e. It makes no difference.

6. In order to compensate for elliptical error when setting a generator, compensation is done
   a. only for the base curve
   b. only for the cross curve
   c. for both base and cross curves

7. Compensation of generator settings for elliptical error is done
   a. when cylinder values are small
   b. when cylinder values are moderate or large
   c. with all cylinders

8. When compensating generator settings for elliptical error
   a. the base curve is strengthened.
   b. the base curve is weakened.
   c. the cross curve is strengthened.
   d. the cross curve is weakened.
   e. both base and cross curves are strengthened.

9. In order to assure that the lens fines from the cen-

ter out, some laboratories set the generator base and cross curves
   a. slightly steeper than calculated values
   b. slightly flatter than calculated values

10. A different fiber ring is used for each base curve lens when generating glass lenses.
    True or False

11. Which of the following are zero-in gauges?
    a. a foursquare gauge
    b. a ball gauge
    c. a sag gauge
    d. a saddle gauge
    e. none of the above

12. On generators that require the use of a zero-in gauge, which part of the generator is moved forward until the lens is separated from the generator wheel by the thickness of the gauge?
    a. the quill
    b. the rotary table
    c. the ring
    d. the tailstock ram
    e. none of the above

13. In generating plastic lenses using an electroplated generator wheel, until the feel of the generator is achieved, how many points of stock removal per pass is it a good idea to begin with?
    a. 1 to 2 pts
    b. 10 to 20 pts
    c. 20 to 30 pts
    d. 30 to 40 pts
    e. 40 to 50 pts

14. A "point" is the same as
    a. 1/10th mm
    b. 1 mm
    c. 10 mm
    d. 2 mm
    e. none of the above

15. When a back cut is used, it is for the purpose of
    a. keeping the lens from having generator marks
    b. keeping the edge of the lens from breaking off
    c. keeping the surface smooth
    d. increasing the life of the generator wheel

16. All but one of the following are disadvantages of using oil as a generator coolant. Which one does not belong?
    a. Oil-based coolants are a fire hazard.
    b. Oil-based coolants are messy to work with.
    c. Oil-based coolants are more expensive than water-based coolants.
    d. Oil-based coolants present a waste disposal problem.
    e. Oil-based coolants have a tendency to foam.

17. Which is the least effective system for keeping coolant clean?
    a. a settling tank
    b. a centrifuge
    c. a filtration system

18. Even though a refrigeration unit does not come with a generator when purchased, coolant refrigeration is necessary in order to generate all types of lenses.
    True or False

19. Which products may reduce skin reactions to the generator coolant?
    a. Kerodex
    b. Lysol
    c. vinegar
    d. Cepacol
    e. none of the above

20. Which procedures can lead to uneven wheel wear and thus decrease wheel life?
    a. Removing large amounts of lens stock all at once
    b. Taking only small amounts of lens stock off with each pass
    c. Grouping together all lenses that have the same back curve

21. The amount of extra thickness needed during generating to allow for thickness loss during fining and polishing is the same amount for all lens materials.
    True or False

22. At the present time, generating a polycarbonate lens "wet" is preferred over the dry method.
    True or False

23. Explain how a 3-inch generator wheel can be used when the generator has been calibrated for a 3½-inch wheel. What might be done to ensure that the correct curves result?

24. Toothed PCD fly cutter wheels can be retrued.
    True or False

25. Prism rings are marked according to prism dioptric values. These values are independent of the index of refraction of the material and can be used for glass, plastic, or high-index materials.
    True or False

26. Generating of polycarbonate lenses can be done with the same generator wheel as is used for standard plastic lenses, as long as regular CR-39 lenses are interspersed between polycarbonate, so that the wheel does not begin to "load" with ground-up polycarbonate material.
    True or False

27. Generator wheels intended for polycarbonate can be used to generate standard CR-39 plastic lenses.
    True or False

28. As generator wheel size becomes smaller, the dioptric range of curves that can be cut

a. increases

b. decreases

c. stays the same

29. As the size of the generator wheel becomes smaller, the lens blank size that may be generated

a. increases

b. decreases

c. stays the same

30. The Gerber Optical SG-8 surface generator cannot cut which lens material(s)?

a. Glass.

b. CR-39 plastic.

c. Polycarbonate.

d. High-index plastic.

e. The SG-8 can cut all of the above lens materials.

31. The SG-8 generator works best with disposable laps and should not be used in conjunction with aluminum laps.

True or False

32. When using the SG-8 generator, the lens should be marked for both cylinder axis and prism axis as with other lens generators.

True or False

33. The SG-8 generator can cut a plano curve.

True or False

References

1. Bennett, A. G. Basic Manufacturing Optics, Part 2, Ophthalmic Lens Production. *Manufacturing Optics International,* February 1974, p. 69.

2. Acknowledgment to Don Adams, Coburn Optical, Jill Mattingly and Sharon Hamontree, Indiana University Optical Laboratory.

3. Nova Communications, Inc. *Lens Learning System.* Tetmus Optical, Petersburg, Va., 1976, p. 82.

4. *How to Surface Lenses Made from CR-39 Monomer for Prescription Eyewear,* 3rd ed., PPG Industries, Pittsburgh, Pa., 1981.

5. *Titmus Polycristyl™ Comprehensive Processing Guide for Polycarbonate Lenses.* Titmus Optical Co., Petersburg, Va., p. 3.

6. *Thin & Lite 1.6 High-Index Lenses Technical Guide,* Silor Optical, St. Petersburg, Fla, 1990, p. 5.

7. *PSI Technical Bulletin 1102-A.* PSI, Tarpon Springs, Fla., Undated.

8. Horne, *Spectacle Lens Technology,* Adam Hilger, Bristol, England, 1978, p. 172.

9. *Coburn Optical Industries Operation and Maintenance Manual, Manual and Semi-Automatic Generators.* Coburn Optical Industries, Muskogee, Okla., Series 108, undated, p. 11.

10. Product information sheet. CDP Diamond Products, Inc., Livonia, Mich., undated.

11. *SG-8 Surface Generator User's Manual,* Gerber Optical, South Windsor, Conn., March 14, 1989, Document no. 104761, Version B.10.

11 Lap Tools

Introduction

Once a lens has been generated, it must be fined and polished. In order to do the fining and polishing, an identically shaped tool surface is needed on which the lens can be worked. Tools that are used for this purpose are called *lap tools*.

There are two basic types of lap tools. One type is used for processing spherical surfaces only. These are used with sphere machines. A *sphere machine* turns a tool rapidly on a spindle. The blocked lens is held against the tool with a single pin. This allows both the lens and the tool to spin so that the lens surface may be smoothed or polished. See Figure 11-1.

Tools that are used with sphere machines are either mushroom tools or hollow tools. *Mushroom tools* resemble a mushroom and have a convex surface. They are used for the purpose of grinding concave spherical surfaces. *Hollow tools* are concave and are used for grinding convex (usually front) spherical surfaces.

In the past, spherical lens surfaces were ground exclusively on sphere machines using sphere tools, and toric surfaces were ground on cylinder machines. Now, instead of using sphere machines to grind spherical surfaces, most laboratories use cylinder machines, as shown in Figure 11-2. Cylinder machines were not used before because the motion of the machine would not produce a good spherical surface.

Cylinder machines use another type of lap tool. This tool does not have a stem. Instead it clamps

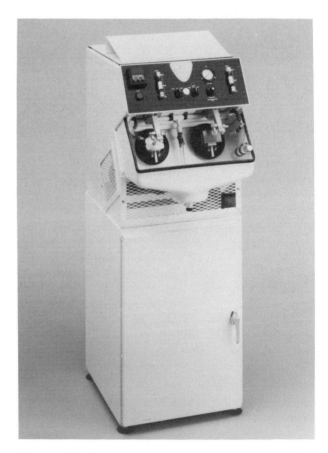

Figure 11-2 The cylinder machine holds the lens against the lap so that it does not rotate. Both the tool and the lens move in complex patterns. The motion is designed to assure an even fine and polish across the entire lens surface. (Photo courtesy FB Optical, St. Cloud, Minn.)

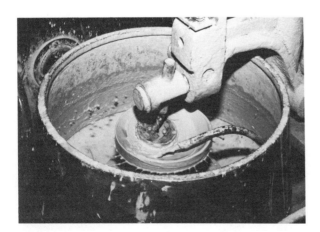

Figure 11-1 Sphere machines move the rapidly spinning lens back and forth on the rotating sphere tool.

into place on the machine. See Figure 11-3. The surface of the tool is toric (which means that it has two different curves) and will produce a lens with a cylinder component in the prescription.

Tool Materials

In the past, lap tools were made only of cast iron. When lenses were made exclusively from glass, all steps preceding lens polishing were performed directly on the bare surface of the cast-iron lap tool. With the advent of metal pads, which are placed directly on the surface of the tool, however, tools made from softer materials could be used.

Speeding the decline of the cast-iron tool was the plastic lens. Because cast iron rusts, pieces of rust could contaminate the polish, increasing the risk of lens scratching for the softer, more vulnerable plastic lens. This necessitated the use of other materials.

Aluminum can be successfully used for lap tools, as long as the tool is padded so that the lens does not rub directly against the lap surface. Aluminum is too soft to allow for lens grinding directly on the tool. The tool would wear quickly and unevenly.

Aluminum has several advantages over cast iron:

1. It has greater dimensional stability than cast iron and is less liable to warp.
2. It can be trued* much more quickly on the lap cutter.
3. It conducts heat away from the lens more quickly, an important factor when surfacing plastic lenses.[1]

In an attempt to develop an even lighter and less costly tool, hard resin was introduced. The lightness of the material adds to the lifetime of lens cylinder surfacing machinery and the lap cutters used to give the tool its curve. The major problem with first generation lap tools made exclusively from hard resin was that they would flex or bend somewhat. Flexing would occur when the tool was being clamped to have its surface cut. After cutting, when the tool was removed from the lap cutter, it would flex back. Then the curve would no longer be the same as it was.

Another possibility for error occurred during fin-

Trueing a lap tool refers to recutting the surface after it has become worn and lost the correct curve. *Lap cutting* is the generating of new curves on a semifinished tool or changing the curve on an existing tool.

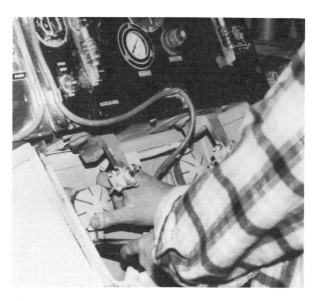

Figure 11-3 The toric tool is used to smooth a lens surface with cylinder power. Both lens and tool move in a complex pattern, but neither will rotate. The axis of the cylinder must remain horizontal.

ing. The tool may have been cut as it should have been, but when it was clamped solidly into place on a cylinder surfacing machine, the tool flexed and the curve was distorted. Thus, in spite of recent efforts that have largely overcome many of these difficulties, laps made exclusively from hard resin are not as popular as might be anticipated.

A solution that has proven acceptable for many has been the metal resin combination lap. Mixing finely shredded or ground aluminum with an epoxy resin material adds the stability to the tool that is required if it is to withstand the rigors of tool clamping and lens surfacing.

Metal/resin laps cut much more easily on lap cutters. They make high-speed lap cutters even more efficient. In addition, they are half the weight of aluminum tools.

For truly high performance and durability in maintaining correct surface curves on lens after lens, diamond-impregnated lap tools are outstanding. Yet because of the very large number of tools required, cost makes using this option prohibitive for surfacing laboratories. For lens blank manufacturers who must produce surface after surface of exactly the same curvature, diamond tools are the method of choice. High production volume offsets the otherwise prohibitive costs.

Diamond tools can be made in one of two ways:

1. The entire surface may be impregnated with diamond material. When the lens surface is smoothed, high pressure is required, but the curve produced is reliable, lens after lens.
2. Diamond "buttons" may be mounted on the surface of the tool. Once the small, round buttons are in place, the tool is trued. (Actually the buttons are trued, not the tool itself.) Lens smoothing takes place directly on the button surface. This means that the process does not require operating pressures as high as those needed for solid surface diamond-impregnated tools.

Diamond tools give a much more consistent curve on the lenses because the laps do not wear like cast iron or metal padded tools. Because the abrasive is "in the tool," slurry problems are reduced.

Brass Lap Gauges

As mentioned when discussing tools made from cast iron, glass fining (smoothing) has been and can be done on the bare tool. However, this results in rapid wearing of the tool, causing it to be out of true. In order to check tools to see if they are correct or not, a set of standard *brass lap gauges* can be used. See Figure 11-4. In using a lap gauge, the following procedure should be followed:

1. Choose the gauge having the correct curve and hold it against the tool.

2. Hold the lap gauge straight up and down (perpendicular to the tool) for an accurate reading.
3. Hold both tool and lap gauge in front of a light source. If the tool allows light to pass at the edges or in the center, the tool must be retrued. See Figure 11-5.

Sphere tools can be retrued by hand. The tool is placed on the spindle in a hand pan. Either a *trueing disk* or a *trueing stick* can be used. If the trueing stick is used, it is held against the spinning tool and drawn across the area where the lap tool needs to be shaved down. If a trueing disk is used, it is held in place by the pin on the arm of the hand pan. This is done just as if the trueing disk were a lens. See Figure 11-6. The area of the tool to be ground off is worked with the disk. There are two types of disks. One is made for a plus surface, the other for a minus.

One helpful hint that has been offered for those using mushroom and hollow sphere tools to obtain better accuracy is to rub freshly cut plus and minus tool surfaces together with a fine abrasive between the pair until a perfect match is obtained.

Brass gauges can also be used to check each of the two curves of a toric tool. The correct brass lap gauge is held up to the base curve (the long dimension of the tool). A second brass gauge is used to check the cross curve (the short dimension of the

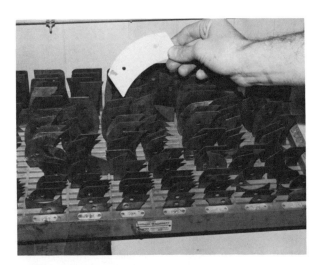

Figure 11-4 Lap gauges come as sets and allow visual evaluation of a tool across its entire surface.

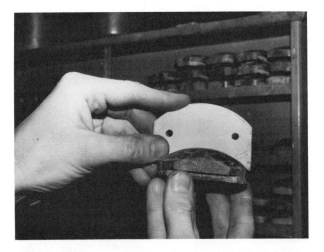

Figure 11-5 When checking the curvature of a lap tool with a lap gauge, there can be no gap between the center of the tool and the center of the gauge. Neither can the gauge touch in the center only. Note that the curvature of the tool is being checked with the metal pad in place.

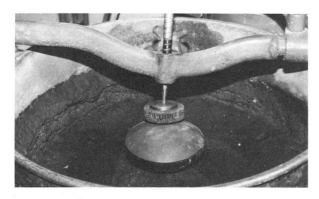

Figure 11-6 A trueing disk is used together with the hand pan. It is handled in the same way as a lens that is being hand-surfaced. A hollow or concave tool is trued using a convex disk. The mushroom or convex tool shown here is trued using a concave disk.

tool). Brass gauges can be used even on tools that have metal pads, although unevenness of pad wear will usually be enough to indicate that the tool is going out of true.

Lap Scoring

Tools with toric surfaces are trued on a lap cutter. If the lens is being fined without a pad on the tool, the tool is *scored*. A tool that has been scored has a number of grooves cut into the surface of the tool at regular intervals. The purpose of the grooves is to allow the slurry to flow under the lens more easily.

A secondary benefit of scoring is that it allows a person to know quickly if the tool needs retrueing. A scored tool that needs retrueing will show a difference in the depth of the grooves. When using scored cast-iron lap tools, a person may expect to surface approximately six lenses before the tool needs to be retrued.

Tools may be scored diagonally, in a criss-crossed fashion, or with score marks perpendicular to the long axis of the tool. See Figure 11-7. Tools may be scored by hand, using a vise to hold the tool in place, and a file. Or they may be scored with a scoring device, such as the Score-O-Matic. The reader must remember that, although lap scoring and bare tool grinding can give excellent optical results, it is very labor-intensive and in the long run will be quite expensive.

Metal Padding

When fining glass lenses on aluminum or other soft laps, the lap surface must be protected. Therefore the tool is padded with a metal or foil pad. The metal pad practically eliminates the need for re-trueing. Pads vary considerably in design, from screen meshes to solid. Some are covered with small holes, while others are shaped like daisies. See Figure 11-8. Pads must be either glued onto the tool or attached with their own adhesive backing. In either case they must be pressed under extremely high pressure using a pad press. Assuming that good-quality metal pads are used, one may expect to surface approximately ten lenses with the tool before it needs to be repadded. Metal pads may be either glued to the tool or are self-adhesive.

Glueing on Pads

To glue on pads, the pads are first placed on wax paper. Next an adhesive is brushed on the pad and on the lap surface. See Figure 11-9. The pad is placed on the tool and allowed to sit. See Figure 11-10.

Before putting the tool and pad in the pad press, talcum powder is sprinkled liberally into the press where the tool will be placed. See Figure 11-11. The tool is put in the press upside down so that when excess glue is squeezed out from between the

Figure 11-7 Whenever lenses are fined directly on a bare cast-iron cylinder lap tool, the tool must be scored. Tool may be scored perpendicular to the long axis (left), or diagonally in a criss-cross fashion (right).

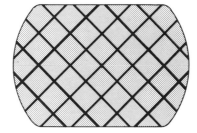
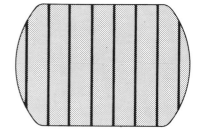

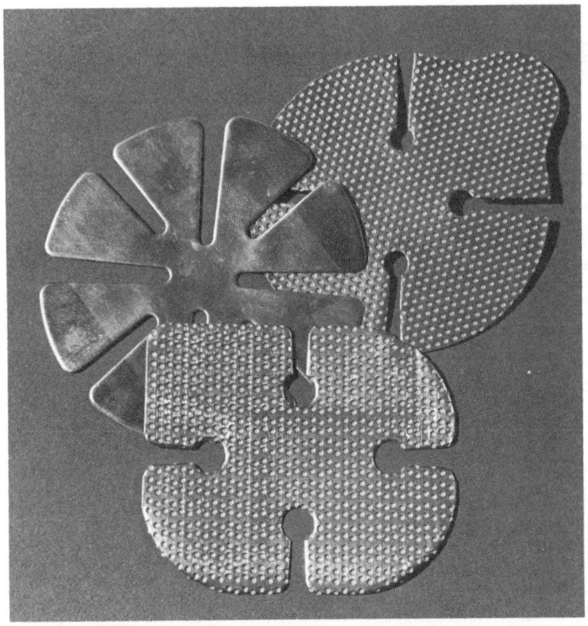

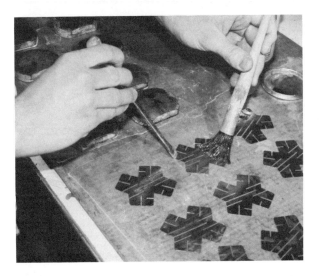

Figure 11-8 Metal lap pads, used in fining glass lenses, come in a variety of configurations. A few samples are shown here.

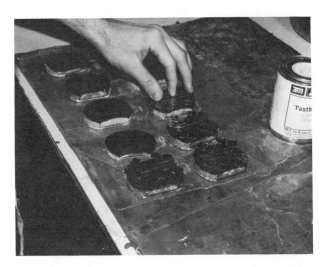

Figure 11-10 After glueing, the pads are placed on the tool in preparation for pressing. Using a self-adhesive pad is mush faster, especially when only a few tools need to be padded.

Figure 11-9 Using metal pads that are not self-adhesive means that the adhesive must first be brushed on the pad, then on the tool.

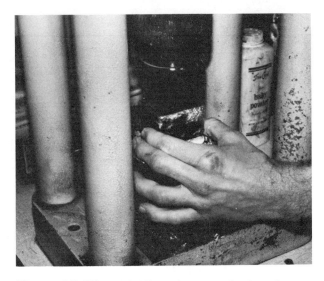

Figure 11-11 Sprinkling talcum powder into the pad press helps absorb excess glue, saving clean-up time. Regular talc or baby powder works well. Here the tool is placed in the press upside down against a hard, compressible pad.

pad and the lap tool, it will not "goop up" the press. Once the lap tool has been placed in the press, the press is activated and begins to squeeze the tool onto the metal pad against a thick, hard, but compressible, resilient pad. See Figure 11-12. Opinions

vary about how much pressure is needed, ranging from 1800 to 7000 pounds per square inch. The higher the pressure, the better the pad will stay in place. However, it may also be more difficult to remove later. The excess glue is cleaned from the

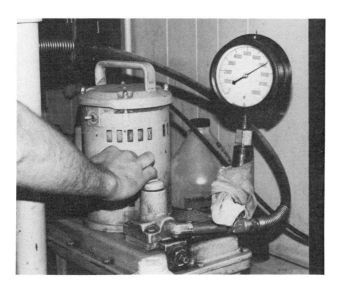

Figure 11-12 The pressure achieved with a press used for applying metal lap pads is much higher than the smaller press used for applying plastic lens fining pads.

tool with a solvent such as lacquer thinner. Tools padded with non-self-adhesive pads should be allowed to sit an hour or so before using.

Adhesive-Backed Pads

Self-adhesive pads may cost somewhat more, but they are much less messy to deal with. The backing is stripped from the pad and the pad is placed on the tool. It is pressed into place in the pad press in exactly the same manner as the glue-on type. Talc is also used in the press, but not in as great a quantity.

Determining When a Tool Is Out of True

It is usually possible to tell when a tool is beginning to wear just by looking at the tool.

Inspecting Scored Tools for Uneven Wear

When glass lenses are being fined directly on a scored tool surface, the scores on the tool will begin to become more shallow. They will not wear away evenly, but rather the outer portions of the tool will wear first. This makes the outer scores more shallow than the central scores and resembles unevenly worn tire treads. Uneven wear can cause the cylinder power to become too strong.

Inspecting Metal-Padded Tools for Uneven Wear

When the lap is protected by a metal pad, the pad may show wear in one of the following ways.

1. If the pad is solid (with no holes or daisy petals), the edge of the pad will become extremely thin in certain areas.
2. If the pad is dotted with small holes, the depth of the holes near the edges will become more shallow than the centrally located holes.
3. If the pad is daisy shaped, the outer areas of some of the daisy edges may visibly thin.

In all of the above cases the pad needs replacing. If visibly worn pads are not replaced in a timely manner, both freshly ground lens *and* pad must be replaced.

Atypical Wearing of Pads or Laps

If tools or tool pads are showing more wear in a slightly oblique direction instead of 90–180, the generator or cylinder machines should be checked for the accuracy of their axis setting.

Removing Worn Metal Pads

Adhesive-backed pads can be stripped from a lap tool using a paring knife. See Figure 11-13. Any remaining adhesive that still sticks to the tool is removed using a solvent.

Pads that have been glued in place can be removed most easily if they are first soaked overnight in lacquer thinner. The next day the pads will come off easily. Some laboratories tape the lap with lens surface-saver tape before applying the pad. This makes the metal pad much easier to strip from the lap.

How Tools Are Marked

Because lens surfaces are specified in diopters, lap tools are marked in diopters of power. Yet dioptric power depends on the refractive index of the lens material and the radius of curvature of the surface (*r*). It can be seen that if lap tools are marked in diopters, the power marked is index specific. It will give the refractive power marked only if it is used to grind a lens having the right refractive index. That is, if a tool is to be used for crown glass of

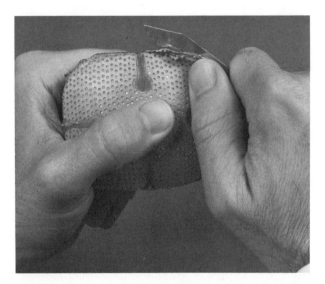

Figure 11-13 Stripping a self-adhesive pad from a tool can be a difficult job. The knife used need not (in fact, should not) be very sharp.

index 1.523, then for the tool to grind a curve that will yield that refractive power every time, it must be cut so that, for the equation

$$D = \frac{n - 1}{r}$$

the refractive index n is 1.523. In the United States, however, this is *not* the way lap tools are marked. Instead they are marked using a reference refractive index of 1.53.*

In optical laboratories in the United States, all instruments that are calibrated to read surface powers in diopters assume an index of 1.53. The index 1.53 is very close to the refractive index of crown glass (1.523). This means that when grinding crown-glass lens surfaces of low powers, tools will grind exactly as marked. However, when crown-glass lens surface powers are high (or when a lens material of a different refractive index is used), compensation must be made to make the lens grind right.

To summarize, tools are marked as if they were grinding 1.53-index material. These markings are reference markings and cannot be expected always to yield these refractive powers for all types of

lenses.† Compensations are made according to procedures discussed in Chapter 7.

Relationship Between Radius of Curvature and Dioptric Power

As has been mentioned, the relationship between the dioptric surface power and the radius of curvature of the surface also depends on the refractive index of the material. This relationship is

$$D = \frac{n' - n}{r}$$

where D is the dioptric surface power, r is the radius of curvature of the surface in meters, n' is the refractive index of the lens material, and n is the refractive index of the surround. Air is the surround and its refractive index is 1. So

$$D = \frac{n' - 1}{r}$$

Since there is only one n in the equation, the prime (') is normally dropped and the equation becomes

$$D = \frac{n - 1}{r}$$

This formula requires that the radius of curvature, r, be in meters. It is really easier to work with millimeters than meters. To make it possible to work in millimeters, the formula can be written

$$D = \frac{(n - 1) \times 1000}{r}$$

For the lap tool this is

$$D = \frac{(1.53 - 1) \times 1000}{r}$$

$$= \frac{530}{r}$$

EXAMPLE 11-1

If we want a tool with a surface dioptric power of 6.00 D, what radius of curvature should the tool have?

---

*In Britain and some British Commonwealth countries, tools are cut to a 1.523 index. However, because so much 1.530-calibrated equipment is manufactured, those using 1.523-indexed tools need to be sure of how their equipment is calibrated.

†Once the surface is ground, however, it will yield the value marked on the tool if the tool has been compensated correctly and the lens has been measured with a lens clock. The lens clock, like most laboratory equipment made for measuring lens surfaces, is also calibrated for an index of 1.53.

SOLUTION

The answer is quick to find, since we have only one unknown, namely, *r*. We know that

$$D = \frac{(n - 1) \times 1000}{r}$$

We also know that this is the same as

$$r = \frac{(n - 1) \times 1000}{D}$$

For our example, *D* = 6.00 D and *n* = 1.53. The equation now reads

$$r = \frac{(1.53 - 1) \times 1000}{6}$$

$$= 83.3 \text{ mm}$$

So the tool radius of curvature needed is 83.3 mm.

Most Tools Are Used with a Pad

Most of the time, lap tools are padded for grinding and polishing operations. The use of metal pads for glass fining has already been mentioned. During the glass polishing operation, a soft polishing pad is placed on top of the metal pad.

For fining plastic, usually an abrasive first fine pad is attached to the surface of a tool. Then a second, somewhat less abrasive pad is placed over the first pad, giving two thicknesses. Lastly, *both* these pads are peeled off and a polishing pad is pressed onto the tool to polish the lens. The polishing pad has a thickness equal to the two fining pads combined.

Polishing pads may perform better when pressed onto the tool with a pad press. The press is smaller and easier to use than the one used for metal pads. See Figure 11-14. Polishing pads that are pressed on will be smoother and will not cause the lens to "wave" as easily. (Waviness can be due to an unevenness in the surface of the lens.) Many laboratories also press first fine pads on the tool for better adherence and a smoother surface.

Pads Change the Power of the Lap Tool

Fining and polishing pads have a definite, measurable thickness. This thickness changes the radius of curvature of the lap surface. What this means is that

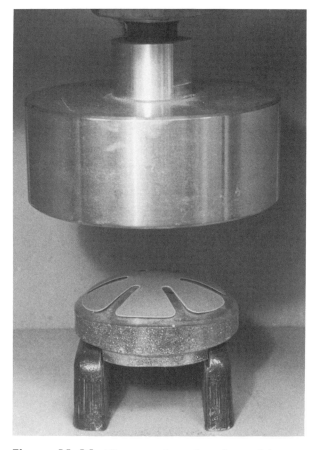

Figure 11-14 The press shown here for applying nonmetal pads to laps works quickly and easily. It cannot do the job of a metal pad press, nor can the more cumbersome metal pad press substitute on this light-duty work.

the radius of curvature of the lap tool is different with a pad on than it was without a pad.

For example, suppose a polishing pad used for plastic lenses has a thickness of 0.018 inches (0.4572 mm). With the polishing pad in place, the radius of curvature of the tool will change by 0.018 inches. If this change is not taken into account, the power of the lens may not come out as expected. The curve of the tool must be cut so that with the lap pad in place, the final curvature of the padded tool will be correct. Tools that are cut to allow for pad thickness are called *compensated tools*. Tools that do not allow for pad thickness are called *uncompensated tools*.

Calculating Tool Curves

The machine used to cut the needed curve on a lap tool is called a *lap cutter*. Most lap cutters have base* and cross-curve scales marked in diopters and indexed for 1.53. Other lap cutters have base and cross-curve scales in millimeters of radius of curvature. Although lap cutters can usually be ordered with either a diopter or a millimeter scale, most people prefer that the scale be in diopters because they are more familiar with this system.

Relation Between Diopters and Radius of Curvature

EXAMPLE 11-2

Suppose a lap cutter has a base and cross-curve scale marked in millimeters. If the tool is not being compensated for pad thickness, how should the radius of curvature of the lap cutter be set in order to cut a -10.00 D surface?

SOLUTION
Use the equation

$$r = \frac{(n - 1) \times 1000}{D}$$

Since the tool is 1.53-indexed, $n = 1.53$. D is -10.00 D. So the equation for the problem is

$$r = \frac{(1.53 - 1) \times 1000}{10}$$

$$= 53 \text{ mm}$$

In practice, a calculator, a computer, or a set of tables would be used rather than this "long-hand" calculation. Not all lap cutters require radius of curvature. Lap cutters can be ordered with either a radius of curvature or a diopter scale. If the lap cutter scale is in diopters, the scale is simply set for -10.00 D.

Determining Compensated Tool Curves for Radius of Curvature in Millimeters

If a tool is to be padded, the thickness of the pads that will be used must be known before the tool can be cut. For plastic lenses fined using a two-step process, the amount of thickness that must be allowed for is the first fine pad thickness plus the second fine pad thickness.

---

*Technically we are speaking of *back* base curve here.

EXAMPLE 11-3

A tool is needed that will fine and polish a -10.00 D surface.

The lab is using fining pads with a total thickness of 0.018 inch for the first and second pads. Assume that the lap cutter scale is marked for radius of curvature in millimeters. What must the radius of curvature of the compensated tool be so that, when the fining pads are in place, the tool will grind a -10.00 D surface?

SOLUTION
We first need to know what the radius of the tool and pad combined will be. If no pads are used, the tool will be uncompensated. Its radius will equal the radius of a compensated tool, plus pad thickness. In Example 11-2 we determined the *uncompensated* tool curve for a -10.00 D surface. The uncompensated tool's radius of curvature was found to be 53 mm.

To find the *compensated* radius for the tool we need to remember that *for convex tools, the uncompensated tool curve radius equals the compensated tool curve radius plus the pad thickness.* See Figure 11-15. Expressed as an equation,

$$r_{(uncomp)} = r_{(comp)} + t_{(pad)}$$

We need to know the pad thickness in millimeters, but it is given in inches. Since 1 inch equals 2.54 cm (or 25.4 mm), 0.018 inch equals 0.4572 or 0.46 mm. Referring back to Figure 11-15 and the above equation, we see that since the uncompensated radius is 53 mm and the pad thickness is 0.4572 mm,

$$53 \text{ mm} = r_{(comp)} + 0.46 \text{ mm}$$

Written another way,

$$r_{(comp)} = 53 \text{ mm} - 0.46 \text{ mm}$$
$$= 52.54 \text{ mm}$$

The compensated tool must be ground more steeply to allow for the pad thickness. Instead of being ground for 53 mm, the tool should be ground with a radius of curvature of 52.54 mm.

Determining Compensated Tool Curves in Diopters

As seen in the previous section, compensating a *convex* tool to work a concave lens surface means cutting it with a *shorter* radius. In terms of diopters, this means cutting a *steeper* curve with a *stronger* dioptric value. *Convex tools are steepened to compensate for pad thickness.*

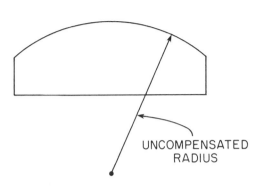
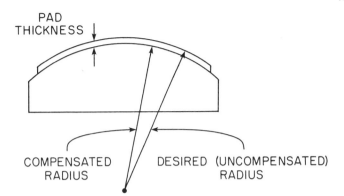

Figure 11-15 The tool on the left is uncompensated. The tool on the right has a shorter radius of curvature and is compensated so that, with a pad in place, $r_{(comp)} = r_{(uncomp)} - t_{(pad)}$.

Now let us consider how a compensated tool curve is calculated in 1.53-referenced diopters.

EXAMPLE 11-4

For the −10.00 D surface in Example 11-3, what is the compensated tool curve expressed in diopters instead of millimeters? Use the same pad thickness.

SOLUTION

In order to find the new compensated tool's dioptric value, we must use the compensated tool radius found in Example 11-3. The radius in millimeters for the compensated tool is 52.54 mm. We use the same lensmaker's formula,

$$D = \frac{(n - 1) \times 1000}{r}$$

So now the equation becomes

$$D = \frac{(1.53 - 1) \times 1000}{52.54}$$
$$= 10.09 \text{ D}$$

To cut the tool for this pad thickness, the lap cutter is set at 10.09 D.

Fortunately, there are both tables and computer programs that tell what compensated powers to use for each pad thickness. An example of such a table is found in the appendix as Appendix 5-1. It is considerably easier to use a table than to calculate each tool individually. Some lap cutter dials are also designed so that compensation can be made right on the dial. See Figure 11-16.

Uncompensated Tools

Some laboratories already have a complete set of tools. If these tools are uncompensated for pad thickness, using a pad may cause the power to be off. When *un*compensated tools are used *with* pads, all convex tools will give slightly weaker powers than what they are marked. Fortunately, tables (or layout computers) can be used to help choose the best tool.

EXAMPLE 11-5

Consider again the example we have been using of a lens with a −10.00 D surface. What uncompensated tool should be chosen when using a pad thickness of 0.018 inch?

SOLUTION

Using the 0.018-inch pad, either calculate or look up in Appendix 5.1 to see what power should be chosen. That tool is a 10.09 D tool.* If the uncompensated tools on hand are cut in 0.12 D steps, the closest uncompensated tool is a 10.12 D tool. Padding this tool causes it to be 0.09 D flatter. The padded tool now smooths (fines) the lens to a 10.03 D power. This is very close to the desired −10.00 D surface.

The −10.00 D surface example is for a lens with a fairly steep back surface and a short radius of curvature. A flat surface will have a longer radius of curvature. This

---

*We are really trying to find the *un*compensated tool that is closest to what *would* be cut if we were going to make a *compensated* tool.

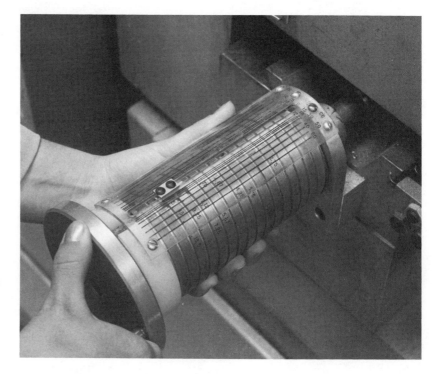

Figure 11-16 When cutting lap tools, tool compensation can be done directly, without using tables. When this is done, the actual curve power is not known. Therefore, when lap tool curves are checked with the sag gauge, either the compensated power must be looked up, or compensated sag charts must be used.

means that for surfaces that are very flat, an uncompensated tool will most likely work, even if it is padded.

Summary: Compensating for Pad Thickness

The easiest situation is to decide what pads will be used and compensate the tool accordingly. Following is a summary of the steps to be taken in determining the required compensated tool curve.

1. Decide what pads will be used and determine how thick they are. For glass lenses the thickness will be the total pad thickness at fining. Ask yourself: "How thick is the metal pad I will be using?" For plastic lenses the thickness will be the total pad thickness at the second fine. Ask yourself: "How thick are the first and second fining pads combined?"
2. Convert this thickness from inches to millimeters, if necessary.
3. Find the uncompensated tool curve radius using the lensmaker's formula:

$$r_{(uncomp)} = \frac{(1.53 - 1) \times 1000}{D}$$

4. Find the compensated tool curve radius needed. Since

$$r_{(uncomp)} = r_{(comp)} + t_{(pad)}$$

find the *compensated* tool curve radius by subtracting the pad thickness from the *uncompensated* tool curve radius:

$$r_{(comp)} = r_{(uncomp)} - t_{(pad)}$$

5. Now change back to dioptric power using the lensmaker's formula again:

$$D_{(comp)} = \frac{(1.53 - 1) \times 1000}{r_{(comp)}}$$

EXAMPLE 11-6
As an example of how this works, what compensated tool curve should be cut for a 7.00 D convex tool if the total pad thickness to be used is 0.022 inches?

SOLUTION
Step 1. The pad thickness is 0.022 inch.
Step 2. Converting the pad thickness from inches to millimeters,

$$\frac{1 \text{ inch}}{25.4 \text{ mm}} = \frac{0.022 \text{ inch}}{\text{pad thickness in millimeters}}$$

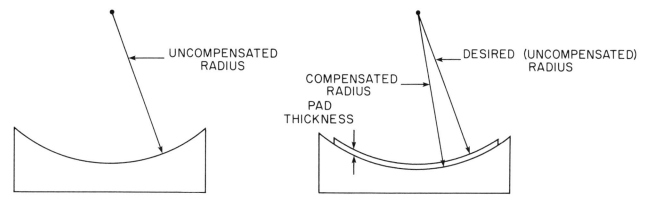

Figure 11-17 The concave tool on the left is uncompensated for pad thickness. The tool on the right has a *longer* radius of curvature, so when the pad is added to the tool, $r_{(comp)} = r_{(uncomp)} + t_{(pad)}$.

Pad thickness in millimeters is $t_{(pad)}$:

$$t_{(pad)} = \frac{(0.022)(25.4)}{1}$$

$$= 0.56 \text{ mm}$$

Step 3. Pad thickness is 0.56 mm. To find the uncompensated tool curve radius, use the lensmaker's formula,

$$r_{(uncomp)} = \frac{(1.53 - 1) \times 1000}{7}$$

$$= 75.71 \text{ mm}$$

Step 4. Now find the compensated tool curve radius:

$$r_{(comp)} = r_{(uncomp)} - t_{(pad)}$$
$$= 75.71 - 0.56$$
$$= 75.15 \text{ mm}$$

Step 5. Reconverting to diopters for tool-cutting purposes:

$$D_{(comp)} = \frac{(1.53 - 1) \times 1000}{75.15 \text{ mm}} = 7.05 \text{ D}$$

Thus, for a tool having an 0.022-inch pad, the lap cutter should be set for 7.05 D. It is necessary to know how tool curves are derived, but it is safer to use tables or a computer. The same result can be obtained using a precalculated table, reducing the risk of making a simple mathematical error.

Note: If a laboratory is using uncompensated tools, the tool *closest* to the uncompensated value should be chosen. In example 11-6, the tool that is closest to a 7.05 should be chosen when a pad having a

thickness of 0.022 inch is used. It can be seen that the closest tool to 7.05 D is still a 7.00 D tool. This means that when using uncompensated tools, the power of the tool will automatically be off by 0.05 D for this particular lens surface.

Tool Curves for Concave Tools

In explaining tool curve compensation for pad thickness, we used examples of convex tools used to grind concave surfaces. These tools are the ones used every day in the laboratory. Concave tools are hardly ever used.* However, it sometimes becomes necessary to grind plus (front) surfaces. When a pad is added to the surface of the concave tool, the radius of the surface of the pad is *shorter* than the bare tool radius. This causes the padded tool to grind a steeper curve. See Figure 11-17.

Compensated tool curves for concave tools are found in basically the same way as are compensated tool curves for convex tools. The only difference is that with concave tools, pad thickness is added to uncompensated tool curve. With convex tools, the pad thickness was *subtracted* from the uncompensated tool curve radius. With concave tools, the pad thickness is *added* to the uncompensated tool curve. In other words, in Step 4 of the procedure,

$$r_{(comp)} = r_{(uncomp)} + t_{(pad)}$$

---

*Concave tools are used with plus cylinder lenses. Plus cylinders are used more often in Germany (Zeiss lenses) and in Great Britain.

EXAMPLE 11-7

Find the dioptric value of the compensated tool for a concave tool that is supposed to grind a +10.00 D surface. The pads that will be used will have a thickness of 0.018 inch.

SOLUTION

Step 1. Pad thickness is 0.018 inch.

Step 2. From previous examples, an 0.018-inch-thick pad is 0.4572 mm thick.

Step 3.

$$r_{(uncomp)} = \frac{(1.53 - 1) \times 1000}{10}$$

$$= 53 \text{ mm}$$

Step 4. (This is the step where there is a difference for concave tools.) For concave tools,

$$r_{(comp)} = r_{(uncomp)} + t_{(pad)}$$

In this example,

$$r_{(comp)} = 53 \text{ mm} + 0.4572 \text{ mm}$$

$$= 53.4572 \text{ mm}$$

Step 5. Now the power of the tool in diopters can be found.

$$D_{(comp)} = \frac{(1.53 - 1) \times 1000}{53.4572} = 9.91 \text{ D}$$

Thus it can be seen that in order to make the surface grind correctly, concave tools must be cut *more flat* if lap pads are to be used.

Using the Same Tools for Both Glass and Plastic

In very small surfacing laboratories, the same tools are sometimes used for both glass and plastic lenses. The tools are padded with metal pads, which are used for glass lenses. When plastic lenses are surfaced, the first and second fine pads are placed on top of the metal pad. If this practice is followed, certain precautions need to be taken.

First, the tool must be thoroughly rinsed after being used for glass lenses, so that there is no contamination of plastic polishing compounds. Contamination with small glass particles introduce scratching problems.

Tool compensation becomes a bit more of a problem. The same tool cannot be compensated for two different thicknesses at the same time. A metal pad

is generally 0.018 inch thick. A metal pad combined with first and second fine plastic pads would give a thickness of 0.018 + 0.022 = 0.040 inch. There are several ways to deal with this problem.

1. Do not compensate at all. If this is done, glass lenses must be compensated for the metal pad thickness of 0.018 inch every time, and plastic lenses must be compensated for a thickness of 0.040 inch every time.
2. Compensate the tool for the metal pads. In this manner glass lenses are compensated. When grinding plastic lenses, the metal-padded tool is treated as an uncompensated tool. For higher curves an allowance for the 0.022-inch pad thickness must be considered.
3. Compensate the tool for an amount halfway between the glass and plastic compensation values. This is a compromise. When this compromise is made, the tools are generally compensated for 0.030 inch. For flatter curves, very little error is thus introduced. For steeper curves, however, accuracy drops. Fortunately, if only a limited number of people are working in the area, a skilled person at layout should know when to pick a slightly steeper tool, once the surface power is strong enough.

EXAMPLE 11-8

A set of tools is used for both glass and plastic lenses. The tools are compensated for the 0.018-inch thickness of the metal pad. The laboratory is using pads for fining plastic lenses that total 0.022 inch when both first and second fining pads are on the tool. It is necessary to grind a −8.50 D surface on a plastic lens for the right eye, and a −6.00 D surface for the left. Which tool powers should be selected?

SOLUTION

The tool with the metal pad in place can now be considered an "uncompensated" tool, since fining pads will be added to the tool. From Appendix 5-1, for an 8.50 D curve, adding pad thickness of 0.022 inch flattens the actual curve by 0.08 D. This will cause the surface to be −8.42 D. To compensate, an 8.62 D tool should be chosen. This tool, when flattened by the pad, will yield a −8.54 D surface, which is much closer to what is needed.

For the −6.00 D surface, Appendix 5-1 shows only an 0.04 D flattening. Therefore the −6.00 D tool will be the closest tool and should be used.

Finished Versus Semifinished Tools

It is possible to buy tools that are already cut to specification. These are called *finished tools*. If a new laboratory must be fully operational rapidly, there will not be time to cut a complete set of tools in-house. It then makes sense to buy a basic set ordered to specification.

Because of the large number of possible curve combinations, a laboratory cannot possibly stock every single lap that might be needed. As unusual prescriptions come in, the tools for these must be either ordered or cut as needed.

Tools on which curves have not yet been cut are called *semifinished tools*. See Figure 11-18. These tools have approximate base and cross curves already molded onto the tool. As a result, much less of the lap surface needs to be removed in cutting a tool. The semifinished lap tool with rough curves closest to the needed finished curves is chosen.

Semifinished tools come stamped with two numbers. The first number is the rough base curve and the second number is the rough cylinder power (*not* the cross curve). Thus, a semifinished (rough) tool marked "82" has a rough base curve of 8 and a

rough cylinder power of 2. The rough cross curve equals 10.

When a tool with an unusual curve has been cut and the lens worked, the lap tool is placed in the lap rack for future use. In the future this lap tool may be used for smoothing and polishing another lens with exactly the same curves. If the surface is unusual, the tool will more likely be recut for another lens with different but similar curves.

Cutting the Tool

Tools are cut on *lap cutters*. Lap cutters that are used exclusively for making *sphere* tools are much like a lathe. The tool spins against a cutter blade as the blade swings an arc equal to the desired tool curve. A spheric lap cutter generally produces a better sphere surface than a toric lap cutter used to cut a spherical surface.

Lap cutters that are used to cut tools with a *toric* surface swing the cutter blade back and forth in an arc. See Figure 11-19. Several brands of lap cutters are available. Following are some basic instructions, which are generally applicable to most brands.

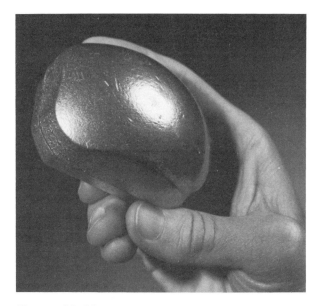

Figure 11-18 Semifinished lap tools are ordered by base curve and cylinder. Having a tool that is close to the desired finished shape reduces the time needed to cut tools. Semifinished lap tools are usually available in 2-diopter base-curve intervals.

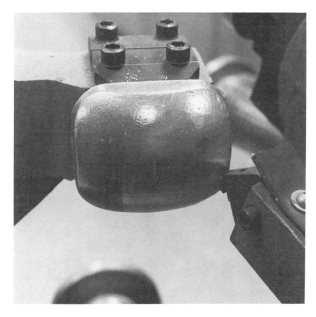

Figure 11-19 The cutter blade swings back and forth across a lap tool, cutting a curve on the surface.

Lap cutters may have settings that allow for pad thickness compensation without having to calculate or look up anything.

If pad thickness compensation is made for the cross curve, it may not be necessary to compensate for the base curve. Compensation may have been made for the base curve when the setting for the cross curve was made.

If the cutter arm is exposed and not shielded by a safety guard, it can be dangerous as it swings back and forth. *Never* reach across the cutter arm to turn the machine on! Stay clear of the arm and blade at all times.

When setting the lap cutter for the thickness to be removed from the surface of the tool on the first cut, if the tool is to be cut flatter than it already is, "zero" the cutting blade on the center of the tool. If the tool is to be made steeper than it already is, zero the blade on the edge of the tool. The blade is zeroed on that area of the tool where the most material will be removed.

When cutting cast-iron tools, oxidation called *scale* will be present on the tool. Because of this scale, the first cut must be smaller. After the first cut, the next cuts may be deeper. Because aluminum and metal/resin laps do not scale, the first cut on these tools can be heavy. Cuts of 1/16 inch or 1½ mm can be made easily with aluminum laps.[2] After several deep "passes" with the cutter, when more and more material has been removed from the lap surface, the whole lap surface will have been changed to the new curve. (A deep cut is called a *rough cut.*) Previous passes will have been deep to remove material and will leave the surface too rough. To smooth the surface, cut a thinner layer for the final cut. This last, thinner cut is called a *smooth cut.*

The speed at which the cutting arm moves back and forth is called the *sweep speed.* The sweep speed of the cutting arm will vary depending on the steepness of the curve being cut. Flatter curves will require slower speed settings.

Using a lap wax or oil on the tool surface will result in smoother cutting and make the cutting blade last longer.

Lap tools used to smooth high-minus lens surfaces will be highly curved. The steep curve

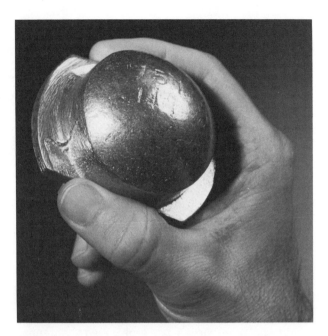

Figure 11-20 Because the curve of a highly convex surface is so steep, the tool is too wide to use its full size. A ledge is created so that less surface area is used.

will not cover the full surface of the tool. This means that the rest of the tool will have a ledge or lip on the side. See Figure 11-20. If the back-and-forth motion of the lap cutter arm is allowed to cover its full stroke width, the arm will hit the ledge on the edge of the tool. To keep this from happening, the cutting stroke of the cutter must be set short.

Save the shavings from aluminum tools. These accumulate quickly and can be sold as scrap.

Tools with especially low base curves and "saddleback" tools* may not cut on most standard lap cutters. They require the use of a *template cutter,* which is a lap cutter that uses individual templates to produce the desired surface curve. See Figure 11-21.

Cleaning the Tool After It Has Been Cut

Once the lap tool has been cut, its rough edges should be filed. See Figure 11-22. The edge of a freshly cut lap tool surface is sharp and has small

---

*A saddleback surface is shaped like a saddle, with a plus surface in one meridian and a minus surface in the other.

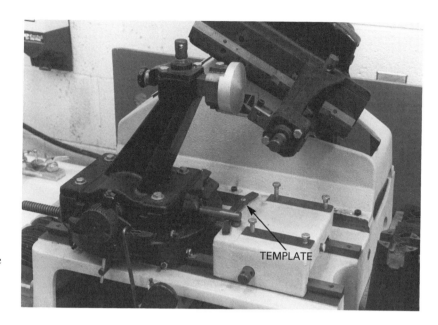

Figure 11-21 Template cutters are lap cutters that use templates like the one shown to cut the correct curve on a lap tool.

burrs. Those who work with lap tools can easily get long, shallow cuts on the hands unless the edges are filed smooth.

At the same time as the edges are being filed, it is advisable to check the bottom of the tool and, if necessary, square up the base of the tool where it is grasped in the cylinder machine. See Figure 11-23. A tool base that is free of burrs and unevenness

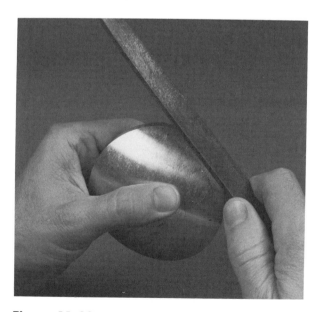

Figure 11-22 If the edge of a freshly cut lap tool is not filed, it will be sharp enough to make long, shallow cuts on the hands.

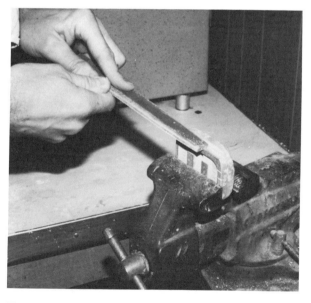

Figure 11-23 It may be necessary to square up the base of the tool where it is grasped in the cylinder machine. This assures that the tool will be less likely to come out of place during fining and polishing.

keeps the tool from jumping out of place during fining and polishing.

If the surface of a freshly trued tool is somewhat rough, it can be buffed with a wire brush to help remove the roughness. The best solution, though, is to find the root problem in lap cutting and follow proper procedures.

Laps that have been retrued many times may become knife-edged. If a grinder (*not* a hand stone used for lenses) is available, the sharpness may be smoothed down. Sharp tools are extremely dangerous, however, and if they cannot be blunted, they must be discarded.

Marking the Tool

After the tool has been cut, it must be clearly marked for future reference. As soon as it comes from the cutter, the fresh surface should be temporarily marked with a grease pencil. Write the base and cross curves on it. See Figure 11-24.

Once all tools have been cut, the tools should be permanently marked. This is done on the underside or edge of the tool with a set of stamps and a hammer. See Figure 11-25. Two areas on the bottom of the tool are used for marking. The upper area is for the base curve, the lower is for the cross curve.

If a master list of tools is kept, the new tool should be entered on that list.

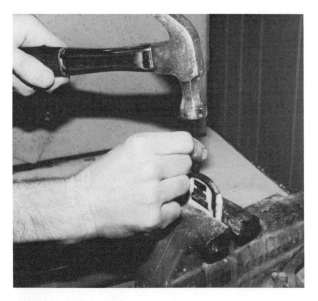

Figure 11-25 The lap tool is stamped using a hammer and metal number stamps.

Disposable Lap Tools

Gerber Optical makes a disposable styrofoam lap tool blank that is cut in their generator. It is used with fining and polishing pads and can be especially handy for unusual lens curves for which a tool may be used only rarely. For more information, see Chapter 10 on generating.

Retrueing Aluminum Tools on the Generator

It is possible to retrue aluminum tools on a Gerber Optical generator. The generator is not meant to replace the lap cutter, but it can be useful once the tool has been initially cut. For more information, see Chapter 10.

Checking Lap Tools for Accuracy

Once a lap tool has been cut or trued, it should be checked for accuracy before being used. One of the oldest methods is to use a brass lap gauge. However, regular uncompensated lap gauges will not measure compensated tools. Although brass lap gauges can be extremely accurate for their respective curves, a special compensated set of gauges is required for compensated tools. (It should be noted that brass lap gauges will wear with repeated use, and should themselves be checked from time to time.)

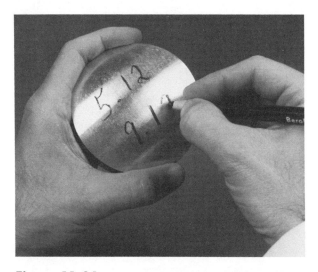

Figure 11-24 As soon as a tool has been cut, it should be marked—at least temporarily. Here the base and cross curves are written on the freshly cut surface with a grease pencil until the tool can be permanently stamped.

The Sagitta Gauge

The instrument of choice for lap tool checking is the sagitta gauge. The *sagitta gauge* measures the dioptric value of a surface indirectly by finding the *sagittal depth* or *sag* of the curve. To visualize the concept of sagittal depth, imagine a circle like the one shown in Figure 11-26. A straight line is drawn horizontally across the circle at or above the center. This horizontal line is called a *chord.* The depth from the top of the circle to the middle of the chord is the sagittal depth. It should be immediately evident that the sagittal depth of a circle having a given radius of curvature depends on (1) the position of the chord and (2) its length or *diameter,* as it is most often referred to.* Simply knowing a sagittal depth does not help much, however, unless the chord diameter that was used to find the sagittal depth is also known.

The most commonly used chord diameter for instruments in the optical laboratory is 50 mm. Sagittal depth is found by placing a gauge with three legs on the surface of the lap tool. The two outer legs do not move and are separated by a distance of 50 mm. The center leg moves up and down and gives a direct measure of the sagittal depth of the surface.

Lap tools are slipped into the base of the sagittal depth gauge. This keeps the tool from turning so that the base curve of the lap will be measured accurately along its meridian. See Figure 11-27. The lap or the gauge (depending on the type of gauge being used) can then be rotated by 90 degrees to measure the cross curve.

The Sag Formula

Sagittal depths are related to the radius of curvature of a tool or lens surface by the *sag formula:*

$$s = r - \sqrt{(r^2 - y^2)}$$

where

s = sagittal depth
r = radius of curvature of the surface
y = semidiameter of the chord (one-half the chord length)

---

*The chord "diameter" is not to be confused with the diameter of the main circle. Sagittal depth may be measured using an instrument with a circular base that fits onto the surface being measured. The chord *diameter* corresponds to the bell-like base of the gauge.

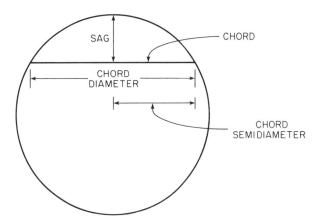

Figure 11-26 Sagittal depth (sag) will vary depending on the radius of curvature of the circle and the chord length (chord diameter).

The sag formula is sometimes written as

$$s = r - \sqrt{r^2 - (d/2)^2}$$

where d is the diameter of the chord. An approximation for finding r in millimeters is

$$r = \frac{530}{D} + 0.445$$

Rather than first finding the radius of curvature of the surface and then converting it to diopters, tables can be used to convert sagittal depth into dioptric values. Such a table is shown as Appendix 5-2. Appendix 5-2 is an "uncompensated" sag chart. (For more on sagittal depth and the sag formula see Chapter 7.)

Compensated Sag Charts

As discussed previously, some lap cutter dials allow pad compensations to be made directly. (This means that a so-called 10.00 D tool will really measure 10.09 D.) A sag gauge reads the actual sag of the lap tool surface. If regular "uncompensated" 50-mm sag charts are used to look up the sag/diopter value, the real 1.53-indexed dioptric tool value is found. In other words, the sag gauge used with uncompensated charts will say that the surface is 10.09 D, not 10.00 D.

If the tools have been compensated for pad thickness, the person measuring will not know if the tool curve is correct or not. In this case the regular (uncompensated) sag chart will not tell us what we need to know. For this reason there are compen-

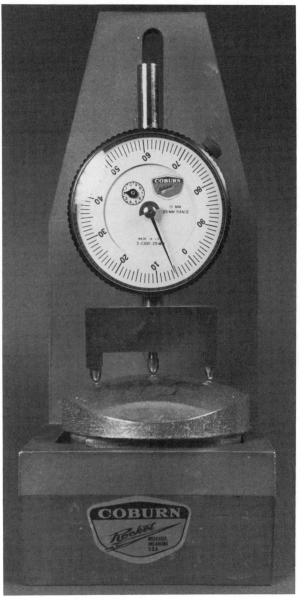

(A)

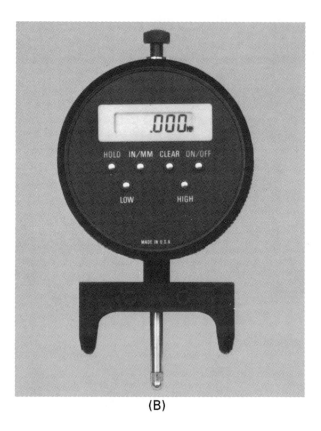

(B)

Figure 11-27 (A) The sagometer shown is a standard dial gauge mounted in a stand for ease of use when measuring lap tools. (B) Sagometers are also available in electronic digital versions offering high-contrast displays, which are easier to read. [Photo (B) courtesy of Coburn Optical, Muskogee, Okla.]

sated sag charts that are corrected for pad thickness. There is a chart for each individual pad thickness. If a sag reading is 6.07 mm, a sag chart made for tools compensated for 0.018 inch will show a "corrected" value of 10.00 D instead of the actual 10.09 D bare tool value. (See Appendix 5-3; charts for other pad thicknesses are also given in the appendix.) When compensated sag charts are used, it is possible to tell if the tool has been cut correctly for a given pad thickness.

Differences in Sag Gauges

If a sag gauge had sharply pointed contact tips, the chord length would be highly accurate for every lap measured—that is, until the tips began to dull. For this reason, and to prevent lens scratching, most sag gauge contact tips are intentionally rounded.

Some sag gauges have ball tips. When it is measured with a ball-tipped gauge, a highly curved surface will have a shorter chord length than a flatter

Figure 11-28 A sag gauge with
5/32-inch ball tips may have a 50-mm
separation between the two outer
balls. However, on steeply curved surfaces, such as the one on the right,
the actual points of contact (*C* and *D*)
will be less than 50 mm. This must be
taken into consideration when con-
structing sag tables and when attempting to use a table for one gauge that
may have been designed for another.
Because of this effect, sag charts for
ball gauges will be different for concave surfaces than they are for convex
surfaces.

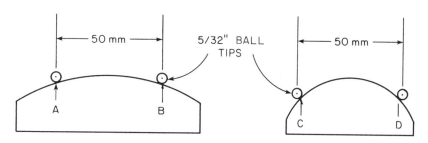

surface. See Figure 11-28. Because of this, sag charts
for ball gauges cannot be used interchangeably with
charts intended for gauges having rounded contact
points. In fact, two ball gauges with different sized
balls on the tips would require two different sag
charts! (A common ball tip size is a 5/32 inch diameter
ball.) Fortunately most of these differences don't
show up until the surface is steeply curved.

Sag gauges that have three contact points, all
lined up in a row, are called *bar gauges* because the
three legs pass through a bar. The bar gauge is used
for toric surfaces.

Another type of sag gauge, called a *bell gauge,* is
used to measure spherical surfaces. A bell gauge
will not work on toric surfaces. A 50-mm bell gauge
has a domelike outer rim that is 50 mm from one
side of the round rim to the other. To use the gauge,
the "bell" or dome is lowered onto the spherical
surface. Exactly in the middle of the "bell," where
the clapper would be, is a movable leg. This movable leg measures the sagittal depth of the surface.
The chord diameter is defined by the bell's circular
rim.

Storing Lap Tools

Lap tools can be a problem to store because of
weight and sheer numbers. Lap tools need to be
reasonably accessible. This means that in most cases
they need to be near the cylinder surfacers so that
they can be retrieved by the person working that
area.

A commonly used storage system consists of rotating racks, as shown in Figure 11-29. Tools can

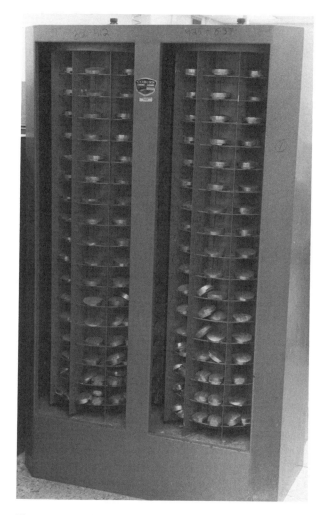

Figure 11-29 Rotating lap storage racks can be constructed from metal, like the Coburn rack shown here,
or from wood, which makes them less expensive.

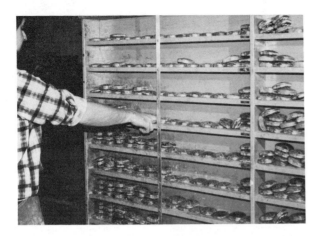

Figure 11-30 Laps do not have to be stored in rotating racks, but can be kept on shallow shelves.

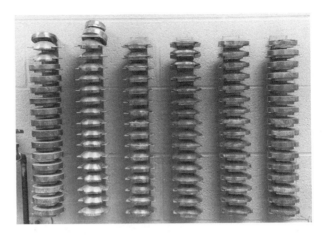

Figure 11-31 Mounting laps on the wall helps to use every available space.

be pulled from the racks from at least two sides if necessary. However, simple shallow shelving, as shown in Figure 11-30, can be constructed at a very reasonable cost. Shelves can be with or without "pigeon holes" separating each tool location. As the number of tools expand, pigeon holes will allow duplicate or triplicate tools to be stacked on top of one another without having them slide out of place.

Another storage method, shown in Figure 11-31, uses wall-mounted racks. Wall racks for mushroom and hollow-sphere tools can be made using metal piping.

Order of the Tools on the Racks

Tools must be placed on the racks or shelves in some sort of logical order. Whatever lap storage system is chosen must allow for expansion in diop-

tric range for sphere and cylinder powers. It is not uncommon to have left and right eyes with identical lens powers. With two identical lenses being processed at the same time, most laboratories will want to increase their tool selection to include at least two of the more commonly used tools.

In most storage systems, tools are classified first by sphere power (back base curve), then by cross curve. Some laboratories mark the tool with its sphere curve and cylinder power. This is handy for crown glass or 1.498-index plastic, but it can be confusing when using materials of higher index. With high-index materials the cylinder power will not correspond to the marked values on the tools. Most laboratories use the more versatile system of marking both base and cross curves by their 1.53-indexed values. Tools are placed on shelves or racks in the order shown below:

6.00/6.00	6.00/6.25	6.00/6.50	6.00/6.75	6.00/7.00	6.00/7.25
6.25/6.25	6.25/6.50	6.25/6.75	6.25/7.00	6.25/7.25	6.25/7.50
6.50/6.50	6.50/6.75	6.50/7.00	6.50/7.25	6.50/7.50	6.50/7.75
6.75/6.75	6.75/7.00	6.75/7.25	6.75/7.50	6.75/7.75	6.75/8.00
7.00/7.00	7.00/7.25	7.00/7.50	7.00/7.75	7.00/8.00	7.00/8.25
7.25/7.25	7.25/7.50	7.25/7.75	7.25/8.00	7.25/8.25	7.25/8.50

Some laboratories store sphere tools separately from tools with cylinder. Tools continue to increase in cylinder power to the right. Labs may keep tools in one-eighth-diopter back-base steps, especially if the set is used for working plastic lenses. See Figure 11-32. This is especially true where laps are used for both glass and plastic lenses.

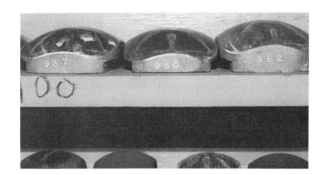

Figure 11-32 Tools that progress in one-eighth-diopter steps allow more accuracy in surfacing, especially in the more commonly used curvatures.

Questions and Problems

1. What must the sag of a convex 5.00 D tool be if it is correctly compensated for a pad having a thickness of 0.45 mm? (Assume the tool's index to be 1.53.) The sag is taken for a 50-mm-diameter section.

2. The thickness of two fining pads stacked on top of each other, as used on a lap tool in the production of plastic lenses, is 0.4572 mm. In order to cut a lap tool of 1.53-index tooling so that an 11.00 D convex tool curve results after padding, to what radius of curvature must the compensated tool be cut? What would this be in diopters (1.53-index reference)?

3. What is the name of the tool shapes that are used in conjunction with the sphere machine?

4. Which type of sagittal depth gauge is only used on spherical surfaces?
   a. a bar gauge
   b. a bell gauge

5. a. What must the compensated dioptric value of a convex 7.00 D tool be if it is correctly compensated for a pad having a thickness of 0.45 mm? (Assume the tool's index to be 1.53.)

   b. What is the sag of the tool if taken for a 50-mm-diameter section?

6. A tool is to be cut so that the curve, including the pad, will produce a 1.53-index tool curve of 7.00 D. (The tool is convex to grind concave.) A standard plastic polishing pad is 0.4572 mm thick.
   a. What radius of curvature should be cut on the tool in order to produce the desired finished curve?
   b. If the lap cutter is not calibrated in millimeters, but only in 1.53-referenced diopters, what dioptric value should it be set to?

7. What are the three most commonly used materials from which lap tools are made?

8. A "hollow" lap tool produces
   a. a plus spherical surface
   b. a plus toric surface
   c. a minus spherical surface
   d. a minus toric surface

9. Aluminum lap tools should not be used for surfacing glass lenses.
   True or False

10. It is not possible to use brass lap gauges to check lap tools that have been compensated for pad thickness. Lap gauge sets are available only in uncompensated curve powers.
    True or False

11. Lap scoring is
    a. a rating system for judging the quality of lap tools
    b. cutting grooves in the surface of a lap
    c. smoothing the surface of a lap so that the pad will adhere to the surface more easily

12. Metal lap pads are pressed on the surface of a tool with the same type of pad press used for pressing on first and second fining pads.
    True or False

13. Under normal circumstances, metal lap pads begin to show wear
    a. first in the center of the pad
    b. first on the edges of the pad
    c. unpredictably

14. Lap tools are always marked with the 1.53-index referenced value they will give to a lens surface, regardless of whether they have been cut as compensated or uncompensated.
    True or False

15. If a convex lap tool is to be cut for a 6.50 D curve, what radius of curvature should the tool have? (Assume that the tool is uncompensated.)

16. A laboratory uses a two-step fining system for plastic lenses. Each of the pads has a thickness of 0.011 inch. How should the convex lap tool be compensated?
    a. The radius of curvature should be shortened by 0.011 inch.
    b. The radius of curvature should be lengthened by 0.011 inch.
    c. The radius of curvature should be shortened by 0.022 inch.
    d. The radius of curvature should be lengthened by 0.022 inch.

17. A convex lap tool is to be cut for an 8.75 D surface. The pad thickness value to be used for com-

pensation is 0.4572 mm. What should the radius of curvature be for the compensated tool curve?

18. The lap cutter being used to cut the tool in Problem 17 has a dioptric scale that does not allow for automatic thickness compensation. What should the dioptric value of the setting be in order to produce a properly compensated tool?

19. Padding an uncompensated tool will probably not throw the lens power off if the curve being cut is fairly flat.
   True or False

20. A concave tool is to be cut to produce an 8.25 D

surface. If the total pad thickness is 0.018 inch (0.4572 mm), for what power should the compensated curve be cut?

References

1. Woodcock, F. R. Prescription Shop Machinery, Part 6: Lap Cutting Machines. *Manufacturing Optics International*, 27(6):296–301 (June 1974).

2. *How to Cut Aluma-Laps.* PSI Technical Bulletin, Practical Systems, Inc., Tarpon Springs, Fla., undated.

12

Fining and Polishing

Introduction

Once lenses have been generated and the correct lap tool chosen, the lens is ready to have the roughened surface *smoothed* or *fined*. After it is fined, it is *polished* to an optical-quality finish. Before generators were used, the surface was roughed in using an extremely coarse abrasive. Thus the final surface was created in a manner similar to that of beginning with rough sandpaper and progressing through continually finer grits until a polish (extremely fine "grit") was used to give the material its finished luster.

Optical Abrasives

Grades of Abrasives

Abrasives are classed by various systems according to the size of the particles. Abrasives, like gravel, may be of one particular material. They can be thought of as a mixture of "large rocks" and "tiny pebbles." In order to separate gravel into particles of the same size, the gravel can be *screened*. This consists of feeding the gravel through screens of increasingly smaller mesh. Only the gravel larger than the mesh size is screened out. All other falls through. An easy way to classify the size of the gravel is by indicating how many wires there are per inch on the screen. As the number of wires per inch increases, the particle size that drops through decreases.

Screen sizes for abrasive are given by U.S. Department of Commerce Commercial Standard CS 271-65 and correspond to abrasives numbered 8 through 240. But optical abrasives can be considerably smaller than these. Abrasives smaller than No. 280 are not standardized, so there are variations in numbering. Numbers greater than No. 280 are too small to run through a sieve system and are called subsieve sizes. In order to define the system, though, theoretical sieve numbers may be used.[1] These, with corresponding particle sizes, are shown in Table 12-1. Optical abrasives are classified by a variety of systems. Here are definitions of the terms used in Table 12-1.

Theoretical Mesh Size The theoretical number of wires which would be used to screen this size abrasive.

Micron Equivalent The size of the grit particles measured in microns. A micron is one one-thousandth of a millimeter.

Microgrit Number A grading system used for the abrasive product "Micro Grit."

Industrial Size Number These size numbers correspond to what are referred to as "Pad Grit" numbers. However, there may not be an exactly equivalent relationship in abrasiveness between pad grit number and micron number.

Typical Optical Powder Number These are grading numbers used by K.C. (Kansas City) Abrasives and other suppliers for their optical powders. Many refer to this number as the "emery number," though it is not necessarily made from emery.

Garnet Powder Number A number used to grade abrasives made from garnet. As the number becomes larger, the powder becomes finer.

Corundum Powder Number A system of grading corundum powder. Corundum is a natural abrasive which is extremely durable and produces a good optical finish.

The theoretical mesh size does not correspond to the typical *optical powder number* (sometimes referred to as the *emery number*). In fact, as the

Table 12-1 Grading of Optical Abrasives*

Theoretical Mesh Size	Micron Equiv.	Microgrit No.	Industrial Size No.	Typical Opt. Pwdr. No.	Garnet Pwdr. No.	Corundum Pwdr. No.
270	53					
325	44					
	42		280			
	35	35	320			
400	30	30			W0	
	27		400	275	W1	
500	25	25		250		500
	23				W2	600
	22			225		
600	20	20	500	200	W3	750
	18	18		175	W4	850
	16				W5	1000
	15	15	600	145	W6	1100
	12	12	800	125	W7	1200
1,250	10	9	1000	95		1600
	9				W8	2100
2,500	5	5		50	W10	2600
	3	3		30	W14	
12,500	1	1		10		

*This is a slightly modified version of a table taken from "A Guide to Optical Abrasives," Practical Systems, Inc., Tarpon Springs, Fla., and is used by permission.

theoretical mesh number becomes larger, the optical powder or "emery" number becomes smaller. Thus a coarse optical powder has a large number and a fine optical powder has a small number.

Abrasive fining pads are numbered with a pad "grit" number, which corresponds to the industrial size number as shown in Table 12-1. They may also be specified according to the average size of the grit particles. This is referred to as the *micron equivalent*. The *microgrit number* is a grading system used for the abrasive product, "Micro grit," and is also based on the micron equivalent.

Garnet powders used in fining and polishing are preceded by a "W." As the garnet number becomes larger, the powder becomes finer and finer.

It is often possible to use either an abrasive pad, garnet powder, or optical powder such as aluminum oxide to perform the same operation. This does not mean that, knowing the abrasive pad grit size, one can automatically look across the rows in Table 12-1 and pick the correct number for the other pow-

ders, as the aggressiveness of the pad will vary depending on the abrasive used. This is true even if both abrasives have the same average size in microns. However, the table gives a fairly good idea as to how the abrasives relate.

Slurries

For glass fining and polishing and for plastic polishing, optical abrasives are suspended in a liquid and pumped over the surface of the lap tool. Abrasive particles suspended in a liquid are called a *slurry*. In order to know how concentrated the abrasive is and, hence, how a slurry can be expected to perform, a concentration numbering system of some kind is required. The system most commonly used measures slurries in terms of *degrees Baumé (°Bé)*.

Degrees Baumé are measured using a *hydrometer*, which is a hollow glass bulb attached to a narrow glass stem. When the hydrometer is placed in a liquid, it sinks until it has displaced its own weight of liquid. The stem floats out of the water and is marked as to degrees Baumé. The relationship between specific gravity and degrees Baumé is

$$°Bé = 145 - \frac{145}{SG}$$

where SG is specific gravity.[2] *Specific gravity* is the mass or weight of a substance compared to water, or

$$SG = \frac{\text{mass (or weight) of a substance}}{\text{mass (or weight) of water}}$$

With *central slurry systems*, which supply a number of cylinder machines and continually recirculate slurry, Baumé readings should be checked often—perhaps every hour—to assure optimum performance.

To measure the degrees Baumé of small quantities of slurry, a hydrometer can be placed inside what appears to be an ordinary glass kitchen baster. The slurry is sucked into the baster using the rubber bulb on the top until the hydrometer inside floats. The hydrometer scale is read at the surface of the slurry. This apparatus is called a *bulb-type hydrometer*.

In order to obtain accurate Baumé readings, one must be certain of the following:[3]

1. The slurry must be uniformly dispersed. If some of the abrasive has settled out, readings will be too low.
2. The slurry must not contain trapped air or foam. Otherwise the reading will again be artificially low.
3. The temperature must not be too high. (For every 10 degrees Fahrenheit above 60 degrees, add 0.1 degree Baumé to the measured value.)

Mixing Abrasive and Water for the Desired Degrees Baumé

Manufacturers of abrasive powders may provide charts or nomograms that allow the surfacing laboratory to mix up any volume of water to obtain any desired Baumé reading. One such nomogram for a polishing compound is shown in Figure 12-1.

When slurries are mixed for one machine only, Baumé readings can be checked as the operator senses a problem. (Most often operators develop a "feel" for the slurry and seldom take an actual Baumé reading.)

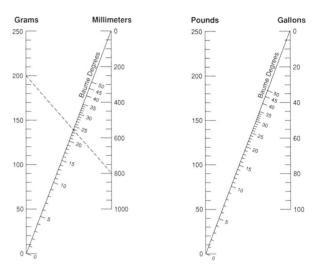

Figure 12-1   Using a nomogram such as this one, it is possible to create a slurry (in this case a Reopol polishing slurry) of any quantity for any desired Baumé reading. The weight of the dry polishing compound is shown in grams or pounds. The volume of water is shown in milliliters or gallons. (From *Reopol Cerium Oxide Glass Polishing Powders*, Shieldalloy Corporation, Newfield, N.J. Used by permission.)

The Effect of pH

Acidity or alkalinity of a liquid is measured in terms of its pH value. The term pH stands for "potential of hydrogen." The pH scale is from 0 to 14. The lower the number, the more acid the solution is. The higher the number, the more alkaline it is. A pH of 7 is neutral (neither acid nor alkaline).

Much attention has been given to maintaining a certain pH value for the slurry, and it is certainly advisable to follow the instructions of the manufacturer, if any. For glass polishing compounds, however, Walter L. Silvernail has made some interesting observations, which are given in his own words in the following paragraphs.

It is likely that there is more speculation and less understanding concerning pH control in polishing operations than any other aspect except for the actual mechanism of polishing itself. This does not imply that pH does not play some role in the polishing process. But over the years attempts to optimize polishing activity by pH control simply have not proven to be very fruitful. Nonetheless, there are some observations that have been made that should be kept in mind. First of all, if the pH of a slurry is lowered to less than about 4, a very rapid decline in speed occurs. . . . Another more pertinent observation is that with continued use, the pH of a slurry will rise to the value of 9 to 9.5 and level off. This is readily explained as being due to the hydrolysis of the glass degradation products. The initial pH may vary anywhere from 5 to 10 depending on the nature of the polish and on any additives.

Although the increase of the pH to the value of 9 to 9.5 does not appear to be detrimental to the polishing activity, nonetheless some users persist in adding acids to decrease the value to 5 to 7. Whereas with a fresh slurry this probably is not harmful, provided the value is not taken lower, in a used slurry it can cause the precipitation of silicic acid formed by the reaction of the hydrogen and silicate ions. This silicic acid in turn, may behave as a diluent with a corresponding decrease in speed.[4]

Glass Roughing

Most of the time lenses are never roughed, as this is now a function of generating. However, when glass lenses are roughed to obtain special curves, a coarse abrasive is used. This abrasive is often called "rough emery," but it is really carborundum. *Emery* is an impure form of aluminum oxide containing iron oxides. Emery itself has not been used for years, yet the name remains, just as "shell" is used to describe plastic frames because frames were once made from tortoise shell!

When working with a hand pan and "rough emery," extreme caution must be taken to avoid contaminating the fining or polishing areas. One grain of this rough abrasive can produce a bad scratch in a glass surface.

Glass Fining

Glass fining is done using an aluminum oxide in slurry form on a metal fining pad or on a bare cast-iron tool. The cylinder machine is set to exert a fining pressure of approximately 20 pounds per square inch (psi) on the lens during surfacing. Pressure may vary depending on the type of machine being used,* the type of slurry, and the Baumé reading of the slurry.

Fining slurry is made very thick and heavy. A Baumé reading of 25 is about average. Slurry mixed for a single cylinder machine will generally last one 8-hour working day. Over time throughout the day the particles of abrasive break up, becoming smaller and losing their cutting power.

In the morning or when first mixing fining slurry, the water used should be 90 to 95 degrees Fahrenheit. If cold water is used, the mixture has a tendency to lump up, like buttermilk.

It is not advisable just to throw a handful of abrasive powder into the slurry, adding water alternately, and seldom changing the slurry throughout the week. Slurry should be changed regularly and the machine washed down each time. This will keep slurry fresh, remove glass sludge, and prolong the life of the machine. If the slurry concentration (Baumé reading) drops, rather than just throwing in dry abrasive powder, add premixed concentrated slurry. This works better than adding abrasive in powder form to slurry already in the cylinder machine.

It can be expected that water will evaporate during the day. If lens stock is not being removed adequately, water can be added to bring the slurry back to the correct Baumé reading.

Preventing Edge Chipping

Before fining a glass lens it may be advisable to remove any sharpness between the back surface of the lens and the lens edge. This is done using a hand edger, as shown in Figure 12-2. If sharpness is not removed, the pad may tear or the lens may chip along the edge.

If a lens edge must be ground thin, or if there is a danger of chipping as sometimes occurs with Franklin-style lenses, the lens can be reinforced. This can be done by taping around the edge of the lens before fining. If the lens is taped so that the tape forms a rim around the convex side of the lens,

---

*Some air gauges are poorly calibrated and should be checked for accuracy against a force gauge such as the Semi-Tech Model ST-45 or the Coburn Durometer. Especially thin lenses may also require lower pressures.

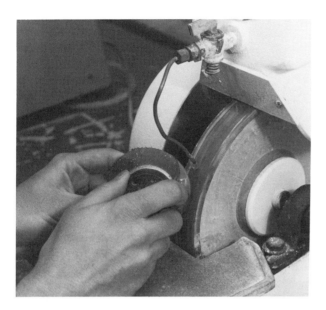

Figure 12-2 Removing the sharp edge from a generated lens blank will keep it from chipping. It also prevents tearing of fining or polishing pads during cylinder surfacing. Hand edging may not need to be done on every lens. Rather, it needs to be done only on those lenses whose edges are especially thin or especially sharp.

metal alloy can be spooned onto the front lens surface around the block. (Pitch dripped onto the lens works too, but this is more of a bother.) Once the alloy hardens, it reinforces the lens edge against surfacing pressure and prevents chipping. See Figure 12-3.

Checking for a Well-Fined Surface

After fining, a lens should be checked for the surface quality of the fine. However, if a glass lens makes a different or unusual sound during fining, it should be checked immediately, even before the fining cycle finishes. An unusual noise during fining could result from the wrong tool being used. Or the tool may be correct, but the lens may be improperly generated due to operator error. Or the generator might not be cutting a true curve.

The surface of the lens will indicate whether the lens is too steep or too flat for the tool. One can tell which it is just by looking at the lens surface. If a lens surface begins to fine from the outside of the lens, the lens is steep in comparison to the tool.

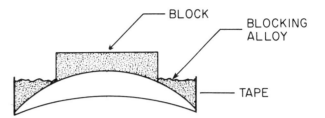

Figure 12-3 Some plus lenses have a thin edge that can chip easily during cylinder surfacing. Such a lens can be reinforced by taking masking tape and taping around the outer edge of the lens. This forms a reservoir area. Metal alloy can then be spooned from the blocker's holding tank onto the front surface of the lens. The alloy hardens and gives the lens edge the necessary reinforcement.

If the lens begins fining from the center, the lens is flat compared to the tool.

At the end of the fining process, the lens should show no evidence of generator marks or other surface irregularities. Generator marks are curved lines extending across the surface of the lens, as shown in Figure 12-4. Their presence after fining may indicate that the lens was generated too fast, or that an attempt was made to remove too much lens stock in the last pass of the diamond generator wheel across the lens.

Glass Polishing
Glass Polishing Theories

There are three main theories as to how glass polishing occurs. Each has merit, and perhaps a combination of the mechanisms is what really takes place. At this point no one knows for sure. The three theories are (1) mechanical abrasion, (2) thermal flow, and (3) chemical action. Phillip Whitman has described these well, and his presentation is given below.[5]

The *mechanical abrasion theory* claims that polishing is merely an extension of fine grinding or smoothing on a submicron scale. The glass is thereby removed by fracturing off small chunks. If this theory were exclusively true, then (1) stock removal rates would depend on glass hardness and (2) the particles removed would all be solid.

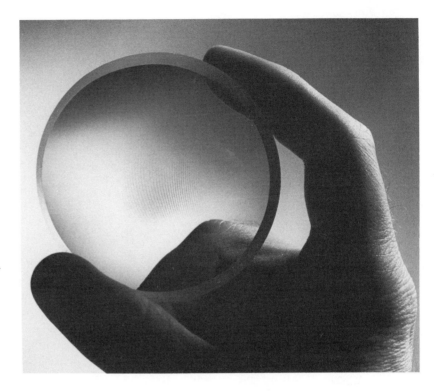

Figure 12-4 Generator marks are curved and run in parallel across the surface of the lens. When a lens is removed from the generator, light generator marks are considered normal and should disappear after the lens is fined. The marks shown here are not light. They are seen centrally even after the lens has been fined and polished.

The *thermal flow theory* also claims a purely mechanical action in which pressure causes the glass to get hot enough to flow into the valleys or to form a hydrated layer that is then smeared over the scratches. If this theory were exclusively true, then (1) the polishing rate would depend on the softening point, (2) there would be glass products in solution, and (3) glass should polish with other abrasives. All three of these factors have been shown to be invalid.

The *chemical action theory* claims that molecular displacement takes place as a result of the chemical reaction between the oxide and the glass. If this theory were exclusively true, the polishing rate would depend upon the durability (percent of silica) of the glass. There would be no glass fines in the slurry, and there would be glass in solution.

It is generally agreed that polishing rate and surface quality do in fact depend upon the chemical durability of the glass and that chemical reaction is a most important factor in glass polishing. It is, however, not the only factor.

Combined theories, of which there are now several, claim that (1) initial stock removal is purely mechanical, as peaks are fractured off

and can be found as solids in the slurry; (2) a hydrated layer is formed on the glass surface, as the surface contact area increases, by the loss of sodium ions from the glass; and (3) the hydrated layer is swept away by abrasive action of the polishing particles.

It is likely that polishing rates and surface quality are most dependent upon the speed of formation of the hydrated layer, particle size, particle density, and particle structure.[5]

Slurries Used in Glass Polishing

Formerly, the main material used in the polishing of ophthalmic glass was iron oxide. Because of its reddish hue, it was referred to as "polishing rouge." It seemed to color every corner of the surfacing lab and even followed the workers home at night! Its replacement with cerium oxide was a welcome improvement.

Cerium is one of the rare earth elements. It must be processed and used in conjunction with some additives. Additives assist in keeping it from caking and help keep it in suspension while in liquid (slurry) form.

A third polishing compound that can be used in polishing lenses is zirconium oxide. Zirconium oxide is a faster polishing agent than iron oxide, but it is not as fast as cerium. Because it is slower than cerium and is fairly expensive, it is not commonly used for polishing glass lenses.

Mixing Polishing Slurries

In mixing powdered polishing compound with water, it is best to use very warm (90–95 degrees Fahrenheit) water.[6] This helps the material go into suspension faster. Slurries can be mixed for single machines for a single day, or in a special mixing tank using a propellorlike device to assist in maintaining a homogeneous suspension. The stirrer is positioned in the bottom of the tank to discourage the abrasive compound from precipitating out.

Baumé Readings, Pressures, and Times for Glass Polishing

As might be expected, glass polishing times vary. Times depend on (1) the speed and design of the cylinder machine, (2) the size of the lap compared to the lens size, (3) the type of polish, and (4) the concentration (Baumé reading) of the polish. A 4- or 5-minute polishing time is average. Lenses with especially high cylinders require longer polishing times. Because of the hardness of the lens material, photochromic lenses also require a longer polishing cycle.

Baumé readings for polishing slurries are considerably less than fining-slurry Baumé readings. Whereas fining slurries may have Baumé readings in the mid-20s, a 5-degree Baumé reading for a cerium oxide polishing compound is normal.

By the time a lens gets to the place where it is ready to be polished, the curves have been worked down to a good tool match. Polishing abrasive particles are very fine. There is also a soft polishing pad on the tool. All these factors mean that glass polishing pressures can be higher than glass fining pressures. Polishing pressures ranging in the mid-30s are average.

Additives for Polishing Slurries

Cerium is expensive. Because of the cost factor, polishing compounds using cerium are made in a variety of grades. (The polishing of eyeglass lenses is only one of the many uses for cerium polishing compound.)

When cerium is found in its natural state in a mixture of rare earths, cerium oxide makes up 45% to 50% of the total rare earth oxide content.[7] Polishes made from this natural mixture are called "low" cerium polishes. If the product is upgraded so that the percentage of cerium is greater, it is known as a "high" cerium polish.

It is possible to add other substances to cerium compounds to reduce the percentage of cerium needed or to increase efficiency. Additives used to reduce the amount of cerium needed are called *extenders*. Additives used to increase efficiency are known as *accelerators*.

Extenders have to be added early in the manufacturing process in order to be effective. Attempting to add them later causes them to have the effect of diluting the cerium, making it perform less efficiently. Examples of extenders are didymium oxide and wallastonite.

Accelerators have little or no polishing abilities by themselves. However, if they are used together with a polishing agent such as cerium oxide, an accelerator will cause the polishing agent to perform better than it would alone. An example of an accelerator is ceric hydroxide. The effectiveness a polish will have when used with an accelerator may vary somewhat, depending on the type of pad used for polishing.

Other additives may be used to (1) hinder settling of the polishing material in suspension and increase the ease of redispersion (remixing) after settling has occurred, (2) control foaming, or (3) maintain a desired pH level.

When using additives to control settling and promote redispersion, it should be kept in mind that lens material may be hindered from settling as well, and the chance of lens scratching may be increased.

In using *foam-control additives*, a little goes a long way. Too much will lead to saponification (the chemical conversion of fats into soap), causing loss of effectiveness. Foam controllers may have to be added from time to time. Adding just enough foam controller to handle the problem each time foam appears is best.

Additives *to control pH* are used primarily for operator comfort when slurry comes into contact with skin. (See the previous section on the effect of pH.)

Fining CR-39 Plastic Lenses

When fining plastic lenses, most laboratories do not use a slurry. Instead, rather sandpaperlike pads that have the abrasive material right on them are used once, then discarded. Instead of slurry being pumped over the lap surface as the lens is being worked, plain water is used. The water cools and lubricates the contact surfaces while flushing out loose abrasive and ground lens material. If the water is continually recirculated, it needs to be changed often or filtered. Where water is abundant and inexpensive, fresh water can be used and not recirculated.

When applying lens fining pads, it is helpful to use a pad press. This will eliminate (well, *almost* eliminate) the possibility of wrinkles in the pad surface. If the pad wrinkles, it will produce a wavy lens surface.

One-Step Versus Two-Step Fining Systems

CR-39 plastic lenses can be fined with either a one- or two-step process. When plastic lens fining takes place in a *two-step process,* the *first fine* is done using a pad with a 15-micrometer silicon carbide-coated surface. See Figure 12-5. The pad is generally black in color or, when its abrasive is slightly finer, it is gray. First fines are run at 15 to 20 psi of pressure, and the fining time is between 1 and 1½ minutes.*

Some types of curves may require a longer first fine. These include very high curves (above 10 diopters) or very high cylinders. If the fine runs longer than the normal time, it will probably be necessary to strip the black pad off and replace it with another, since the normal life of these pads is 1 to 1½ minutes.

The *second fine* is run on a pad with a 12 micron aluminum oxide film on the surface. The pad is placed directly on top of the first fine pad. (The first fine pad is already on the lap.) See Figure 12-6. Before placing the second fine pad on the lap, the lap with the first pad on it should be thoroughly rinsed. (This is also true for the lens itself.) All possibility of contamination with coarse abrasive material should be eliminated.

Unless there is a continuous flow of fresh water through the cylinder machine, separate bowls should be used for first and second fines. Otherwise the

*Fining times and pressures may vary.

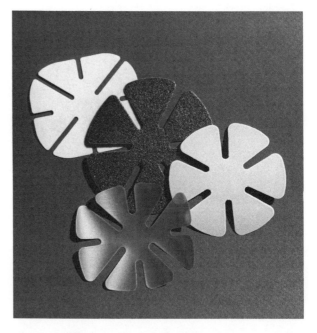

Figure 12-5 Fining and polishing pads come in a variety of shapes and sizes. The first fine for CR-39 plastic lenses is generally a 600 grit pad having a silicon carbide abrasive with a 15-micron particle size.

dislodged silicon carbide abrasive from the first fine may recirculate during the second fine and scratch the surface of the lens.

The second fine is run for 2 minutes at the same pressure as was used for the first fine. This two-step process produces a very smooth surface, nicely prepared for polishing.

To save time, pads (especially second fine pads) can be prepeeled from the roll and stuck to the lap rack, the top of the cylinder machine, or in another convenient place until they are needed.

It is possible to fine lenses in a *one-step process* using a pad with a 15-micron aluminum oxide-coated surface.† Pressure is set at 20 psi and fining time at 1 minute. Newer one-step pads may use a 4-micron pad and fine the lenses from 1 to 3 minutes. Newer generator wheels and changing grinding technology is producing lenses that are generated more smooth than was previously possible. This, coupled with improved one-step fining pads, are making the one-step process more than simply a time-saving com-

†Note that the one-step pad is the same size grit as the first-fine two-step pad. The difference is in the abrasive. The two-step first-fine pad has a silicon carbide abrasive.

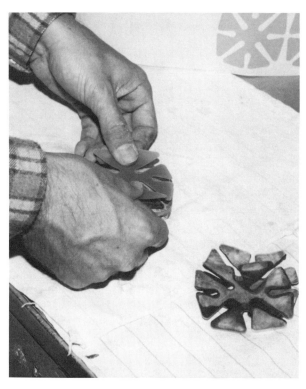

Figure 12-6 The second fine pad is placed directly on top of the first fine pad.

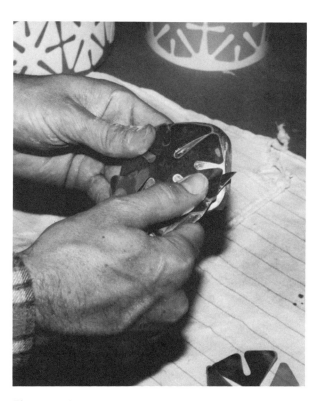

Figure 12-7 Here first and second fining pads are being stripped from a lap tool before the tool is repadded with a polishing pad. A paring knife works well.

promise. However, it is usually necessary to increase polishing times after only a single fine.

Removing Fining Pads

Once the lens has been fined, the pads are stripped off the tool. Most often this is done using a paring knife to get each daisy petal started. See Figure 12-7. Then the pad can be pulled off.

Using Slurries for Fining CR-39 Plastic Lenses

It is possible to use a fining slurry instead of abrasive pads on plastic lenses. To do this, a two-step fine is required. The results are good, but the process is more involved than using abrasive pads.

The first fine uses a heavy Pellon pad and #95 or #125 optical powder in slurry form.* Fining time is 4 to 6 minutes.

---

*For difficult lenses such as those having greater than 2 diopters of cylinder, greater than 3 diopters of prism, or that are blocked considerably off center, a foil or wire mesh pad is used first, instead of a pellon pad. After this preliminary step is completed the pellon pad is used.

The same Pellon pad can be used for the second fine, as long as it has been well washed off. The second fine slurry is made from W14 garnet† or #30 optical powder. The finish on the lens after this second fine is better than that obtained by using a yellow abrasive pad for the second fine. Because of this, some laboratories like to use a combination abrasive pad/slurry process. They use a black abrasive pad for the first fine and a slurry for the second fine. This makes use of both the convenience and aggressiveness of the black pad and the ability of the second fine slurry to produce a smooth, almost lustrous prepolish surface.

Polishing CR-39 Plastic Lenses

After the lens has been fined, the fining pads are stripped from the tool. The tool is rinsed well to assure that no grains of abrasive are still present,

---

†A W12 or W16 garnet will also work.

then checked for any adhesive or abrasive that might still be on the tool. Next the polishing pad is placed on the surface. Dipping the pad in water first will make it conform to the curvature of the tool nicely. However, to get best adherence of the pad to the tool, leave the pad dry. Leaving the pad dry is advisable when two lenses have the same curve and can be run one after the other on the same pad.

Polishing time is approximately 3 minutes at 20 psi pressure, but depends on the type of machine used, the size of the polishing pad, and the kind of polishing compound used. Polishing compound is usually purchased premixed. With plastic, the lens does much better when the polish is kept cool. A 55- to 60-degree Fahrenheit temperature is optimum. If the polishing compound becomes too warm, it begins to break down, the lenses become wavy, and rejection rates increase quickly. Therefore a chiller is recommended.

Plastic lenses that are to be AR (antireflection)-coated demand an especially well-polished surface. Antireflection coatings are applied at thicknesses that have a tolerance of ¼ wavelength. Surface irregularities give rise to slight depth variations, which adversely affect the coating's ability to quench surface reflections. If AR coating is a factor, then the polishing compound should be of the highest quality, with sufficient time devoted to polishing and a careful inspection of the polished surface.

In polishing plastic lenses, the concentration of the polish (degrees Baumé) is important, even though most polish comes premixed. If the concentration thickens, it will begin to act a little like a second fine. If the concentration becomes too watery (low Baumé reading), the lens will begin to acquire what is sometimes referred to as a "water polish." A water polish results in an orange peel-like surface defect.

As with any slurry (suspension of particles in a liquid), there is a tendency for settling to occur, even though settling time may be slow. To help keep particles from settling, some slurry flow through the machine is helpful. The slurry can be kept flowing even when no actual polishing is going on.

Removing Polishing Pads

Polishing pads can be removed from the lap tool using a paring knife in the same way fining pads are removed. If it is hard to get the pad off, it may help to immerse the tool in hot water or to run hot water over the surface.

One-Step Plastic Lens Processing

FB Optical Mfg., Inc. advocates a one-step processing system which skips fining altogether and goes directly from generating to polishing. One-step processing requires the use of the Tiger Tooth™ generator wheel in combination with a generator that cuts with extreme accuracy (within 0.02 D over the full curve range). The generator should also be equipped with a power sweep capable of making a 15- to 30-second last cut. To keep the surface smooth, FB recommends removing 1.5 mm of lens stock during the last cut. The last cut must be made "wet," using a good quality coolant.

Because no fining takes place, the surface curve will polish out exactly as removed from the generator. To ensure a complete polish across the entire lens surface, laps are permanently padded with a soft, resilient pad. The specially designed "One Step" polishing pad adheres to the resilient pad without adhesive. Because of the softness of this pad combination, no unevenness of polishing results even when the generator manifests elliptical error. FB Optical also states that, "The resilient pad masks up to 0.125 D of power. Therefore lens laps, for any lens material, need only be stocked in 0.25 D increments. No special laps are needed for polycarbonate or high index lenses."[8] Polishing is done for 4 minutes at 40-psi pressure using Micronal Supreme polish or the equivalent. (For more on pad hardness, see the section on "Polishing Pad Materials and Hardness" later in this chapter.)

Fining and Polishing of Polycarbonate Lenses

Polycarbonate is a soft material and must be generated with a flycutter wheel, a coarse-grit diamond cutting wheel, or a wheel that combines both methods. When polycarbonates were first used, the polycarbonate lens surface was not as smooth after generating as a lens made from conventional plastic lens material. To make up for this an extra step in fining, referred to as *rough-in*, was needed.[9] For roughing-in, a 320-grit, 3-inch, notched fining pad was used. The next stage used a 600-grit pad placed on top of the rough-in pad. This was followed by a 15-micron pad stacked on top of the other two, making a total of 3 pads.

At the time of this writing most polycarbonate lenses are fined using a two-step process. Before the fining process begins, the back edge of the generated lens should be hand bevelled. This will remove the sharp edge and allow for a better coolant flow between the lens and the pad. Some polycarbonate lenses have extra tags of material on the edge from the molding process. These will also need to be removed with a hand edger.

For polycarbonates the first fine is done using a 280-grit (40-micron) pad for 2 minutes at 18 to 20 psi. To avoid pad wrinkles, the pad is pressed onto the lap tool (an aluminum or other non-cast-iron-type tool) using the type of pad press normally used for nonmetallic fining pads. After first fine, the lens should be rinsed in fresh water so as not to contaminate the fining process. The second fine is done with a 1200-grit (13- to 15-micron) pad. Fining time is again 2 minutes at 18 to 20 psi. After fining, a polycarbonate lens may look more cloudy than a CR-39 lens. This cloudiness is not unusual and should clear up during the polishing process.

To avoid scratching, the water should not be recirculated. However, if it is to be recirculated, a filter with a 5- to 10-micron particle size should be used to trap any particles of pad abrasive or polycarbonate material. Recirculated water may require an antifoaming additive to prevent foaming and to keep the fining pads from loading up with lens material. After the second fine, the lens is rinsed once more.

For *polishing*, the pads are now stripped from the lap tool and thrown away. A new polishing pad is put on the lap. The pressure is 20 psi and polishing time is 4 to 6 minutes. The quality of the polish must be excellent, as the use of an inferior polishing compound with a low particle size tolerance* can produce more trouble than anticipated. It may be advisable to filter the polish to remove unwanted lens material (swarf) produced during polishing or left on the lens from fining. As in regular plastic polishing, the polish should be chilled to 65 to 70 degrees Fahrenheit to achieve the best possible surface.[10]

Because of the changing technology for polycarbonate and high-index plastic lenses, it is likely that procedures will change rapidly in this area, and may well be different by the time this text is in print.

Because of the ease with which uncoated polycarbonate lenses scratch, wash the lens with diluted mild detergent and rinse it in fresh, running water. Dry with a Hyperclean™ tissue or the equivalent. Never let water or polish dry on the lens and do not use an air dryer on the lens.

Fining and Polishing Polyurethane Lenses

Some high-index plastics are made from polyurethane material. Polyurethane, like polycarbonate, is softer than CR-39. This means that polyurethane lenses require more attention to detail during the surfacing process. One disadvantage of these softer materials is that they require a hard coating to prevent scratching. Fortunately the same softness that requires a special hard coating also results in a lens that is less brittle and thus more impact resistant.

Polyurethane is fined and polished at a lower pressure than CR-39. The Varilux Corporation recommends a method for determining just how low that pressure should be. The method consists of using the amount of lens material removed during fining as a gauge. They suggest that if the amount of lens thickness removed exceeds 2.5 mm, fining and polishing pressure should be reduced by 2 to 3 psi. In most instances pressure ends up being 15 to 17 psi.

When using a two-step process, the first fine is done with a 600-grit pad for 1 minute, and the second fine with a 1200-grit pad for 1½ to 2 minutes. The stroke on the cylinder machine is set at a maximum and fresh nonrecirculating water is recommended. If water is recirculated, it should be filtered and changed frequently.

A one-step fining process is possible if the generator is very accurate and the generator wheel cuts smooth enough. One-step fining may be attempted using a 1200-grit seven-leaf pad for 1½ minutes.

Immediately after fining some manufacturers recommend that polyurethane lenses be dipped in an alcohol bath to prevent surface oxidation. After being dipped in alcohol, the lens can be permitted to air dry.

Polishing polyurethane is done using a good quality, chilled polish at 15 to 17 psi for 6 minutes. A low polishing pressure enables the polish to get into the pad and stay between the pad and lens during polishing. The key to a well-polished polyurethane lens is how thoroughly the pad is flooded with pol-

---

*A low particle size tolerance means that there may be more particles in the polish that are larger than the indicated particle size than is desirable.

ish. All spouts on the cylinder machine must be directed onto the pad with a full, rapid, unrestricted flow of polish.

The lens should be rinsed with warm water immediately after the polish cycle. Varilux recommends using natural sponges. Since touching the uncoated back surface introduces oils and greatly increases the possibility of surface scratches, polyurethane lenses should always be handled by their edges.

Fining and Polishing Transitions Photochromic Plastic

"Transitions" is the trade name for a photochromic plastic developed by PPG Industries and marketed through Essilor and Orcolite. A Transitions lens is fined using a two-step process which starts with a 600-grit first fine for ½ minute, followed by a 12-micron second fine for 1 minute. If the lens leaves the generator smooth enough, a one-step fining process using a 1200-grit pad for 1 minute is possible.

Recommended cylinder machine pressures are 15 psi for both fining and polishing. Essilor recommends a 4-minute polishing time using a good quality polish that has been chilled to between 50 and 60 degrees. At the present time it is not recommended that the lens be tinted or coated in any way.

Polishing Pad Materials and Hardness

Polishing pads can be made from a great variety of materials. They have been made from wool, felt, and synthetic mixtures such as polypropylene, rayon, and polyester mixtures.

How well a polishing pad works is not related directly to how soft the pad is. It might be thought that the softer the pad, the better the polish. Actually, the less exact the curvature of the fined surface, the softer the pad must be. Soft pads are more "forgiving" and will polish a surface that may not quite fit the tool.

The beauty of a hard polishing material is that it produces a very well-polished surface and may be used over and over again. To use a hard pad, a laboratory must have lap tools of the same curve, one for fining and the other for polishing.

One kind of hard polishing pad is made from polyurethane. In mass production situations it is possible to polish as many as 1000 surfaces on the same pad. Then, when the pad is worn smooth, it can be trued with a diamond tool and used again.

Very hard polishing pads work only when the tool used for fining the lens is exactly true to curve. Maintaining such an exact curve match is hard to do, but can be done when diamond lap tools are used to fine the lens.

Pellon is a brand of material used for polishing pads. It is available in different thicknesses. Pellon is a popular material and is reputed to hold polish within the pad microstructure while still allowing the individual polishing particles to roll and polish.

Special Types of Surfacing Pads

Many different types of pads are available to the surfacing laboratory. A few types that have not yet been mentioned are described in the following paragraphs. Some pads are for general use, while others are appropriate only in specific instances.

Gripper Pads

One of the small but time-consuming jobs that has to be repeated many times over during the surfacing process is stripping adhesive fining and polishing pads off the lap. It is possible to greatly reduce the time involved by using gripper pads instead of adhesive-backed pads. *Gripper pads* use a friction grip system that requires a special backing on the tool. The pad sticks to the backing. Once the backing has been put on the tool, it seldom needs to be replaced. The backing is self-adhesive and shaped like the fining and polishing pads. The backing holds the specially made fining and polishing pads. Fining and polishing pads stay in place from the pressure of the cylinder machines, but can be simply lifted off after fining or polishing operations. Because pads are so easy to peel off, the second fine pad is not stacked on top of the first fine pad. Consequently first fine, second fine, and polishing pad thicknesses are all the same. This means that the fined lens surface curve is closer to the curvature of the lap with the polishing pad in place. (For steeper curves this may even reduce the polishing time slightly.)

Because glass polishing uses metal pads for fining, glass lens gripper systems are not commonly used at present, even though such systems are available.

With glass lenses the gripper system's metal pad is removed and replaced by the polishing pad during processing.

Power-Compensating Pads

Sometimes a tool curve is needed that is halfway between two tools. Instead of cutting a new tool, it may be possible to place a *tool-compensating pad* on the steeper tool. This pad lengthens a convex tool's radius of curvature, flattening the tool and causing it to grind a slightly weaker minus curve. Exactly how much this weakens the dioptric power of the curve depends on the thickness of the pad and how steep the tool is to begin with. The tool-compensating pad is placed directly on the tool. Then the fining or polishing pad is placed on top of it. See Figure 12-8.

Diamond Pads

As has been noted, diamond tools are excellent for exact fining of optical surfaces. For the surfacing laboratory the main problem with diamond tools is their cost. When a diamond-impregnated pad is used with a gripper pad system, the same diamond pad can be used on a whole range of tool curves. Such a system keeps the tool from wearing and gives exact curves. Diamond pad systems have, as yet, not reduced production time. Therefore, since conventional fining methods are producing acceptable lens curves, the popularity of diamond pads has not been great.

Polish-Impregnated Pads

As will be remembered from previous sections, the fining pads used in the production of plastic lenses have the abrasive on the pad, not in a slurry. This is quite advantageous because it is so convenient.

There is no slurry to prepare, and cleanup of both the machinery and the laboratory itself is much easier. If fining is easier with abrasive-coated pads, why not do the same for polishing pads?

Polish-impregnated pads have indeed been developed and sold commercially. Yet they have not been widely used, mainly because of the cost factor and because of the increased polishing time required. The potential for such pads is good, however, since they are especially suited for small laboratories. Laboratories that produce only a very limited number of lenses must spend just as much time preparing slurry and cleaning up afterward as laboratories with higher volumes. Such a pad would certainly encourage the smaller operator to enter or stay in surfacing by reducing time requirements.

Pitch Polishing

Pitch polishing, seldom used for eyeglass lenses, consists of applying softer pitch, or pitch and wax, to a metal support. While the pitch is still soft, the fined surface of the lens is pressed into the pitch to create the exact curve to be polished. When the pitch hardens, the pitch surface is scored to help in the flow of the polishing slurry.

Although the pitch surface is hard, polishing is successful because of the exact match between lens surface and polishing surface. Pitch polishing's primary usage in ophthalmic lenses has been for the polishing of very-high-powered surfaces.

Checking for a Well-Polished Surface

A lens surface should be inspected using a clear (unfrosted) incandescent light. The lens is held as if it were a mirror, and the reflection of the bulb

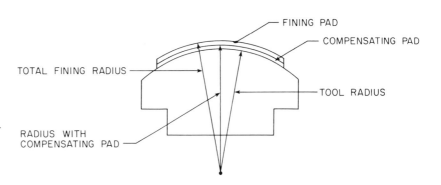

Figure 12-8 A tool-compensation pad increases the radius of curvature of the tool. When the radius of curvature changes, the power changes. If the tool is convex, the power will be weakened slightly.

looked at on the surface of the lens. The lens is tilted first one way, then another. The bulb filament should look sharp no matter where on the surface it appears. *Haziness* in any part of the surface shows an incomplete polish.

Grayness

Grayness may be caused by incomplete polishing. This grayness is a result of some of the roughness from the fining operation showing through. Grayness may be due to several different causes, the most obvious being that the lens has simply not been polished long enough. Other problems in polishing can be a result of:

1. an incorrect Baumé reading for the polishing slurry
2. a polishing slurry temperature that is too high for the plastic lenses being polished
3. incorrectly positioned slurry tubes, which are not directed on the lap well enough
4. an inadequate volume of slurry or water on the lap tool
5. a wrong match between the fining and polishing pad thicknesses for plastic lenses

An incomplete polish, especially when it appears in only certain areas of the lens, may have originated in an incomplete fine. An incomplete fine may have been caused by:

1. using the wrong lap tool
2. using a lap tool that is slightly off-curve
3. a generator that is not cutting an exactly correct curve

If there is a grayness at the top and bottom* of the lens, the cylinder power has been ground inaccurately. This could be a tool problem, a generator problem, or just plain human error.

Grayness at two obliquely opposite positions on the lens indicates an axis problem. See Figure 12-9. Either the pins that hold the lens on axis in the generator are wearing, or the axis in either the generator or the cylinder machine is off.

For plastic lenses, grayness may result from allowing the lens to sit too long between processing steps. For plastic lenses that have high curves, the

---

*The top and bottom of the lens referred to here is with reference to the three horizontal holes in the lens block. These correspond to the minus cylinder axis.

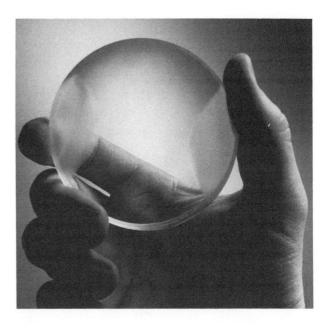

Figure 12-9 Grayness in a lens. When grayness is found in a meridian oblique to the cylinder axis, an axis problem is indicated. The problem could be in the generator or in the cylinder machine.

pressure of the generating or fining process compresses the lens slightly. If the next process is initiated quickly, there is no problem. However, if the lens sits too long, it will relax (the *relaxation effect*), and the curve will change slightly. This will result in a slightly inaccurate match between the lens surface and lap tool and can sometimes produce grayness. If a long interval between processes is anticipated, this problem can be avoided by making small cuts during generating or by using lower fining pressures.

Polishing Burn

Another surface defect related to the polishing process is polishing burn. A *polishing burn* looks like a blister or a small group of blisters on the lens surface. Polishing burn may be caused by a polishing pad that was not sufficiently wetted with polish.

Scratches, Sleeks, and Swirls

Distinct marks on the lens surface cannot always be identified and traced until the mark is looked at more carefully. Not all surface marks are scratches. A *scratch* is a furrowed-out line that has jagged edges, whereas a *sleek* is a furrowed-out line whose edges are smooth instead of jagged.

The cause of scratching may be obvious mishandling of lenses at a certain phase in production and therefore easy to trace. On the other hand, it can also be very difficult to identify. If scratching is a problem, here are some of the places to begin looking.

1. Look for problems with the slurry, or when fining plastic, the coolant. If the slurry or coolant has become contaminated, it should be changed and the equipment thoroughly cleaned.
2. On glass lenses, scratching may occur because of bad fining pads.
3. If scratching occurs when fining lenses on a bare tool, the tool may not be scored properly.
4. If the cylinder machine is loose or wobbly in its motion, the lens may rock on the surface of the tool and incur scratches.

Specific patterns may help in distinguishing where the marks on a lens surface came from. *Swirl marks* on a lens indicate that a larger grain of abrasive material was trapped in the pad and has scratched the surface. The swirls show the rotational motion of the machine. With plastic lenses, such swirl marks are less common when using a two-step fining system than when using a one-step system, as the second fining step usually removes such marks.

Removing Scratches

Small hairline scratches on glass lenses are sometimes removed by using a rubber ball mounted on a spindle. The outer layer is peeled off and the inner part used with polishing compound to buff out the scratch. Such methods always run the risk of causing aberrations in the surface and a waviness in the optical characteristics of the lens.

On plastic lenses, hairline sleeks or scratches are sometimes removed using a spindle-mounted buffing sponge and a concentrated polishing compound, such as PSI-Lite Concentrate No. 375. Again, caution must be exercised, as the wholesale removal of lens scratches in this manner masks the root problem and is sure to lead to some instances of viewing-area aberration.

Other Distinct Marks

When other distinct marks (not just grayness or scratches) are observed on the lens after polishing, the problem stems back one or two steps previously. Either the generator is cutting too coarsely or inaccurately, or the fining operation has been insufficient. The answer is *not* just to polish longer.

The most common type of unwanted patterned surface marks are *generator marks*. Generator marks are parallel, curved marks across the surface of the lens. See Figure 12-4. They are caused by the generator wheel. Light generator marks are normal after generating. After fining and polishing, they should not be visible. If generator marks do not disappear after fining and polishing, it is usually because of one of three problems:

1. incomplete fining
2. a lap tool that does not match the curve of the lens
3. a generator that is cutting off curve

Another type of undesirable surface mark is the *block mark*. These marks are visible on plastic lenses after the lens has been deblocked. They appear on the front surface of the lens and are caused by pressure from the block or heat from the blocking alloy. It is sometimes possible to bake or boil the mark out by heating the lens to approximately 212 degrees Fahrenheit.

Waves

A surface defect that does not show up because of an unpolished or marked area on the surface, but that must nevertheless be watched for, is a wave. A *wave* is due to the curvature of the surface changing somewhat in one particular area of a lens. It can be seen by viewing a line through the lens while slowly moving the lens from side to side. The lens should be held at from 20 to 40 cm from the eye. A wave may also be seen by moving the lens across the lensmeter stop while looking through the lensmeter. The lensmeter should be set for the proper power. If waves are present, the lensmeter target will change focus and/or move in an irregular manner.

If waviness is present in the surface, the lens must be re-fined in order to get rid of it. A further polishing of the lens just leaves the wave in place, or makes it even worse. In fact, some waves are caused by overpolishing. Other causes of waves include an improper slurry mixture (incorrect Baumé reading) or a cylinder machine that is either worn or is not adjusted correctly. Examples of adjustment problems are incorrect stroke setting, wrong head pressure, or loose belts.

A defect that is closely related to a wave is called an *orange-peel* defect. Some say that this type of defective surface has a *water polish*. The defect is really a type of wave and looks like the peel of an orange. Most often it occurs because the polish is not dense enough (hence the name "water polish"). It may be, though, that the polishing pads are not absorbing the polish sufficiently, or that the polish is not getting far enough up on the pad. This could occur because a hose on the cylinder machine is pointed in the wrong direction and is not squirting polish directly onto the lap pad.

Special Adjustments and Precautions

Cylinder Machine Stroke

In order to produce an evenly fined and polished lens, the path a lens travels over the lap during fining or polishing should not often duplicate itself. Excessive tracking over one area of the lens will tend to produce an irregular surface.[11]

The length (pattern size) of the stroke on the cylinder surfacer can be adjusted. The lens is made to move by the upper machine assembly. The lap tool moves too, but independently of the lens. The tool moves by means of the lower machine assembly. This means that there are two stroke lengths that can be adjusted: the upper and the lower stroke.

Stroke length called for in the fining process is different from that used for polishing. Fining stroke pattern size recommendations may vary by machine manufacturer and personal philosophy. For fining, Coburn Optical Company recommends a long stroke for the upper pattern and a medium stroke for the lower pattern. For polishing, a long stroke is recommended for both the upper and lower strokes.[11] Thus, if the function of a machine is changed from smoothing (fining) to polishing, or vice versa, the stroke pattern for the machine should also be reset.

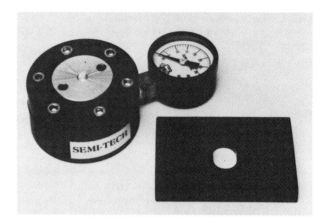

Figure 12-10 A head pressure gauge measures the pressure of the cylinder machine pins on the blocked lens. The cylinder head pins fit directly onto the gauge. (Photo courtesy of Semi-Tech, Garland, Texas.)

Checking Head Pressure and Cylinder Axis

Almost any piece of machinery tends to get out of adjustment with continuous use. Thus, when the gauge on a cylinder machine shows 30 psi of pressure, this does not guarantee that there is actually 30 psi of pressure on the lens. To be certain that the pressure is as indicated, a *head pressure gauge*, as shown in Figure 12-10, must be used. The gauge is placed in the surfacer where the blocked lens would normally be. The pins are positioned in the appropriate holes on the gauge and pressure is applied. The head pressure gauge shows actual pressure compared to what the cylinder machine shows. If there is a difference, the cylinder machine dial can be recalibrated or compensated for.

The accuracy of the *cylinder machine axis* can be checked with a gauge designed just for this purpose as well. Although the machine itself may lose its axis adjustment, this is not the only source of error. Inaccuracies in cylinder axis may be due to pin wear. When the three pins that hold the blocked lens on the lap during surfacing become rounded, the axis may not be exact. Even though the pins may be new and sharp, if the centers in the lens block are worn and hollowed out, they too can cause the cylinder axis in the prescription to be wrong.

Working Spherical Lenses on Cylinder Instead of Sphere Machines

The question of using cylinder machines to fine and polish spherical surfaces was discussed in Chapter

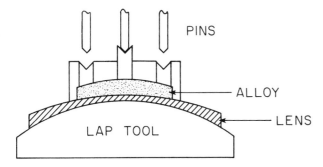

Figure 12-11 When an extra long center is used in the middle hole of a lens block, the two outer pins on the cylinder machine are not used. This allows the lens to rotate and can help in producing a more spherical surface.

11. Most laboratories use cylinder surfaces for all their sphere lenses, processing both spheres and cylinders in exactly the same manner. However, some laboratories use a lens block with a raised center for processing sphere lenses. If such a raised center is used, as the pins in the cylinder machine are lowered onto the lens block, the high middle block center prevents the two outer pins from touching. See Figure 12-11. This allows the lens to rotate on the lap tool during fining and polishing. The rotational movement bears a slight resemblance to the action of the sphere machine.

If spheres are to be surfaced on cylinder machines, it is also helpful to cut the tools on a sphere lap cutter. Sphere lap cutters spin the tool while cutting and can cut a surface that is more truly spherical.

Questions and Problems

1. One method of grading the size of an optical abrasive uses screen size. This means that an abrasive numbered by screen size has been physically run through a screen corresponding to that particular size.
   True or False

2. The concentration of polishing slurry is measured in degrees Baumé using a
   a. hydrometer
   b. barometer
   c. thermometer
   d. pachometer
   e. none of the above

3. Degrees Baumé is an expression of specific gravity. Specific gravity of a substance is equal to

   a. $\dfrac{\text{mass of mercury}}{\text{mass of the substance}}$

   b. $\dfrac{\text{mass of the substance}}{\text{mass of mercury}}$

   c. $\dfrac{\text{mass of water}}{\text{mass of the substance}}$

   d. $\dfrac{\text{mass of the substance}}{\text{mass of water}}$

   e. none of the above

4. A central slurry system is
   a. a system consisting of a central tank and pipes that lead to each cylinder machine for continuous recycling of the slurry
   b. the recycling reservoir in a cylinder machine
   c. the mixing tank found in a central area of the lab from which premixed slurry is drained and carried to individual cylinder machines as needed

5. Which of the following is an incorrect statement concerning the precautions necessary in order to obtain accurate Baumé readings.
   a. The slurry must be uniformly dispersed. If some of the abrasive has settled out, the reading will be too low.
   b. The slurry must be somewhat aereated (i.e., slightly foamy). Otherwise the reading will be artificially high.
   c. The temperature must not be too high. (For every 10 degrees Fahrenheit above 60 degrees, add 0.1 degree Baumé to the value measured.)

6. If polishing slurry has a pH value of 10, the liquid is
   a. more acid than alkaline
   b. more alkaline than acid
   c. neutral

7. Adding acid to a slurry to bring down the alkalinity
   a. is harmful for new slurry
   b. causes the formation of silicic acid when the slurry has already been used and acts as a diluent

8. Glass fining is done on a metal fining pad or on a bare cast iron tool using
   a. iron oxide in slurry form
   b. cerium oxide in slurry form
   c. aluminum oxide in slurry form
   d. none of the above

9. When working with a single cylinder machine for the fining of glass lenses, the best policy is to add dry abrasive powder when the slurry concentration drops, or water when the concentration increases. This should be done for approximately 1 week, and then the slurry changed.
   True or False

10. During the fining process, if the lens begins to fine from the center out, the tool is
    a. steeper than the lens
    b. flatter than the lens

11. Which is not a theory of how glass polishing occurs?
    a. physical collusion
    b. chemical action
    c. thermal flow
    d. mechanical abrasion

12. Which polishing compound is commonly referred to as "polishing rouge"?
    a. zirconium oxide
    b. iron oxide
    c. cerium oxide
    d. none of the above

13. Which is not a polishing compound?
    a. zirconium oxide
    b. iron oxide
    c. cerium oxide
    d. All of the above are polishing compounds.

14. In mixing powdered polishing compound, it is best to use
    a. boiling water
    b. very warm water
    c. room-temperature water
    d. cold water
    e. ice water

15. Which of the following does not have an effect on glass polishing time?
    a. the speed and design of the cylinder machine
    b. the size of the lap compared to the lens size
    c. the type of polish
    d. the concentration (Baumé reading) of the polish
    e. All of the above have an effect on glass polishing time.

16. Cylinder machine pressures for glass polishing can be higher than for glass fining.
    True or False

17. Cerium found in its natural state and made into a polish with a natural mixture of rare earths is called
    a. an extended polish
    b. an accelerated polish
    c. a high-cerium polish
    d. a low-cerium polish
    e. polishes are not made this way

18. If used with a polishing agent such as cerium oxide, which of the following will cause the polishing agent to perform better than it would have alone?
    a. antifoaming agent
    b. extender
    c. accelerator
    d. energizer
    e. none of the above

19. Foam-controlling agents are best added to polishing compounds
    a. during manufacture, before the polish is processed
    b. when dry, before the compound is mixed into its slurry form
    c. after the slurry is mixed, but before the polishing process begins. Once the foaming starts it is difficult to keep under control
    d. after foaming appears

20. For plastic lens fining, longer fining times may be required for
    a. especially flat curves
    b. especially steep curves
    c. especially high cylinders
    d. all of the above
    e. both b and c

21. When only water is used in combination with abrasive pads in the fining of plastic lenses, the same cylinder machine may be used for first and second fines, as long as the recirculated water is kept cool.
    True or False

22. Why might a polishing pad be dipped in water before putting it on the lap?
    a. to cause it to stick more firmly to the surface
    b. to cause it to conform better to the surface curvature
    c. to cause it to absorb the polish better
    d. to cause it to polish more rapidly
    e. all of the above

23. Which plastic lens demands an especially high-quality surface?
    a. a lens that will be ultraviolet dyed
    b. a lens that will be tinted to a solid color
    c. a lens that will be antireflection-coated
    d. a lens that will be antiscratch-coated
    e. all of the above

24. When polishing plastic lenses, if the slurry concentration becomes high:
    a. The lenses will polish a lot faster.
    b. The lenses will polish a lot more slowly.
    c. The polish will act somewhat like a second fine.
    d. The lens surface will begin to manifest an "orange-peel" defect.

25. When polishing plastic lenses, if the slurry concentration becomes low:
    a. The lenses will polish a lot faster.
    b. The lenses will polish a lot more slowly.
    c. The polish will act somewhat like a second fine.
    d. The lens surface will begin to manifest an "orange-peel" defect.

26. Unless a high-grade generator wheel is used for polycarbonate lenses, there is an extra step in the fining process called "rough-in."
    True or False

27. A soft polishing pad gives a more highly polished surface than a hard polishing pad.
    True or False

28. Which is the hardest type of polishing pad?
    a. a Pellon pad
    b. a gripper pad
    c. a polyurethane pad
    d. a felt pad

29. A power-compensating pad will cause the tool to
    a. *increase* the power of a minus (concave) lens surface
    b. *decrease* the power of a minus (concave) lens surface
    c. either increase or decrease surface power, depending on how thick the pad is

30. Polish-impregnated polishing pads are potentially an excellent idea, and have been produced commercially.
    True or False

31. Surface grayness can be due to several reasons. Which of the following is *not* a reason for surface grayness?
    a. The lens was simply not polished long enough.
    b. The polishing slurry had an incorrect Baumé reading.
    c. The polishing slurry was at too high a temperature for the plastic lens being polished.
    d. The slurry tubes were positioned incorrectly and were not directed on the lap well enough.
    e. *All* of the above may cause surface grayness on a lens.

32. Grayness at two obliquely opposite positions on the lens indicates what?
    a. The wrong tool was chosen.
    b. The lens was ground too steep.
    c. There is an axis problem with the generator or cylinder machine.
    d. The cylinder power has been ground inaccurately.
    e. None of the above is the source of the problem.

33. A *sleek* is
    a. an area of dried polish on a lens surface that is difficult to remove
    b. a furrowed-out line on a lens surface whose edges are smooth instead of jagged
    c. a furrowed-out line on a lens surface whose edges are jagged
    d. an area within the lens that has a different refractive index than the rest of the lens
    e. none of the above

34. Swirl marks are caused by
    a. a larger grain of abrasive trapped in the pad
    b. a faulty generator wheel
    c. slurry whose pH value has been allowed to get too high

d. a slurry whose Baumé reading (concentration) has been allowed to get too high
    e. all of the above

35. Which of the following may *not* be the cause of generator marks on a lens after fining?
    a. incomplete fining
    b. a lap tool that does not match the curve of the lens
    c. a generator that is cutting off-curve
    d. Generating a glass lens too fast
    e. All of the above are possible causes of generator marks on a lens.

36. It may be possible to remove block marks from a plastic lens by baking or boiling the lens at 212 degrees Fahrenheit.
    True or False

37. A localized change in surface curvature that does not disappear with further polishing, but which requires that the lens be re-fined, is called
    a. an orange peel defect
    b. a polishing burn
    c. grayness
    d. a wave
    e. None of the above is localized, and none fits the description.

38. Which of the following do not affect cylinder axis accuracy during surfacing?
    a. block center wear
    b. cylinder machine stroke length
    c. cylinder machine pin wear
    d. the adjustment of the cylinder machine itself (which can be measured with an axis gauge)
    e. All of the above affect axis accuracy.

39. There is no value in having sphere tools that will be used on a cylinder machine cut on a sphere lap cutter. Sphere tools cut using a cylinder lap cutter are just as good.
    True of False.

40. A lens has been blocked off-center and now overhang exists. List three ways to prevent the overhang from causing unwanted prism or an uneven fine and polish of the back surface.

41. Compared to the traditional way of processing CR-39 lenses, pressures used in fining and polishing polyurethane lenses are:
    a. higher
    b. lower
    c. the same

42. For what purpose is a 320-grit silicon carbide pad most commonly used?

43. What is the name for the polyurethane pad that is most commonly used by manufacturers of uncut lenses?

44. Which glass polishing compound is better known as "rouge"?

45. a 1200-grit silicon carbide pad is rougher than a 600-grit silicon carbide pad.
True or False

46. Name the three theories of glass lens polishing.

47. In many laboratories, metal pads are used in the process of fining glass lenses. Name three other methods that can be used in the fining process of glass instead of metal pads.

48. What rust-red compound was used almost exclusively for polishing glass lenses before cerium oxide began to be used? Give both the name and the material from which it was made.

49. For what purposes are additives to glass polishing slurry used?

50. What is a gripper pad?

51. Could you use a polyurethane polishing pad in almost any optical laboratory? Why or why not?

References

1. *A Guide to Optical Abrasives.* Practical Systems, Inc., Tarpon Springs, Fla., n.d.

2. Silvernail, W.L. The Use of Slurry Specific Gravity as a Measure of Concentration. *Reopal Technical Bulletin #2.* Shieldalloy Corporation, Newfield, N.J., 1979, p. 3.

3. Silvernail. The Use of Slurry Specific Gravity, p. 4.

4. Silvernail, W.L. The Use of Additives and Their Effects on Optical Polishes. Shieldalloy Corporation, Newfield, N.J., 1978, p. 6.

5. Whitman, P.C. Fundamentals of Glass Polishing for the Prescription Laboratory—Part 2: Polishing Theory and Cerium Oxide. *The Optical Index,* 54 (12): 58–60 (December 1979), presented at the Manufacturing Opticians International Symposium, Amsterdam, The Netherlands, June 28, 1979. Used by permission.

6. *Standard Glass Procedure,* Coburn System Bulletin. Coburn Optical Industries, Muskogee, Okla., revised 1980.

7. Silvernail, W.L., and Silvernail, B.L. The Mechanism of Glass Polishing. *Reopol Technical Bulletin #3.* Shieldalloy Corporation, Newfield, N.J., 1979, p. 13.

8. *Introducing One Step Plastic Lens Polishing,* FB Optical Manufacturing, Inc., Saint Cloud, Minn., undated.

9. *Titmus Polycristyl™ Comprehensive Processing Guide for Polycarbonate Lenses.* Titmus Optical Co., Petersburg, Va.

10. *Coburnsystem Procedure for Processing Polycarbonate Lenses.* Coburn Optical Industries, Muskogee, Okla. Copyright 1989, February, 1990.

11. Woodcock, F.R. Prescription Shop Machinery, Part 3: Automatic Cylinder Surfacing Machines. *Manufacturing Optics International,* 27 (3): 105 (March 1974).

12. *Coburnsystem Bulletins No. 4 and 9.* Coburn Optical Industries, Muskogee, Okla.

13 Deblocking, Verifying, and Hard Coating

Deblocking

When a lens has been blocked using a metal alloy, it can be deblocked through shock deblocking or hot-water deblocking.

Shock Deblocking

Shock deblocking of plastic lenses is done with a ring that is placed around the outside of the lens block on the front surface of the lens. It is deeper than the block, so when the lens and block are turned block side down, the ring may be struck against a flat surface. See Figure 13-1. The block drops off the lens from the shock. This is generally used when the block is formed completely from alloy material. Then the complete alloy block may be dropped back into the lens blocker's melting pot. Lenses which have been blocked with a conventional block held in place by low melting point alloy material may be successfully deblocked using such a method. However, the alloy would still have to be melted from the block. The deblocker should have a rubber ring at the upper rim, otherwise shock deblocking risks indenting the front surface of a plastic lens. Shock deblockers come in different diameters, depending upon lens blank/lens block sizes being used.

Shock deblocking is the method of choice for polycarbonates, high-index plastics and plastic photochromics. It should be used even if a hot-water deblocker is available.

Hot-Water Deblocking

Hot-water deblocking is a commonly used technique that utilizes a hot-water bath. The temperature of the water is kept below the boiling point. The blocked lenses are placed on a rack, which is lowered into the water (usually simultaneously with the lowering of the lid on the deblocking unit). See Figure 13-2. With the lens under water, the alloy begins to melt and drips to the bottom of the tank. There is a valve at the bottom of the tank through which the liquid alloy can be drained off from time to time. The liquid alloy should be drained into a flexible container. When using alloy for plastic lenses, allow

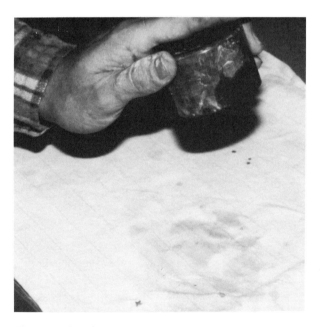

Figure 13-1 When plastic lenses are blocked using a lens block made entirely from alloy, the cost of a lens deblocking unit can be avoided by shock deblocking the lenses. Here the lens is placed block side down in the hollow deblocker. The deblocker is slapped firmly on a flat surface, so that the block drops off.

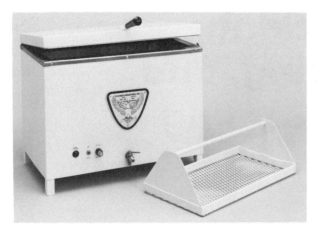

Figure 13-2 Lenses to be deblocked are placed in the tray that normally resides inside the tank. As the lid is closed, the tank is lowered into the hot water. When the alloy melts, it sinks to the bottom and can be drained out into a flexible container using the stopcock in the front. It is then allowed to cool. The hardened alloy is removed from its container and placed back into the blocking unit to be used again. (Photo courtesy FB Optical Manufacturing, Inc., Saint Cloud, Minn.)

the alloy to harden before returning it to the blocking unit. This assures that the liquid alloy passing through the blocker will not be hotter than the 122–125 degree temperature produced by the blocker. Inadvertently using overheated alloy will cause problems for all types of plastic lenses. (These problems were discussed in Chapter 12.)

After deblocking, the blocks and lenses are removed from the rack, the surface tape removed, and the lenses cleaned. (The blocks must also be inspected to assure that they are clean as well, since any foreign matter can cause an error in the next lens that is processed on the block.)

Ultrasonic Deblocking

Ultrasonic deblocking is really a combination deblocking-and-cleaning process. One such machine is manufactured by Autoflow Engineering Ltd. (Warwickshire, England) and employs a hot-water deblocking tank that is also an ultrasonic unit. The blocked lenses are placed in clips. As the alloy begins to melt, the ultrasonic unit speeds its removal and the block drops off into a catch tray. The process takes approximately 2 minutes, except when there are stubborn contaminants.[1]

Cleaning of Surfaced Lenses

Once the lenses have been deblocked, they must be cleaned before they can be verified. If the lenses have been taped for surfacing, the surfacing tape is peeled off. Generally, spray coatings will also peel off nicely. The best cleaning method available is an ultrasonic bath using a detergent or other solvent, but this may not always be cost-effective for smaller laboratories.

Glass lenses can be cleaned with a detergent solution. Acetone is used extensively for cleaning CR-39 plastic lenses, but detergent can be used to clean CR-39 lenses as well. Acetone has been used in the optical laboratory for quite some time. Lenses have been "washed" in it and individuals have continually dipped their fingers into and out of the acetone. However, it is now recognized that acetone is quickly absorbed through the skin and, in sufficient quantity, can cause a health hazard. If acetone or other similar agents are used in the cleaning of lenses, care should be taken to avoid skin contact.

Because polycarbonate and many types of high-index plastic materials are soft, they must be coated to protect the lens surface from scratching. Polycarbonate material is susceptible to damage by several different kinds of solvents. Under no circumstances should methylene chloride, methyl ethyl ketone, any other members of the ketone family, or acetone be used. Highly volatile chlorinated or aromatic hydrocarbons must also be avoided.[2]

Polycarbonate or high-index lenses which must be hard-coated need to be cleaned right after polishing. Failure to immediately clean these lenses will result in a stubborn residue. Even if such a residue seems to have been cleaned off, remaining traces may mix with the coating and occasionally cause problems. Because these problems are only periodic, they are difficult to track down. Here is one method for cleaning polycarbonate lenses which has proven effective.[3]

1. After polishing, rinse the lens with water.
2. Shock deblock the lens and rinse it again in running water. (Using a bucket of water promotes the transfer of contaminants from one lens to the next.)
3. Using a HyperClean tissue, dry the lens. Do not dry the lens with compressed air or with an air blower, especially if the water in your area is hard. Do not save the HyperClean

tissue for later. Using the tissue again may just transfer the contaminants to another lens.

4. For polycarbonates, use a mild liquid detergent like Joy (one capful in 1 gallon of water), and a natural sponge to remove any remaining residue. For high-index plastics or CR-39 lenses, use Soft Scrub instead of a liquid detergent.

5. Rinse the lens in running water and dry it with a HyperClean tissue.

This procedure cleans the lens well enough to prevent problems later, but does not get the lens clean enough to actually coat.

Progressive-addition lenses may still have markings on the front surface that denote the location of the near portion, the 180-degree line, and the major reference point. If these markings are still clear, the laboratory may wish to leave them intact. Most often, though, the surfacing laboratory replaces these markings. Progressive lenses are re-marked with a rubber template stamp and non-water-soluble ink for aid in the lens edging process. Progressive lens manufacturers provide these stamps and appropriate instructions on how they are applied. To remove progressive-add lens markings (or regular lens markings when applied with non-water-soluble ink), a solvent such as alcohol or acetone is used.

Checking Surfaced Lenses Before Edging

When lenses will be edged elsewhere, the lenses must be checked for accuracy before being sent out. (Of course, the procedure for checking these surfaced lenses is the same procedure as will be used by the receiving individual.) The sections that follow explain the procedures to use in verifying the accuracy of a surfaced lens before it has been edged.

Remember that polycarbonates or other soft, high-index plastic lenses should be coated before being verified. Chances of scratching the uncoated lens are extremely high. More time and money will be saved by verifying after coating, even though some coated lenses will end up being rejected.

Verifying Single-Vision Lenses

For single-vision lenses, the first step is to set the lensmeter power wheel at the prescribed sphere power. Set the axis wheel for the desired cylinder axis. Begin with the right lens. Place the right lens in the lensmeter and find the optical center by moving the lens until the illuminated lensmeter target centers. See Figure 13-3. (If there is Rx prism in the prescription, move the lens until the correct amount of prism is present in the lensmeter.)

Because the cylinder axis is already set in the lensmeter, the lens can be rotated to find the optical center. Rotate the lens until the illuminated sphere line(s) of the lensmeter target are smooth and unbroken. This indicates that the cylinder is oriented correctly. See Figure 13-3.

At this point the sphere line(s) should also be clear and crisp. If they are not, turn the power wheel until the line(s) become clear. The difference between what was ordered and what the instrument now reads is the error in the sphere power. To determine if the error is within tolerance, check the American National Standard Recommendation for Prescription Eyewear. A summary of these standards is given in Appendix 7.

Now turn the power wheel in the minus direction until the cylinder lines are clear. This will cause the

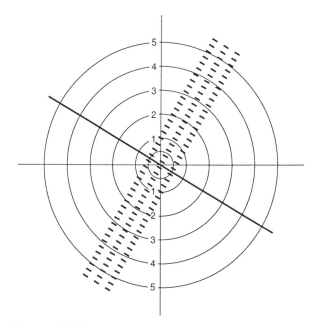

Figure 13-3 If there is no prism in the prescription, the surfaced lens is moved in the lensmeter until the target centers, as shown here. With the sphere and cylinder axis preset to the prescribed amount, the lens may have to be rotated until the sphere line comes into clear focus.

sphere line to blur. The difference between the sphere power previously read and what the instrument now reads is the cylinder power and is a negative number. If the cylinder power found differs from the prescribed cylinder power, ANSI standards should be used to determine whether the difference is small enough to be acceptable.

With the lens now centered and the sphere and cylinder powers verified, spot the lens with the spotting device in the lensmeter.

If the frame is available, hold the lens up to the frame. The center dot of the three lensmeter dots marks the location of the optical center (or major reference point when prescribed prism is present). With the optical center (or major reference point) decentered to where the eye will be, the lens should completely cover the frame's lens opening. If it covers the lens opening, the blank is big enough.

The entire procedure is repeated for the left lens. A summary of the procedure is given in Table 13-1.

Verifying Multifocal Lenses

Checking Sphere, Cylinder, and Axis

To verify multifocal lenses, begin by performing the steps described for the verification of single-vision lenses. Again start with the right lens. If the lens is a flat-top bi- or trifocal, note whether the segment tops are straight or crooked before removing the lens from the lensmeter. The segment tops must be exactly horizontal, that is, parallel to the lensmeter table. If the top is not straight and the lens has a cylinder in the prescription, the cylinder will be off-axis.

To find out just how far off the axis is, first turn the lens until the seg top is horizontal. Next, readjust the lensmeter axis wheel until the target lines

Table 13-1 Verifying Surfaced Single Vision Lenses

1. Set the lensmeter power wheel to the sphere power and the axis wheel to the cylinder axis.
2. Turn the lens until the sphere line(s) are clear, indicating that the axis is correct.
3. Move the lens until the optical center is centered (or until the target is at the correct prism position if Rx prism is present).
4. Verify the sphere power.
5. Turn the power wheel until the cylinder lines clear and verify the cylinder power.

are clear again. The difference between what the cylinder axis now reads and what the prescription calls for is the axis error. Look up the amount of error in the ANSI standards to determine if it is within tolerance.

Checking Add Power

When measuring the power of the near portion of a bi- or trifocal lens, it is important to remember that the lensmeter will read the *sum* of the power of the distance lens and the power of the near add. In other words,

$$\left(\begin{array}{c} \text{distance} \\ \text{lens power} \end{array}\right) + \left(\begin{array}{c} \text{add} \\ \text{power} \end{array}\right) = \left(\begin{array}{c} \text{total} \\ \text{near power} \end{array}\right)$$

For example, if there is no power in the distance lens and the add power of the segment is $+1.50$ D, then

$$(0.00) + (+1.50) = +1.50$$

so the lensmeter will read $+1.50$ D. If the distance lens has a power of $+2.00$ and the same add, then

$$(+2.00) + (+1.50) = +3.50$$

and the lensmeter will read $+3.50$ D.

Any cylinder that is in the distance lens will be in the add as well. If the distance prescription is $+0.50 -0.75 \times 35$ and the add is $+1.00$, then the total near power through the segment portion will be

$$\begin{array}{c} +0.50\ -0.75\ \times\ 35 \\ \underline{+1.50\ \text{sph}} \\ +2.00\ -0.75\ \times\ 35 \end{array}$$

The lensmeter reading will be $+2.00 -0.75 \times 35$.

Here is the procedure:

1. Turn the lens around backwards in the lensmeter. Since the segment is on the front of the lens, the concave side of the lens must face the operator in order to measure the add power.
2. Read the distance power again from the back. The distance power should be read at a point on the lens that is as far above the major reference point of the lens as the segment is below the major reference point.
3. Note the distance power of the sphere.
4. Move the lens upward in the lensmeter and read the near sphere power through the add.
5. Subtract the distance sphere from the near sphere. The difference between these two

values is the add power. (It should be noted that when there is an oblique cylinder in the prescription, the cylinder axis will not be the same as it was from the front: It will be the mirror image of what it was before. For example, if it was Axis 30, it will now read Axis 150.)

Although the above procedure for turning the lens around in the lensmeter is correct, it is not always followed. When the distance power and the near-add power are both small, most operators do not bother to turn the lens around. For small powers the results will be almost identical. When powers are larger, there will be significantly measurable differences.

Remove the lens from the lensmeter and repeat the above steps for the left lens. A summary of the procedure is given in Table 13-2.

Checking Horizontal and Vertical Prism

One of the easiest ways to check for prism is to use a lens marking device. If a lens marker is not available, prism can be checked another way.

Using a Lens Marking Device Using a lens marking device, position the lens in the device in the same manner as would be done if it were still a semifinished blank and had not yet been marked for sur-

facing. See Chapter 4. This is done by positioning the seg at the seg drop and seg inset called for in the prescription. If the lens has been surfaced correctly, the center lensmeter dot will now be right in the center of the grid. If it is not, the amount of horizontal and/or vertical error in millimeters can be easily seen.

According to ANSI standards for *high-powered lenses,* both the seg inset and the seg drop should be within 1 mm of what was ordered. However, if it is not within 1 mm, this does not mean that the lens is unacceptable.

If the major reference point (MRP) of the lens is not within 1 mm of the expected location horizontally and/or vertically, mark the lens with the lens marking device. It should already be in position and should be marked just as if it were a semifinished lens.

After it has been marked (stamped), the lens is put back in the lensmeter. The place on the lens where the stamp is located is where the optical center or MRP should be. Center this new mark in the lensmeter. See Figure 13-4. Look through the lensmeter and see how much prism is present. (The lensmeter should be set to the correct sphere and cylinder axis.) For the lens to be within ANSI standards, there should be less than one-third of a prism diopter difference, either vertically or horizontally, from what was ordered.

Table 13-2 Verifying Surfaced Multifocal Lenses for Sphere, Cylinder, Axis, and Add Power

---

Part I—Sphere, Cylinder, and Axis

1. Perform the verification procedure for surfaced single-vision lenses.
2. For flat-top lenses with cylinder, check to see if the segment top is exactly horizontal.
3. If the seg top is crooked, turn the lens until the segment top is straight. Turn the cylinder axis wheel to find the actual cylinder axis. Compare and see how far the axis is from what was prescribed.

Part II—Add Power

1. Turn the lens around backwards in the lensmeter.
2. Read the distance power again from the back.
3. Note the distance power of the sphere.
4. Move the lens upward in the lensmeter and read the near sphere power through the add.
5. Subtract the distance sphere from the near sphere to find the correct add power.

Checking Prism Without a Lens Marking Device An uncut lens can be checked for prism without the aid of a lens marking device. This is done by measuring the distance from the center of the seg top to the optical center or MRP by hand.

Before trying to make any measurements, mark the center of the seg top with a lens marking pen. Next, draw a perfectly straight vertical line. Draw it upward from the center of the segment top until it crosses the horizontal plane where the three lensmeter dots are found. See Figure 13-5. Now measure the horizontal distance from this newly drawn vertical line over to the center lensmeter dot. This is the actual seg inset.

Next, measure the distance from the center lensmeter dot down to the top of the segment. This is the actual seg drop. As stated previously, both should be within 1 mm of what was ordered for high-powered lenses.

To find out if the lens is within tolerance if it failed the above test or is a low-powered lens, dot the lens where the optical center (or MRP) *ought*

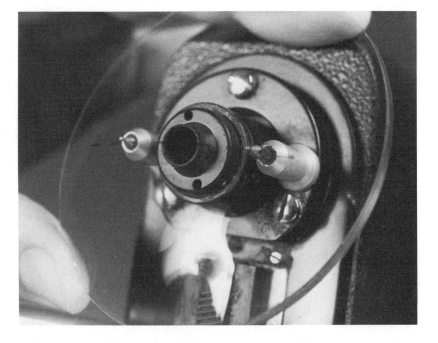

Figure 13-4 When there is a question of unwanted prism in the semifinished multifocal lens, the lens can be layed out with the prescribed seg inset and drop. (The seg inset is one-half the difference between the distance and near PDs.) The lens is lightly stamped and then transferred to the lensmeter. With the stamp centered over the lensmeter aperture, the target is viewed to see if unwanted prism is present, and how much there is.

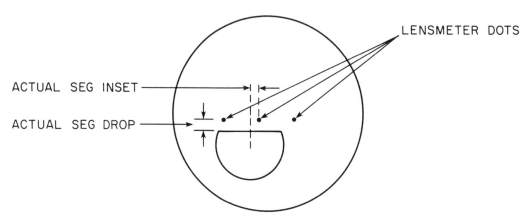

Figure 13-5 If the major reference point of the lens is spotted, the actual seg drop and inset can be measured and compared to what was ordered in the prescription.

to be using a millimeter rule and felt-tip pen. This is done by measuring up from the center of the seg line by an amount equal to the seg drop, then over by an amount equal to the seg inset. Mark this spot and center it in the lensmeter. Check for the one-third-diopter vertical and horizontal tolerances with the lensmeter as described above. The illuminated target should be within one-third diopter of the center when there is no Rx prism.

Even if both lenses pass this test, the pair may still fail if the lenses manifest vertical prism in *opposite* directions from one another. The *total* amount of vertical prism allowable is one-third prism diopter for both lenses together.

Checking Prism of Lenses That Will Be Edged In-House A somewhat quicker verification method may be used if the lenses are to be processed in-house. This method is as follows:

First, hold the two lenses back to back, viewing the lenses using a background that permits the segments to be seen easily. Position the lenses so that their segments exactly overlap each other. The lensmeter spots should also exactly overlap each other.

See Figure 13-6. If the dots do not overlap, tolerance problems are likely.

If one set of lensmeter dots is higher than the other, choose the weaker lens.* With the lenses still back to back, place a dot on the weaker lens. The dot must correspond exactly to the location of the center dot on the stronger lens. Now put the freshly dotted weaker lens in the lensmeter and center it using the new dot. Read the amount of vertical prism shown in the lensmeter. The amount of vertical prism that is present will also be present in the finished pair of glasses. (This assumes, of course, that both seg heights were ordered at the same height.)

To check for PD (horizontal prism), begin by measuring each of the two seg insets. These seg insets may be found by measuring the horizontal distance from the center of the seg top to the center lensmeter dot. Next, add the sum of these two seg insets to the prescribed near PD. This is what the distance PD is likely to be once the lenses are edged. If the difference between this calculated distance PD and the ordered distance PD is less than 2.5 mm, the lenses will pass ANSI standards once they are edged. If the difference is greater than 2.5 mm, then horizontal prism tolerances must be checked by the conventional methods described earlier to see if the lenses will still fail. A summary of the procedure used for verifying multifocal lenses for unwanted prism is given in Table 13-3.

Rechecking Blank Size If the frame is available, the finished lens can be checked to determine if it will be large enough. With multifocal lenses, the seg is used for reference. The lens is held up to the frame so that the seg height and near PD are correct. This can be estimated or determined more exactly by using a millimeter ruler. If a ruler is used, measure first from the center of the bridge to the center of the seg top (half the near PD). Next, measure the seg height from the lowest portion of the inside bevel of the lower eyewire to the seg top. (When you first try this, you may wish you had three hands.) If the seg height and near PD are correct, the lens blank should cover the frame's lens opening.

Checking Thickness
If the thickness of a lens is not specified, the minimum center thickness of a glass or CR-39 plastic,

*The "weaker" lens refers to the lens with the least power in the vertical meridian, since we are concerned with vertical prism.

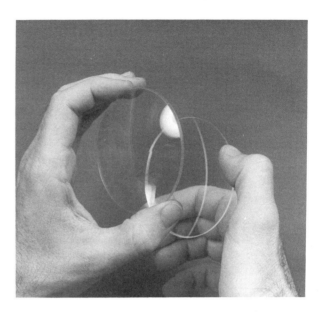

Figure 13-6 Once the lenses have been spotted for MRP location in the lensmeter, they can be held back to back to see if the locations of the major reference points coincide.

Table 13-3 Verifying Surfaced Multifocal Lenses for Unwanted Prism

Using a Lens Marking Device

1. Lay out the surfaced lens as if it were to be resurfaced.
2. The center lensmeter dot should be within 1 mm of the center of the target. If it is, verification is complete. If it is not, proceed to step 3.
3. Stamp the lens.
4. Center the stamp in the lensmeter.
5. Check for unwanted horizontal and vertical prism.

Using an In-House Method

1. Hold the surfaced and lensmeter-spotted lenses back to back, with the segments overlapping one another.
2. The lensmeter dots should overlap. If they do, verification is complete. If they do not, proceed to step 3.
3. With both lenses still back to back, dot the weaker lens at the place where the center lensmeter dot on the other lens falls.
4. Place this new dot in front of the lensmeter aperture and see how much unwanted vertical prism is present.
5. If the seg inset looks incorrect, measure the seg inset for the right and left lenses and add to the near PD. This is what the distance PD will be.

minus lens is generally 2.2 mm. The expected average edge thickness of a plus lens will be 1.8 or 1.9 mm. Edge thickness is not simply measured at the edge of the finished blank. Edge thickness is where the edge of the lens will be once the blank has been edged for the frame.

Sources of Errors*

Errors in Lens Power

If the refractive power of a lens is incorrect, there are a number of possible sources for the problem. For example, one of the most likely places to look is the lens layout.

Incorrect Lens Layout   In laying out lenses there are a great many points where an error can cause the power to be off. This is especially true if back curve powers for plastic lenses are figured without the use of a computer. Many of the possible sources can be eliminated by using a good layout computer. Remember, however, that a computer is only as good as the software program that runs it. More attention needs to be paid to the quality of the program than to the cost or reputation of the computer hardware that runs the program.

Inconsistent Base Curves   Power may also be off because it was assumed that the base curve of the lens equaled what was marked on the box. Unfortunately, base curves may be inconsistent. Front curves on semifinished blanks may not be exactly the same from lens to lens and should be checked using a sag gauge.

Individual glass lenses do not need to be checked each time at lens layout unless a problem is occurring. However, because plastic lenses can have some variation in their front curves, the base curves of each individual lens should be checked. If the front curve varies, the correct choice for a back tool curve may also change.

Lap Tool Errors   Another source of power error can originate in the individual tool used to grind the surface. If a particular tool is going out of true, the sphere or cylinder power of the lens will be thrown off. If this is the case, the tool should either be retrued, or if the metal pad on the tool is all that is worn, the pad should be replaced.

---

*Much of the material on power and axis errors has been adapted from *Coburnsystem Bulletins 7* and *11* (Coburn Optical Industries, Muskogee, Okla.).

Another possible cause of incorrect power may have to do with tool pad thickness. It could be that the tools being used have not been properly compensated for the pads that are being used on the tools.

Excessive Blocking Pressure   Too much pressure applied to plastic lenses while blocking will cause a power error. If the lens is pressed on too heavily while blocking, it will flex and be held in a flexed position for surfacing. (This is especially true for high-minus powers.) It is better to hold the lens lightly in place with the fingers than to use a hold-down arm on the blocker.

Errors in Cylinder Axis

Cylinder axis problems may arise from lens layout, cylinder machine problems, or difficulty with the lens block. Here are some things to check.

Incorrect Lens Layout   The layout marker could be stamping off axis. To check for this, set the cylinder axis of the layout marker for 90 or 180. Next, stamp a lens (or the face of the marker grid itself) and, without moving the lens, look to see if the mark is exactly on the 90 or 180 line. If it is not, readjust the stamping mechanism in the layout marker.

Cylinder Machine Errors   The axis of each cylinder machine can be checked with an axis alignment device. See Chapter 12. This should be done often—even daily.

Another source of error could be loose belts. Such belts should be tightened or replaced.

Cylinder machine pins, which hold the blocked lens in place, become worn with time. If these pins become rounded, they will not hold an accurate axis.

Worn Block Centers   Although the three block centers in the lens blocks look to be a permanent part of the block, they are not. When new, the tops of these centers are sharply V-shaped to accept the pointed cylinder pins. If the centers become rounded, the axis will stray even if the pins are new and sharp.

Errors in Prism

One of the most frustrating aspects of surfacing is producing a lens that is perfect in every way except for one "small" defect: The lens contains unwanted prism. To help in avoiding this frustration, several factors can be considered.

Errors in Off-Center Blocking When a lens is blocked off center (see Chapter 3), one side of the lens may extend out from the block a fair distance. This means that during surfacing there is more pressure on the one side, where the block is, than on the side that extends out beyond the block. This uneven pressure can cause more lens stock to be removed from one side of the lens than from the other, resulting in an unwanted prismatic effect.

To avoid prism from this lens overhang,

1. Reduce the fining pressure by one-half and increase the run time slightly (about 30 seconds longer).
2. Use an offset block adapter, which mounts to the lens block and shifts the pressure toward the lens center (see Chapter 9).
3. If there are extra pin positions in the block, offset the position of the pins on the block by using one of these smaller sets of noncentral holes (see Chapter 9).

Problems Related to Foreign Matter (Dirt) Another possible source of prism may be a small piece of matter that has been trapped under the fining pad. This lifts one side of the lens surface ever so slightly. Because of the speed with which the lens is fined, stock removal will be very uneven. To avoid this problem the laboratory must make sure that laps are thoroughly cleaned before each use.

Problems Related to the Generator Occasionally the source of unwanted prism will be associated with the generator. If prism is only appearing from time to time, the problem is not the generator itself. If the generator is causing the problem, it will cut the same amount of prism in the same direction for every lens. If this does happen, the generator requires a prism adjustment.

When generating glass lenses using standard-size glass blocks, a fiber ring must be used. If this fiber ring wears or becomes damaged, it acts like a prism ring and can become the source of unwanted prism. Fiber rings are not made to last a lifetime and should be periodically replaced as they become worn.

When the slide gibs* that regulate base curve, plus–minus, and tailstock amounts loosen, they fail to keep the machine securely set during operation. When this happens, unwanted prism can result. To avoid loosening, set screws should be checked

---

*A *gib* is an adjustable piece of metal for keeping the moving parts of the machine in place.

and tightened if necessary. (Check the generator manual.)

If the hydraulic pressure in the generator is low, prism can be a consequence.

Finally, prism can be caused by simply not placing the lens in the generator chuck squarely. If the lens is angled even slightly in chucking, prism will result.

Coating of Lens Surfaces

Many specialized plastic lens materials, such as polycarbonates and high-index lenses, are made from relatively soft materials. These materials need to be coated in order to prevent scratching. This *antiscratch coating* is not used just to make the lens more appealing to the wearer. For materials such as polycarbonate and for most high-index plastics, an antiscratch coating is a necessity. Without the coating, the lens simply cannot be used for ophthalmic purposes.

Coating Qualities

A great variety of antiscratch coatings are available. Many of the processes are intended primarily for standard CR-39 material. Coatings intended for use with CR-39 increase the scratch resistance of a surface that is already fairly hard. However, CR-39 lenses can be used without an antiscratch coating; most other plastics cannot.

Application of Antiscratch Coatings

Coatings for CR-39 lenses can be applied during the molding process. The coating is applied to the lens mold. After the liquid plastic resin is poured into the mold, it hardens into a lens. When the lens has fully hardened or "cured," it has the coating on it. Such *in-mold* coating systems are, on the whole, excellent.

For semifinished lenses, however, the back surface still has to be ground. This means that any coating for the back surface must be applied *after* the surfacing process. Such processes vary considerably. The most basic type of coating unit uses a bottle of coating material and a small oven. First the coating material is applied to the surface. Next the lens is cured in the oven. Other systems are more elaborate. The better systems necessitate a dust-free area kept clean through positive air pressure as used in "clean rooms." Quality varies considerably.

It should be evident that lenses must be immaculately clean before coating. Earlier in the chapter, in the section entitled "Cleaning of Surfaced Lenses," the cleaning procedure needed after polishing and deblocking was explained. However, before a lens can be coated it must be cleaned even more thoroughly. This time cleaning is done using isopropyl alcohol—but not the ordinary drugstore variety. Ordinary isopropyl alcohol may cause the coating to fog, so 97% isopropyl alcohol[4] or filtered isopropyl alcohol[5] is used. (For exact cleaning procedures, consult the coating unit manual.)

Curing is done either with ultraviolet light or thermally. Ultraviolet curing is considerably faster than thermal curing. Thermal cures are not limited to ovens, but may be done using a heat transfer method employing vapor that has been generated by boiling an optical curing fluid.

For polycarbonate and high-index plastic, a top-quality system is imperative. Anything less will not work. If the coating is poor or for the wrong type of lens material, the lenses will not hold up under ordinary use. Lenses that *require* a coating are so easily scratched that even verification is difficult to perform without scratching the uncoated surface. Because a coating is so important, a laboratory must be careful about which type of system is purchased. It is essential that other laboratories be questioned about their experience with given systems before a final decision is made.

Hard Coating and the Tinting Process

Once a lens is hard-coated, it is more difficult to tint. The coating not only keeps scratches off the lens, in many instances it is relatively successful in keeping dye off the lens. It is possible to tint a lens before it is coated. The tint is easily accepted by the lens, but unfortunately cannot be removed from the lens once the lens has been coated. Because tinting is not done in the surfacing lab, this is not really a good option. There are simply too many opportunities to scratch the lens before it has been coated.

A coating unit may allow for the use of more than one type of coating material. There are coatings that are very hard but also very dye resistant. Such coatings, generally referred to as "nontintable coatings," can be used only for lenses that do not have to be dyed any darker than a light fashion tint. Other "tintable" coatings will accept sunglass tints

more readily but are not as scratch resistant. As dye chemistry and coating technology improve, this difficulty should disappear.

Even if a coating is classified as "tintable," the time required to tint a lens is still longer than for uncoated lenses. Dyes designed especially for polycarbonate lenses may be needed for certain coatings. Other coatings allow lenses to be dyed using conventional dyes. One thing which is not interchangeable is neutralizing fluid. Neutralizing fluid used to remove the tint from a CR-39 lens cannot be used with hard-coated lenses, as it causes the coating to craze. A specially formulated neutralizer must be used instead.

Polyurethane lenses also require specific changes in the normal tinting procedure. For best results, stringently follow the manufacturer's recommendations.

Summary

Any laboratory that intends to process polycarbonate or high-index plastic lenses must have hard-coating facilities. Hard coating should not be confused with color coating or antireflection coating. These are different processes. A complete color/antireflection system is not required in order to hard-coat a lens. Nevertheless, a hard-coating unit is not a small investment. It is perhaps one of the largest hurdles a small laboratory faces before embarking on polycarbonate and high-index plastic processing.

Resurfacing of Lenses

Even when the best precautions are taken, there are times when a surfaced lens comes out wrong. The axis may be off, or the power somewhat in error. Whatever the reason, no one likes to simply throw away an expensive lens blank and start over. Being able to resurface a lens can save not only the price of a replacement lens, but also eliminate the necessity of breaking up a pair of blanks.

Choosing Lenses for Resurfacing

It is much easier to resurface a lens before it has been edged. Once a lens has been edged, the size is so small that it becomes more difficult to work with.

With any lens, whether it is uncut or edged, there must be sufficient center and edge thickness remaining to permit a regrind. To successfully regrind a lens without getting it too thin, remember these factors:

1. Most axis error corrections can be done without removing much thickness.
2. If minus sphere or minus cylinder power must be increased, the lens will be thinned most in the center.
3. If plus sphere power must be increased, the lens will be thinned most at the edges.

For example, suppose that a plus lens was verified and found to be weak. If the lens has a thin edge to begin with, the chances are great that regrinding will cause the edge of the lens to become unacceptably thin.

Resurfacing an Uncut Lens

Because power, axis, and prism errors are discovered after the lens has been deblocked and cleaned, the process must be started over again. There are, however, certain important differences between first-time surfacing and resurfacing of lenses. Here is the procedure for resurfacing a lens.

1. Re-mark the lens. Mark the lens just as if it had never been surfaced. The only difference may be in marking prism. If the error is such that the generating step may be skipped, then there is no need to mark a prism axis. A prism axis must be marked and the lens generated a second time if there is a prism or PD error, or if there is a large error in sphere or cylinder power.

2. Tape the lens. One of the problems in resurfacing plastic lenses is the heat factor. Because the lens is so thin compared to the thickness of a semifinished blank, liquid alloy can heat up a thin lens enough to cause uneven lens flexure. This results in waviness. To help avoid waves, tape the lens twice. Two layers of tape will better insulate the lens from the heat of the alloy during blocking.

3. Block the lens. It is here that a lens can easily be ruined. Heat is not the only danger for plastic lenses during the blocking process. Plastic lenses are so flexible that it takes very little pressure to warp the lens. During blocking, hold the lens *very* lightly in place with the fingers while carefully filling the cavity between the block and the lens with alloy. If

the lens is flexed during blocking, it will hold its flexed shape. This means that new curves will be cut into a flexed lens. When the lens unflexes, the power may be even farther off than it was before.

Use a smaller block when resurfacing. This may seem backward, since a plastic lens will need support to keep it from warping. However, a small block will require less hot alloy. Less alloy will also reduce the possibility of a wavy lens surface.

4. Regenerate the lens (sometimes). If the power is off only slightly, this step can be skipped. If the lens has unwanted prism or incorrect prism, it cannot. When regenerating is necessary, begin by zero-cutting the lens. *Zero-cutting* is done by setting the generator for no stock removal. Skim over the surface of the lens very slowly. It may be preferable to sweep the generator over the lens manually. After the first cut, check the lens surface. The beginning of a change in curve will be easy to see. Remove more stock a point* or two at a time until the surface has been reshaped.

5. Fine and polish the lens. When refining and repolishing, both pressures and times should be reduced. This is especially true when the lens has not been regenerated.

For plastic lenses, the water and the slurry should be as cold as possible. Many operators find that their success rate increases if they add ice to the water for fining and to the polishing slurry.

6. Deblock and check the lens for accuracy.

Resurfacing an Edged Lens

The procedure for resurfacing an edged lens is much the same as that described for an uncut lens. If a plastic lens has already been edged, it may not be possible to reblock it on the larger, plastic-style blocks. Instead, the standard glass 43-mm blocks are used. (Remember that a fiber ring must be used in conjunction with a glass block during generating.)

Sometimes even the 43-mm block is too large for an edged lens. The small lens may allow the alloy to leak out during blocking. If this happens, using an O-ring with the 43-mm block may work. An *O-ring* is a round, rubber ring that, in keeping with its name, looks like the letter "O." Place the O-ring between the block and the lens. The alloy is trapped by the O-ring and allows the lens to be blocked.

---

*A *point* is one-tenth of a millimeter (0.1 mm).

Questions and Problems

1. Lenses should be dried off immediately after deblocking in order to avoid water spots.
True or False

2. The use of facial tissues on a *clean* CR-39 lens for purposes of drying the lens will result in scratching.
True or False

3. The use of facial tissues on a *dirty* CR-39 lens for purposes of cleaning the lens may result in scratching.
True or False

4. Ultrasonic deblocking in surfacing is done using hot water to melt the block. The main advantages of ultrasonic deblocking are speed and a cleaner lens and block.
True or False

5. Polycarbonate lenses are best cleaned using
   a. methylene chloride
   b. methyl ethyl ketone
   c. dishwashing liquid
   d. acetone

6. For the distance PD of a single, uncut bifocal lens to be within the American National Standards Institute's recommendations for horizontal prism tolerance:
   a. The major reference point must be horizontally within 1 mm of where it was ordered.
   b. There must be less than one-third prism diopter of unprescribed horizontal prism at the desired major reference point location.
   c. The conditions listed in *both* a and b must be met.
   d. If *either* condition is met, the bifocal lens is considered to be within tolerance.

7. To check for vertical prism with bifocals that are to be edged in house, hold the two spotted lenses back to back. If the lensmeter dots on one lens are higher than they are on the other lens, a vertical prism problem may be present. To see how much vertical prism there will be in the edged lenses:
   a. With the lenses still held back to back, dot the *right* lens exactly over the location of the center dot found on the *left* lens. Place the newly dotted lens in the lensmeter with the dot centered over the lensmeter aperture. Read the amount of prism present.
   b. With the lenses still held back to back, dot the *left* lens exactly over the location of the center dot found on the *right* lens. Place the newly dotted lens in the lensmeter with the dot centered over the lensmeter aperture. Read the amount of prism present.
   c. With the lenses still held back to back, dot the *stronger* lens exactly over the location of the center dot found on the *weaker* lens. Place the newly dotted lens in the lensmeter with the dot centered over the lensmeter aperture. Read the amount of prism present.
   d. With the lenses still held back to back, dot the *weaker* lens exactly over the location of the center dot found on the *stronger* lens. Place the newly dotted lens in the lensmeter with the dot centered over the lensmeter aperture. Read the amount of prism present.

8. During the layout process, errors in lens power are best avoided by
   a. routinely checking every *plastic* lens base curve individually with a sag gauge
   b. routinely checking every *glass* lens base curve individually with a sag gauge
   c. Both a and b are necessary

9. Which is *not* a possible source of power error when surfacing plastic lenses?
   a. worn pins on the cylinder machine
   b. slight variations in base curve from lens to lens
   c. a lap tool that has been improperly compensated for pad thickness
   d. excessive pressure applied when holding the lens in place while blocking

10. Which of the following are *not* a possible source of unwanted prism in a surfaced lens?
    a. off-center blocking of plastic lenses
    b. dirt under the fining pad
    c. a worn generator fiber ring
    d. chucking the lens unevenly in the generator
    e. all of the above are possible sources of unwanted prism.

References

1. Mullins, P. Accurately Measuring Lens Surfaces During Manufacturing. *Optical Index*, 56 (2):39 (February 1981).

2. Optical Laboratory Marketing Plan, Section 4, Finishing and Glazing, Gentex Corporation, Dudley, Mass., 1980.

3. Coating Bulletin #1, Section 9-1, *Coburn/LTI Coating System Owner's Manual*, Coburn Optical Industries, Muskagee, Okla., August, 1990.

4. *Coating Manual*, Gentex Corporation, Dudley, Mass., 1988, p. 7.

5. *Coburn/LTI Coating System Owner's Manual*, Coburn Optical Industries, Muskagee, Okla., August, 1990, p. 9-1.

14 High-Powered Lenses

High-Powered Plus Lenses

When the power of a plus lens is especially high, any additional reduction in thickness is especially important. There are a few ways of reducing thickness that have not yet been considered in previous chapters.

High-plus lenses can be divided into several types, each addressing a certain aspect of the problem:

1. high-plus spherical base lenses
2. lenticulars
3. aspheric lenticulars
4. full-field aspherics
5. multidrop aspherics

High-Plus Spherical Base Lenses

The most basic type of high-plus lens simply has a spherical base curve like any other semifinished lens. As plus lens power increases, the recommended base curve steepens in curvature and the lens becomes thicker and thicker. Because thickness becomes such a critical factor, ways of reducing thickness should be considered.

A Smaller Chord Diameter

Lens diameter is commonly determined using a formula similar to the minimum blank size formula for single-vision lenses, except for a breakage factor. This formula is

Chord diameter = ED + (A + DBL − PD)

where ED is the effective diameter, A is the eyesize, DBL is the distance between lenses, and PD is the wearer's interpupillary distance. This is really the same as the effective diameter plus two times the decentration per lens and could be written as

chord diameter = ED + (dec × 2)

It will be recalled from Chapter 7 that this formula is an estimate only, since it does not include the angle of the longest radius for the effective diameter.

Effective Diameter Angle

If the angle of the effective diameter is considered, thickness can usually be reduced even further. The effective diameter is twice the longest radius of the edged lens as measured from the boxing center. Using the right lens as a reference, the angle from the zero-degree side of the 180-degree line to the effective diameter axis is referred to as X. See Figure 14-1.

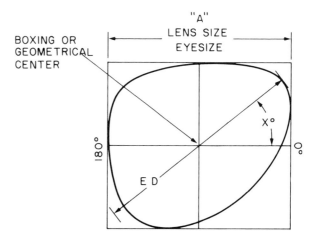

Figure 14-1 In the boxing system, ED is the abbreviation for effective diameter, which is twice the longest radius of the shape as measured from the boxing (geometrical) center. The angle from the zero-degree side of the 180-degree line to the effective diameter axis is X for the right lens. The measure is used in accurate calculation of the minimum lens blank size and blank thickness required to fabricate the prescription. (From C.W. Brooks, *Essentials for Ophthalmic Lens Work*, Butterworth-Heinemann, Boston, 1983), p. 224.

The simplest case is a lens shape that is round or oval. With a round or oval lens, the effective diameter is exactly the same as the eyesize (or *A* measure) of the shape. But as the lens starts to deviate from a round or oval shape, the distance from the boxing center of the shape to the farthest edge begins to increase. The effective diameter of a lens can become greater than the *A* dimension only if the lens shape expands in some direction *other than* the horizontal. Yet the chord diameter formula assumes that the lens is getting bigger in the 180. (It assumes the worst.) This means that when the frame ED is greater than the frame *A* dimension, the formula used to estimate lens chord diameter will always yield a slightly larger size than needed. See Figure 14-2.

A Modified Chord Diameter Formula

Because the ED meridian is usually not in the 180, the formula for chord diameter can be modified to produce a smaller estimated lens blank diameter. (If we can reduce the minimum lens blank size, we will end up with a thinner lens.) Therefore, the formula is modified by reducing the decentration factor to three-quarters of its actual size. The lens chord diameter becomes

$$\frac{\text{Chord}}{\text{diameter}} = ED + [0.75 \times (A + DBL - PD)]$$

The Effect of a Minus Cylinder on Lens Thickness

Up to this point, all plus-lens thickness calculations have been done assuming that the lens is a sphere. And, to avoid grinding a lens too thin, this is the safest assumption.

EXAMPLE 14-1

In order to compare a sphere lens with a spherocylinder lens, suppose that a prescription is ordered as follows:

R: +5.00 D
L: +5.00 D
A = 50 mm
B = 30 mm
DBL = 20 mm
ED = 50 mm
Wearer's PD = 64 mm

If the lens is made of crown glass, ground to an oval shape and decentered inward, the thinnest edge will be found temporally. See Figure 14-3. No lens can be ground thinner than a knife edge. Therefore the limiting factor for reducing center thickness is the temporal edge.

Here's how the thickness calculations would go. Since the lens is oval, the chord diameter of the lens is

Chord diameter = 50 + (50 + 20 − 64) = 56 mm

For simplicity we can assume that the lens is plano convex. Looking up the sag of a +5.00 D surface for a 56-mm chord in Appendix 4-1, we find a value of 3.8 mm. This means that the lens can have a center thickness of no less than 3.8 mm.

Yet what would happen if the prescription included a cylinder component whose axis was in the 90-degree meridian? Because the power meridian of a cylinder is 90 degrees away from the axis meridian, the lens will have an increased thickness both temporally and nasally (but not at the top or bottom). Since the temporal thickness is thicker, this means that the whole lens can now be thinned.

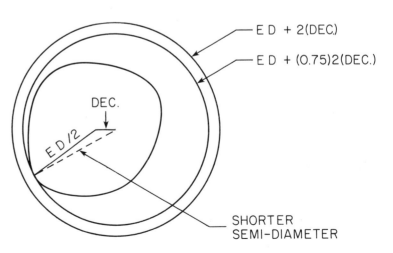

Figure 14-2 It can be seen that the formula ED + (0.75) (2) (decentration) is closer to the shorter semidiameter needed than the worst-case estimation of ED + (2) (decentration). The first formula will result in a smaller estimate of blank size, and as a result, a thinner lens.

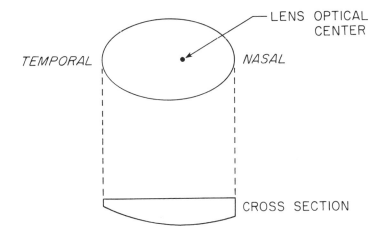

Figure 14-3 When an oval-shaped plus lens is decentered nasally, the thinnest point will be the temporal edge in the 180-degree meridian. This is the area of the lens that limits how thin the entire lens may be ground.

How Much Can a Lens Be Thinned Because of Cylinder Power?

The amount of thinning possible because a lens has a minus cylinder depends on both the power and the axis of the cylinder. To see how this works, think of what would have happened if the cylinder in Example 14-1 was at 180 degrees. There would have been no thinning of the temporal edge at all, and thus no reduction in overall lens thickness. However, suppose the lens has a power of $+5.00$ -1.50×90. How would the amount of lens thinning be determined in this case?

In this case, the power in the 180-degree meridian is equal to the sum of the sphere and the cylinder combined. This is $+3.50$ D. Therefore the center thickness of the lens can now be based on $+3.50$ D instead of $+5.00$ D. In figuring the sag of a $+3.50$ D surface based on a 56-mm chord diameter, we find a value of 2.6 mm. This is a considerably thinner lens.

A Short Summary

In our example we have seen that if the cylinder axis and ED meridian had both been in the 180, there would have been no thickness increase in the 180 due to the minus cylinder. Since the thinnest portions of both sphere and cylinder components are in the 180-degree meridian, no additional thinning is possible. However, if the *power* meridian of the minus cylinder corresponds to the thinnest part of a spherical lens, the full edge thickness of the minus cylinder would fall on what would otherwise be the thinnest part of the lens. If this happens, then maximum thinning is possible.

For plus spheres, the thinnest edge of the lens is most likely to be in the ED meridian. Therefore it can be said that

1. if the axis of a lens is in the ED meridian, no lens thinning is possible, but
2. if the power meridian of the cylinder falls in the ED meridian, maximum thinning is possible.

What If Either the ED Meridian or the Cylinder Axis Is Placed Obliquely?

A minus cylinder lens has two different curves on the back surface. These curves may be found by placing a lens clock on the back surface and slowly turning the lens. The maximum and minimum values are found in what are referred to as the *major meridians*. It is obvious from the gentle swing of the needle on the lens clock as the lens is turned that the change in curvature is gradual. Since lens curvature changes gradually, we can expect edge thickness to change in a gradual, predictable manner as well. Here's how it happens.

Edge thickness depends on the sag of the surface. And if we know the radius of curvature of the surface, we can use the sine-squared method. (The sine-squared method was introduced in Chapter 3.) Therefore we assume that

$$D_\theta = D_{cyl} (\sin^2 \theta)$$

The angle θ we are interested in is the angle from the cylinder axis to the ED meridian. See Figure 14-4. D_θ is the "power" value that the cylinder has in the ED meridian. Once found by using either a calculator or tables, D_θ is added to the sphere power. This new value is used to calculate thickness.

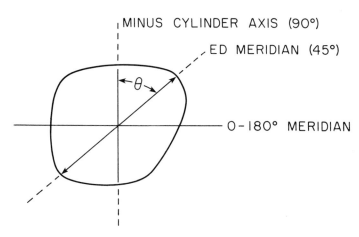

Figure 14-4 To figure the "power" of the cylinder in the ED meridian, we need to know the angle between the minus cylinder axis and the ED meridian. This angle is referred to as angle θ. Here angle θ is equal to 45 degrees. If the cylinder had an axis of 105, what would angle θ be? (Ans.: 60 degrees.)

EXAMPLE 14-2

Suppose a prescription for a right lens is as follows:

R: +6.00 −1.50 × 90
A = 47 mm
DBL = 18 mm
ED = 51 mm
X of the ED = 45 degrees
Wearer's PD = 61 mm

The lens is made from crown glass having an index of 1.523.

If a knife edge on the thinnest edge were desired, how would the center thickness be calculated?

SOLUTION

Step 1. Find the chord size diameter.

Chord size = ED + [(A + DBL − PD)] (0.75)
= 51 + (47 + 18 − 61)(0.75)
= 54 mm

Step 2. Find the angle between the cylinder axis and the ED meridian.

θ = |cyl axis − ED meridian|
= 90 − 45
= 45 degrees

Step 3. Find the "power" of the cyl in the ED meridian. Using the formula, this is

$$D_\theta = D_{cyl} \,(\sin^2 45)$$
$$= -1.50(0.5)$$
$$= -0.75 \text{ D}$$

In Appendix 3-1, we look up the angle 45 under "Cyl Axis" and 1.50 under "Cyl Power." The table shows the answer to be 0.75 D.

Step 4. Add the "power" of the cyl in the ED meridian to the sphere.

$$+6.00 + (-0.75) = +5.25 \text{ D}$$

Step 5. Find the sag of the lens in the ED meridian using either sag tables (Appendix 3-1) or the sag formula.

The sag of +5.25 D for a chord size of 54 mm is 3.7 mm. (This is in contrast to the thickness of 4.2 mm that would have been obtained without considering the minus cylinder.)

Lenticulars

Lenticular lenses have a steeply curved optic zone of approximately 40 mm diameter. This small optically usable portion is termed the *aperture*. High plus power is limited to the area of the aperture. Beyond this zone the lens surface abruptly changes to a much flatter curve, which is usually on the order of approximately +3.00 D. See Figure 14-5. This design is used in order to reduce lens thickness and weight.

Lenticular lenses are surfaced to the same thickness for a given power regardless of what the A, ED, or decentration dimensions are.

The outermost portion of a lenticular lens bordering the central aperture is called the *carrier portion*. The front curve of the carrier portion is shaped so that it will have approximately the same radius of curvature as the back surface of the lens once the lens is ground. This makes the carrier have close to a zero refractive power. To achieve a nearly plano-powered carrier, it is necessary to remain within the recommended base curve limits as spec-

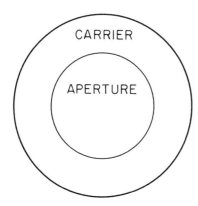

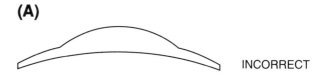

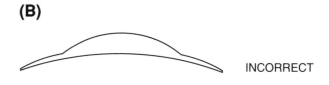

Figure 14-5 A lenticular lens design, when viewed from the front, looks like two concentric circles. The inner circle contains the power called for in the prescription. The outer portion simply carries the optically sound inner portion and is usually near zero in power.

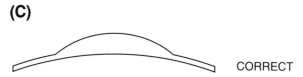

ified in the manufacturer's surfacing charts. Choosing a lens blank with a base curve that is *flatter* than recommended produces a finished lens that is either too thick in the center or that has edges that are too thin. See Figure 14-6. Using a semifinished lens blank that is *steeper* than recommended means that the edges must be ground thicker than desired or the lens may break at the aperture–carrier border. See Figure 14-7.

Aspheric Lenticulars

A lenticular lens having a spherical aperture surface is called a *spheric lenticular*. (Spheres have only one

Figure 14-6 It is important that the correct base curve be used for lenses of lenticular design. If the base curve chosen is too flat, the back curve must be ground too flat. If correct carrier edge thicknesses are adhered to, the lens will be thicker in the center than it was designed to be, as in (A). If it is ground so that the center will be thinner, the carrier edge will end up thin, unstable, and unsafe, as in (B). The base curve is designed so that the back curve will nearly parallel the front curve of the carrier, as in (C).

Figure 14-7 If a base curve that is too steep is chosen for a lens having a lenticular design, it must be ground thicker so that the carrier maintains a minimum thickness, as in (A). Often, though, when the lens is generated the carrier is measured at its outer edge, as in (B). When the base curve is too steep, the area immediately surrounding the lens aperture becomes so thin that it breaks off, leaving a donut-shaped carrier with an empty aperture.

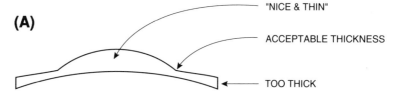

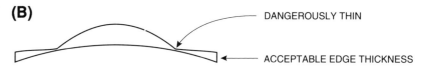

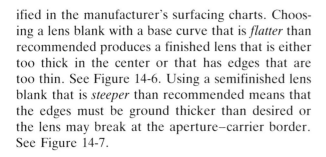

radius of curvature over the whole surface.) If a lens is over + 7.00 D in refractive power and is designed to correct aberrations, the front surface cannot be kept completely spherical. Instead, at 12 to 14 mm from the optical center, the front surface will begin to drop in power. See Figure 14-8. When a lens is designed in this manner it ceases to be spheric, so it is termed an *aspheric* lens. (The prefix "a" means "without," so aspheric means without sphericity.) A lens may be simultaneously lenticular and aspheric. Such lenses are termed *aspheric lenticulars.*

There are differences in carrier curves and the amount of asphericity in each lens depending on design philosophy. Because of this, manufacturers' tables or computer programs individualized for the specific brand should be used to find the correct curves. In other words, it is not a good idea to try and use one manufacturer's tables to grind another's lenses.

Full-Field Aspherics

When the wearer may use the entire lens for viewing, the lens is referred to as being *full field.* A lens may be aspheric without being lenticular in design. When a lens is aspheric beginning where the small central spheric region leaves off and continuing in its asphericity all the way to the edge of the lens, it is termed a *full-field aspheric.*

Full-field aspherics have been used for quite a number of years. Since then a lens type has been introduced in which the surface power drops much more rapidly as the edge of the lens is approached.

This lens surface may drop as much as 4 diopters in power from the center to the edge of the lens. In other words, the lens may clock as being +14.00 D at the center and only +10.00 D at the edge. Such a lens is referred to as a *multidrop lens.* Multidrops are not inherently better than regular aspherics. They simply reflect a different philosophy of lens design.

As with other lenses described previously, the manufacturer's own tables should be used when working with these lenses. This point is perhaps even more important for multidrop lenses.

The surfacing guide will lead the reader through a series of calculations and compensations to take into account the factors that have been mentioned here. Out of the necessity for keeping things as simple as possible, some factors may be ignored. Thus each set of charts for finding thicknesses and tool curves may have certain strengths and certain weaknesses. Yet all will include some of the considerations we have described.

Multidrop Aspherics

A regular aspheric lens that is designed primarily for the purpose of reducing peripheral lens aberrations will cause the lens to be only slightly thinner. To thin the lens further, the aspheric is combined with the lenticular design. Robert C. Welsh, M.D., broke with tradition and designed an aspheric lens with the primary purpose of reducing lens thickness. This lens, the first multidrop aspheric, was originally named the *Welsh 4 Drop.*

The Welsh 4 Drop lens had a spheric central front

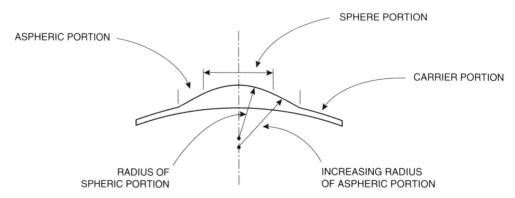

Figure 14-8 Aspheric lenticular lenses will be slightly thinner than spheric lenticulars, because the optical portion begins flattening as the edge of the aperture is approached. An aspheric lenticular will be both thinner and optically better than a simple spheric lenticular.

High-Powered Lenses / **241**

surface. Beginning 13 to 14 mm from the center of the lens, the front surface dropped in power by 1 diopter. By the time the edge of the blank was reached, the front surface had dropped off four times. Each drop was 1.00 D, hence the name "4 drop." A lens with a 14.00 D base curve would have dropped to a +10.00 D at the edge. This made the lens considerably thinner.

As the multidrop lens was improved, the abrupt drops in power were smoothed out and the amount of drop was tailored to the strength of the base curve. Yet the multidrop was still not addressing the issue of peripheral aberrations such as oblique astigmatism and curvature of field, as the original aspheric designs did. The considerations remained lens thickness, lens weight, and the elimination of the visible lenticular circle.

American Optical was one of the first to address both issues with its Ful-Vue lens. The Ful-Vue multidrop aspheric lens was designed to drop more slowly in power closer in toward the center of the lens. This slower drop addressed the problem of peripheral aberrations. At about a 50-mm diameter, the lens very suddenly dropped in power, resulting in what could almost be considered a blended lenticular design. See Figure 14-9. It accomplished all the cosmetic and thickness aspects of the previous multidrop designs and eliminated the visible lenticular circle as well. Other lens manufacturers have also incorporated this design philosophy into their multidrop product line.

Moderate- and Low-Powered Aspheric Lenses

Because of the increase in ease of manufacturing aspheric surfaces, it is becoming increasingly practical to design moderate- and low-powered lenses with aspheric surfaces. Aspheric surfaces result in lenses that are thinner, flatter, and lighter in weight than lenses with conventional spheric base curves. Properly designed, aspherics will also be better optically. Examples of aspheric lens designs include Silor's Hyperal, Signet Armorlite's RLX Lite Aspheric, and Rodenstock's Cosmolit. Because these lenses are aspheric, the major reference point has a fixed location in the lens blank—even for single vision lenses. As with high-plus aspherics, no prism for decentration may be ground.

A sagometer which measures for a 50-mm diameter will not give accurate results on an aspheric

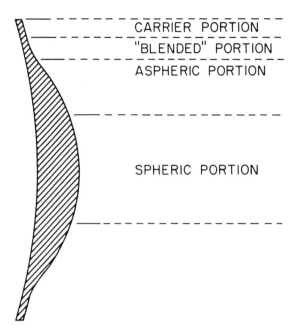

Figure 14-9 A well-designed multidrop lens will incorporate corrections for oblique astigmatism and curvature of field in the midperiphery of the lens before making a rapid drop in surface power at about a 50-mm diameter.

lens. When working with aspherics, do not use a sagometer reading. Instead use the manufacturer's tables or a computer program designed specifically for that brand of aspheric lenses. The true base curve and any sag value listed by the manufacturer are useful in calculating tool curves, but not for lens thicknesses.

In the future, aspheric lens designs will become increasingly commonplace. Progressive-addition lenses with their nonspherical front surfaces have paved the way for aspheric lens designs by making both laboratories and dispensers more comfortable in working with aspheric lenses. Although aspheric lenses require a higher degree of skill in both laboratory and dispensary, both are rising to meet the challenge.

Compensating for Changes in Vertex Distance

Often a prescription for high-plus lenses is written by the doctor and given to the patient to be dispensed by another. Since the doctor does not know what frame is to be used, it is appropriate to write the *vertex distance* at which the refraction took place. (The vertex distance is the distance from the back surface of the lens to the front of the eye.) The effective power of a lens changes, depending on the distance from lens to the eye. If the lenses are to be worn at a distance other than the refracting distance, the lens power must be changed to give the same effect as the original prescription gave during the refraction. Refracting distance is usually equal to a 14-mm vertex distance.

After the eye examination is finished, the patient goes to have the prescription filled. A frame is picked out and the new vertex distance measured. If the dispenser does not wish to recalculate the new lens power needed for the new vertex distance, or is unable to, the prescription will be sent to the laboratory with the request that the laboratory make the necessary power compensations. Compensation for vertex distance is not really that difficult. It can be calculated, looked up in tables, or found using a computer program. Here is how it is done.

Calculating Changes in Vertex Distance for Sphere Lenses

When the prescription to be fitted at a new vertex distance is a sphere, the first thing that is necessary is to determine the focal length of the lens. The *focal length* is the reciprocal or inverse of the focal power. Focal length is designated with a small f.

$$f = \frac{1}{D}$$

For illustration purposes, assume that light is traveling from left to right. When light coming from infinity enters a plus lens from the left, the focal point will be to the right of the lens. The focal point

is located at a distance f from the lens. See Figure 14-10.

Suppose the person will be wearing their lenses closer to the eye than the refracting distance. If we imagine the eye as being to the right of the lens, we can think of the lens as moving to the right. This means that in order to keep the net effect of the prescription the same, the focal point should not move. In other words, the focal length must be shorter. Just how much shorter depends on how far the lens is moved. To find the new focal length, subtract the distance the lens moves toward the eye from the old focal length. See Figure 14-11.

EXAMPLE 14-3

Suppose a prescription calls for a +12.00 D lens. The new glasses will be worn at a 10-mm vertex distance, but the prescription was written for a 14-mm refracting distance. What should the power of the lens be at the new vertex distance so that it will have the same effect as the prescribed power at the original refracting distance?

SOLUTION

The focal length for the +12.00 D lens is

$$f = \frac{1}{12}$$

$$= 0.0833 \text{ m or } 83.3 \text{ mm}$$

The distance the lens moves is 14 mm minus 10 mm, or 4 mm closer to the eye. To find the new focal length, this change in lens position is subtracted from the old focal length.

$$f_{new} = 83.3 - 4$$
$$= 79.3 \text{ mm}$$

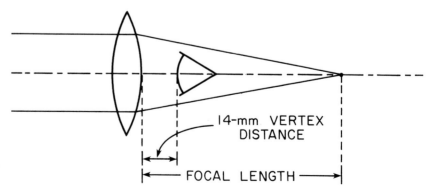

Figure 14-10 The focal length of a lens is the reciprocal of its power. The vertex distance of a lens is the distance from the back surface of the lens to the front surface of the eye.

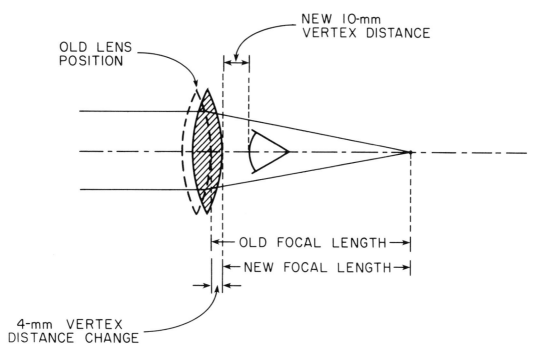

Figure 14-11 Moving a plus lens closer to the eye requires an increase in lens power to obtain the same effective power. In this figure the new focal length must be 4 mm shorter than the old focal length.

To find the new lens power, we now convert back to diopters. If

$$f = \frac{1}{D}$$

then

$$D = \frac{1}{f}$$

so

$$D_{\text{new}} = \frac{1}{f_{\text{new}}} = \frac{1}{0.0793}$$

$$= +12.61\ D$$

To the nearest quarter diopter, this is +12.50 D.

The correct power to use for this prescription at a 10-mm vertex distance will be +12.50 D.

What If the Lens Is a High-Minus Sphere?

If a lens is minus in power, its focal point will be in front of the lens instead of behind the lens. Now what happens when a high-*minus* lens is worn at a shorter vertex distance?

When a high-minus lens is worn closer to the eye, in order to achieve the same effect as during the refraction, a longer focal length is needed. See Figure 14-12. Therefore, to find this new focal length, in absolute terms the change in vertex distance is added to the original focal length. (Actually, the focal length of the minus lens is a minus distance. If the vertex distance change is still subtracted from this minus number, a longer minus focal length results.)

Can This Be Written as a Formula?

Vertex distance power compensation can be written as

$$D_{\text{new}} = \frac{1000}{f_{\text{old}} - d}$$

where D_{new} is the new power needed for the new vertex distance, f_{old} is the focal length of the original prescription in millimeters, and d is the change in vertex distance in millimeters. If the vertex distance

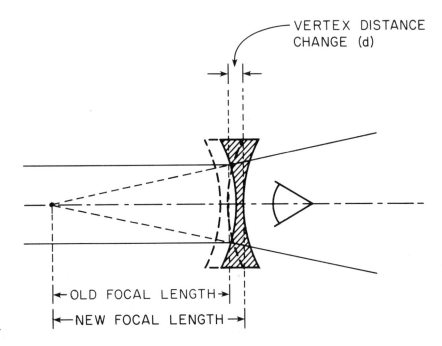

Figure 14-12 When a high-powered minus lens is worn at a shorter vertex distance, the power of the lens must be decreased to obtain the same effective power for the eye.

VERTEX DISTANCE CHANGE (d)

←OLD FOCAL LENGTH→

←NEW FOCAL LENGTH→

change is closer to the eye, d is a positive number. If the vertex distance change is in a direction that is farther from the eye, d is a negative number.

EXAMPLE 14-4

For a $+12.00$ D lens (see Example 14-3) the original focal length in millimeters is 83.3 mm, and the change in vertex distance is $+4$ mm. Therefore

$$D_{new} = \frac{1000}{83.3 - 4}$$

$$= \frac{1000}{79.3}$$

$$= +12.61 \text{ D}$$

EXAMPLE 14-5

As another example, suppose the lens were a -12.00 D lens. If all else were the same, the solution would be

$$D_{new} = \frac{1000}{-83.3 - 4}$$

$$= \frac{1000}{-87.3}$$

$$= -11.45 \text{ D}$$

This means that a high-minus lens would need to be reduced in power if its vertex distance were made smaller.

Changes in Vertex Distance with Spherocylinder Lenses

Spherocylinder lenses are handled in exactly the same manner as are sphere lenses, except that each meridian is considered separately. The cylinder is not calculated separately, but each meridian in the power cross is written separately.

EXAMPLE 14-6

A lens was refracted at a vertex distance of 14 mm, resulting in a prescription of $+14.00 -2.00 \times 90$. What is the new power required if the new vertex distance is 10 mm?

SOLUTION

To solve this problem, we need to know the power in the two meridians. On a power cross, the prescription would appear as shown in Figure 14-13A. The two meridians are calculated as if they were spheres. As we have seen, the $+12.00$ meridian will calculate out to be $+12.61$ D. The $+14.00$ D meridian will be $+14.83$ D. On the power cross this now appears as shown in Figure 14-13B. The new cylinder is the difference between the two meridians.

$$\text{New cyl} = 14.83 - 12.61$$
$$= 2.22 \text{ D}$$

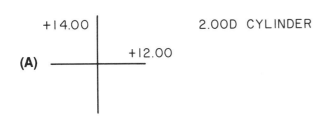

+14.00   2.00D CYLINDER
(A) ———————— +12.00

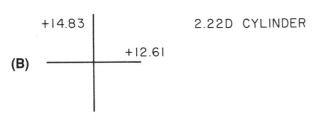

+14.83   2.22D CYLINDER
(B) ———————— +12.61

Figure 14-13 (A) The power of the lens in each of its two major meridians. When calculating out the needed power for this prescription at a new vertex distance, each meridian is treated separately. (B) The power the lens should have if it is to be worn at a vertex distance that is 4 mm shorter than the prescribed or previously worn position.

Written in minus cylinder form to the nearest quarter-diopter, the prescription becomes

$$+14.75 \ -2.25 \times 90$$

Can All This Be Done with Tables?

Fortunately, these calculations can be done with either a computer program or a table. Yet the basic understanding of the concept and how it is done mathematically is important. It prevents easily made errors and enables the individual to have the understanding necessary for the important overview of the optical process. Steps in using vertex distance difference tables are summarized in Table 14-1.

Vertex distance difference tables given in Appendixes 3-4 and 3-5. They are useful not only when changing spectacle lens vertex distances, but also when figuring what contact lens power would be appropriate when a spectacle lens refractive power is given.

EXAMPLE 14-7
Using the appropriate vertex distance difference table, tell what power lens should be used for the following situation:

Table 14-1 Steps in Finding Vertex Difference Power Changes

1. Find the difference between the old and new vertex distances.
2. Look up the sphere power in the chart and find out what it becomes at the changed vertex distance.
3. Add the sphere and cylinder powers for the prescriptions. This is the power in the second meridian.
4. Look up this second meridian power in the chart and find out what it becomes at the changed vertex distance.
5. Find the difference between the new powers in the two meridians (those powers which were found in steps 2 and 4). This is the new cylinder power.
6. Write the new prescription and round to the nearest quarter diopter.

Refracting distance: 14 mm
Prescribed lens power for this distance: +13.50
  −2.25 × 85
Vertex distance for the new frame: 9 mm

SOLUTION
Step 1. The vertex distance difference is

$$14 - 9 = 5 \text{ mm}$$

Step 2. Looking up +13.50 D in Appendix 3-4 for a 5-mm vertex distance change, we find +14.48 D.

Step 3. We find the second meridian power by adding:

$$+13.50 - 2.25 = +11.25 \text{ D}$$

Step 4. Using the same table we look up +11.25 D for a 5-mm vertex distance change, and find +11.92 D.

Step 5. The new cylinder power is

$$14.48 - 11.92 = 2.56$$

Step 6. The theoretical prescription is +14.48 − 2.56 × 85. The rounded prescription is

$$+14.50 - 2.50 \times 85$$

This is considerably different from the +13.50 − 2.25 × 85 power we started with.

High-Powered Minus Lenses

High-powered minus lenses are a challenge for the optical laboratory. There are many techniques used in edging and in the selection of materials that help to reduce both actual edge thickness and the noticeability of edge thickness for high-minus lenses. Some of these methods

use high-index glass, high-index plastic, or polycarbonate (which has a somewhat higher index and also allows a thinner center)

use a slight pink or rose tint in the lenses

antireflection-coat the lenses

choose a frame with a smaller eyesize and smaller ED

use a facet edge design

move the bevel farther back on the lens

use a frame with thick rims

for an especially high-powered minus lens, use a minus carrier design

Much can be accomplished by advising accounts as to what alternatives are available for high-minus wearers. Often the most productive results can be produced in the frame selection area.[1]

Lenticular Minus Designs

One of the last options that people choose is the lenticular design, because it clearly lets the world know that the lenses being worn are *strong*. In some instances, however, the power is so strong that such a design is the best option.

A lenticular design for a high-minus lens uses the same idea as the lenticular design for high-plus lenses. The central area of the lens contains the prescribed refractive power of the lens, while the peripheral area serves only to extend the physical size of the lens, without increasing its thickness.

Lenticular minus lenses can be found in a variety of forms. The most common are the myodisc, the so-called minus lenticular, and the Younger blended myodisc lens.

The Myodisc

According to the traditional definition, the myodisc design has a front curve that is either plano in power or very close to plano. The front usually contains the cylinder component of the prescription. A myodisc also has a plano back carrier area with a high-minus bowl in the center of the back of the lens.

In a myodisc, the thickness of the carrier is basically the final edge thickness. Because a minus lens is thicker as it is made bigger, if the size of the central bowl is increased, so also is the thickness of the carrier. And, for lenses with the same sized bowl areas, the lens with the greater refractive power will also have the thicker carrier. See Figure 14-14.

The myodisc is ground by beginning with a plano-base lens blank. The front of the lens is ground close to plano, incorporating the cylinder. The front curve may be made minus in power. Next the optics of the bowl are ground on the back of the lens and polished out. It is advisable to fill the polished center of the bowl with wax, pitch, or an easily removeable epoxy resin to protect it from scratches and to give a clean-looking, sharply demarcated bowl line. Lastly, the back plano carrier is ground. This can be done using a hand pan and a plano lap so that the size of the bowl can be easily watched.

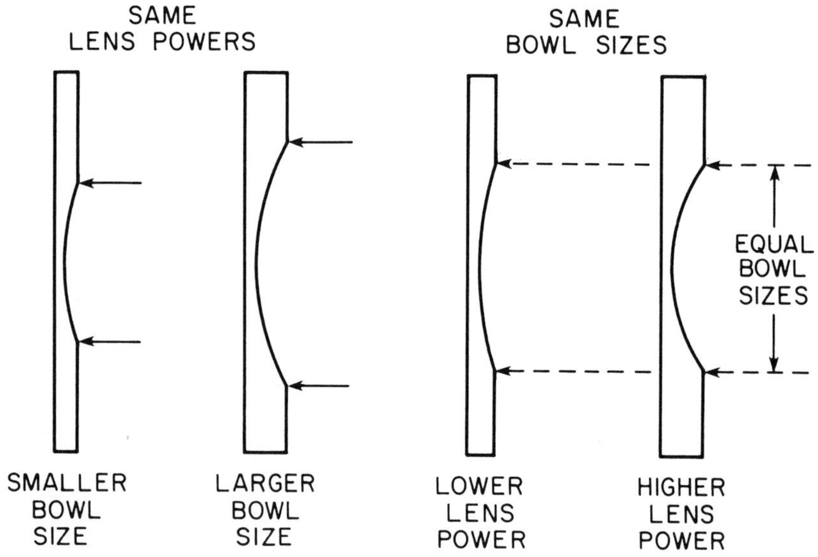

SAME LENS POWERS

SAME BOWL SIZES

EQUAL BOWL SIZES

SMALLER BOWL SIZE

LARGER BOWL SIZE

LOWER LENS POWER

HIGHER LENS POWER

Figure 14-14 Edge thickness on negative lenticular lenses varies depending on both lens power and bowl size. As the bowl size increases, so does the edge thickness. For lenses of equal bowl size, the edge thickness increases with an increase in lens power.

The carrier is roughed down until the bowl size is just slightly oversized. It is then fined to the requested or desired size and polished.

In spite of the advantageous design, edge thickness with a myodisc may still be somewhat greater than hoped for. If this is the case, the lens can be ground using a variation on the myodisc, called the minus lenticular.

The Minus Lenticular Design

A thinner edge can be obtained on a lenticular-type minus lens by making a lens with a carrier that has plus power. Since a plus lens becomes progressively thinner toward the edge, if a minus lens is designed with a plus carrier, it too will end up with a thin edge. See Figure 14-15.

There are specific formulas that allow the power of this plus carrier to be calculated. However, calculations may not always be necessary—adequate results have been obtained by experience. Unlike the myodisc lens, it is not necessary to grind the carrier curve for a minus lenticular. Instead a high-plus, full-field spheric lens can be chosen to match the desired curve of the plus carrier. This semifinished plus lens is used backward. The bowl is ground into the front of the high-plus semifinished blank. This becomes the back of the minus lenticular lens. In deciding what power to grind for the bowl, keep in mind that the front curve should be close to minus 6 diopters.

The front curve is ground on last. To do this the lens is blocked using a lens block that corresponds to the power of the plus carrier curve.

The Younger Blended Myodisc

There is a lens that has the advantages of a lenticular design but is not obviously lenticular. This is called a *blended myodisc* and is made by Younger. The lens has a lenticular bowl, but the edges of the bowl are blended so that they are not obvious to someone looking at the wearer's glasses.

Blended myodiscs come as semifinished blanks with the bowl and carrier already finished. There are two options. One is a semifinished blank with the carrier and bowl on the front. The other is a semifinished blank with the carrier and bowl on the back. In the strict sense of the word this lens is really more of a minus lenticular than a myodisc design. Technically, a myodisc has a plano carrier. Yet this blended lens thins toward the edge, resembling a minus lenticular design. The reason this lens is termed myodisc is because the word "myodisc"

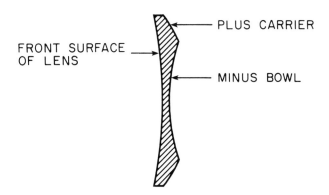

Figure 14-15 A minus lenticular design uses a concave front surface that normally includes the cylinder. The minus bowl is surrounded by a plus carrier to help reduce edge thickness.

is often used to describe any minus-powered lens that has a lenticular design, even though it does not fit the strict definition.

Questions and Problems

1. A right lens has an effective diameter angle of 45 degrees. The effective diameter is larger than the frame *A* dimension. Which lens shape is most likely to be the shape described?
   a. an oval shape
   b. a harlequin shape (upswept temporal corners)
   c. a round shape
   d. an aviator shape (long lower temporal and upper nasal corners)

2. A frame has the following dimensions:

   > *A* = 47 mm
   > ED = 49 mm
   > DBL = 19 mm
   > Wearer's PD = 62 mm

   Using the modified chord diameter formula, what chord diameter would be used to determine lens thickness?

3. **a.** A lens has a power of $+6.50 -1.50 \times 180$. If the lens is a right lens and has a 40-degree ED meridian, what power can be used to calculate lens thickness?

   b. If the lens in part **a** had a power of $+6.50 -1.50 \times 150$, what power could be used to calculate lens thickness? (Note: The only change is in the axis of the cylinder.)

4. Which of the following powers would result in the thinnest lens when placed in a frame with an ED meridian at 50?

a. $+7.00 -2.00 \times 180$
b. $+7.00 -2.00 \times 50$
c. $+7.00 -2.00 \times 90$
d. $+7.00 -2.00 \times 140$

5. The outermost area of a lenticular lens is called the
   a. aperture
   b. closure
   c. carrier
   d. cortex
   e. none of the above

6. All lenticular lenses have an aspheric central portion.
   True or False

7. The thickness of a lenticular lens will vary according to the effective diameter and decentration of the lens.
   True or False

8. Which type of lens design is likely to end up with the smallest center thickness, assuming that all are of the same refractive power?
   a. A spherical-based full-field lens.
   b. A spheric lenticular.
   c. An aspheric lenticular.
   d. All three will have the same center thickness.

9. A prescription is written as

   R: $+10.25$ sph
   L: $+9.75$ sph
     14 mm refracting distance

   What is the correct prescription if the order indicates that the lens is to be used at a 9-mm vertex distance?

10. A prescription is written as

    R: $+11.50 - 2.00 \times 75$
    L: $+12.00 - 2.50 \times 105$

    The order also indicates that the refraction was done at a 14-mm vertex distance, but that the prescription should be altered so that it will be correct for an 8-mm vertex distance. What should the new prescription be?

11. For a myodisc, the thickness of the carrier portion increases with
    a. a decrease in bowl diameter
    b. an increase in bowl diameter
    c. an increase in minus lens power when there is no change in bowl size
    d. a decrease in minus lens power when there is no change in bowl size

12. In a minus lenticular design, the carrier power is
    a. plus in power
    b. minus in power
    c. plano in power

13. The Younger blended myodisc comes with the bowl
    a. on the front of the lens
    b. on the back of the lens
    c. on either the front or the back of the lens
    d. on both the front and back of the same lens

14. What diameter would you use to calculate thickness for the following prescription in order to achieve maximum thinness?

    $+5.75$ D sphere
    $+5.75$ D sphere
    $A = 49$ mm
    DBL $= 19$ mm
    ED $= 51$ mm
    Wearer's PD $= 61$ mm

15. What power would you use for the following lens in calculating thickness in order to achieve maximum thinness?

    R: $+5.75 -1.00 \times 005$
    X of ED meridian $= 40$ degrees

16. A single-vision prescription for a person with a 62-mm PD is to be placed in a frame with

    $A = 50$ mm
    DBL $= 20$ mm
    ED $= 56$ mm

    a. What is the smallest uncut lens that can be used?
    b. What is the smallest semifinished lens that can be used?
    c. What is the chord diameter that you would use for a low-plus lens in calculating center thickness?
    d. What is the chord diameter you would use for a higher-plus lens in calculating to get the thinnest possible lens?

17. A person is wearing the following Rx at a 14-mm vertex distance: $+12.50 -2.00 \times 015$. A new frame is chosen to reduce magnification and increase field of view. The new vertex distance is 8 mm. What should the new lens power be to achieve the same refractive effect?

Reference

1. Brooks, C.W., and Borish, I.M. *System for Ophthalmic Dispensing*. Butterworth-Heinemann, Boston, 1979.

15 Progressive Addition Lenses

Introduction

As a person grows older, the eye's ability to focus for close work decreases. When this happens, two different lens powers may be needed, one for distance and a second for close work. The usual way to correct this problem is to use bifocals. Bifocal lenses cause light to focus at two places, one in the distance (infinity) and one near (usually at 40 cm). When the power of the bifocal near-add power is more than +1.50, the focusing ability of the eye has decreased to the point where bifocals do not allow for clear vision at all distances. There is an intermediate area of vision just beyond arm's length that will not be clear through either the distance portion of the lens or the bifocal. This in-between area can be cleared up by using a trifocal lens, which has a small intermediate segment area just above the bifocal area. It can also be corrected by using a progressive-addition lens.

Progressive-addition lenses, like bifocals, have distance power in the upper part of the lens. But starting at the major reference point (MRP), a progressive-addition lens begins to increase in plus power until the full near power is reached at a level 10 to 14 mm below the MRP. See Figure 15-1. This means that there is a continuous increase in power from the MRP to the near reading point, so that somewhere in the progressive corridor there is a place where clear vision can be obtained at any viewing distance.

Progressive lenses have the added benefit of being invisible to an untrained observer. However, because of changing optical power and blending of these power changes, there are areas of optical distortion on either side of the progressive zone and near area.

It should be understood that progressive-addition lenses are not used solely as a replacement for trifocals. They are also used for add powers of +1.50 and less, being preferred by many over a conventional bifocal lens.

Two Major Progressive-Addition Design Types

A large number of progressive-addition lens designs are currently marketed, all with their own individual characteristics. For surfacing purposes, however, there are two major types.

Figure 15-1 One basic philosophy of progressive-addition lens construction is shown. (OC = optical center, N = near visual point, h = length of progressive zone, d = inset of the near portion). (From C.W. Brooks and I.M. Borish, *System for Ophthalmic Dispensing,* Butterworth-Heinemann, Boston, 1979, p. 268.)

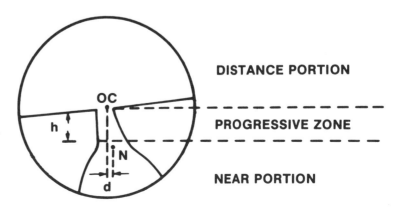

DISTANCE PORTION

PROGRESSIVE ZONE

NEAR PORTION

1. The first type includes those lenses with a front surface that is spherical in the upper half of the lens. See Figure 15-2. These lenses have surfacing characteristics somewhat similar to the Franklin-style lens. They are blocked like a Franklin-style lens.

2. The second type of progressive-addition lens allows the asphericity that is always present in the lower part of the front surface of the lens to extend above the middle and into the upper half. See Figure 15-3. This means that special procedures need to be used during blocking to keep the lens from tipping on its uneven surface.

Surfacing Progressive-Addition Lenses with Spherical Upper Halves

As was just stated, progressive-addition lenses can be made with the upper half of the front surface of the lens as a sphere, as in all other multifocal lenses. In thinking about the design of these lenses, it may be helpful to consider how much they are like Franklin (Executive)-style lenses. Both have spherical upper halves. Both have a different curve (or curves) in the lower half of the lens.

The steps used in processing this type of progressive lens begins with verifying that the lens will cut out by using the spectacle frame and a progressive-

addition lens reference card provided by the lens blank manufacturer. See Figure 15-4. Next, using a computer program designed especially for the brand of lenses being used, or the manufacturer's base curve selection charts, the appropriate base curve is chosen.

After the blank has been selected, the lens thickness and back surface tool curves that will be required are determined. (If no specific charts are provided by the manufacturer, thickness and tool curves may be determined in the same manner as for Franklin-style bifocals.)

Most lens blanks come right–left specific. That is, they are for either a right eye or a left eye, but cannot be used for either. However, a few progressive-addition lenses are based on a lens blank that can serve as either a right or a left lens. If this is the case, the lens blank must be rotated. This is done by turning the segment area nasally in the same manner as with the round-segment semifinished bifocal lens.

In either case, the major reference point on the semifinished blank must be located. (Remember, the MRP is *not* the fitting cross.) Fortunately, in most cases the MRP is already stamped on the lens. See Figure 15-5. If the lens has not been stamped, the MRP can be located with the help of hidden reference marks on the front surface of the lens. These marks may be visible as slight etchings or

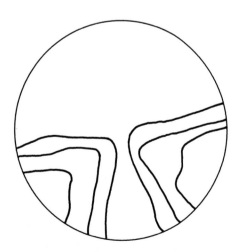

Figure 15-2 A representation of a progressive-addition lens with a spherical upper front surface. The concentric lines in the lower half represent areas of changing surface curvature.

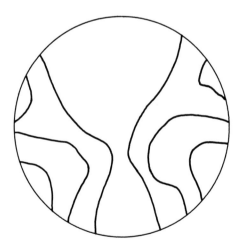

Figure 15-3 A representation of a progressive-addition lens with an upper front surface that is not entirely spherical. The asphericity always present in the lower half of a progressive-add lens has here been designed to extend into the upper portion. This is done in an effort to reduce the amount of unwanted aberration found in any one area of the lens.

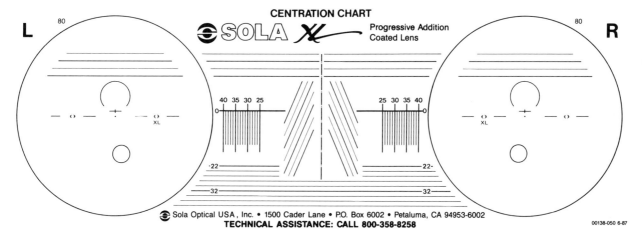

Figure 15-4 To use the centration chart shown, start by marking the fitting cross position on the dummy lens that comes with the frame or on a piece of transparent tape spanning the frame's lens opening. The fitting cross position can be located by first centering the frame bridge on the middle series of "upside-down Vs." Next, move the frame up or down until the fitting cross height on the order shows correctly at the bottom of the lens opening. Start with the left eye. The "lens" or tape is dotted or marked with a small + for the fitting cross. Now move the frame to the left. The dot or + on the left "lens" is placed over the fitting cross on the left. The lens blank picture must completely encircle the frame's lens opening. This procedure is repeated for the right eye. In actual practice it should be obvious if the lens will or will not cut out. Dotting need be done only when cutout is too close to call. (Courtesy of Sola Optical USA, Inc., Petaluma, Calif.)

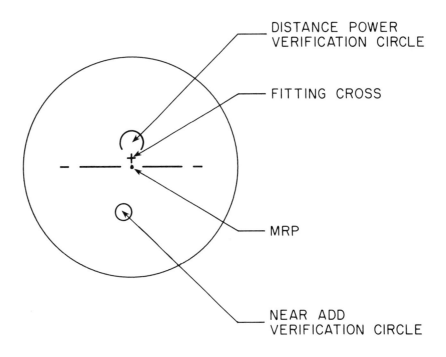

Figure 15-5 Progressive-add lenses come with certain marks already stamped on the lens. These marks aid in lens layout.

may show up under ultraviolet light. It is not unusual to find clear orientation marks toward the very edge of the semifinished lens blank. In the rare instances where a lens blank is used as either a right or a left lens, the blank must be rotated on the protractor a specified number of degrees before it can be marked. (In some cases rotation may have already been done in using a template to re-mark the lens.)

Now the lens must be marked at the major reference point. This includes marking for the correct cylinder axis and, when prism has been prescribed, the base direction of the prism. *Do not grind prism for decentration.* Grinding prism for decentration will move the MRP away from its proper location at the top of the progressive zone, rendering the lens useless. In addition to the standard cylinder axis, prism axis, and tray number markings, hand-mark an X on the lens in the 90-degree meridian at a point midway between the MRP and the top of the lens. This will allow the top of the lens to be immediately indentified and will be used for blocking orientation.

Now that the lens has been marked correctly, it is taped to protect the surface, to make blocking easier, and to preserve factory markings for edging and dispensing. (If special tape is used to cover only certain parts of the lens, this tape should not extend over the area where the block will rest on the lens. This would induce unwanted prism.)

In blocking a progressive-add lens, the same care is used as with Executives. The X-marked top of the lens must be turned downward so that liquid alloy does not leak out during blocking. Hold the upside-down lens against the block using the previously marked X as the pressure point for light finger pressure.

Lens generating is done in the normal manner. The main thing to remember is that if glass blocks are used, the lens is chucked in the same manner as would be done for Executive lenses, holding the upper part of the lens against the fiber ring. (If the lower half of the lens is held against the fiber ring, the lens will tilt, resulting in unwanted prism.)

Afterwards the lens is fined, polished, and deblocked. In order to preserve lens markings, cleanup is done with water and a mild detergent. But even if the markings are removed accidentally (or intentionally by cleaning with alcohol or acetone), they may be re-marked with either a special stamp or by using a template. When re-marking, the hidden etchings on the front surface of the lens are used.

Surfacing Progressive-Addition Lenses with Aspheric Upper Halves

Because of the nature of the lens, all progressive-add lenses are aspheric in the lower half. However, the second type of progressive-add lens is designed so that the asphericity extends into the upper half of the lens. This is done in order to reduce the intensity of unwanted distortions. Unfortunately, unevenly aspheric surfaces in *both* the lower and upper portions will prevent the lens from resting on a surfacing block without rocking. To keep the lens from having unwanted prism, some system of steadying the lens is needed. This stability can be obtained by using blocking tabs or a vinyl blocking *shim* for plastic lenses. For glass lenses that are blocked using regular glass blocks, a specially designed fiber generator ring is needed. This ring compensates for the unevenness of the aspheric lens surface and prevents unwanted prism from being ground during the generating process.

The steps in the processing of lenses with aspheric upper halves are similar to those for progressive lenses with spheric upper halves. As before, begin by verifying that the lenses will cut out, choosing the appropriate base curve and obtaining the blanks. Determine lens thickness and tool curves using a computer program or surfacing charts. Using the guide markings on the lenses, position the lens on the protractor or layout marker on the 180 line and the MRP. Mark the lens for axis, Rx prism, and calipering points as needed. See Figure 15-6. (Calipering points allow the lens thickness to be measured without removing it from the lens block.) Remember, *never grind prism for decentration.*

When 3M Surface Saver tape is being used, original lens markings need no additional protection. They will be intact when the tape is removed. However, if another system of lens protection is used, marks should still be protected by some sort of tape. (Such tape is often provided by the lens blank manufacturer.)

Up to this point, procedures have been much the same for both types of lenses. In processing plastic lenses with aspheric upper halves, blocking tabs or shims need to be placed on the lens. Blocking tabs come in different thicknesses, depending on how large the block is and where on the lens the tape is placed. Naturally, one should place the tabs on the lens as specified by the manufacturer. See Figure

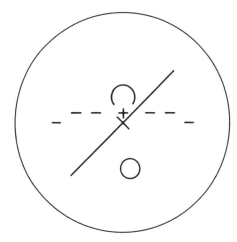

Figure 15-6 This lens is marked on the MRP location and is shown convex side up for the right eye. The cylinder is marked for Axis 45. Note that the fitting cross is *not* the MRP; it is *above* the MRP.

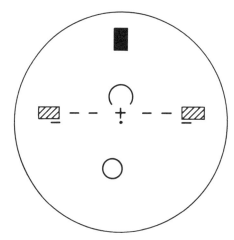

Figure 15-7 For lenses with aspheric upper surfaces, blocking tabs are placed so that they are between the lens block and the lens surface. Because lens surface curvature is not spherical, the block will not sit on the aspheric lens surface evenly unless the tabs are used to keep the lens from rocking.

15-7. Proper placement is currently along the 180-degree line at the points where the lens block rests on the lens surface. Sometimes an additional tab is placed in the upper 90-degree meridian. (For a 55-mm block, the tabs would be 27.5 mm from the centrally located MRP.) Blocking shims look like a modified letter T with arms angled upward slightly, halfway between a T and a Y. This T shim is placed on the lens either before the lens is sprayed, or after it has been taped with surface saver tape. In most cases the T shim is oriented upside down with the trunk of the T upward. The trunk and arms of the T overlap the same points where blocking tabs would be placed and serve the same function.

Once more, the lens is blocked in the same manner as Executive-style multifocals, that is, by lightly applying pressure on the top half of the lens. This way there is no tipping of the lens and subsequent unwanted prism. (An exception would be the AO Technica lens where pressure is applied at the bottom, where the trunk of the shim is located.)

In generating plastic lenses, the procedure is identical to that which is normally used. For glass lenses, using small glass blocks, a specially furnished fiber ring may be required to avoid prism since blocking tabs are not used. When glass lenses are blocked using a blocking method that does not require a fiber ring for generating, blocking tabs are used too.

During fining and polishing of lenses that are not blocked on center, some laboratories suggest that times and pressures be reduced. This helps to lessen

the chance of unwanted prism caused by uneven pressure.

Spotting and Verifying Progressive-Addition Lenses

The procedure for verification of progressive-addition lenses is slightly different from that for conventional multifocals. Because of the nature of the progressive-add lens, the power begins to increase at the level of the major reference point. This power increase continues in the plus direction until the full add power is reached. Normally this is at a point somewhere between 10 and 14 mm below the MRP.

Because add power starts to change right at the MRP, when verifying the lens in the lensmeter the centered lensmeter target will not look the same as usual. Instead the illuminated target will look clear at the top and blurry at the bottom. To get an accurate power reading, the distance power must be checked by dropping the lens slightly and using a point above the MRP. Yet in order to center the lens to spot for PD, the lensmeter target must be positioned right on the MRP. This is true even if the illuminated target looks somewhat blurry.

The near power of a progressive lens is checked at a point well into the near zone. If the lens is still marked, this near point is usually circled.

When checking a progressive-power lens for internal deficiencies, remember that peripheral distortions in the lower (and sometimes upper) peripheral portions of the lens are normal. These are not to be mistaken for inferior quality. The individual should become familiar with each lens design in order to be able to tell the difference between normal design characteristics and deficiencies in quality.

Grinding Base-Down Prism to Reduce Lens Thickness

Progressive-addition lenses gain their near power by increasing the steepness of the front surface of the lens. The principle is much the same as a Franklin-style lens. The steeper the lens curve, the thicker the lens must be in order to maintain the same size lens diameter. Figure 15-8A shows a progressive-addition lens in cross section. It has been surfaced as thin as possible. Because the lower half of the lens is more plus in power than the upper half, the lower edge limits how thin the lens may be ground. This means that for plus lenses and low-minus lenses, the entire lens will be thicker than a single-vision lens of equal power.

In order to better understand how one can reduce the overall thickness of the lens, imagine adding base-down prism to the lens. Adding base-down prism will thicken the lower lens edge without thickening the upper lens edge. This is shown in Figure 15-8B. Figure 15-8C shows the same lens as Figure 15-8B. It is now evident that the overall thickness of the lens can be reduced evenly, as is being done in Figure 15-8D. The end result is seen in Figure 15-8E. The lens is thinner and lighter in weight with base-down prism than it was without.

If such an option were used on one lens only, the glasses would be unwearable. The individual would either see double or have tremendous headaches. However, if moderate amounts of equal base-down prism are used in *both* lenses, the net difference between the two eyes is zero and no discomfort is experienced. This use of bilateral *yoked prism*, as it is called, has proven successful. When used in low amounts, studies have shown that "the subject population could not significantly differentiate between 2^Δ base down and 0^Δ. There was nearly unanimous rejection of 4^Δ base down. Postural changes were significant during 4^Δ wear, but not during 2^Δ wear. The results suggest the 2^Δ may be accepted by most patients, but 4^Δ will not."[1]

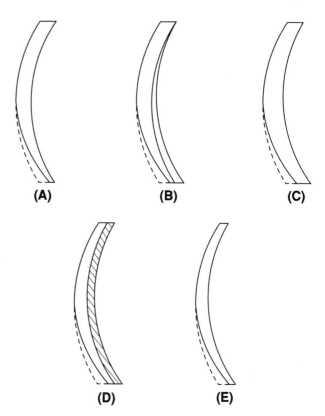

Figure 15-8 The concept of progressive-addition lens thinning through the use of base-down prism. Lens A shows the lens as normally ground. Lenses B and C show the effect of added base-down prism before removing excess thickness. Lenses C and D show the effect of thinning achieved.

Determining How Much Vertical Yoked Prism to Grind

Varilux recommends the use of vertical yoked prism, which it calls Equithin. The company suggests using a rule of thumb that calls for an amount of base-down prism equal to approximately two-thirds of the add power. Amounts are shown in tabular form in Table 15-1.

Use of vertical yoked prism to thin other progressive-addition lenses and Franklin-style lenses will work just as well.

Questions and Problems

1. Progressive-addition lenses are used primarily as a replacement for trifocals, making them appropriate for powers only above a +1.50 D add.
   True or False

Table 15-1 Yoked Base-Down (Equithin) Prism for Varilux Lenses*

Varilux	0.75	1.25	1.50	2.00	2.25	2.75	3.00	3.50
Addition		1.00		1.75		2.50		3.25
BD prism	0.50	0.75	1.00	1.25	1.50	1.75	2.00	2.25

*The base-down prism required is equal to approximately two-thirds of the Varilux addition power.
From *Laboratory Manual for Processing Varilux Lenses,* The Varilux Corporation, Foster City, Calif., undated, p. 25B. Used by permission.

2. Which type of progressive-addition lens is blocked in a manner similar to a Franklin-style bifocal lens?
   a. a progressive-add lens with asphericity in the lower half only and a spherical upper distance portion
   b. a progressive-add lens with most of the asphericity in the lower half, but with some of that asphericity spilling into the upper half of the lens
   c. both
   d. neither

3. Progressive-add lenses are all made so that they can be rotated and used for either a left or a right eye, even though most are marked as right or left.
   True or False

4. On progressive-add lenses, the major reference point is
   a. at the fitting cross
   b. above the fitting cross
   c. below the fitting cross

5. When the lens blank for a progressive-add lens is slightly small for the frame's eyesize,
   a. It is possible to make it cut out by moving the distance PD outward without making the lens unwearable.
   b. It is possible to make it cut out by grinding prism for decentration without making the lens unwearable.
   c. Both a and b are possible.
   d. Neither a nor b is possible.

6. "Blocking tabs" or shims are needed for processing
   a. all progressive-add lenses
   b. progressive-add lenses that have spheric upper halves
   c. progressive-add lenses that have aspheric upper halves
   d. all plastic progressive-add lenses
   e. all glass progressive-add lenses

7. In verifying a progressive-add lens, the distance refractive power is verified
   a. above the MRP
   b. at the MRP
   c. just below the MRP
   d. well below the MRP and slightly nasalward

8. In verifying a progressive-add lens, the prismatic effect of the lens is verified
   a. above the MRP
   b. at the MRP
   c. just below the MRP
   d. well below the MRP and slightly nasalward

9. When surfacing a plus-powered spherical progressive-add lens with a moderate amount of distance decentration, the center thickness of the lens is limited by
   a. the nasal edge of the lens
   b. the upper edge of the lens
   c. the lower edge of the lens

10. It is possible to grind a low-minus or a plus-powered progressive lens thinner by
    a. grinding base-down prism on the lens
    b. grinding base-up prism on the lens
    c. grinding either base-up or base-down prism on the lens, depending on which lens it is
    d. grinding neither base-up nor base-down prism on the lens

11. Bilateral yoked prism utilized for thickness considerations
    a. is well tolerated by the wearer if the amount is approximately 2^Δ or below
    b. is well tolerated by the wearer if the amount is approximately 4^Δ or below
    c. is well tolerated by the wearer if the amount is approximately 6^Δ or below
    d. is tolerated well by the wearer in any amount
    e. is never well tolerated by the wearer in any amount

12. The makers of Varilux lenses advocate the use of vertical yoked prism for lens thickness reduction in cases of low-minus and plus-powered progressive lenses. They recommend using
    a. a prism amount equal to approximately one-third of the add power
    b. a prism amount equal to approximately one-half of the add power
    c. a prism amount equal to approximately two-thirds of the add power
    d. a prism amount that is approximately equal to the add power

13. Using "Equithin" guidelines, how much prism in what base direction would you use to thin the following progressive-add lens?

> R: +2.50 −0.50 × 180
> L: +2.50 −0.50 × 180
>   Add = +2.25

Reference

1. Sheedy, J.E., and Parsons, S.D. Vertical Yoked Prism—Patient Acceptance and Postural Adjustment. *Ophthalmic and Physiological Optics*, 7(3): 255, 1987.

16 Creating Horizontal Prism with the Near Addition

Introduction

Bifocals are actually two distinct lenses: one small lens placed on a larger lens. When a person looks through the bifocal segment, the powers of both lenses come into effect. The combination of the distance lens power and the near-segment power are additive. This is why the segment is called an addition or "add."

By the same reasoning, it can be seen that both the distance lens and the near-segment "lens" will each have its own *prismatic* effects. How much prismatic effect is manifested depends on which part of the lens a person is looking through. The prismatic effects of the distance lens and the bifocal "lens" are also additive.

In this chapter we will see how this phenomenon can be used to advantage. Because of this combination of prismatic effects, it is possible to:

1. Produce a prescribed horizontal prismatic effect only in the near portion of a bifocal without having to use a special prism segment lens.
2. Produce a zero horizontal prismatic effect at the reading center. To produce a zero horizontal prismatic effect, the prismatic effect at the reading center created by the distance lens must be counteracted. This is done by moving the segment left or right.

Why might an individual need prism only at near? Although the situation does not arise often, there are occasions when it can be advantageous to create a horizontal (base-in or base-out) prismatic effect

at near viewing only. This means that there is no prescribed prism in the distance portion of the lens. Here are some examples of situations in which this might occur.

1. The AC/A ratio is either high or low. Some individuals have an abnormally high or low AC/A ratio. The *AC/A ratio* is "the ratio of accommodative convergence (AC) to accommodation (A), usually expressed as the quotient of accommodative convergence in prism diopters."[1] People with this problem do not lose binocular vision. Both eyes still accurately point at the object being viewed. However, the fusion required to keep from seeing double makes concentrated viewing at near a strain.
2. There is a periodic strabismus (tropia) at near only. *Strabismus* is an eye condition where one eye looks at the object being viewed, but the other eye does not. (Such an individual is often referred to as being "cross-eyed" or "wall-eyed." Sometimes a tropia exists during near viewing only. When this is the case, base-in or base-out prism at near may enable the individual to see with both eyes simultaneously.
3. Nonconcomitant strabismus is present. With *nonconcomitant strabismus*, the angle of deviation varies. The eye turns at a different angle when the person looks at distant objects compared to when he or she looks at near objects. Using one amount of prism for both distance and near may solve the prob-

lem for distance, but not for near. For such cases, creating a different amount of prism at near could provide the answer.

4. A desire to neutralize prism that has been caused by the distance lens at the near point. When a spectacle lens wearer views an object in the distance, she is looking through the distance optical centers of the lenses. There is no prismatic effect at the distance OCs. But when she looks at a near object, she is no longer looking through the lens OCs. This creates a prismatic effect at near. For low-powered prescriptions, this is seldom of any consequence. But when the distance Rx is increased in power, the horizontal prismatic effect at near that is caused by the distance lenses increases as well. In certain instances the prescriber may wish to counteract this prismatic effect. This can be done by repositioning the bi- or trifocal segment.

Horizontal Prismatic Effects Caused by the Near Addition

Normally a bifocal segment is set so that it corresponds precisely to the near PD. Because the segment optical center is inset for the near PD, when the wearer is looking at near objects the segment "lens" creates no horizontal prismatic effect. As the person looks through the lenses at near, he is either looking through the seg OC, or directly above or below it. See Figure 16-1. This means that any horizontal prismatic effect present will be caused by the distance lens alone.

Suppose the bifocal segment were mistakenly inset farther nasally than was called for. What would be the result?

Because bifocal additions are plus in power, moving the segment "lens" off the line of sight nasally will produce a base-in prismatic effect. See Figure 16-2. However, if the lenses were not decentered enough, the prism induced by the seg would be base out.

Suppose, for example, that a lens with an add power of +2.00 D mistakenly had the segment placed at a seg inset of 4 mm instead of the 2 mm called for in the prescription. What would be the result?

First, if the lens had been decentered the required 2 mm, no prismatic effect would be produced by the segment. The wearer would be looking directly through the segment optical center. In this case, though, we see that the seg is moved 2 mm *past* the place where it should be. Therefore the horizontal prismatic effect is

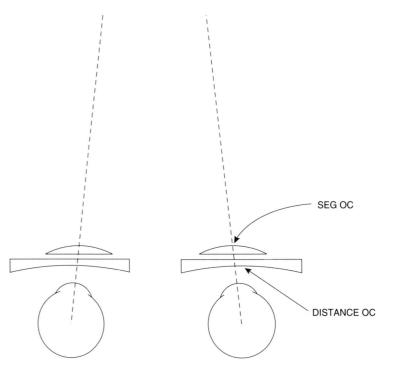

Figure 16-1 When individuals turn their eyes inward to read, they are no longer looking through the distance optical centers of their lenses. However, the customary placement of the near bifocal segment centers equals the near PD. This means that since they are looking either directly through the seg center, or slightly above or below it, there is zero horizontal prism due to the seg.

Figure 16-2 Bifocal segments are really small plus lenses. This means that if the segment optical centers are moved nasalward, they will cause a base-in prismatic effect. This prismatic effect occurs only in the near position.

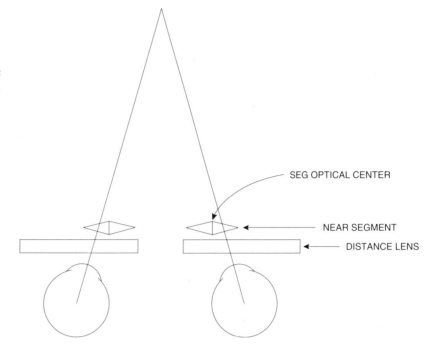

SEG OPTICAL CENTER

NEAR SEGMENT

DISTANCE LENS

Horizontal prism = (0.2)(2)
= 0.4 prism diopter

The amount of prism induced is 0.4 prism diopter of base-in prism.

Creating Prism at Near by Using the Segment

There are times when a prismatic effect is desired for near vision but not for distance. When this is the case, the segment must either be a special one containing prism, or a conventional segment that has been intentionally decentered away from the near PD position.

The most popular prism segment currently in use looks like a ribbon seg that has been extended nasalward. See Figure 16-3. Using such a segment, 1.00 through 3.50 diopters of prism per lens can be created in the segment area only.

As seen earlier, if a segment is placed too far inward or outward, it will produce a horizontal prismatic effect. Therefore, if a horizontal prismatic effect in the seg is desired, then intentionally moving the segment horizontally may be sufficient to produce the amount of prism called for in the segment area.

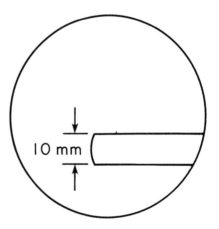

10 mm

Figure 16-3 The Vision-Ease prism segment may be ordered with horizontal prism ranging in strength from 1.00 to 3.50 prism diopters.

EXAMPLE 16-1

Suppose a prescription reads (in part) as follows:

R: +0.50 D
L: +0.50 D
+2.00 add
PD = 62/58
Flat-top 35 segment

Special instructions: 1 base-in prism per eye for near only.

How could this amount of prism be created simply by moving the segment away from its normal location?

Solution

The first question that must be asked is *how far* away from its normal location the seg must be moved in order to produce 1 prism diopter. The unknown factor in the Prentice's rule equation is the distance c. Since this is in addition to the normal amount of seg inset, we will use c_a, or *additional seg inset*. The equation then reads

$$Prism = c_a \times (add\ power)$$

or

$$1 = c_a \times 2$$

which is the same as

$$c_a = \tfrac{1}{2} \text{ or } 0.5 \text{ cm}$$

Therefore the segment must be displaced 5 mm from the position it normally occupies.*

The next element that must be determined is *the direction of the displacement.* In figuring direction of displacement, one must remember that, in plus lenses, decentration inward produces base-in and decentration outward produces base-out prism. This means that our segment must be decentered 5 mm farther inward than it would be normally.

The last consideration is the *net seg inset* actually required and its effect on the measured near PD. If the normal seg inset is $(62 - 58)/2 = 2$, then the amount required to produce 1 prism diopter Base In is $2 + 5 = 7$ mm. The net segment inset is 7 mm.

What Happens to the Traditional "Near PD"?

When a segment is decentered, the distance between seg centers no longer corresponds to the wearer's near PD. In Example 16-1, there is 5-mm *additional* inset per lens. Instead of measuring a "near PD" of 58 mm, we will end up with 10 mm less overall, or a distance between seg centers of only 48 mm.

---

*The question may arise as to the role of the prismatic effect induced by the distance lens. The answer is that when prism is prescribed for near, the prism induced by the distance lens has already been taken into account. It need not be considered.

What Special Precautions Must Be Taken into Consideration Because of the Larger or Smaller Distance Between Seg Centers?

Because of the especially small (or large) near PDs that will be produced by this process, it is possible for a small seg to be decentered so far that there is not enough room left in front of the eye to read. Imagine what would happen if a 22-mm segment were decentered 11 mm. The wearer would end up looking right into the side line of the segment. Therefore a segment with large enough dimensions to allow for extra decentration must be chosen.

How Large Must the Segment Be?

In order for the segment to be large enough to use comfortably, it should at least be the size of the smallest segment that has been used successfully. This is a 20-mm segment. To assure that this size is duplicated, there must be 10 mm of segment on either side of the near reading point. Thus, for each 1 mm of additional segment decentration required beyond the normal seg inset, the seg size should be increased by 2 mm. Written as a formula, this is

$$Seg\ size = 2(10 + additional\ seg\ inset)$$

Generally, a segment of not less than 28 mm should be used for this type of prescription. If a 28-mm seg is chosen, only a small amount of decentration will be possible. More often a 35-, 40- or 45-mm seg, or a Franklin-style lens, is chosen.

What Happens When Considerable Outset Is Required?

When a considerable amount of seg outset is required, there will come a point where there is not enough lens material on the nasal portion of the lens blank to allow the lens to cut out. When this is the case, it may be possible to use a left lens blank instead of a right, or vice versa. Because lens manufacturers know that bifocals are always moved nasally, the lens is made with a nasal blank seg inset. However, if very much *outset* is required when creating prism by seg decentration, then the blank for the opposite lens should be used. A lens blank that is used on the "wrong" eye will already have "outset."

In general, the practice of swapping a left for a right blank or vice versa will be used only in the

Table 16-1 Creating Prism at Near by Decentering the Segment

1. Find the customary seg inset.

$$\text{Seg inset} = \frac{\text{distance PD} - \text{near PD}}{2}$$

2. Find the additional seg inset needed to produce the prism prescribed for near using a transposed form of Prentice's rule.

$$c_a = \frac{\text{near prism}}{D_a}$$

where c_a = additional set inset, and D_a = the add power.

3. Determine if the additional seg inset is inward or outward. If the prescribed near prism is base in, the additional seg inset is inward. If the prescribed near prism is base out, the additional seg inset is outward.

4. Find the net seg inset.

Net seg inset = seg inset + additional seg inset

5. Find the minimum segment size needed to give the wearer enough area to read with.

Seg size = 2(10 + additional seg inset)

case of Franklin-style bifocals, since these have the largest available seg and a relatively small blank seg inset.

As mentioned before, lenses having small segs (such as the flat-top 25) cannot be used to create a prismatic effect. Bifocals with a large seg will work unless the center of the seg is outset past the center of the edged lens. (Flat-top segs that are outset beyond the center of the edged lens will look as funny as wearing shoes on the wrong feet.)

The procedure for determining the amount of segment decentration needed to create prism at near is summarized in Table 16-1.

EXAMPLE 16-2

A prescription calls for the following:

−1.50 −1.00 × 180   2.0 Base In at near only
−1.50 −1.00 × 180   2.0 Base In at near only
add = +2.50
PD = 65/61
Seg style: flat top

How much net seg inset is needed to create the prism at near? What is the smallest segment size which can be used successfully?

SOLUTION

We will use the steps outlined in Table 16-1 to solve the example.

Step 1. $\text{Seg inset} = \dfrac{\text{distance PD} - \text{near PD}}{2}$

$$= \frac{65 - 61}{2}$$

$$= 2 \text{ mm}$$

Step 2. Additional seg inset is

$$c_a = \frac{\text{near prism}}{D_a}$$

$$= \frac{2}{2.5}$$

$$= 0.8 \text{ cm or 8 mm}$$

Step 3. Because the prescribed near prism is base in, the direction of additional seg inset is inward.

Step 4. Since

Net seg inset = seg inset + additional seg inset

then for this example

Net seg inset = 2 + 8
= 10 mm

Each segment must be inset a total of 10 mm.

Step 5. The minimum segment size needed is found using:

Seg size = 2(10 + additional seg inset)

The amount of additional seg inset was found to be 8 mm. Therefore,

Seg size = 2(10 + 8)
= 36 mm

There are no flat top 36 segments made. The closest manufactured flat tops are 35 and 40. Since 36 is the smallest we should use, the flat top 40 segment is chosen.

Achieving a Zero Horizontal Prismatic Effect at the Near Reading Center

It is possible to *neutralize* the horizontal prism induced by the distance prescription at near. In other words, the prism caused by the distance prescription at the near reading center can be calculated and the seg moved in or out to produce an effect equal but opposite to that of the distance lens. The reasons for doing this are

1. so that the amount the eyes must turn inward for near work will be the same as when no glasses at all are worn.
2. so that the near PD for Franklin-style bifocals may be measured with a lensmeter.

This practice is not as common today as it used to be, but may be requested from time to time.

Determining the Amount of Seg Decentration Required

The amount the bifocal segment must be moved in order to create an equal but opposite prism compensation is determined by first finding the horizontal prismatic effect of the distance prescription at the near reading center of the lens. This can be calculated by finding the power of the distance lens in the 180-degree meridian. The calculation is straightforward for spheres and for cylinders which have their axis in either the 90- or 180-degree meridian. Cylinders with oblique axes require an extra step.

Determining the Amount of Horizontal Prism Created by the Distance Prescription

When the wearer looks at a near object, the line of sight passes through the lens at a point below and nasal to the distance optical center. This point is called the *near reading center*. The horizontal distance between the distance optical center and the near reading center is the seg inset.

If the distance prescription is a sphere, the amount of horizontal prism produced by the distance lens at the near reading center can be found simply by multiplying the seg inset by the power of the distance lens.

As the wearer looks through the near reading center, the distance lens causes a prismatic effect. The amount of horizontal prism that will be induced is

$$P_{180} = c_i D_{180}$$

where

c_i = seg inset in centimeters
D_{180} = power of the distance lens in the horizontal

EXAMPLE 16-3

If a lens has a distance power of -3.00 D and the wearer's PD is 65/61, how much horizontal prismatic effect will be produced by the distance lens when the wearer looks at a near object?

SOLUTION

First find the seg inset. The seg inset is $(65 - 61)/2 = 2$ mm or 0.2 cm. Using Prentice's rule, the horizontal prismatic effect is

$$\text{Prismatic effect} = cD$$
$$= (0.2)(3)$$
$$= 0.6 \text{ prism diopters}$$

Because we are looking nasal to the optical center of a minus lens, the base direction is base in.

Determining Horizontal Prismatic Effect in Spherocylinders

In order to calculate the horizontal prismatic effect of a spherocylinder lens, it is necessary to know the power of that lens in the 180-degree meridian. For spherocylinder lenses with an axis at 90 or 180 degrees, the power of the lens in the horizontal meridian can be found by drawing a power cross. The powers in the 90- and 180-degree meridians are entered on the power cross. The power in the 180-degree meridian is used with Prentice's rule to calculate the prism.

EXAMPLE 16-4

If a lens has a power of $+4.50 - 1.00 \times 90$ and the wearer's PD is 64/60, how much prismatic effect is caused by the distance lens when the wearer looks at a near object?

SOLUTION

Enter the lens powers on a power cross as shown in Figure 16-4. The power in the 180-degree meridian is $+3.50$. The seg inset is $(64-60)/2 = 2$ mm. The horizontal prismatic effect is

$$P_{180} = (0.2)(3.50)$$
$$= 0.7 \text{ prism diopter}$$

When a lens has an oblique cylinder, finding the power in the 180-degree meridian is not as straightforward. To calculate the horizontal prismatic effect, find the power of the cylinder in the 180-degree

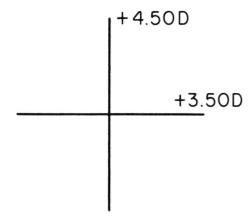

Figure 16-4 When entering $+4.50 - 1.00 \times 90$ on a power cross, the sphere power ($+4.50$) is entered on the axis meridian (90). The other meridian contains the sum of the sphere and cylinder powers ($+4.50 - 1.00 = +3.50$).

meridian using sine-squared tables.* Add this value to the sphere power. The sum of these two lens power values is plugged into the Prentice's rule formula. (This procedure was explained in detail in Chapter 3 in the discussion of on-center blocking for spherocylinder lenses with oblique axes.)

Calculating Additional Seg Inset

In the last section we calculated horizontal prism produced by the distance lens. We have also seen that in order to counteract the prismatic effect induced by the distance lens, the segment is moved. (Remember, the object is to produce an equal but opposite amount of prism with the add so as to neutralize the prismatic effect caused by the distance prescription.) This was explained earlier in this chapter. To express needed segment decentration as a formula, we can say that

$$P_{180} = c_a D_a$$

where c_a is the *additional* seg inset required (an amount beyond the normal seg inset), P_{180} is the amount of prism needed to counteract the distance prism (the amount of prism in the 180-degree meridian of the distance portion), and D_a is the power of the add. Rearranging the equation, the needed additional segment displacement is

---

*This method does not give results that are entirely accurate, but for these purposes will work acceptably well.

$$c_a = \frac{P_{180}}{D_a}$$

Since P_{180} appears in the above formula and in the formula for figuring seg decentration, the two formulas may be combined. Using one formula, the additional seg inset can be found directly. This is done as follows. If

$$P_{180} = c_i D_{180}$$

and

$$P_{180} = c_a D_a$$

then

$$c_a D_a = c_i D_{180}$$

Therefore

$$c_a = \frac{c_i D_{180}}{D_a}$$

Remember, the c_a value is the *additional seg inset*.

Calculating the Net Seg Inset

We have just shown how to calculate how far the seg must be moved from its normal near-PD position in order to neutralize the horizontal prismatic effect of the distance lens. This was called the additional seg inset. For lens layout, though, the normal seg inset must be taken into consideration. We need the sum of the additional segment inset plus the regular seg inset. This is termed *net seg inset*.

We now know that

Net seg inset = seg inset + additional seg inset

or

$$\text{Net seg inset} = c_i + c_a$$

Combining

$$c_a = \frac{c_i D_{180}}{D_a}$$

and

$$\text{Net seg inset} = c_i + c_a$$

a direct formula for calculating net seg inset may be found as

$$\text{Net seg inset} = c_i + \frac{c_i D_{180}}{D_a}$$

A Note on Plus and Minus Signs

When designating inset or outset, inset will be considered as positive and outset as negative. To work the formula, be sure to include plus and minus signs when referring to the power of the lens. If the result is positive, the net seg inset is inward. If the result is negative, the net seg inset is outward.

Remember, just using the formula without understanding what is going on will not help. The concept is more important. An answer may be arrived at by understanding the concept even *without* a formula. However, a formula memorized, then forgotten, brings no understanding.

EXAMPLE 16-5

Suppose a zero horizontal prismatic effect is desired at the near reading center. The lens chosen is a Franklin-style bifocal. The prescription information is

R: +4.00 D sph
L: +1.00 D sph
+2.00 add
PD = 65/61

What is the net seg inset required for each lens?

SOLUTION

For the right lens, the net seg inset is

$$\text{Net seg inset} = c_i + \frac{c_i D_{180}}{D_a}$$

$$= 0.2 + \frac{0.2 \times 4}{2} = 0.6 \text{ cm}$$

Thus the net seg inset is 6 mm. By insetting the seg 6 mm, there will be no horizontal prismatic effect at the reading center.

For the left lens,

$$\text{Net seg inset} = 0.2 + \frac{0.2 \times 1}{2} = 0.3 \text{ cm}$$

which means that the net seg inset for the left lens will be 3 mm inward.

EXAMPLE 16-6

A prescription reads as follows:

R: −2.00 −1.00 × 90
L: −2.00 −1.00 × 70
Add = +2.50
PD = 67/64

A zero horizontal prismatic effect is desired at the near reading center. How much net seg inset is required per lens?

SOLUTION

For the right lens, the power of D_{180} is −3.00 D. The seg inset is $(67 − 64)/2 = 1.5$ mm. Because

$$\text{Net seg inset} = c_i + \frac{c_i D_{180}}{D_a}$$

we substitute the values just determined:

$$\text{Net seg inset} = 0.15 + \frac{0.15 \times -3}{2.5} = -0.03 \text{ cm}$$

A net seg inset of −0.3 mm is really an outset of 0.3 mm.

For the left lens, the D_{180} must be determined by taking the "power" of the cylinder in the 180-degree meridian. Using $\sin^2$ tables, we find that for a −1.00 cylinder of axis 70 degrees, the "power" in the 180-degree meridian is −0.88 D. This is added to the sphere for a total D_{180} value of −2.88 D. All else in the calculation remains the same. Thus,

$$\text{Net seg inset} = 0.15 + \frac{0.15 \times -2.88}{2.5}$$

$$= 0.15 + (-0.1728)$$

$$= -0.0228 \text{ cm or } -0.228 \text{ mm}$$

The net seg inset is an outset of 0.2 mm. (The difference between the two lenses is imperceptibly small.)

Lens Layout

When laying out a Franklin-style bifocal to produce a zero prismatic effect at near, the blank seg inset must be known. Franklin-style lenses may have blank seg insets of 0, 3, 4, 5, or even 6.5 mm, depending on the manufacturer. If the blank seg inset is zero, the blank geometric center is right above the seg optical center. The blank geometric center is used for reference and, when using traditional off-center blocking, is moved the amount of the net seg inset. However, if the blank geometric center is used for reference when the lens has blank seg inset, then the blank seg inset must be subtracted from the net seg inset if the seg center is to end up in the right place.

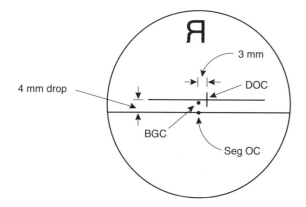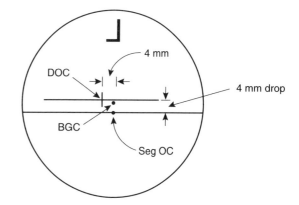

Figure 16-5 A Franklin-style lens with a zero blank seg inset. To neutralize the base-out effect of a minus lens, the segment optical center is displaced in an outward direction. Although the seg OCs are farther apart than the near PD, since the reading center has a zero prismatic effect, the lensmeter may be used to find the near PD.

EXAMPLE 16-7

Calculate the net seg inset needed to produce a zero horizontal prismatic effect at near for the following prescription. Show how the lenses would look when marked for surfacing.

R: −5.00 sph
L: −6.00 sph
Add +2.00
Seg drop = 4 mm
PD = 64/60

The semifinished blanks to be used have a blank seg inset of zero.

SOLUTION

For the right lens,

$$\text{Net seg inset} = c_1 + \frac{c_1 D_{180}}{D_a}$$

$$= (0.2) + \frac{0.2 \times (-5.00)}{2}$$

$$= -0.3 \text{ cm} = -3 \text{ mm}$$

For the left lens,

$$\text{Net seg inset} = (0.2) + \frac{0.2 \times (-6.00)}{2}$$

$$= -0.4 \text{ cm} = -4 \text{ mm}$$

The right lens has a net seg outset of 3 mm and the left lens has a net seg outset of 4 mm. If the semifinished blanks have a zero blank seg inset, they should be marked as shown in Figure 16-5.

EXAMPLE 16-8

In Example 16-6 we saw that since the net seg inset was negative, we moved the segment optical center outward. For Franklin-style lenses with decentered optics, if a seg outset is required, the blanks may be swapped. The left blank may be used for the right lens and the right blank for the left lens. Suppose a 78-mm Franklin-style lens with a 5-mm blank seg drop and a 3-mm blank seg inset is chosen. How should the lens be marked for the prescription in Example 16-6?

SOLUTION

The correctly marked lens is shown in Figure 16-6.

Using Surfacing Charts to Determine a Zero Horizontal Prismatic Effect at the Near Reading Center

As might be expected, surfacing charts are available to reduce the necessary calculations for achieving a zero horizontal prismatic effect at the near reading center. These charts, such as those furnished by Sola Optical, give the precalculated lens decentration needed. They also give prism grind required so

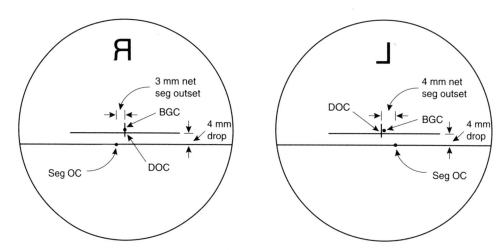

Figure 16-6 A 78-mm Franklin-style lens with a 3-mm blank seg inset. Because the net seg inset is minus, calling for an *outset* of the segment optical center, the decentered blanks are swapped, left for right. This layout will give exactly the same optical result as shown in Figure 16-5.

that the lens may be blocked using on-center blocking. A section of one such chart is shown as Table 16-2.

It should be noted that the Sola charts take into account the 3-mm blank seg inset that is standard for the larger Sola lenses. Therefore the amount of lens decentration found in the Sola charts will be 3 mm different from the calculated net seg inset.

Questions and Problems

1. a. A pair of glasses has a plano distance portion and a +2.50 add. The near PD should be 58 mm. Instead the near PD is found to be 62 mm. How much total prismatic effect is caused by the incorrect near PD?
(1) 0.50 prism diopter
(2) 1.00 prism diopter
(3) 1.50 prism diopters
(4) 2.00 prism diopters
(5) none of the above

b. What is the base direction of this prism?
(1) Base in
(2) Base out
(3) It depends upon which eye is being spoken of.

2. A Vision-Ease prism segment looks most like which of the following:
a. a flat-top seg
b. a Franklin-style lens
c. a panoptic seg
d. a ribbon seg
e. none of the above

3. a. A prismatic effect at near of 1.50 Base In per lens is desired for near only. The seg has an add power of +3.00 D. How far and in which direction should the segment be decentered in order to achieve this result? (In other words, what is the additional seg inset required?)

b. If the wearer's PD is 64/60, what should be the net seg inset per lens?

c. What should the "Near PD" for the wearer's glasses be if measured with a PD ruler in the usual manner?

4. A prescription calls for 2 prism diopters Base In per lens at near only. The add power is +1.50 D. The prismatic effect is to be achieved by decentering the seg. What is the smallest flat-top bifocal segment that can be used to accomplish this without cutting off too much of the reading area?

5. Of the following segment types, which is most likely to be used for swapping left for right and right for left blanks when seg outset for prism at near is required?
a. flat-top 22
b. Franklin style
c. curve-top 25
d. ribbon seg
e. none of the above

6. A person who is wearing single-vision lenses will experience a prismatic effect when looking anywhere in the lens. This is true unless the lens has no power (is plano) or unless the person is looking exactly through the optical center.
a. For the following single-vision prescription, how much horizontal prismatic effect is experienced

Table 16-2 A Section from the Prism/Decentration Table for the Sola E-Line Surfacing Chart for Decentering 68-mm Blanks

Distance Power at 180 Degrees	Add	Decentration	Prism Diopters	Prism Difference at 68 mm	Distance Power at 180 Degrees	Add	Decentration	Prism Diopters	Prism Difference at 68 mm
2.50	1.00	4.0	1.00	1.3	1.75	1.00	2.5	0.43	0.5
2.50	1.25	3.0	0.75	1.0	1.75	1.25	1.8	0.31	0.4
2.50	1.50	2.3	0.58	0.7	1.75	1.50	1.3	0.23	0.3
2.50	1.75	1.8	0.46	0.6	1.75	1.75	1.0	0.17	0.2
2.50	2.00	1.5	0.37	0.5	1.75	2.00	0.7	0.13	0.1
2.50	2.25	1.2	0.30	0.4	1.75	2.25	0.5	0.09	0.1
2.50	2.50	1.0	0.25	0.3	1.75	2.50	0.4	0.07	0.0
2.50	2.75	0.8	0.20	0.2	1.75	2.75	0.2	0.04	0.0
2.50	3.00	0.6	0.16	0.2	1.75	3.00	0.1	0.02	0.0
2.25	1.00	3.5	0.78	1.0	1.50	1.00	2.0	0.30	0.4
2.25	1.25	2.6	0.58	0.7	1.50	1.25	1.4	0.21	0.2
2.25	1.50	2.0	0.45	0.6	1.50	1.50	1.0	0.15	0.2
2.25	1.75	1.5	0.35	0.4	1.50	1.75	0.7	0.10	0.1
2.25	2.00	1.2	0.28	0.3	1.50	2.00	0.5	0.07	0.1
2.25	2.25	1.0	0.22	0.3	1.50	2.25	0.3	0.04	0.0
2.25	2.50	0.8	0.18	0.2	1.50	2.50	0.2	0.03	0.0
2.25	2.75	0.6	0.14	0.1	1.50	2.75	0.0	0.01	0.0
2.25	3.00	0.5	0.11	0.1	1.50	3.00	0.0	0.00	0.0
2.00	1.00	3.0	0.60	0.8	1.25	1.00	1.5	0.18	0.2
2.00	1.25	2.2	0.44	0.5	1.25	1.25	1.0	0.12	0.1
2.00	1.50	1.6	0.33	0.4	1.25	1.50	0.6	0.08	0.1
2.00	1.75	1.2	0.25	0.3	1.25	1.75	0.4	0.05	0.0
2.00	2.00	1.0	0.20	0.2	1.25	2.00	0.2	0.03	0.0
2.00	2.25	0.7	0.15	0.2	1.25	2.25	0.1	0.01	0.0
2.00	2.50	0.6	0.12	0.1	1.25	2.50	0.0	0.00	0.0
2.00	2.75	0.4	0.09	0.1	1.25	2.75	−0.0	−0.01	−0.0
2.00	3.00	0.3	0.06	0.0	1.25	3.00	−0.1	−0.02	−0.0

Using the chart: From the lens power in the 180 meridian and the add power in the first two columns, the decentration needed for off-center blocking, the prism needed for on-center blocking, and the prism difference at 68 mm for calipering thickness differences along the 180 can be found. (Courtesy Sola Optical USA, Inc., Petaluma, Calif.)

when the individual converges the eyes to look at a near object? The object is located at the normal 40-cm reading distance. (Consider the right lens only for this problem.)

   R: −5.00 sphere
   PD = 64/60

(1) 5 prism diopters
(2) 2.50 prism diopters
(3) 1.50 prism diopters
(4) 1.00 prism diopter

(5) 0.50 prism diopter
(6) none of the above

b. What is the base direction for the above problem?
(1) Base in
(2) Base out

7. An individual converges the eyes to look at a near object located at the normal 40-cm reading distance. How much combined horizontal prismatic effect is experienced for both right and left eyes

together if the individual is wearing the following single-vision prescription? Be sure and give the base direction as well.

> R: −5.00 sphere
> L: −4.00 sphere
> PD = 64/60

8. How much combined horizontal prismatic effect is experienced with this prescription when the wearer is working at the normal reading distance? Remember to give base direction.

> R: +2.75 sphere
> L: +3.25 sphere
> PD = 66/62

9. How much combined horizontal prismatic effect is experienced at the normal reading distance with this spherocylinder prescription? Remember to give base direction.

> R: −1.00 −2.50 × 90
> L: −1.00 −2.50 × 90
> PD = 66/62

10. Using the sine squared method for finding the power of a cylinder in the horizontal meridian, calculate the combined horizontal prismatic effect experienced with this single-vision prescription at the normal reading distance. Remember to give base direction.

> R: −2.00 −3.00 × 35
> L: −2.00 −3.00 × 145
> PD = 66/62

11. To grind a pair of Franklin-style lenses so that the near PD can be measured using a lensmeter, the horizontal prismatic effect of the distance lenses must be neutralized. This is done by moving the segment optical center to produce an equal but opposite prismatic effect. How much net seg inset per lens is required in order to accomplish this for each of the following prescriptions? (For simplicity, assume that the lens blank being used has a blank seg inset of zero.)

a. +2.50 sphere
   +2.50 sphere
   +2.00 add
   PD = 62/58

b. −2.00 −0.50 × 90
   −2.00 −0.75 × 180
   +2.25 add
   PD = 60/57

c. +4.25 −1.75 × 55
   +4.25 −1.75 × 100
   +2.50 add
   PD = 65/61

12. It is desired that a pair of Franklin-style lenses have a zero horizontal prismatic effect at the near reading center. *The lenses have a blank seg inset of 5 mm.* To lay out the lenses, the blank geometric centers are spotted and used as reference points for decentration. How far in or out should the blank geometric center be moved for each lens? (Remember to figure net seg inset first, then compensate for how far the seg centers are *already* decentered as a result of the blank seg inset.)

a. +5.00 sphere
   +4.50 sphere
   +2.00 add
   PD = 61/57

b. −7.00 −2.50 × 30
   −7.50 −1.75 × 150
   +2.50 add
   PD = 64/60

Reference

1. Cline, D., Hofstetter, H.W., and Griffin, J.R. *The Dictionary of Visual Science* 4th ed. Chilton Trade Book Publishing, Radnor, PA, 1989, p. 573.

17

Vertical Imbalance Corrections

The Nature of Vertical Imbalance

An unwanted difference in the amount of vertical prism in the right and left eyeglass lenses is especially difficult for the wearer to overcome. It can easily result in visual discomfort and a rejection of the glasses. Recognizing how critical this is, the American National Standards Institute allows only a difference of one-third prism diopter between the two eyes, or 1 mm difference in major reference point (MRP) levels. An individual may experience difficulties caused by vertical prism differences between the two eyes at near only. The purpose of this chapter is to discover how these problems originate, and how they may be overcome.

Prismatic Effects of Ordinary Lens Prescriptions

When the eyes work together as a team, they can turn in unison easily. Both can look to the right, to the left, up, or down. They must also work as a team to see objects close up. In this case, the eyes must turn inward, or *converge*. Because convergence is a normal eye movement, the eyes can also turn inward to overcome base-out or sometimes even base-in prismatic effects caused by a pair of glasses.

For example, consider a person who wears a pair of −5.00 D lenses. We can assume that the optical centers are set correctly for the distance PD. When this individual looks off into the distance, the lenses cause no prismatic effect. In this situation the eyes are looking directly through the centers of the lenses

and incoming light is parallel. See Figure 17-1. But if the person looks to the right, the lenses cause prismatic effects. The right lens causes a base-out prismatic effect and the left lens causes a base-in prismatic effect. Fortunately, since these two prismatic effects have equal but opposite values, the net result is no prismatic effect. Incoming light is still parallel. This is shown in Figure 17-2.

When a spectacle lens wearer looks down and in to see an object up close, the lenses cause *two* prismatic effects. One is a horizontal prismatic effect caused by the eyes looking inward. The other is a vertical prismatic effect caused by the eyes looking downward.

Unless the lens powers are especially high, the wearer can usually compensate for these horizontal prismatic effects. (Details on how to overcome unwanted horizontal prism at near were presented in Chapter 16.)

The second prismatic effect experienced when looking down and inward is a vertical prismatic effect. For minus lenses, the vertical prismatic effect is base down. Since both lenses are equal in power, both lenses exert the same amount of base-down effect. Thus, both eyes angle downward the same amount. This is illustrated in Figure 17-3.

Lenses of Unequal Power

When the left eye requires a different lens power than the right eye, the condition is referred to as *anisometropia*. In some cases, the left eye may require a plus lens, while the right requires a minus lens, or vice versa. This is a specialized instance of anisometropia known as mixed anisometropia or *antimetropia*.

TOP VIEW

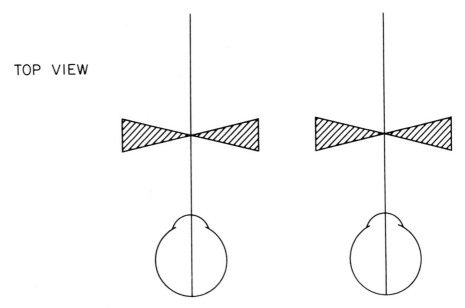

Figure 17-1 When the eyes look directly through the optical centers of a pair of glasses, the wearer experiences no prismatic effect.

TOP VIEW

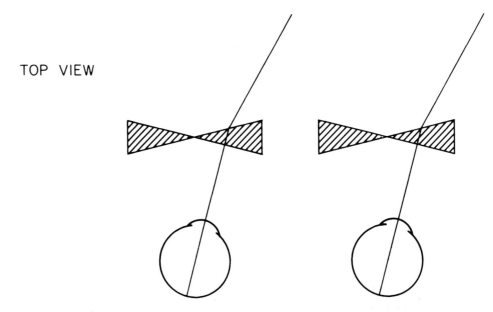

Figure 17-2 Light from an object at infinity when viewed through the periphery of prescription spectacle lenses is deviated by the prismatic effect of the lenses. When both lenses are of the same power, the deviation is symmetrical. Both rays emerging from the lenses, though deviated, are still parallel. Therefore the eyes neither converge nor diverge relative to one another. (From C.W. Brooks and I.M. Borish, *System for Ophthalmic Dispensing,* Butterworth-Heinemann, Boston, 1979, p. 423.)

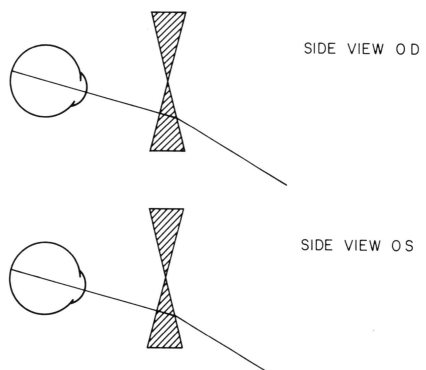

SIDE VIEW O D

SIDE VIEW O S

Figure 17-3 When both eyes turn downward and both lenses have the same refractive power, the two vertical prismatic effects are the same. The eyes turn downward at the same angle. (Here the eyes are shown one above the other so that each can be seen individually.)

Suppose the right and left lenses in a pair are not of the same power. As the person looks to the left or to the right, each lens exerts its own base-in or base-out prismatic effect, but now the two effects are not equal.

Horizontal Prismatic Effects of Looking Sideways

Now let us take another look at our spectacle lens-wearing myope. What happens if the wearer looks to the right? Consider the situation where the right lens has a higher minus power than the left. As the wearer looks to the right, the right lens still causes a base-out effect. But now, because the right lens is stronger, the base-out effect of the right lens is greater than the base-in effect of the weaker left lens. See Figure 17-4. This forces the eyes to converge somewhat, even though the wearer is looking off into the distance.

What if the wearer looks to the left? If this particular spectacle lens wearer looks to the left, the eyes will have to diverge. Even so, people in these situations do not usually experience difficulty, because sustained viewing through the sides of the lenses is not often required. If people must look at an object off to one side for a long period of time, they turn their heads toward that object, not just their eyes.

Unequal Vertical Prismatic Effects of Downward Gazing

When sustained viewing through the upper or lower area of the lenses is required and the right and left lenses are significantly different in power, there can be a problem. Unequal powers in the right and left lenses create unequal amounts of vertical prism when a person must look down. See Figure 17-5. Obviously, it is not a natural situation for one eye to look farther up or down than the other. Because this is an unnatural situation, the eyes are not as readily adaptable. When spectacle lenses force one eye to turn up- or downward farther than the other in certain areas of gaze, the condition is referred to as *vertical imbalance.*

Occurrence of Vertical Imbalance Problems

The single-vision lens wearer can escape the vertical imbalance problem when reading by simply drop-

Figure 17-4 When parallel light from a peripherally viewed object at infinity strikes a pair of spectacle lenses whose powers are unequal, the prismatic effects created at these non-central lens positions are unequal, causing more deviation of light entering through one lens than through the other. This in turn causes either a con- or divergence of the eyes, depending on the lens powers. (From C.W. Brooks and I.M. Borish, *System for Ophthalmic Dispensing,* Butterworth-Heinemann, Boston, 1979, p. 424.)

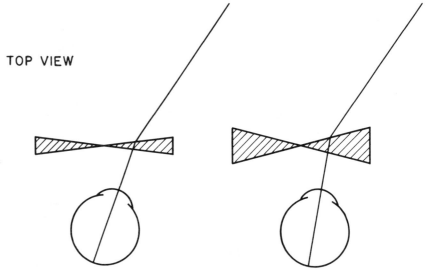

TOP VIEW

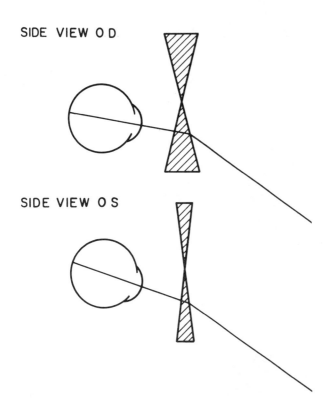

SIDE VIEW O D

SIDE VIEW O S

Figure 17-5 Unequal lens powers cause the same type of prismatic effect for objects viewed through tops and bottoms of spectacle lenses as is caused when looking through the sides. Unfortunately, the problem created is harder for the eyes to overcome, since turning one eye farther up or down than the other is not a natural paired eye movement. (From C.W. Brooks and I.M. Borish, *System for Ophthalmic Dispensing,* Butterworth-Heinemann, Boston, 1979, p. 425.)

ping the head. The eyes look through a point closer to the optical centers of the lenses, and the prism difference is drastically reduced. But most people do not wear single-vision lenses forever. When multifocals are required, the location of the reading segment forces the wearer to look through the lower parts of the lenses. Even so, life-long wearers of unequal prescriptions are either surprisingly adaptable to or tolerant of vertical imbalance, even when wearing bifocals.

Problems can appear more suddenly for individuals with developing cataracts. A *cataract* occurs when the crystalline lens in the eye loses its clarity, making vision difficult or impossible. Developing cataracts can cause the eyes to change refractively. There is a decrease in plus or an increase in minus lens power. If one eye develops a cataract more rapidly than the other, there will be a difference between the right and left lens powers that was not there earlier. Such an individual may need a correction for vertical imbalance.

Vertical imbalance problems can also develop after cataract surgery. Cataract surgery today often involves replacing the clouded natural lens with a permanent plastic lens. Such *intraocular lens implants* can change the power in the operated eye so that very little, if any, distance correction is required. Persons who have had a cataract removed from one eye and previously were myopic or hyperopic in both eyes may suddenly find themselves with a new problem: For these individuals, this strange new vertical prismatic effect caused by spectacle lenses of different powers may present major difficulties.

Options Available for Correcting Vertical Imbalance

Several options are available to overcome the problem of vertical imbalance:

1. two pairs of glasses
2. dropping the MRP height
3. slab-off (bicentric grind)
4. dissimilar segs
5. R-compensated segs
6. Fresnel press-on prism
7. contact lenses

Two Pairs of Glasses

When anisometropes wear single-vision lenses, vertical imbalance seldom surfaces as a problem. This is because single-vision lens wearers have the option of dropping the head and looking through the lens optical centers instead of just dropping the eyes and looking below the OCs. This means that if an anisometrope decides against multifocal lenses, he or she is not forced to look below the OCs where the near segment is located. Thus, one option for overcoming vertical imbalance is to have *two pairs of single-vision glasses*—one for distance and one for near. When using two pairs of glasses, the reading glasses should be ordered with the OCs lower than normal. This way the wearer looks through the lens OCs. A separate pair of single-vision glasses for near does not *correct* for vertical imbalance—it *avoids* vertical imbalance. Ordinarily the near Rx

optical centers are positioned 5 mm below the vertical center of the frames.

Instead of using a regular frame for the near Rx and lowering the OCs, a pair of half-eye frames can be used. In this way the Ocs are lower, even at their normal locations. They do not have to be lowered further.

Dropping the MRP Height

Reducing the amount of vertical imbalance at near by dropping the OC or MRP of a multifocal lens pair is used in practice, but is not as optically sound as other options. By dropping the OC, the distance from the OC to the reading depth is reduced, and so is the prismatic effect at near. However, lowering the OC will transfer imbalance from the near portion to the distance portion, as gain at near is offset by an increase in imbalance in the upper portion of the lens. Dropping the MRP in multifocals might be successful in borderline cases of imbalance but is not the best option available.

Slab-off

The most common option produces a vertical prismatic effect in the entire lower half of one lens only, beginning at the level of the bifocal segment line. This type of correction is called a *slab-off* or *bicentric grind*. It is identified by the presence of a horizontal line across one lens at the level of the segment top. See Figure 17-6.

Slab-off is almost always used unless the amount of correction required is less than 1.50 prism diopters or greater than 5.00 prism diopters. Below 1.50 prism diopters it is difficult to control the appear-

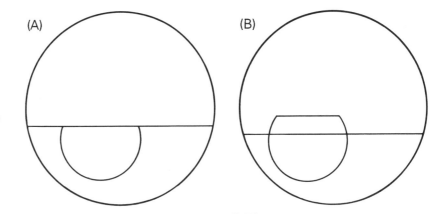

Figure 17-6 Slab-off prism produces a thin line that is easily concealed by a flat-top seg. The wider the seg, the more inconspicuous the line will be. (A) shows a bifocal lens, while (B) shows the correct position for slab-off prism on a flat-top trifocal. (From C.W. Brooks and I.M. Borish, *System for Ophthalmic Dispensing*, Butterworth-Heinemann, Boston, 1979, p. 428.)

(A)

(B)

ance and placement of the slab line. Fortunately, problems with vertical imbalance do not occur as frequently once vertical imbalance drops below 1.50. Slab-offs greater than 5.00 prism diopters are generally considered to be cosmetically unacceptable.[1]

Dissimilar Segments

A fourth method of dealing with vertical imbalance creates a difference in vertical prism between the two eyes in the reading area. This is done by using two differently shaped bifocal segments—one shape for one eye and another for the second. This method of correction is called *dissimilar segs*. See Figure 17-7. Differing shapes mean that the segment OCs are located at different heights. By carefully choosing two shapes for the relative location of their segment OCs, an equal but opposite vertical prismatic effect can be created.

When cost is a factor, the dispenser or prescriber may choose dissimilar segments. If the account specifies the combination of dissimilar segments desired, the cost will most likely be equal to the cost of two half-pairs of lenses.

R-Compensated Segments

A fifth method of correcting vertical imbalance uses R-compensated segments. See Figure 17-8. *R-compensated segments* are ribbon-style segments that have been modified so that the segment OC for one lens is higher than in the other. The principle is the same as in using dissimilar segs. The only difference is that R-compensated segs are not so obviously different in shape. They do not look as unusual as some dissimilar seg combinations.

The R-compensated seg may be used to correct amounts of vertical imbalance below 1.50 prism

diopters, but the R-compensated segment does not work for high amounts of imbalance.

Fresnel Press-on Prism

A *Fresnel press-on lens* is made from "thin, transparent, flexible, plastic material which adheres to the surface of an ophthalmic lens when pressed in place."[2] Such lenses also are available in prism only. Thus, it is possible to cut a Fresnel press-on prism to fit the lower half of one lens in order to counteract a vertical imbalance. Placed on the back surface of the ophthalmic lens, the Fresnel prism simulates the slab-off lens. Fresnel lenses for such an application are usually not considered to be a permanent solution, but rather are used on a trial basis to see if the wearer's visual difficulties can be alleviated.

Contact Lenses

From a purely optical standpoint, one of the best options available is the contact lens. The optical center of the contact lens moves with the eye. When an individual wears contact lenses, the spectacle lens-induced prismatic difference disappears, and the vertical imbalance problem with it.

Calculating Vertical Imbalance

Ideally, the prescriber should decide the amount of correction needed for vertical imbalance. A specific amount of vertical imbalance is caused by the spectacle lenses. This amount can be calculated exactly for a given reading depth. Yet not everyone may need the full amount corrected. Over the years, some wearers have learned to compensate for at least part of the imbalance while wearing their single-

Figure 17-7 Correcting vertical imbalance with dissimilar segments utilizes prism induced by the segment itself. Prism produced by the segment for a given reading level varies with the position of the seg optical center. Seg optical center location depends on the bifocal shape, so using segs of two different shapes may correct a vertical imbalance at near. (From C.W. Brooks and I.M. Borish, *System for Ophthalmic Dispensing*, Butterworth-Heinemann, Boston, 1979, p. 432.)

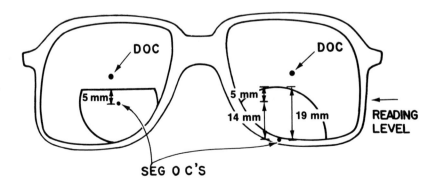

Figure 17-8 R-compensated segments are made from ribbon-style segment lenses. The optical centers can be lowered or raised as in (A) and (C). Optically compensated R segments behave just like dissimilar segments.

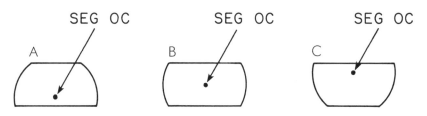

vision lenses. If less than the full imbalance must be corrected, this can be determined through patient response in subjective testing.

If the prescriber does not test for vertical imbalance at near, then the next best person to indicate the amount of compensating prism is the dispenser. The dispenser can determine at what depth in the glasses the wearer will be reading.

The one person who never even sees the wearer is the laboratory optician. Yet often the laboratory is asked to perform the necessary calculations, since either the prescriber and dispenser do not wish to take the time, or do not know how.

When the laboratory is asked to calculate the amount of vertical imbalance correction required, the easiest method is to use a lens layout computer program that includes vertical imbalance calculations. The program asks questions about the nature of the prescription and then provides the answer.

If no program is available, the calculation can be done by hand. This is relatively easy for those who know how to calculate prism for decentration. Prism decentration and vertical imbalance calculations are very similar.

Calculating Vertical Imbalance When Both Lenses Are Spherical

Calculating for vertical imbalance is easiest when both the right and left lenses are spheres. To help understand the concept, the method summarized in Table 17-1 is used. This method will be simplified later on. Here are the steps, with an explanation of each.

1. *Find the reading depth.* The reading depth is that place on the lens through which the wearer looks when reading or doing close work. It is specified in terms of its distance from the major reference point of the lens. To find this distance, first note the distance from the MRP to the seg line. The distance from the MRP to the seg line is equal to the seg drop (unless the MRP height is specified on the order or is moved from its customary location by the surfacing laboratory). When bifocals are worn,

Table 17-1 Conventional Method for Calculating Vertical Imbalance

---

1. Find the reading depth:

    Reading depth = seg drop + 5 mm (usually)

2. Find the power of each lens in the 90-degree meridian.
3. Find the prismatic effect at the reading depth of each lens.
4. Find the prismatic difference (vertical imbalance) between the right and left lenses.

---

reading is generally assumed to take place at a depth 5 mm below the segment line.* Thus the reading-depth distance can be considered to be

$$\text{Reading depth} = \text{seg drop} + 5 \text{ mm}$$

2. *Find the power of each lens in the 90-degree meridian.* Because a *vertical* imbalance is being considered, the power of the lens in the 90-degree meridian is used for calculation purposes. When lenses are spherical, they have the same power in all meridians. Therefore, the power of the lens in the 90-degree meridian is the sphere power.

3. *Find the prismatic effect at the reading depth of each lens.* To find the vertical prismatic effect, use Prentice's rule and multiply the reading-depth distance in centimeters times the power in the 90-degree meridian. Expressed as a formula, this is

Vertical
prism   = (reading-depth distance)(power in 90)

(Instead of using the formula, it is possible to use the Prism Power Decentration Chart, which was first explained in Chapter 3 and also appears as Appendixes 2-3 and 2-4.)

4. *Find the prismatic difference (vertical imbal-*

---

*It is possible to use a different distance below this line for calculation purposes. Three to five millimeters is most common. The closer to the line the reading level is assumed to be, the smaller the vertical imbalance will be.

ance) *between the right and left lenses.* If both lenses are plus powered in the 90-degree meridian, the lenses will have base-up prismatic effects at any point below the distance OC. If both lenses are minus powered in the 90-degree meridian, they will both have base-down prism below their distance OCs. In both cases, differences in prism at the reading depth are in the same direction. The vertical imbalance is the difference between the two prismatic effects at the reading depth for the lenses.

If one lens is plus powered in the 90-degree meridian and one lens is minus powered in the 90-degree meridian, then one will be creating base-up while the other creates base-down prism. If this is the case, the amount of vertical imbalance is the sum of these two amounts.

EXAMPLE 17-1

Suppose a prescription is received as follows:

R: −0.50 sphere
L: −5.50 sphere
  Add +2.50
Frame A = 55 mm
Frame B = 46 mm
Seg height = 20 mm

What is the amount of vertical imbalance at the reading depth?

SOLUTION

Proceed through each step as previously outlined.
  Step 1. Find the reading depth.

$$\text{Reading depth} = \text{seg drop} + 5 \text{ mm}$$

The seg drop is half the frame B dimension minus the seg height,* or

$$\text{Seg drop} = \frac{46}{2} - 20$$

$$= 3 \text{ mm}$$

Therefore

$$\text{Reading depth} = 3 \text{ mm} + 5 \text{ mm}$$
$$= 8 \text{ mm or } 0.8 \text{ cm}$$

Step 2. Find the power of each lens in the 90-degree meridian. In this instance the power of each lens in the

---

*Technically, the seg drop is the seg height minus half the B dimension. This yields a negative number for seg drop, which is technically correct. For these purposes, we will take seg drop as positive.

90-degree meridian is equal to its sphere power. The right lens is −0.50 D and the left lens is −5.50 D.

Step 3. Find the prismatic effect at the reading depth of each lens. For the right lens, the prismatic effect at the reading depth is

Vertical prism = (reading depth distance)(power in 90)
        = (0.8 cm)(0.50)
        = 0.4 prism diopter Base Down

For the left lens,

Vertical prism = (0.8 cm)(5.50)
        = 4.4 prism diopters Base Down

Step 4. Find the prismatic difference (vertical imbalance) between the right and left lenses. Since both the right and left lenses have minus power in the 90-degree meridian, both create base-down prism at the reading depth. Therefore the amount of vertical imbalance is the difference between the two:

Vertical imbalance = 4.4 BD − 0.4 BD
          = 4.0 BD before the left eye

Thus the vertical amount of imbalance created by the spectacle lenses is 4 prism diopters Base Down for the left eye. (It could also be expressed as 4.0 prism diopters Base Up for the right eye.)

In order to counteract this imbalance, the laboratory will need to create just the opposite effect, using base-up prism before the left eye or base-down prism before the right.

Calculating Vertical Imbalance for Lenses with a Cylinder Axis at 90 or 180 Degrees

When a lens pair has cylinder power with the cylinder at Axis 90 or 180, the vertical imbalance calculations are still done in basically the same manner as with sphere lenses. The only difference is that the power in the 90-degree meridian may or may not equal the sphere power.

For a minus cylinder lens with an axis of 180 degrees, the power of the cylinder falls in the 90-degree meridian. For example, if a lens has a power of −5.00 −2.00 × 180, the full power of the cylinder is in the 90. The lens will have a power of −5.00 D in the 180-degree meridian, but a power of

$$(-5.00 \text{ D}) + (-2.00 \text{ D}) \text{ or } -7.00 \text{ D}$$

in the 90-degree meridian. See Figure 17-9.

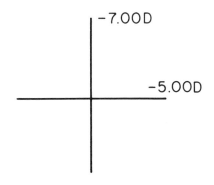

Figure 17-9 For a lens having a power of −5.00 −2.00 × 180, the power in the 90-degree meridian will be −7.00 D.

To demonstrate, calculate the vertical imbalance for the lens pair given in Example 17-2.

EXAMPLE 17-2

If a prescription is as follows, what is the amount of vertical imbalance at the reading depth?

R: +5.00 −2.00 × 180
L: +0.75 −0.50 × 180
   Add +2.50
Frame *A* = 56 mm
Frame *B* = 48 mm
Seg height = 20 mm

SOLUTION

Follow the same steps as were outlined for the spherical lens pair.

Step 1. Find the reading depth.

Reading depth = seg drop + 5 mm
                = 4 mm + 5 mm
                = 9 mm or 0.9 cm

Step 2. Find the power of each lens in the 90-degree meridian. The power of the right lens in the 90-degree meridian is

$$(+5.00) + (-2.00) = +3.00 \text{ D}$$

The power of the left lens in the 90-degree meridian is

$$(+0.75) + (-0.50) = +0.25 \text{ D}$$

Step 3. Find the prismatic effect at the reading depth of each lens. For the right lens, the prismatic effect at the reading depth is

Vertical prism = (reading depth distance)(power in 90)
           = (0.9 cm)(3.00)
           = 2.7 prism diopters Base Up

For the left lens,

Vertical prism = (0.9 cm)(0.25)
           = 0.225 prism diopter Base Up

Step 4. Find the prismatic difference (vertical imbalance) between the right and left lenses. The vertical imbalance between the lenses is

Vertical imbalance = 2.7 BU − 0.225 BU
                = 2.475 BU

Therefore the vertical imbalance created by the lenses is 2.5 prism diopters Base Up for the right eye or 2.5 prism diopters Base Down for the left eye. As before, to compensate for the imbalance, the laboratory uses the exact opposite base direction to correct the problem.

Calculating Vertical Imbalance for Lenses with Oblique Cylinders

For lens pairs having one or both of their cylinders at an oblique axis, the only complication in finding vertical imbalance is in finding the lens power in the 90-degree meridian. The method that will be presented here has been used for quite some time with considerable success. Some computer programs use more exact methods, but many programs still use the original method.

Finding the Power in the 90-Degree Meridian for Spherocylinder Lenses with Oblique Axes

The procedure for finding the "power" of an oblique cylinder in the 90-degree meridian is very close to the procedure described for finding the power of a cylinder in the 180-degree meridian. This was explained in Chapter 3 and was needed for finding decentration prism with spherocylinders. To find the power in the 90-degree meridian for a spherocylinder lens with an oblique axis, follow the procedure outlined in Table 17-2.

EXAMPLE 17-3

What is the power in the 90-degree meridian for the spherocylinder lens −4.50 −2.00 × 10?

SOLUTION

To find the power of the spherocylinder lens in the 90-degree meridian, first find the power contributed by the cylinder in the 90-degree meridian. (Spheres have the same power in any meridian.)

Table 17-2 Finding the Power of a Spherocylinder Lens in the 90-Degree Meridian

1. Find the power of the cylinder in the 90-degree meridian. This can be done in either of two ways. The first is to use the formula

$$F = F_{cyl} \cos^2 \theta$$

where θ is the cylinder axis.* The second is to look up the cylinder power in the 90-degree meridian in a set of tables. Such tables are shown as Appendix 3-2 at the back of the book.†

2. Add this reduced cylinder value to the sphere power of the lens.

$$\text{(Sphere power)} + \text{(cyl power in 90)} = \text{(total power in 90)}$$

---

*Recall that the formula $F = F$ cyl $\sin^2 \theta$ is used to calculate the power in the 180-degree meridian.
†These tables are *cosine-squared tables*. It is also possible to use the sine-squared tables that are normally used for finding power in the 180-degree meridian. If sine-squared tables are used, the only modification that must be made is to add 90 degrees to the cylinder axis before looking up the power in the table.

The power of the -2.00×10 cylinder in the 90-degree meridian is -1.77 D. Because the cylinder axis is close to 180, almost all the power is manifested in the 90-degree meridian.

Next this value is added to the sphere power:

$$-4.50 + -1.77 = -6.27 \text{ D}$$

This means that if vertical imbalance were calculated for a lens having a power of $-4.50 -2.00 \times 10$, the power used to figure the prismatic effect at the reading depth would be -6.27 D.

To find vertical imbalance for oblique-axis spherocyl lenses, the same steps may be followed as were outlined in Table 17-1. The only difference is that Step 2 requires the use of the cosine-squared formula or cosine-squared tables. Following are two examples, worked step by step.

EXAMPLE 17-4

Find the amount of prism needed to correct the vertical imbalance found at the reading depth for the following prescription.

R: $-4.50 -2.00 \times 10$
L: $+0.25 -1.50 \times 155$
  Add $+2.50$
Frame $A = 55$ mm
Frame $B = 46$ mm
Seg height = 18 mm

SOLUTION

To find the imbalance for these spherocylinder lenses with oblique axes, follow the standard steps.
  Step 1. Find the reading depth.

$$\text{Reading depth} = \text{seg drop} + 5 \text{ mm}$$

The seg drop is $46/2 - 18$, or 5 mm. Therefore

$$\text{Reading depth} = 5 \text{ mm} + 5 \text{ mm}$$
$$= 10 \text{ mm or } 1 \text{ cm}$$

  Step 2. Find the power of each lens in the 90-degree meridian. Notice that the *right lens* has the same power as the lens in Example 17-3. In Example 17-3 we found the power of this lens in the 90-degree meridian to be -6.27 D. However, we have not yet found the power of the left lens in the 90-degree meridian.

  The *left lens* is calculated by first finding the power of the *cylinder* component in the 90-degree meridian. The cylinder is -1.50×155. The power of this cylinder in the 90-degree meridian can be found by using either a hand calculator or Appendix 3-2.

  Using a standard hand calculator equipped with trigonometric function, use the formula $(-1.50) \cos^2 155$. The cosine of 155 is -0.9063. This value is squared:

$$(-0.9063)^2 = 0.8214$$

(This means that 82.14% of the cylinder is manifested in the 90-degree meridian.) Because the cylinder has a power of -1.50, multiply -1.50 times 0.8214:

$$(0.8214)(-1.50) = -1.23$$

The power in the 90-degree meridian for the cylinder is -1.23D.

  This mathematical approach may not suit everyone. For those who never liked math very well anyway, the same answer can be found directly from Appendix 3-2.‡

  Now that the power of the cylinder in the 90-degree meridian has been determined, this reduced cylinder value is added to the sphere power of the lens. For the right lens this is

$$\text{(Sphere power)} + \text{(cyl power in 90)} = \text{(power in 90)}$$
$$-4.50 + -1.77 = -6.27 \text{ D}$$

For the left lens this is

$$+0.25 + -1.23 = -0.98 \text{ D}$$

---

‡Again, it is possible to find the cylinder power in the 90-degree meridian by using $\sin^2$ tables. Instead of looking up the axis directly, first add or subtract 90 degrees. In this case, the number to look up is $155 - 90$, that is, 65 degrees. When 65 degrees is looked up for a -1.50 D cylinder, the $\sin^2$ table shows -1.23 D. This is the correct answer.

Step 3. Find the prismatic effect at the reading depth of each lens. For the right lens, the prismatic effect at the reading depth is .

Vertical prism = (reading depth distance)(power in 90)
   = (1 cm)(6.27)
   = 6.27 prism diopters Base Down

For the left lens,

   Vertical prism = (1 cm)(0.98)
      = 0.98 prism diopter Base Down

Step 4. Find the prismatic difference (vertical imbalance) between the right and left lenses. The vertical imbalance between the lenses is

Vertical imbalance = 6.27 BD − 0.98 BD
      = 5.25 prism diopters Base Down

Now let us look at a second example.

EXAMPLE 17-5

Find the prismatic effect needed to correct the vertical imbalance found at the reading depth for the following prescription.

   R: +3.75 −1.75 × 105
   L: −0.75 −1.50 × 35
   Add +1.50
   Frame *A* = 53 mm
   Frame *B* = 42 mm
   Seg height = 19 mm

SOLUTION

To find the imbalance for these spherocylinder lenses with oblique axes, we again follow the steps outlined in Tables 17-1 and 17-2.

Step 1. Find the reading depth.

   Reading depth = seg drop + 5 mm

The seg drop is 42/2 − 19, or 2 mm. Therefore

   Reading depth = 2 mm + 5 mm
      = 7 mm or 0.7 cm

Step 2. Find the power of each lens in the 90-degree meridian. To calculate the cylinder component power in the 90-degree meridian, either a hand calculator or the appropriate tables can be used. The power of a −1.75 × 105 cylinder in the 90 is

   $(-1.75) \cos^2 105 = -0.12$ D

The power of the cylinder component may now be added to the sphere component. This is

$$+3.75 + -0.12 = +3.63 \text{ D}$$

For the left lens, the power of a −1.50 × 35 cylinder in the 90 is

   $(-1.50) \cos^2 35 = -1.01$ D

The power of the cylinder component is added to the sphere component, resulting in

$$-0.75 + -1.01 = -1.76 \text{ D}$$

So, for the right lens, the power in the 90-degree meridian is +3.63 D; and for the left lens, it is −1.76 D.

Step 3. Find the prismatic effect at the reading depth of each lens. For the right lens, the prismatic effect at the reading depth is

Vertical prism = (reading depth distance)(power in 90)
   = (0.7 cm)(3.63)
   = 2.54 prism diopters Base Up

For the left lens,

   Vertical prism = (0.7 cm)(1.76)
      = 1.23 prism diopters Base Down

Step 4. Find the prismatic difference (vertical imbalance) between the right and left lenses. The vertical imbalance between the lenses is

Vertical imbalance = 2.54 BU + 1.23 BD
      = 3.77 prism diopters Base Up

The amount of vertical imbalance is 3.77 BU when referenced to the right eye and 3.77 BD when referenced to the left eye. This imbalance is corrected by using a prism of equal power and opposite base direction.

A Simplified Method of Calculating Vertical Imbalance

There is a shortcut that can be used in figuring vertical imbalance. Using the conventional method we calculate the prismatic effect at the reading depth for first the right, then the left lens. Instead of finding prismatic effects twice, it is possible simply to take the difference in power between the 90-degree meridians for the right and left lenses. Using Prentice's rule, this power difference is multiplied by the reading-depth distance in centimeters, giving the vertical imbalance directly. This method is summarized in Table 17-3.

To see how the simplified method works, we will use it to rework the previous example.

Table 17-3 Simplified Method for Calculating Vertical Imbalance

1. Find the reading depth.

    Reading depth = seg drop + 5 mm (usually)

2. Find the power of each lens in the 90-degree meridian.

3. Find the difference between the right and left 90-degree meridian powers.

4. Find the vertical prism imbalance. Multiply the reading-depth distance in centimeters times the 90-degree meridian power differences (or use Appendix 2-5).

EXAMPLE 17-6

Use the simplified method for calculating vertical imbalance to work Example 17-5.

SOLUTION

In Example 17-5, the powers in the vertical meridian were found to be

R: +3.63 D in the 90
L: −1.76 D in the 90

Instead of multiplying each lens's 90-degree meridian by the reading-depth distance, take the difference between the two meridians:

$$(+3.63 \text{ D}) - (-1.76 \text{ D}) = 5.39 \text{ D}$$

For this pair of glasses, the difference between the two 90-degree meridians is 5.39 D. Therefore, either multiply the reading-depth distance by 5.39 D or use Appendix 2-5, the vertical imbalance prism compensation table:

$$\text{Vertical prism imbalance} = (0.7 \text{ cm})(5.39)$$
$$= 3.77 \text{ prism diopters}$$

This method gives the same result as was found using the conventional method. As before, this prism diopter difference can be written as either 3.77 BU when referenced to the right eye or 3.77 BD when referenced to the left.

EXAMPLE 17-7

Here is a prescription for a person who has just had a cataract extraction and intraocular lens implant for the right eye. Using the simplified method, tell how much vertical imbalance is present at the reading depth for this postsurgical lens correction.

R: −0.75 −0.50 × 80
L: −4.75 −1.25 × 160
  Add = +2.25
Frame *B* = 48 mm
Seg height = 21 mm
Seg style = FT-28

SOLUTION

Step 1. Find the reading depth.

$$\text{Reading depth} = \left(\frac{48}{2} - 21\right) + 5 \text{ mm}$$
$$= 8 \text{ mm}$$

Step 2. Find the power of each lens in the 90-degree meridian. For the right lens, using Appendix 3-2, the power in the 90-degree meridian of a −0.50 × 80 cylinder is only −0.02 D. Therefore the total power in the 90-degree meridian is

$$\text{Sphere + cylinder in 90} = \text{total in 90}$$
$$(-0.75) + (-0.02) = -0.77 \text{ D}$$

For the left lens, using the same tables, for a −1.25 cyl, Axis 160, the power in the 90-degree meridian is −1.10 D. This means that for the left lens, the total power in the 90-degree meridian will be

$$(-4.75) + (-1.10) = -5.85 \text{ D}$$

Step 3. Find the difference between these 90-degree meridian powers. The difference between the two powers is

$$(-0.77) - (-5.85) = 5.08 \text{ D}$$

Step 4. Find the vertical prism imbalance by multiplying the reading-depth distance in centimeters times the 90-degree meridian power differences (or use Appendix 2-5). Multiplying gives

$$\text{Vertical imbalance} = (0.8)(5.08)$$
$$= 4.06 \text{ prism diopters}$$

Using Appendix 2-5 requires rounding 5.08 D to 5.00 D. Looking up 5.00 D in the table, we find an imbalance of 4.0 prism diopters. The difference between 4.00 and 4.06 is not significant

EXAMPLE 17-8

A certain individual has worn +2.00 D lenses with a +2.25 D add for years. He is now developing cataracts, especially in the left eye. The developing cataract is causing a change in his refractive error. Because the refractive error is less than it was before, this person does not need his glasses as much as he did before. The change in refraction has caused him to gain his "second sight," and he is not yet ready to have cataract surgery. The prescription is now

R: $+1.75 -0.50 \times 70$
L: $-0.50 -0.75 \times 150$
  Add $= +2.25$
Frame $B = 48$ mm
Seg height $= 19$ mm
Seg style $=$ FT-35

Use the simplified method to find the amount of vertical imbalance that will be experienced by the wearer when he has his new prescription filled.

SOLUTION

Step 1. Find the reading depth.

$$\text{Reading depth} = \left(\frac{48}{2} - 19\right) + 5$$
$$= 10 \text{ mm or 1 cm}$$

Step 2. Find the power of each lens in the 90.

Sphere + cyl power in 90 = power in 90

For the right lens,

$$(+1.75) + (-0.06) = +1.69 \text{ D}$$

For the left lens,

$$(-0.50) + (-0.56) = -1.06 \text{ D}$$

Step 3. Find the difference between the 90-degree meridian powers.

$$(+1.69) - (-1.06) = 2.75 \text{ D}$$

Step 4. Find the vertical prism imbalance.

$$\text{Vertical imbalance} = (1.0)(2.75)$$
$$= 2.75 \text{ prism diopters}$$

This person will experience 2.75 prism diopters of vertical imbalance at near, whereas before there was no imbalance.

Calculating Vertical Imbalance When MRP Height Is Given

Most dispensers do not specify a major reference point height, especially for bi- or trifocals. But if they do, then the reading-depth distance must be calculated differently. Instead of measuring the reading depth from the middle of the lens (at one-half the *B* dimension), it is measured from the MRP

height. Now, instead of the reading depth being $(B/2 - \text{seg height}) + 5$, it is

Reading depth $=$ (MRP height $-$ seg height) $+ 5$

After the reading depth has been calculated, the steps in finding vertical imbalance are exactly the same.

EXAMPLE 17-9

Find the vertical imbalance for the following Rx.

R: $+1.50 -1.50 \times 175$
L: $+3.50 -1.50 \times 35$
Frame $B = 46$ mm
MRP height $= 26$ mm
Seg height $= 20$ mm
Seg style $=$ FT-28

SOLUTION

Step 1. Find the reading depth.

Reading depth $=$ (MRP height $-$ seg height) $+ 5$
$$= (26 - 20) + 5$$
$$= 11 \text{ mm or 1.1 cm}$$

Step 2. Find the power of each lens in the 90

Sphere + cyl power in 90 = power in 90

For the right lens this is

$$+1.50 -1.49 = +0.01$$

and for the left lens it is

$$3.50 -1.01 = +2.49$$

Step 3. Find the difference between these 90-degree meridian powers.

$$+2.49 -0.01 = 2.48 \text{ D}$$

Step 4. Find the vertical prism imbalance.

$$\text{Vertical imbalance} = (1.1)(2.48)$$
$$= 2.73 \text{ prism diopters}$$

Calculating Vertical Imbalance When Seg Heights Are Unequal

Sometimes a prescription has one bifocal seg higher than the other. When this happens, the MRP heights should also be unequal by the same amount. Suppose, for example, that the right seg height is 2 mm higher than the left. If this is the case, then one eye is probably higher than the other. If one eye *is* higher than the other, then the right MRP will also be 2 mm higher than the left MRP. If MRP heights and seg heights are unequal by the same amount, as they should be, then the reading-depth distances will be equal for the two eyes. Calculations for vertical imbalance will be done the same as was described. Unfortunately, some dispensers are careful in taking each seg height individually, but never measure for MRP height. If this happens, two different measures for reading depth result.

Calculating Vertical Imbalance with Two Different Reading Depths

Sometimes orders give unequal seg heights but no MRP. If the laboratory must calculate vertical imbalance for such a prescription, there will be two different reading depths. With two reading depths, the short method for calculating vertical imbalance as outlined in Table 17-3 will not work. We must return to the original method of Table 17-1.

EXAMPLE 17-10

Find the vertical imbalance for the following Rx.

R: $-8.50 - 1.75 \times 18$
L: $-3.25 - 1.25 \times 164$
Frame $B = 42$ mm
R seg height = 18 mm
L seg height = 20 mm

SOLUTION

Step 1. Find the reading depth. In this example the MRP heights and seg heights do not correspond to one another. The reading depth for the right lens is lower than the reading depth for the left. Since MRP heights are not specified, both are at half the B dimension ($B/2$). This means that one reading-depth distance is 2 mm greater than the other. For the right eye the reading-depth distance is

$$\text{Right reading depth} = \left(\frac{42}{2} - 18\right) + 5$$
$$= 3 + 5$$
$$= 8 \text{ mm or } 0.8 \text{ cm}$$

The left reading-depth distance is

$$\text{Left reading depth} = \left(\frac{42}{2} - 20\right) + 5$$
$$= 1 + 5$$
$$= 6 \text{ mm or } 0.6 \text{ cm}$$

Step 2. Find the power of each lens in the 90-degree meridian. In this example both cylinders have an axis that falls between the 5-degree intervals in Appendix 3-2. There are three possibilities for finding power in the 90-degree meridian:

1. Use the formula.
2. Round to the nearest 5 degrees.
3. Interpolate between the values shown for the nearest 5 degrees on either side.

Using the table and rounding to the nearest 5 degrees for the right lens gives

$$\text{Sphere} + \text{cyl power in the 90} = \text{power in the 90}$$
$$-8.50 + (-1.64) = -10.14$$

For the left lens,

$$-3.25 + (-1.13) = -4.38$$

Step 3. Find the prismatic effect at the reading depth of each lens.

$$\text{Right vertical prism} = (0.8)(10.14)$$
$$= 8.11 \text{ Base Down}$$

$$\text{Left vertical prism} = (0.6)(4.38)$$
$$= 2.63 \text{ Base Down}$$

Step 4. Find the prismatic difference (vertical imbalance) between the right and left lenses. The imbalance is

$$\text{Vertical imbalance} = 8.11 \text{ BD} - 2.63 \text{ BD}$$
$$= 5.48 \text{ BD (right eye)}$$
$$\text{or } 5.48 \text{ BU (left eye)}$$

The *correction* will be 5.48 BU right eye or 5.48 BD left eye.

In practice, many laboratories, knowing that unequal seg heights indicate unequal MRP heights, will set the MRPs the same distance above the seg line. In the majority of cases this will benefit the wearer. But there are pros and cons.

Pros:

1. Setting the MRPs unequally to match the unequal seg heights will mean a zero vertical prismatic effect in the distance Rx during wear.
2. Laboratory-calculated vertical imbalance corrections are trying to bring about a zero imbalance at near. Therefore, there should be no imbalance for distance either.

Cons:

1. The wearer may be used to the distance imbalance in single-vision lenses.
2. The account may object to the vertical prism caused by unequal MRP heights in the distance prescription, which may be noticed while verifying the Rx in the conventional manner.

The safest practice (if done tactfully) is to phone the account, relate the problem, and suggest that matching, unequal MRP heights be used.

Surfacing Lenses that Correct for Vertical Imbalance

Slab-off

The most common and probably the best choice for correcting vertical imbalance is the use of slab-off prism. Formerly there was only one type of lens option available to the slab-off wearer. That option was to use a fused-glass type of bi- or trifocal lens. Options have since expanded considerably. As the demand for plastic lenses has increased, innovative laboratories have developed methods for producing slab-off in plastic.

More recently, premolded plastic lenses with the slab-off correction already on the semifinished blank have been developed. Premolding has simplified the process for the prescription optical laboratory considerably.

Using Slab-off for Single-Vision Lenses

Although most slab-off prescriptions are multifocal lens corrections, it is possible to grind slab-off on a single-vision lens. Slab-off may be appropriate for a single-vision wearer if the prescription contains a very large right and left lens power difference. A large power difference between the right and left eyes is called *anisometropia*. If the single-vision lens wearer is anisometropic and either unable to drop the head far enough or hold the head in a dropped position long enough to work comfortably, a slab-off can be helpful.

Another reason for using a single-vision slab-off correction is because of a paralysis or partial paralysis of an extraocular muscle. Such an eye muscle problem can prevent fusion in one particular field of gaze. If that field of gaze is the lower field,

reading is extremely troublesome. Unless compensating prism is used in one particular area, the wearer experiences double vision.

Segment Styles for Slab-off Lenses

Even though it is possible to grind slab-off prism on any type of fused-glass lens, the most attractive results will be obtained on lenses that camouflage the slab line. Lenses that already have a line, such as the standard flat-top bi- or trifocal or even a Franklin-style lens, are best. (Although the Franklin-style lens is not a fused lens, it can still be made into a slab-off correction.)

If slab-off is prescribed for trifocal lenses, the slab line should be on the second segment line down. If slab-off prism is ground over the intermediate area of the trifocal but calculated for the near area, the wearer will be significantly overcorrected for imbalance when using the intermediate viewing distance.

Grinding Slab-off Prism on a Glass Lens

After the amount of slab-off prism has been determined, the procedure for grinding slab-off prism on a glass lens is as follows. See Figure 17-10.

1. *Choose the most minus or least plus lens.* Select the lens that will have the most minus or least plus power in the 90-degree meridian. The most minus or least plus is chosen because a conventional slab-off grind will result in base-up prism in the lower half of the lens.

2. *Zero-cut the blank to remove unwanted blank prism.* Later on in the slab-off process the lens will be blocked on the back surface. If the lens is the least bit wedge-shaped, the prism, which will be cut on the front of the lens, may be inaccurate. Therefore, as a precaution, some laboratories block the lens as usual, then zero-cut the back surface. The curve used should match the back surface curve on the semifinished blank. If the generator is set for zero thickness removal, any prism in the blank will show up as a partial cut across the back surface. Remove stock very slowly until the full surface is even. Then fine and polish the lens.

3. *Make a cover lens.* A *cover lens* can be made from a single-vision blank. The cover lens should have a back surface that matches the front base curve of the semifinished lens blank. In other words, if the semifinished blank to be used has a base curve of $+8.00$ D, then the cover lens must have a back curve of -8.00 D.

Figure 17-10 Slab-off prism manufacture. (A) A cover lens is manufactured to have the same inside curve as the base curve of the required semifinished lens blank. (B) The cover lens is cemented to the semifinished blank. (In practice, only half a cover lens is required, covering from the center of the lens on down. For instructional purposes, however, the complete cover lens is shown.) (C) Base-down prism is ground on the front surface of the lens. Glass is surfaced off until only the lower half of the cover lens, from the seg line down, remains. The dioptric value of the prism is equal to the prescribed amount needed for compensation. (D) The distance power is surfaced on and the prismatic effect removed during generating. Now the entire lens is once again without prism. (E) Last, the remaining portion of the cover lens is removed. This wedge-shaped portion is a base-down prism whose value equals that surfaced, as shown in (C). The net effect is the addition of base-up prism to the lens from the seg downward. (From C.W. Brooks and I.M. Borish, *System for Ophthalmic Dispensing.* Butterworth-Heinemann, Boston, 1979, pp. 426–427.)

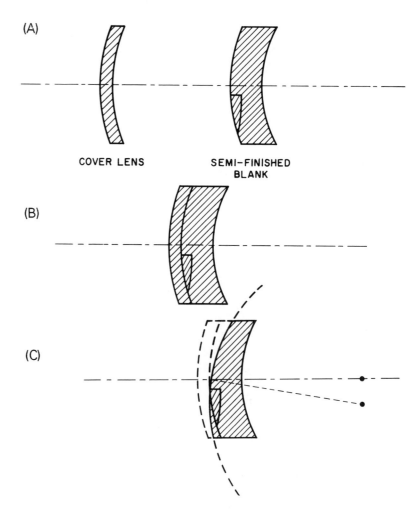

4. *Clean the cover lens and semifinished blank surfaces.*

5. *Stamp the needed lines.* Using a layout marker, stamp a horizontal line directly on the seg line. Stamp a second line 4 or 5 mm above the seg line to help in guiding the slab line. Stamp or draw a vertical prism line on the back of the semifinished lens to indicate base-down prism.

6. *Cement the cover lens in place.* The cover lens is cemented to the front surface of the lens. It serves to protect the lower half of the lens surface during lens surfacing and assures that a sharp, thin, straight slab line will result. The following procedure is used:

a. Heat the semifinished lens and the cover lens on a hot plate until they are hot enough to cause balsam to melt when it is rubbed over the lens surface. Instead of a hot plate, the lenses can be placed in an oven set for 200 degrees Fahrenheit.

b. Coat both the back surface of the cover lens and the front surface of the semifinished lens with Canadian balsam.

c. Place the cover lens on the semifinished lens. Use gloves, a clothespin, or tongs to keep from getting burned.

d. Work out the bubbles from between the lenses. This can be done by moving the cover lens around on the semifinished lens with gloves or using the eraser end of a pencil if no gloves are used. It may be helpful to apply pressure to the lenses during drying. This can be done by weighting them with a heavy object or by using a clamp.

e. Wait until the lens cools completely.

7. *Block the lens.* The semifinished lens is blocked "backwards" so that the front of the lens may be worked.

8. *Generate the front surface of the lens.*

(D)

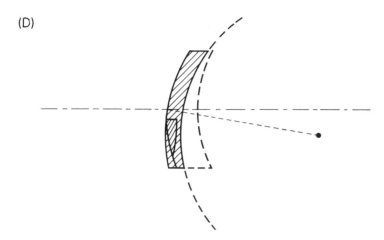

(E)

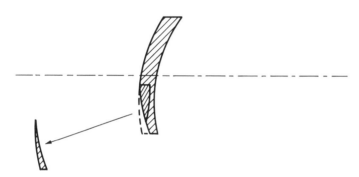

a. Set the generator to grind plus, and use the same curve as the front base curve of the semifinished lens.

b. Select a prism ring for the amount of slab-off needed. The ring should be turned so that it grinds base-down prism. (The thin edge of the *ring* will be at the bottom of the lens.)

c. Thickness should be reduced by very small amounts at a time. As lens stock is cut away, the first sweep will graze the top part of the lens only. The lens is thinned and checked, thinned and checked. As the cover slip is ground away, the lens surface begins to show what will become the slab line. See Figure 17-11. This line should be perfectly horizontal, parallel to the stamped guide lines and to the top of the seg.

d. If the slab line is at an angle, the thin edge of the prism ring should be turned very

slightly toward the low side of the line. This will cause the line to angle toward the horizontal.

e. When this line is parallel to, and about 5 mm from, the top of the bifocal segment, for most lenses the generating process must be halted. Lenses with small amounts of slab-off prism will require that the slab line be left the full 5 mm away from the segment line before fining and polishing. However, for prescriptions with larger amounts of slab prism, the slab line can be brought closer to the bifocal seg line. (The line will move to the desired position right on the bifocal line as the last bit of lens stock is removed during fining and polishing.)

9. *Fine the lens on slow speed, watching the slab line*. If the slab line begins to tilt while fining, put

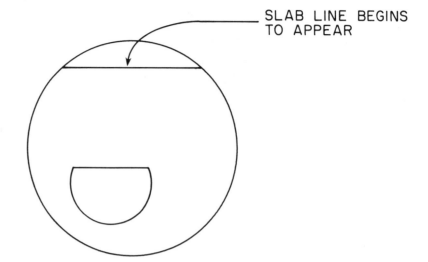

SLAB LINE BEGINS
TO APPEAR

Figure 17-11 As the front surface is generated with prism, the cover lens begins to be ground away, leaving the location of the slab line visible. The slab line will continue to move down the lens as more lens thickness is removed.

pressure on the upper half of the lens where the slab line is highest. This can be done by offsetting the pins on the block to the smaller, peripheral holes, or by using an offset block adapter. Because the speed is slow, finger pressure can be applied on the high side of the line instead of offsetting the pins. Fine until the slab line is right on the segment line.

10. *Polish the lens.*

11. *Remove the block.*

12. *Re-mark the lens in the conventional manner.* Mark the lens a second time, this time in the conventional manner for surfacing the power on the back.

13. *Block and process the lens.* With plus- and low minus-powered lenses, care must be taken not to remove too much lens stock. If too much lens stock is removed, the bottom of the lens may be too thin after the cover lens has been removed.

14. *Remove the remaining portion of the cover lens.* Remove the cover lens from the lower portion of the front of the lens by heating the lens in an oven. Heat until the remaining portion of the cover lens can be pushed off using the eraser end of a pencil.

A summary of how to grind slab-off on a glass lens is given in Table 17-4.

Glass Semifinished Slab-off Lenses

It is possible to avoid the slab-off process entirely by factory-ordering a semifinished glass lens with the slab-off correction already ground on the front surface. These lenses are not "reverse slab," but

Table 17-4 Grinding Slab-off on a Glass Lens

1. Choose the most minus or least plus lens for the grind.
2. Zero-cut the back of the blank (optional).
3. Make a cover lens.
4. Clean both lenses.
5. Stamp the seg line, guide lines, and prism line.
6. Cement the cover lens in place.
7. Block the lens backwards.
8. Generate the front surface until the slab line is 5 mm from the seg line.
9. Fine the lens until the slab line is on the seg line.
10. Polish.
11. Deblock.
12. Re-mark the lens in conventional manner.
13. Block, generate, fine, polish, and deblock the lens.
14. Remove the remaining portion of the cover lens.

have base-down prism over the segment area, as is customary for glass lenses. At present, Vision-Ease offers this option in most colors and multifocal segment sizes and styles.

Using Franklin-Style Glass Lenses for Slab-off

A Franklin-style (Executive) lens can be used for slab-off with only a slight modification in how the slab-off is applied to the lens. When making a cover lens, the back surface of the cover lens must have the same curve as the front surface of the near add portion. The cover lens is then cut in half and cemented onto the lower half of the Franklin-style lens. The cover lens should not actually touch the edge of the bifocal line. All other steps in the manufacturing process are the same.

Slab-off Prism for Plastic Lenses

As more people began to wear plastic lenses, the demand for a plastic slab-off correction grew. Laboratories were quick to develop innovative processes, and two basic methods for grinding slab-off for plastic lenses developed. As with many manufacturing processes, there may be considerable variation, all resulting in a satisfactory end product.

For the plastic lens, the slab-off prism is ground on the *back* surface instead of the front. This is because plastic lenses have a one-piece front-surface design. Yet the slab-off correction itself is still ground on the most minus or least plus lens of the pair.

Blocking Methods for Slab-off Plastic Lenses

It is possible to use either on- or off-center blocking when making a slab-off lens in plastic. With *off-center blocking* the lens is blocked off the geometric center and at the location of the lens optical center. If off-center blocking is chosen, the only prism that must be contended with is the slab prism (and, on rare occasions, Rx prism). This method works satisfactorily if the lens is cribbed or if an overhang adapter is used in fining to prevent unwanted prism.

If *on-center blocking* is used, the process becomes a bit more complicated. This is because the prism that is used for decentration must be combined with the slab prism. This combination yields a resultant prism with a new amount and new prism axis direction. (For a review of on- and off-center blocking, see Chapter 3.)

Grinding Slab-off Prism on the Back Surface of a Plastic Lens

There are two ways to grind slab-off prism on a plastic lens. One method grinds the lower area of the lens, which will be used for near viewing, first. This causes the slab line to begin at the top of the lens during the second phase. This "from-the-top-down" movement of the slab line is like the way the line moves when grinding glass lenses. The other method grinds the upper, distance area of the lens first. This causes the slab line to begin at the bottom of the lens during the second grind.

"From-the-Top-Down" Method The most straightforward way of grinding slab-off for plastic lenses is to begin by first grinding what will be the near portion. The advantage is that since the slab prism is ground on first, the slab line will approach the seg line from the top of the lens during the second phase. The main disadvantage appears if the slab line begins to tilt as it is moving downward. If the line is tilted, it cannot be corrected during generating. A tilted slab line can be corrected only during the fining process. Because the prism is not applied in this first grind, there is no prism ring to tilt. The tilt of the ring controls the slab line angle, so the line cannot be reangled.

To grind slab-off prism "from the top down," these steps are followed:

1. *Choose a lens with a very straight seg line.* Upon careful inspection, it will be noticed that many lenses have a "smile" on their bifocal segment. Choose a lens whose segment top is as straight as possible.

2. *Calculate thickness and tool curves.* Lens thickness is calculated as if the lens had Rx prism. In other words, the lens should be as thick as it would be if it contained Rx prism equal to the amount of slab-off prism needed. Tool curves are calculated assuming this thickness as well.

3. *Mark the cylinder axis, the prism axis, and the seg top.* The lens should be marked for axis in the customary manner. Prism should be marked now and will be ground the first time the lens is generated. In addition, a horizontal line must be marked on the front surface across the seg top.

4. *Block the lens.*

5. *Generate the lens,* including *the slab prism.* The lens should be generated, with prism, to the calculated thickness. Remember that the prism being ground is base up. (If slab prism is combined with prism for decentration, prism will be at an oblique angle.)

6. *Fine and polish the lens.*

7. *Thoroughly clean the back surface of the lens.* Do not deblock the lens.

8. *Spray the back surface with clear precoat.*

9. *Prepare the lens and pour the resin.* Tape around the outside of the lens to form a boat for the liquid resin. See Figure 17-12. Mix the liquid resin and

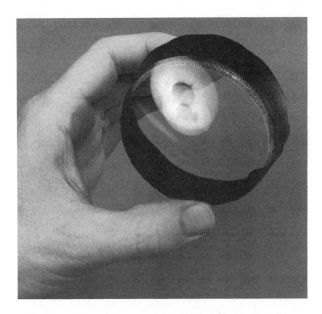

Figure 17-12 A ledge around the lens is created with tape. The epoxy is poured onto the lens surface. Do not completely fill the "boat" up to the rim. Use only enough to cover the surface.

pour it onto the back surface of the lens. Use only enough resin to cover the surface. Too much resin creates heat as it sets up. Some operators recommend propping up the lens "so that the bottom of the lens (where the apex of the prism will be) is higher, and so no extra resin settles in the bottom of the lens."[3]

A number of different types of epoxy resins are used in slab-off grinding and are available through optical supply houses. Some laboratories have chosen to use epoxy resins from other industries, which they have found to be suitable.

10. *Allow to dry for 24 to 48 hours.*

11. *Generate the lens without slab prism.* Remove only 4 or 5 points on each cut until the slab line becomes visible. As the slab line approaches the bifocal line, stop generating.

For small amounts of slab prism, stop generating at a point 4 or 5 mm from the bifocal line. For large amounts of slab prism the line can be brought up to as close as 1 to 2 mm from the bifocal line.

12. *First-fine the lens.* Fine the lens at 15 psi pressure or less, using slow speed. "A good starting point is to use a 600-grit pad."[4] Remember to use the *same lap tool* as was used for fining the lens the first time. Each time the lens is checked, also remove resin from the fining pad with a brush.[5]

If the slab line begins to tilt, either press on the upper half of the lens toward the side where the slab line is highest, or offset the block in that same direction.

For slab-off prism of 2 prism diopters or less, keep fining until the slab line is from 0.25 to 0.50 mm of the seg line. For slab-off prism above 2, some operators may prefer to bring the slab line down to within 0.15 mm of the seg line.

13. *Second-fine and bring the slab line up to the seg line.* Allow just enough for polishing.

14. *Polish the lens normally.*

15. *Remove the remaining resin.* First put the lens in the reclaim tank to soften the epoxy and to remove the block, then, using a knife or optical screwdriver, peel off the epoxy. Start at the nasal edge of the blank, since this area is most likely to be edged off later. Remove any remaining epoxy using a tissue and alcohol. Some operators recommend using a compressed-air hose to remove the remaining resin material.

"From-the-Bottom-Up" Method Slab-off prism can also be ground on a plastic lens beginning with the distance portion. In this case the slab line approaches the seg line from the lower portion of the lens. The advantage to this method is that if the slab line tilts, compensation can be made during generating by changing the prism axis direction. Most of the steps in processing a lens "from the bottom up" are the same as for the previous method. Therefore the following explanation will be a bit more abbreviated. The process is illustrated in Figure 17-13.

1. *Choose a lens with a very straight seg line.*

2. *Calculate thickness and tool curves.* Again, the lens thickness is calculated as if the lens had Rx prism equal in value to the slab prism.

3. *Mark the cylinder axis, the prism axis, the seg top line, and the horizontal guidelines.* The lens should be marked for axis and prism. A horizontal line must be marked on the front surface across the seg top. Since the slab line is to be brought up from the bottom, also mark several horizontal guidelines below and parallel to the seg top for monitoring the straightness of the slab line while the lens is being generated.

4. *Block the lens.*

5. *Generate the lens without slab prism.* Do not generate any prism; generate the lens to the calculated thickness.

6. *Fine and polish the lens.*

Figure 17-13 Bicentric grinding on a plastic lens must be carried out entirely on the rear surface, as the front surface contains the one-piece-construction bifocal segment area. (A) semifinished lens as shown in (A) is surfaced to the required prescription, (B), exclusive of the desired prism at near. A liquid resin material is poured into the concave rear surface and allowed to dry. This resin, shown in (C), serves the same purpose as the cover lens serves in the glass lens technique. The lens is then resurfaced at an angle (shown in D). Surfacing a lens at an angle serves to grind on prism. The surfacing tools used are the same as were used in (B) so that correct power is maintained. The near portion now contains the proper amount of prism base up and the correct power. Lastly, the lens is chilled to make the remaining resin to break away. The upper portion had not been changed since it was originally surfaced. The completed lens is shown in (E). It will be noted that with bicentrically ground plastic lenses, the slab line is on the rear surface instead of the front. (From C.W. Brooks and I.M. Borish, *System for Ophthalmic Dispensing.* Butterworth-Heinemann, Boston, 1979, p. 429.)

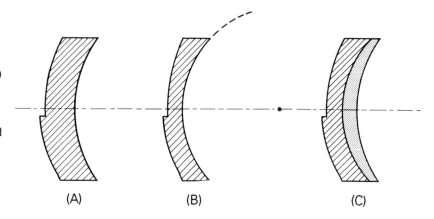

(A)   (B)   (C)

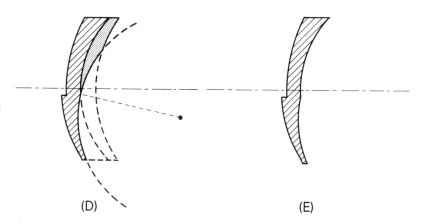

(D)   (E)

8. *Thoroughly clean the back surface of the lens.*

9. *Spray or tape the lens.* Either spray the back surface with clear precoat or tape the upper section of the back surface with 3M Surface Saver tape. If tape is used, the upper section should be taped to within 0.5 mm of the seg top.[6]

9. *Prepare the lens and pour the resin.* Tape around the outside of the lens to form a boat for the liquid resin. Mix liquid resin and pour onto the back surface of the lens until it is covered. Do not use more resin than needed.

10. *Allow to dry for 24 to 48 hours.*

11. *Generate the lens.* Generate the lens with slab prism, removing stock slowly. Once the slab line is halfway up to the bifocal, the maximum stock removal should be 0.2 mm at a time.[7]

Check for straightness of the slab line as it approaches the bifocal line from below. If the slab line is higher on one side than the other, turn the thinnest part of the prism ring toward the high side of the line.

For small amounts of slab prism, stop generating 4 to 5 mm from the bifocal line; for large amounts, 1 to 2 mm.

12. *First-fine the lens.* Fine the lens at 15 psi pressure or less, using slow speed. If the slab line begins to tilt, use the same correcting methods as were described for the "top-down" method. If the slab line begins to "lip up" on one or both sides, cut the side(s) of the pad off.

13. *Second-fine and bring the slab line up to the seg line.* Allow just enough for polishing.

14. *Polish.*

15. *Deblock and remove remaining resin.* Remove the remaining resin in the same manner as previously described.

A summary of how to grind slab-off prism on plastic lenses is given in Table 17-5.

Table 17-5 Grinding Slab-Off Prism on Plastic Lenses

From the Top Down	From the Bottom Up
1. Choose a lens with a very straight seg line.	
2. Calculate thickness and tool curves.	
3. Mark cylinder axis, prism axis, and seg top.	3. Mark cylinder axis, prism axis, seg top, and horizontal guidelines.
4. Block the lens.	
5. Generate the lens including slab prism.	5. Generate the lens without slab prism.
6. Fine and polish.	
7. Clean the lens surface.	
8. Spray the lens.	8. Spray or half-tape the lens.
9. Prepare the lens and pour the resin.	
10. Allow to dry.	
11. Generate the lens without slab prism.	11. Generate the lens with slab prism.
12. First-fine the lens.	
13. Second-fine and bring the slab line up to the seg line.	
14. Polish.	
15. Deblock and remove the remaining resin.	

Precast Slab-off Lenses

A high degree of skill is required to grind plastic slab-offs. The increased need for plastic slab-off lenses and the level of skill required offered an incentive for the development of a suitable precast slab-off that could be surfaced in the normal manner. The first precast CR-39 slab-off lens, developed by Aire-o-Lite in 1973,[8] was for a 25-mm round seg.

This was followed in 1983 by the Younger Optics Slab-Off Lens Series and more recently by Vision-Ease.

The precast slab-off lens is made using a flat-top 28 lens. The lens blank is large and has the segment in the center so that it may be used for either a right or a left lens. See Figure 17-14. Slab-off prism starts at 1.50 and goes up to 5.00 in half-prism-

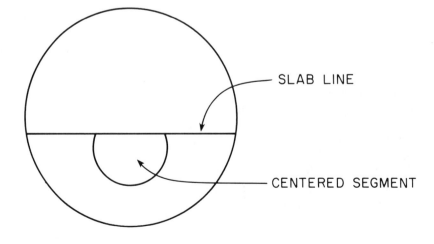

Figure 17-14 The Younger molded slab-off lens has the slab-off prism on the front. Prism is base down, instead of the customary base up. The segment is centered so that the blank will work for either a right or a left lens.

diopter increments. In contrast to conventionally ground slab-off lenses, the precast lenses are a *reverse slab*. This means that instead of having base-up prism in the are a below the slab line, the precast lenses have base-down prism. The slab-off prism is cast-molded on the front of the lens so that the semifinished blank can be surfaced on the rear surface in the normal manner. See Figure 17-15. The end result is a thinner lens.

With back-surface slab grinds, some wearers experience the sensation of seeing two lines. They see the seg line on the front and the slab line on the back. With precast lenses the slab line is on the front *with* the seg line. This eliminates the possibility of the wearer seeing two lines. Because reverse-slab lenses use base-down instead of base-up prism, not only is the prism direction reversed, but also the eye it is worn on. The reverse slab is placed on the most plus or least minus, instead of the most minus or least plus of the custom slab lens.

There appears to be no difficulty switching wearers from conventional slab-off to precast slab-off.[9] However, if a person has more than one pair of glasses, including sunglasses, then all the pairs of glasses should be switched; otherwise, the wearer may have trouble due to the difference in object displacement between the Rx's.

Processing of Precast Slab-off Lenses The entire portion of a precast slab-off lens, from the seg line downward, protrudes farther forward than the distance portion of the lens. This means that unless appropriate procedures are implemented, the lens will be tilted during either the blocking or the generating process. Tilting causes unexpected prismatic effects. Because of this, precast slab lenses should be treated the same way as plastic, front-surface, Ultex-style lenses would be. Here are some ideas provided by the manufacturer on how to obtain the best results.[10]

Sag the lens only on the upper distance portion of its surface. (Normally the true base curve will equal the nominal base curve within ±0.03 D.) Take blank thickness measurements within the distance-portion area as well.

The precast slab-off lens can be ground off center with no prism for decentration, even though it is a plastic lens. It can be ground off center because the segment is centered in the semifinished blank. This means it need only be offset by an amount equal to the seg inset. This is usually only 1.5 or 2 mm.

Use a small, 43-mm Coburn glass lens block and block on the distance optical center. Remember that glass blocks must be used in conjunction with a fiber generating ring. If the normal generating ring is

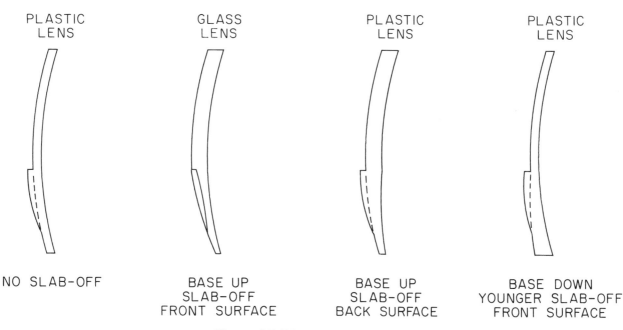

PLASTIC LENS   GLASS LENS   PLASTIC LENS   PLASTIC LENS

NO SLAB-OFF   BASE UP SLAB-OFF FRONT SURFACE   BASE UP SLAB-OFF BACK SURFACE   BASE DOWN YOUNGER SLAB-OFF FRONT SURFACE

Figure 17-15 Slab-off lenses of plano distance power are compared to one another and to a non-slab-off plastic lens. These cross-sectional drawings show the location of the slab-off grind and how that grind affects lens thickness.

used, unwanted prism results. Instead use one of the following:

1. an Ultex ring that has been scooped out so that it does not come in contact with the lower portion of the lens
2. an Executive ring that has been modified as described for the ultex
3. a standard glass fiber ring that has been cut in half

If half a glass fiber ring is used, the ring is placed between the generator chuck and the distance portion of the lens. The ring should not come in contact with any part of the lens that is below the slab line. If the lower lens area touches the ring, the lens will be angled and unwanted prism will be ground on the lens. Because these rings offer so little support to the lens, lens stock should be removed slowly and in small amounts while generating.

The Semi-tech system has a blocking ring that can be modified as well. Laboratories that use the Semi-tech system should also cut a portion of the ring away in the lower area. The Semi-tech Ultex-style ring is used as a guide to determine how the standard ring should be modified so as not to touch the lower half of the lens.

Laboratories that use the Shuron system may use the Executive ring without modification. The lower part of the ring is rubber and will compress enough so that the upper part of the lens will still press evenly against the ring without tilting.

Remember, the precast reverse slab lens places the slab-off correction on the most plus or least minus lens, just the opposite from conventional slab-off corrections.

Using Dissimilar Segs to Correct for Vertical Imbalance

If vertical imbalance is corrected using one style of segment on one eye and a second style of segment on the other, the vertical imbalance is said to be corrected with *dissimilar segs*. Dissimilar segs work this way.

Bifocal segments are like small plus lenses attached to the main lens. These small lenses have the same optics as do normal lenses. The segment lens has an optical center and will create a prismatic effect if objects are viewed through them anywhere than through that optical center. As with normal bifocals of any type, the right and left segments are identical. Even when the wearer looks through the segment area above or below the seg optical center, vertical prismatic effects caused by the segs are the same for both eyes. That is, if a wearer looks through a +2.00 D add at a point 3 mm below the seg OC, the prismatic effect will be 0.6 Base Up for the right eye and 0.6 Base Up for the left eye. The prismatic difference between the two, which is the critical thing, is zero.

Different style bifocals have their segment OCs located at different distances from the segment line, depending on the shape of the segment. For example, a flat-top seg is like a round seg with the top cut off. But this means that the seg OC of the flat-top lens will be a lot closer to the seg line than in a round-seg lens. If two *different* segment styles were used for the same pair of glasses, the segment optical centers would be at different heights. There would be a definite difference between the amount of vertical prism induced by the two segs when the wearer tried to read.

This phenomenon can be used to advantage in counteracting a vertical imbalance created by the distance lenses. Table 17-6 gives the procedure used to choose a correct combination of segment styles to counteract vertical imbalance.*

The chief disadvantage of using dissimilar segments in the correction of vertical imbalance is a cosmetic one. In most cases the two styles are obviously different, producing an unusual looking pair of glasses. If the segments are noticeably different in size, they will create a situation where, at certain angles of gaze, the wearer will be looking through the distance portion of one lens with one eye, and the near portion of the second with the other.

An excellent combination of segments for correction of small amounts of vertical imbalance is obtained using two differently styled flat-top 35s. Some flat-top 35s are made with the seg OC 5 mm below the line. Others are made with the seg OC right on the line. If a flat-top 35 made with its seg OC 5 mm below the seg line is used for one eye, and a flat-top 35 made with its seg OC right on the seg line is used for the other, the segs look very much alike but create a differential vertical prismatic effect. See Figure 17-16. This difference of 5 mm multiplied

---

*For more information on dissimilar segments and how to choose them, see C. W. Brooks and I. M. Borish, *System for Ophthalmic Dispensing*, Butterworth-Heinemann, Boston, 1979, chap. 19.

Table 17-6 Finding Correct Dissimilar Segs

1. Calculate vertical imbalance at the reading depth.
2. Calculate the required distance between seg centers needed to counteract reading-depth imbalance.

$$\Delta = cD_s \quad \text{or} \quad c = \Delta/D_s$$

c = distance between seg centers in centimeters

D_s = add power (*not* near Rx)

Δ = necessary prism

3. Note which lens requires the *higher* seg optical center. (This will be the lens with the most minus or least plus power in the vertical meridian.)
4. Choose two seg styles so that, with seg tops at equal heights, the seg optical centers will be separated by the required amount (i.e., c in step 2).

(From C. W. Brooks and I. M. Borish, *System for Ophthalmic Dispensing*, Butterworth-Heinemann, Boston, 1979, p. 432.

by the power of the add gives the amount of vertical imbalance this combination will correct.

For example, if the add is +2.50, the amount of imbalance this combination will correct is

$$\text{Prism imbalance corrected} = (0.5)(2.50)$$
$$= 1.25 \text{ prism diopters of imbalance}$$

In advising the dispenser on the matter of vertical imbalance correction, this option should be mentioned. It should even be mentioned if the amount of imbalance that it will correct is less than the amount specified on the order. The prescriber may choose to go with a lesser amount of slab-off correction when such a good cosmetic choice is available so inexpensively.

R-Compensated Segments

Another option available for correcting small amounts of vertical imbalance is the R-compensated segment. The R-compensated segment is made by modifying a normal ribbon-style segment. Ribbon segs, like flat-tops, are fused into the blank. The front of this fused-glass blank is resurfaced to a different base curve. This causes the shape of the segment to change. The shape change also changes the location of the segment optical center. (This was seen in Figure 17-8.)

In looking at the changing shapes of the R-compensated segment styles, it does not take long to realize that compensated segs are really just a variation on the dissimilar-seg concept. But because the different shapes of the R-compensated segs are so much alike, the disadvantages of dissimilar segs are overcome.

To move the segment optical center upward, a semifinished blank with a flatter base curve than called for is chosen. The *front* of the lens is then resurfaced with a steeper tool. This removes part of the segment. Because of the tool shape, more of the segment thickness at the lower part of the seg is removed, forcing the seg OC upward. This creates base-up prism in the segment.

To move the segment optical center downward and produce a base-down prismatic effect, a blank with a steeper base curve than called for is chosen. The front of the lens is flattened, removing more of the upper part of the segment and forcing the seg OC down. See Figure 17-17.

Because compensated segs are used so rarely, most laboratories prefer to either order the blanks after the seg OCs have already been moved, or have

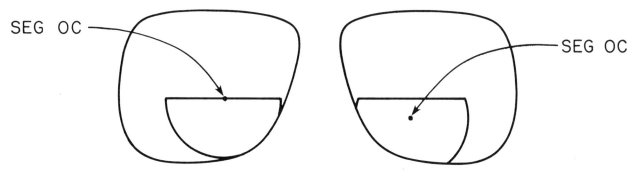

Figure 17-16 Two different styles of flat-top 35 lenses work well together for correcting small amounts of vertical imbalance. The lower the seg height, the less obvious the differences will be.

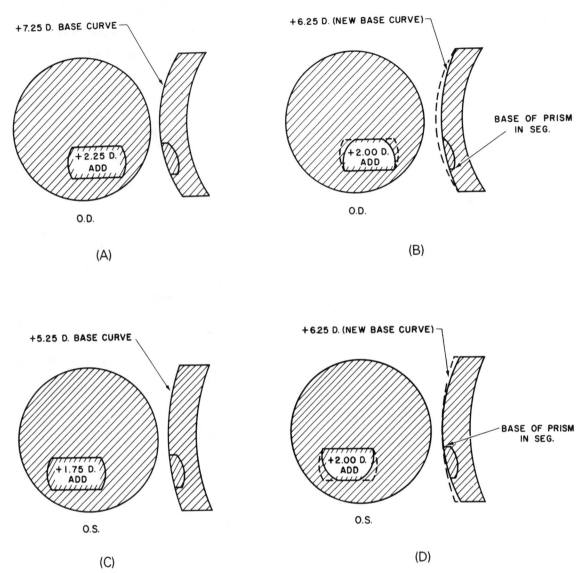

Figure 17-17 Grinding R-compensated segs. (A) To achieve a lens pair with +2.00 D adds and +6.25 D base curves, when base-down prism in the right eye is required, a steeper blank with a slightly higher add is chosen. (B) The finished front surface of this blank is then resurfaced to the desired base curve, thinning the upper edge of the fused-in seg more than the lower edge and creating base-down prism in the seg. Grinding in prism changes the location of the optical center. In this case the seg OC is lowered. The upper seg width narrows since the seg portion, being knife-edge thin, is partially ground away. (C) For the left lens a flatter base curve blank, having a slightly lower add, is chosen. (D) The +6.25 D base curve is surfaced on the finished lens surface, removing more glass peripherally than centrally. This thins the lower seg portion more, creating base-up prism, and raising the seg OC. It may be seen from the illustrations that R-compensated segs are really just a skillful version of the dissimilar principle. (From C.W. Brooks and I.M. Borish, *System for Ophthalmic Dispensing,* Butterworth-Heinemann, Boston, 1979, p. 434.)

the surfacing done by a specialty laboratory or supplier.

Questions and Problems

1. Where is the reading depth for the following Rx?

> R: −3.00 sph
> L: −4.50 −1.50 × 180
> A = 59 mm
> B = 48 mm
> DBL = 16 mm
> Seg height = 20 mm

2. In order to calculate the imbalance between two lenses, the difference in power between the right and left lenses in the 90-degree meridian must be found. Find the power in the 90-degree meridian for each of the following lenses. If the lens has an oblique cylinder, use $\cos^2 \theta$ or the appropriate table to aid in finding the answer.
   a. +5.00 −1.00 × 180
   b. +3.00 −1.00 × 90
   c. −5.00 −1.50 × 180
   d. −5.00 +1.50 × 180
   e. −2.75 D sph
   f. −1.00 −1.00 × 30
   g. +1.75 −0.50 × 10
   h. −7.00 −1.25 × 75
   i. −4.00 +0.50 × 45
   j. −4.00 +0.50 × 135
   k. +2.25 −2.25 × 165
   l. −1.00 +1.00 × 110

3. If the reading depth is 8 mm below the distance optical center for each of the lenses in Problem 2, how much prismatic effect does that lens exert at the reading depth? What is the base direction of the prismatic effect?

4. What is the vertical imbalance to the nearest quarter-diopter for the following Rx, assuming that the reading depth will be 5 mm down into the bifocal?

> R: −0.50 −0.50 × 180
> L: −5.75 −0.75 × 180
> Add = +2.00
> Seg height = 20 mm
> A = 55 mm
> B = 48 mm
> DBL = 18 mm
> PD = 64 mm

   a. 6.25 prism diopters
   b. 5.50 prism diopters
   c. 5.25 prism diopters
   d. 5.00 prism diopters
   e. none of the above

5. If the correction in Problem 4 were to be made using a Younger reverse slab lens, on which eye would the slab-off lens be placed?
   a. right eye
   b. left eye

6. What is the vertical imbalance for the following Rx, assuming that the reading depth will be 4 mm down into the bifocal.

> R: +3.50 −1.50 × 30
> L: −0.75 −2.00 × 150
> Add = +2.00
> Seg height = 21 mm
> A = 55 mm
> B = 48 mm
> DBL = 19 mm
> PD = 64 mm

   a. 0.12
   b. 3.25
   c. 4.25
   d. 4.62
   e. none of the above

7. Here is a prescription for an individual who will be wearing a slab-off correction.

> +0.50 −0.75 × 165
> −3.25 −0.50 × 35
> Add = +2.00

On which eye would the slab-off prism be put for each of the following lenses?
   a. Fused-glass flat-top 28 bifocal
      (1) right
      (2) left
      (3) cannot be made
   b. CR-39 plastic Executive bifocal
      (1) right
      (2) left
      (3) cannot be made
   c. Younger precast slab-off flat-top 28 bifocal
      (1) right
      (2) left
      (3) cannot be made

8. A prescription is as follows:

> +1.50 −2.00 × 180
> +3.50 −1.00 × 180
> Add = +2.25
> Frame A = 54 mm
> B = 48 mm
> DBL = 17 mm
> Seg height = 20 mm

   a. If you were to correct for the full amount of vertical imbalance, how much prism would you use? (Assume the reading level to be 5 mm below the seg line.)

b. What kind of vertical imbalance correction would you use?

c. On which eye would you put the correction?

9. If the prescription in the above problem were

$$+1.50 -2.00 \times 30$$
$$+3.50 -1.00 \times 70$$
$$Add = +2.25$$

how much vertical imbalance would there be at the reading depth?

10. You have an order with a vertical imbalance of 1.50 prism diopters. The account wishes to correct the imbalance using dissimilar segs. The right lens is plus and the left lens is minus. If the add power is +2.50, what combination of segs would you propose using? Which seg style would you use on which eye?

11. An order for the following prescription goes through the laboratory. On which eye should slab-off prism be found? Assume that the lens is a flat-top plastic bifocal and that the slab-off line can be felt on the front of the lens.

$$-2.00 -1.00 \times 35$$
$$-5.75 -1.25 \times 167$$
$$+2.75 \text{ add}$$

12. How much vertical imbalance is present for the following prescription at a point 5 mm below the near segment line? (Careful!)

$$+1.75 -1.00 \times 180$$
$$+4.25 -0.50 \times 180$$
$$Add +2.00$$
Segment height = 20 mm
Wearer's PD = 64/60
Frame A = 50 mm, B = 46 mm, DBL = 18 mm

13. How much vertical imbalance is there for each of the following prescriptions and, using the Younger reverse-slab lens, on which eye would you expect the slab-off grind to be made?

R: -2.00 sph
L: $+5.50$ sph
Reading depth is at the seg OC of a flat-top 28 and the lens has a seg drop of 4 mm.

14. A prescription is found to have a vertical imbalance of 1.50 prism diopters Base Up on the right eye. (Or Base Down on the left eye, however you want to look at it.) If the power of the add is +2.00 D, what two lens segment styles could you use to correct the problem using dissimilar segs? Which seg would go on which eye?

15. Find the vertical imbalance for the following Rx,

assuming that the reading depth is 5 mm below the seg line.

R: $-7.50 -1.00 \times 35$
L: $-0.75 -0.50 \times 85$
MRP height = 27 mm
Seg height = 21 mm
Seg style is a flat-top 35

16. Find the vertical imbalance for the following Rx, assuming that the reading depth is 5 mm below the seg line.

R: $+3.00$ D sph
L: $-0.25 -0.50 \times 180$
right MRP height = 29 mm
left MRP height = 27 mm
Right seg height = 25 mm
Left seg height = 23 mm
Seg style is a flat-top 28

17. Find the vertical imbalance for the following Rx, assuming that the reading depth is 5 mm below the seg line.

R: $-5.25 -0.75 \times 155$
L: $-0.50 -0.50 \times 45$
Frame B = 48 mm
Right seg height = 18 mm
Left seg height = 20 mm

References

1. *Aniso Rx, The Correction of Vertical Imbalance.* Univis, Inc. (now Vision-Ease, St. Cloud, Minn.), 1964, p. 4.

2. Cline, D., Hofstetter, H. W., and Griffin, J. R. *Dictionary of Visual Science,* Chilton Trade Book Publishing, Radnor, Pa., 1989, p. 395.

3. Check, W. Slab-off Grinding. *Optical Index,* 56 (3): 54 (March 1981).

4. *Instructions for "Perfect Slab."* D-Cote, Inc. Distributed by Econ-O-Cloth, Lansing, Ill., n.d., p. 2.

5. Mancusi, R. J. *Ophthalmic Surfacing for Plastic and Glass Lenses.* Butterworth-Heinemann, Boston, 1982, p. 78.

6. Tracy Dunn, Tulsa, Okla., personal communication.

7. Check, W., Slab-off Grinding. *Optical Index,* 56 (3): 56 (March 1981).

8. Drew, R. CR-39 Slab-Off Lenses: Now Ready Cast. *Optical Management,* January 1984, p. 23.

9. Rosen, K. Premolded Slab-offs Bring Results. *Optical Management,* September 1984, p. 32.

10. *Younger Optics Slab-Off Lens Series.* Younger Optics, Los Angeles, undated insert.

18 Alternatives to Lens Surfacing

Introduction

There are a few alternatives to the full surfacing laboratory. These alternatives are viable options in certain situations and should not be dismissed lightly. At this time, however, such options are not a replacement for the traditional surfacing laboratory. Nor are they presented as such. They are meant to fill a certain need for those whose circumstances are especially suited for them.

In-House Lens Casting

Plastic lenses are made using a process that involves pouring liquid resin material into a mold. The mold consists of a front and a back surface made from glass or metal. The front and back of the molds are fastened together with a pliable plastic gasket. See Figure 18-1. This process is basically the same for both semifinished blanks and finished single-vision uncuts. It is therefore logical to conclude that if such a system is successful for mass production, perhaps it is adaptable for individual prescription lenses made up on an in-house basis.

Some commercially available in-house lens-casting systems approach the "surfacing" of lenses in just this manner. These systems are intended primarily for the moderate-volume retailer who already operates a finishing laboratory but may not have the resources, personnel, desire, or volume to be able to undertake a full surfacing operation. The individual or establishment considering in-house casting is generally looking for a faster, more cost-effective way of producing a finished lens.

The Process

Two liquid components are necessary for the molding of plastic lenses.[1] The first is the CR-39 mon-omer. CR-39 is the trade name for PPGs allyldiglycol carbonate (ADC). In order to make ADC harden, a catalyst must be added to it. That catalyst is called isopropyl percarbonate (IPP). Unfortunately, IPP is extremely volatile. It would not be safe for semi-skilled individuals to work with such a substance near high-traffic areas. Nor would it be easy to ship or store the material. In order to overcome the problem, in-house casting systems premix IPP with ADC. Once mixed, the material will harden, even at room temperature. To keep the premixed liquid from hardening, it must be frozen. Premixed packets or cartridges of resin are packed in dry ice and sent to the user. The user stores the packets in a freezer until they are needed.

The correct combination of front and back mold surfaces and lens thickness is found with the help of an on-board computer system. The molds are assembled and the surfaces set in the gasket so that the lens will have the correct thickness. The toric

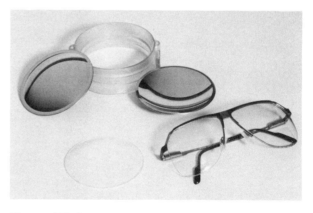

Figure 18-1 The gaskets used for the in-house casting of plastic lenses are basically the same as those used for mass production of plastic lenses. The photo shows a gasket, along with the front and back molds that produce the finished lens. (Photo courtesy of TechnaVision Santee, California.)

mold surface is turned to the prescribed cylinder axis. With such systems, the optical center for multifocal lenses will have a standard segment inset and a standard segment drop. When all is ready, the liquid CR-39 is poured into the mold. Once the resin has been placed in the mold, it is run through a controlled cycle of gradual heating and cooling. This process causes the lens material to harden and cure.

In large manufacturing facilities, lenses of different thicknesses and powers are ordinarily cured at different rates. This is not practical for an in-house system. To further complicate matters, lenses of some powers tend to shrink more than others. When all powers and shapes of lenses are cured in the same batch, in-house systems are challenged to develop processes and additives that will overcome such problems.

Because lens molding is an exacting process, the in-house lens-casting systems use computers to control the process. Nothing is required of the operator once the filled molds have been placed in the unit. See Figure 18-2.

In a factory situation, lens curing takes approximately 17 to 18 hours. An in-house system may take anywhere from 6 to 16 hours for a complete cycle, depending on the kind of system being used.

Advantages

1. In-house systems are small enough for modest-volume retailers. The standard unit will hold 15 pairs in a batch.

2. The systems are adaptable for larger businesses. They allow for additional cure units and can process 200 pairs per day.

3. The number of lenses that must be processed for immediate orders may not fill up the unit. The unit can either be run with fewer than the maximum number of lenses, or it can be filled up with single-vision or spherical bifocal lenses to build current inventory.

4. Several mold styles are available, such as flat-top, round, blended, and progressive-addition, depending on manufacturer.

5. In-house systems are claimed to allow production of up to 90% of all plastic prescription orders.

6. As would be expected, lenses may be tinted. Tinting times are predictable because material content and cure does not vary.

7. The amount of floor space required is small, especially compared to that which is required for the normal surfacing laboratory.

Disadvantages

1. In-house molded lenses do not have to be individually tested for impact resistance after edging. Neither do regular plastic lenses. However, an in-house system is really the "factory." Factory lenses that have been batch-molded have to be batch-tested for impact resistance, according to U.S. Food and Drug Administration regulations.

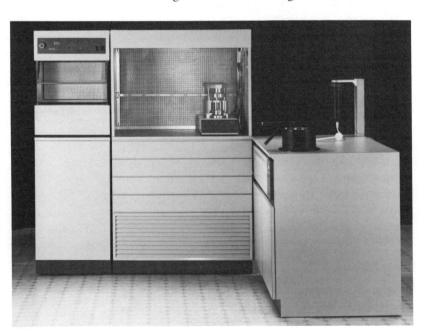

Figure 18-2 One of the advantages of in-house casting is that it does not take a great deal of floor space. (Photo courtesy of Techna-Vision, Santee, California.)

2. Additional bifocal-style molds must be purchased if more bifocal types are to be offered. Availability depends on manufacturer.
3. In-house systems are unable to fulfill all surfacing needs, even in plastic. Lenses have a standard seg inset and seg drop.
4. Even though casting systems have a low cost per lens on the basis of liquid resin alone, the initial cost of the system must be considered. Volume, especially multifocal volume, must justify initial purchase costs.

Laminated Lenses

Another alternative to lens surfacing is *lens lamination*.* There have been, and will continue to be, attempts to produce lenses in front and back halves. Front and back halves can then be glued together to produce the correct lens power. The reason for using this sandwich-type system is to allow for the production of finished bifocal lenses from a relatively small stock of "lens parts."

Construction of Laminated Lenses

The front part of the laminated lens contains the bifocal. The front part is usually plano, but it sometimes includes some sphere power. The back part of the lens provides all or almost all of the sphere power and the cylinder. See Figure 18-3.

When an order arrives, the bifocal style and add power are selected. Then the very thin front half corresponding to this style and add power is pulled from stock. Next the back, spherocylinder portion is selected. The back half is very much like a regular uncut lens. As expected, the back of the bifocal portion must have the same curve as the front of the spherocylinder portion.

The front section of the lens is positioned face down with the segment line horizontal, and glue is applied to the back surface. The spherocylinder portion, marked according to axis, is placed on the front half of the correct axis orientation. The two are pressed together until there is only a thin, even layer of glue between them. If the glue is a type that is activated with ultraviolet light, it can be dried rapidly.

---

*There are many different uses for lamination, or "layering," of lenses. Such uses include tints, safety lenses, combining glass with plastic, etc. Here we are discussing only one aspect of lamination.

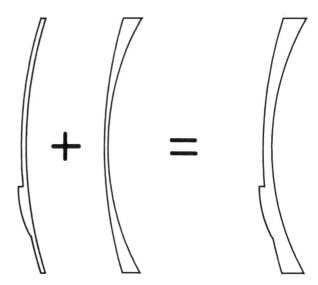

Figure 18-3 Laminated lenses can be used in place of surfaced plastic lenses for some bifocal styles and powers. The front half of the lens shown on the left contains the bifocal. The right half contains the sphere and cylinder powers. The two halves are bonded together to make a "surfaced" lens.

Laminated lenses offer a promising alternative to individual lens surfacing. Most of the hurdles in development have already been overcome. Perhaps the biggest hurdle yet to be conquered is not a technical one. The biggest hurdle is skepticism on the part of the retailer—skepticism that a lens can be glued together from two halves and still be as optically sound and physically strong as a conventional one.

Questions and Problems

1. Which of the following lens styles can be produced as uncuts using an in-house lens-casting system?
   a. single-vision
   b. flat-top 28s
   c. round segs
   d. blended bifocals
   e. progressive-adds
2. In-house lens-casting systems are especially attractive to retailers because they eliminate the need for a lens-edging facility.
   True or False
3. CR-39 liquid resin material is shipped to in-house lens casters in a frozen state because:
   a. Both the CR-39 liquid and the catalyst that makes it harden are extremely volatile in liquid form. They are frozen separately when shipped and mixed on-site in a special mixing vat.

b. Once mixed, the CR-39 material is volatile and must be shipped frozen.

c. The hardening catalyst is volatile until mixed, but causes the material to harden at room temperature after mixing.

4. In-house lens-casting system manufacturers maintain that it is possible to produce up to _____% of all plastic prescription orders in-house.
   a. 98
   b. 90
   c. 70
   d. 50
   e. 35

5. The laminated lens concept produces a bifocal lens by taking a stock single-vision uncut lens and cementing a small bifocal add to the uncut, using ultraviolet light to harden the adhesive.
True or False

Reference

1. Drew, R. In-Office Lens Casting Can Offer a Marketing Edge. *Optometric Management*, 23 (11): 45 (November 1987).

19

Eyewear Safety Standards

Introduction

No area of the eyecare industry is unaffected by regulations of some type. The regulatory aspect that is of special concern to the surfacing laboratory is lens thickness. In the following sections, several aspects of regulations and recommendations are reviewed in order to give an overview. The material in this chapter is not meant to be inclusive, and should not be relied on instead of regulatory documents.

Summary of FDA Regulations for Impact-Resistant Lenses

In 1970 the U.S. Food and Drug Administration (FDA) published a proposal for a regulation requiring that spectacle lenses be made impact-resistant. The regulation became effective in 1971 and has been modified slightly since that time. The main points of the regulation are outlined in the following paragraphs.

Lenses Affected

Eyeglass and sunglass lenses must be impact-resistant, except when the physician or optometrist finds that they will not fulfill the visual requirements of the patient if made impact-resistant. If the practitioner decides that lenses should not be made impact-resistant, then this must be recorded in writing and the patient notified in writing as well.

It should be noted that an agreement by the wearer to assume all responsibility for non-impact-resistant glasses does not allow the practitioner the freedom to dispense lenses that are not in compliance. In rare circumstances and in an extreme emergency the wearer may be dispensed non-impact-

resistant lenses. If this is done, it must be on a temporary basis and with the knowledge and consent of all involved.

With only a very few exceptions, all *glass* lenses must be tested individually for impact resistance after they are edged and before they are put in the frame. The only exceptions are the following

1. raised multifocals lenses (These are generally regarded to be lenses with raised bi- or trifocal segments, or lenses with some kind of a ledge area on the lens.)
2. prism segment multifocals
3. slab-off lenses
4. lenticular cataract lenses
5. iseikonic* lenses
6. depressed-segment one-piece multifocals
7. biconcave, myodisc, and minus lenticular lenses
8. custom laminate lenses
9. cement assembly lenses

None of the above lenses has to be tested individually. Nor do any of them have to be batch-tested. *Batch testing* means testing a statistically significant number of lenses in a manufactured group. Lenses that do have to be batch tested include the following.

1. Plastic lenses. These lenses are tested by the lens blank manufacturer.
2. Nonprescription lenses, such as mass-produced nonprescription sunglass lenses. It should be noted, though, that individually produced glass, plano sunglass lenses must

---

*Iseikonic lenses are lenses which equalize magnification differences between the right and left eyes. They do this by using special thicknesses, base curves, and bitoric designs. (*Bitorics* have two curves on the front and two curves on the back of the lens.) Iseikonic lenses are also known as *size lenses*.

be hardened and tested in the same manner as any other glass prescription lenses.

Determination of Impact Resistance

The test used to determine impact resistance consists of dropping a 5/8ths-inch steel ball on the lens from a height of 50 inches. Tests for Occupational and Educational (Safety) lenses use a 1-inch steel ball. The FDA does not limit the manufacturer 'o this test only. If other methods will test the lens with equal accuracy, they may be used.

Record Keeping

People who sell any kind of eyewear must keep certain records for 3 years. These records include

1. copies of invoices
2. shipping documents
3. records of sale or distribution (meaning the names and addresses of those who bought the glasses)

People who sell nonprescription eyeglasses and sunglasses to the public do not have to keep a record of the names and addresses of those who bought them.

Those persons who conduct the impact-resistance tests must maintain a record of the results of those tests. Again, the records must be kept for 3 years.

Physical Characteristics of Lenses

The FDA does not stipulate how lenses must be made impact-resistant. This is to allow for future developments and improvements in methodology.

It should also be noted that there is no minimum thickness for regular "dress-wear" lenses. Some lens materials or hardening methods will allow for lenses that are thinner than others. Manufacturers of plastic semifinished lens blanks assume a certain thickness when conducting their batch testing. Those choosing to grind thinner than the semi-finished blank manufacturer warrants should be aware that they become responsible for batch testing the product at this new reduced thickness.

An additional point worthy of note is that any glass lens that has been re-edged or hand-edged after being made impact-resistant will lose a measure of its impact resistance. Such lenses should be rehardened and retested to assure safety.

Summary of OSHA Requirements for Eye Protection[1]

The federal agency that regulates safety in industrial and educational settings is the Occupational Safety and Health Administration (OSHA). OSHA's requirements for when eye protection must be worn are purposely vague. It is simply not possible to list every situation in every setting that would require a certain type of protection. Instead, the requirement states: "Protective eye and face equipment shall be required where there is a reasonable probability of injury that can be prevented by such equipment."

In such instances the employer is required to have protectors "conveniently available" and "employees shall use such protectors."

Minimum Requirements for Protectors

Requirements of the protective devices are outlined generally. They are as follows:

1. They shall provide adequate protection against the particular hazards for which they are designed.
2. They shall be reasonably comfortable when worn under the designated conditions.
3. They shall fit snugly and shall not unduly interfere with the movements of the wearer.
4. They shall be durable.
5. They shall be capable of being disinfected.
6. They shall be easily cleanable.
7. Protectors should be kept clean and in good repair.

However general these requirements appear, the last paragraph in the section states that "design, construction, testing, and use of devices for eye and face protection shall be in accordance with American National Standard Practice for Occupational and Educational Eye and Face Protection. . . ." This effectively makes the ANSI Z87.1 standards a specific requirement for OSHA.

Summary of ANSI Z87.1 Standards

What follows is a summary of some of the ANSI Z87.1 standards which are related directly or indirectly to the surfacing laboratory. The document is entitled "Z87.1-1989, American National Standard Practice for Occupational and Educational Eye and Face Protection," and is available from the American National Standards Institute, Inc., 1430 Broadway, New York, NY 10018. This document should be referred to by those producing safety eyewear.

In contrast to earlier versions, the Z87.1-1989 standard is intended to be performance oriented. This means that there are less specific rules about how the protective eyewear should be designed or what the device should look like. Instead more information is provided by ANSI on how the eyewear or protective device should function.

Z87.1 Frame and Lens Requirements

Frames which are to be used for safety purposes must be capable of withstanding specific stress tests and must be clearly marked. These required markings are summarized in Table 19-1. A frame without the required markings is not considered to be a safety frame, no matter how strong it is.

According to Z87 standards, corrective (prescription) lenses have a minimum thickness of 3.0 mm. Most laboratories grind safety lenses 3.2 mm thick so that they are sure not to accidentally produce a lens which would cause a potential legal liability

Table 19-1 ANSI Z87.1-1989 Safety Frame Marking Requirements

Fronts

1. A-dimension (eye size)
2. DBL (Distance Between Lenses)
3. "Z87" to indicate compliance with Z87 standards
4. Manufacturer's identifying trademark

Temples

1. Overall length
2. "Z87" to indicate compliance with Z87 standards
3. Manufacturer's identifying trademark

Source: American National Standard Practice for Occupational and Educational Eye and Face Protection (ANSI Z87.1-1989).

should it break and allow injury. High-plus lenses above +3.00 D can be made as thin as 2.5 mm on the thinnest edge. This is because a high-plus lens is so thick in the center that it will end up being just as strong as a lower-powered lens anyway. Plano (nonprescription) safety lenses can be as thin as 2.0 mm if they are capable of withstanding a more stringent impact resistance test. Impact resistancy testing requirements are summarized in Table 19-2. Lens thickness requirements for safety eyewear are summarized in Table 19-3.

Table 19-2 ANSI Z87.1-1989 Lens Impact Resistance Requirements for Prescription and Plano Safety Glasses

Test	*Requirement*
Drop Ball Impact Test All types of lenses	Withstand impact of 1-in. (25.4-mm) diameter steel ball dropped from 50 in. (127 mm). Lenses which might sustain surface damage may be batch tested.

High Velocity Impact Test
  For plano lenses which are
  to be made less than 3.0
  mm thick. (These lenses
  must still be >2 mm thick.)
	Capable of withstanding impact of 6.35 mm (¼-in.) diameter steel ball weighing 1.06 gm (0.04 oz) and travelling at a velocity of 45.7 mps (150 fps). Impact angles are 15° nasal, straight ahead center, 15, 30, 45, 60, 75, and 90° temporal, and straight ahead 10 mm above and below center.

Penetration Test
  (Plastic nonprescription
  lenses only)
	Capable of resisting a penetration from a pointed projectile weighing 44.2 gm (1.56 oz) dropped from a height of 127 cm (50 in.).

Source: American National Standard Practice for Occupational and Educational Eye and Face Protection (ANSI Z87.1-1989.)

Table 19-3 ANSI Z87.1-1989 Lens Thickness Requirements

Lens Type	Requirement
Corrective (prescription) lenses used in safety frame	Not less than 3.0 mm thick except lenses of power $> +3.00$ D in the most plus meridian. Lenses $> +3.00$ shall have a minimum thickness no less than 2.5 mm.
Plano safety spectacle lenses	Not less than 3.0 mm thick unless capable of withstanding High Velocity Impact Test. Lenses withstanding High Velocity Impact Test must be not less than 2.0 mm. All spectacle lenses must withstand Drop Ball Impact Test.
Goggle lenses	Not less than 3.0 mm thick. Plastic: Not less than 1.27 mm thick
Cover plates	No thickness requirements
Safety plates Welding helmets, hand shields	Removable welding helmet lenses: Not less than 2.0 mm thick. Nonremovable lenses: Not less than 2.0 mm thick except plastic, which shall not be less than 1.0 mm thick

Source: American National Standard Practice for Occupational and Educational Eye and Face Protection (ANSI Z87.1-1989).

Table 19-4 ANSI Z87.1-1989 Marking Requirements for Lenses

Lens Type	Requirement
Clear lenses	Manufacturer's monogram Example: K
Tinted (absorptive) lenses except for special purpose lenses	Manufacturer's monogram; shade number Example: K-2.5
Photochromic lenses	Manufacturer's monogram; "V" for variable shade Example: K-V
Special purpose lenses* Special purpose lenses provide eye protection while performing visual tasks which require unusual filtering of light. Examples: Didymium-containing Cobalt-containing Uniformly tinted lenses Photochromic lenses (see above) Lenses prescribed by an eye specialist for particular vision problems	Manufacturer's monogram; "S" for special purpose Example: K-S

All markings must be legible and permanent and placed so that interference with the vision of the wearer is minimal.

*"Many such (special purpose) lenses offer inadequate ultraviolet and/or infrared protection; caution shall be exercised in their use. For each application, the responsible individual shall ensure that the proper ultraviolet, infrared, and visible protection is provided. Spectral transmittance data shall be available to buyers upon request." (ANSI Z87.1-1989 American National Standard Practice for Occupational and Educational Eye and Face Protection, American National Standards Institute, Inc., 1430 Broadway, New York, NY 10018, 1989, p. 14.)

Table 19-5 ANSI Z87.1-1989 Nonprecsription Optical Quality Requirements (Plano Safety Spectacles and Goggles)

Lens Type	Requirement
Prismatic power	The prismatic power shall not exceed ½ prism diopter in any direction. Vertical prism imbalance shall not exceed ¼ prism diopter. Horizontal prism shall not exceed ¼ prism diopter Base In or ½ prism diopter Base Out.
Refractive power*	Shall not exceed ±¹⁄₁₆ diopter in any meridian.
Astigmatic refractive power	Difference in refractive power between any two meridians must be ¹⁄₁₆ D or less.

*Cover lenses or plates are exempt from all requirements. (Exception—Luminous transmission must not be less than 85%.)
Source: American National Standard Practice for Occupational and Educational Eye and Face Protection (ANSI Z87.1-1989).

Like safety frames, a lens is not a safety lens until it is properly marked, even if the lens is of safety thickness. Marking is done by sandblasting a company logo or abbreviated name on the lens after edging. The usual positioning of the marking is at the top of the lens or in the top, outside corner. An additional marking is required for certain specialized lens types. These marking requirements are summarized in Table 19-4.

We can see that safety eyewear includes both the lenses and the frame. Safety lenses in a regular frame (called a dress frame) do not constitute a pair of safety glasses. Regular thickness lenses (dress thickness) placed in a safety frame do not constitute a pair of safety glasses. This is true regardless of the strength of the lens material.

Corrective lenses made for safety eyewear fall under the same optical tolerance recommendations as do all prescription lenses. These are the Z80.1 American National Standard Recommendations for Prescription Ophthalmic Lenses and are found in Appendix 7.

It is important to note that optical tolerances such as refractive power and prismatic effect are more strict for nonprescription (plano) lenses than they are for prescription lenses. These nonprescription optical quality requirements are summarized in Table 19-5.

Many other aspects of the ANSI Z87.1 standards have to do with edging and with plano-powered or tinted protective eyewear. As mentioned earlier, the original document should be consulted to assure compliance.

Questions and Problems

1. According to FDA regulations, all glass lenses must be made impact-resistant by treating them in some manner. However, it is possible to have the wearer sign a waiver acknowledging that the lenses are not impact-resistant. If an injury occurred to an individual who had signed a waiver, would the doctor or dispenser be free of liability?
   a. yes
   b. no

2. Which of the following lenses below do not have to be individually drop-ball tested after they are manufactured?
   a. All lenses have to be drop-ball tested.
   b. Plastic single-vision prescription lenses.
   c. Plastic multifocal prescription lenses.
   d. Plastic mass-produced plano sunglass lenses.
   e. Glass single-vision prescription lenses.
   f. Glass fused multifocal prescription lenses.
   g. Glass Executive bifocals.
   h. Glass mass-produced plano sunglasses lenses.
   i. Corlon laminated lenses.

3. If a pair of prescription glasses is sold to an individual, how long do records have to be kept on those lenses for FDA purposes?
   a. No records need to be kept.
   b. One year.
   c. Two years.
   d. Three years.
   e. Four years.
   f. Five years.
   g. Six years.
   h. Seven years.

i. Ten years.

j. As long as an individual is in business.

4. Which government agency has made the standards set forth in the American National Standard Practice for Occupational and Educational Eye and Face Protection a requirement for those areas under their jurisdication?

a. No agency has ever done this.

b. The American National Standards Institute *is* a government agency.

c. The FAA.

d. The FDA.

e. OSHA.

5. Suppose a doctor or dispenser does edging in the office. He wishes to make a pair of industrial-thickness lenses that will be put in a frame that conforms to ANSI Z87 standards. The glasses are for a person who needs them for his job in a local factory. Does the doctor or dispenser need to mark the lenses, since he is a private practitioner?

a. yes

b. no

6. All dress lenses must be at least 2.2 mm thick at their thinnest point, except for high-plus lenses, which may be as thin as 1.8 mm at the thinnest edge.

True or False

7. What is the standard test for testing the impact resistance of corrective lenses that are made to be in compliance with the American National Standard Practice for Occupational and Educational Eye and Face Protection? Describe how this test is carried out.

Reference

1. Requirements referred to here are from *General Industry*, OSHA Safety and Health Standards (29 CFR 1910), U.S. Department of Labor, Occupational Safety and Health Administration, OSHA 2206, revised June 1981, p. 292.

Appendix
1

Base Curves

1-1 Base Curves for Spheres and Minus Cylinder Form Lenses, Glass (Index 1.523)

If the spherical equivalent $\left(sphere\ power + \dfrac{cylinder\ power}{2} \right)$ is	Then use this base curve (± 1.00 D)
Greater than $+7.50$	Use an aspheric design
Between $+6.37$ and $+7.50$	Use $+12.50$
Between $+4.37$ and $+6.37$	Use $+10.50$
Between $+1.50$ and $+4.37$	Use $+8.50$
Between -2.12 and $+1.50$	Use $+6.50$
Between -5.82 and -2.12	Use $+4.50$
Between -10.50 and -5.82	Use $+2.50$
Greater than -10.50	Use $+0.50$

Source: G.A. Fry, The Optometrist's New Role in the Use of Corrected Curve Lenses, *Journal of the American Optometric Association,* 50 (5): 562 (May 1979).

1-2 Base Curve Selection Chart

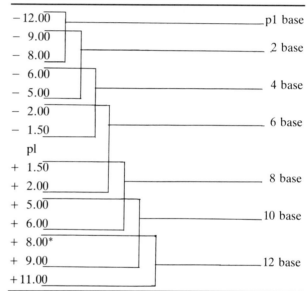

*Beyond $+7.00$ D of refractive power, a lens with an aspheric base curve should be used.

This base curve chart shows a great deal of overlap among base curves. It is designed to help in choosing the correct compromise curve when left and right lens powers are unequal. It is not meant as a replacement for manufacturers' recommendations.

Adapted from R.L. Mancusi, *Ophthalmic Surfacing for Plastic and Glass Lenses,* Butterworth-Heinemann, Boston, 1982, p. 7.

Appendix
2

Prism

Explanation of Chart

From center of circle outward, both lines and circles are gradated in prism diopters ($^\Delta$). Radial lines are in degrees of meridian.

EXAMPLE

To find resultant prism of an Rx calling for R E 3$^\Delta$ In and 4$^\Delta$ Down, proceed as follows:

a. Checking legend at top of chart, determine which side of center is to be used.

b. Then locate the horizontal line below center marked 4. This represents 4$^\Delta$ Base Down.

c. Then, in this case, move to the right to the vertical line marked 3, representing 3$^\Delta$ Base In. Note this point.

d. This point falls on the circle marked 5, which represents 5$^\Delta$ (5 prism diopters).

e. The meridian of the base is located by means of the radial lines. You will note that the 5$^\Delta$ falls between the radial 125° and 130° lines at about 127°. This indicates a resultant prism of 5$^\Delta$ Base Down at 127°.

From *Coburn Equipment Catalog*, Coburn Optical Industries, Muskogee, Okla. Used with permission.

2-1 Handy Resultant Prism Chart.

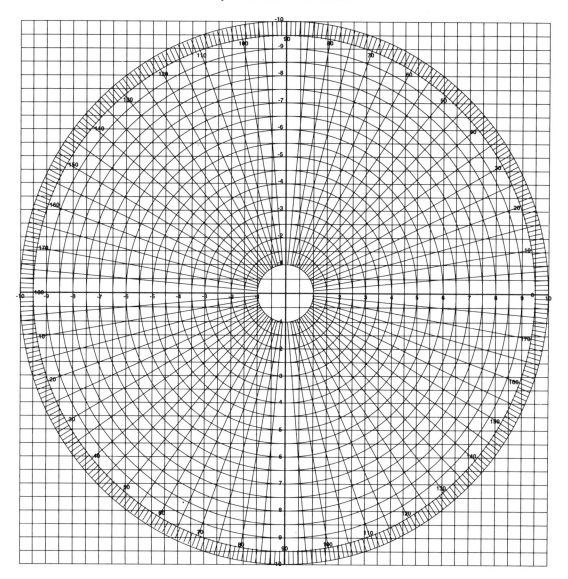

2-2 Resultant Prism and Measure in Degrees of the Resultant Prism Axis from the 180-Degree Meridian

Base Up or Base Down (rows) / Base In or Base Out (columns). Each cell lists the resultant prism value over the resultant axis in degrees.

Base Up or Base Down	0.25	0.50	0.75	1.00	1.25	1.50	1.75	2.00	2.25	2.50	2.75	3.00	3.25	3.50	3.75	4.00	4.25	4.50	4.75	5.00	5.25	5.50	5.75	6.00	6.25	6.50
0.25	0.35 / 45	0.56 / 27	0.79 / 18	1.03 / 14	1.27 / 11	1.52 / 9	1.77 / 8	2.02 / 7	2.26 / 6	2.51 / 6	2.76 / 5	3.01 / 5	3.26 / 4	3.51 / 4	3.76 / 4	4.01 / 4	4.26 / 3	4.51 / 3	4.76 / 3	5.01 / 3	5.26 / 3	5.51 / 3	5.76 / 2	6.01 / 2	6.25 / 2	6.50 / 2
0.50	0.56 / 63	0.71 / 45	0.90 / 34	1.12 / 27	1.35 / 22	1.58 / 18	1.82 / 16	2.06 / 14	2.30 / 13	2.55 / 11	2.80 / 10	3.04 / 9	3.29 / 9	3.54 / 8	3.78 / 8	4.03 / 7	4.28 / 7	4.53 / 6	4.78 / 6	5.02 / 6	5.27 / 5	5.52 / 5	5.77 / 5	6.02 / 5	6.27 / 5	6.52 / 4
0.75	0.79 / 72	0.90 / 56	1.06 / 45	1.25 / 37	1.46 / 31	1.68 / 27	1.90 / 23	2.14 / 21	2.37 / 18	2.61 / 17	2.85 / 15	3.09 / 14	3.34 / 13	3.58 / 12	3.82 / 11	4.07 / 11	4.32 / 10	4.56 / 9	4.81 / 9	5.06 / 9	5.30 / 8	5.55 / 8	5.80 / 7	6.05 / 7	6.29 / 7	6.54 / 7
1.00	1.03 / 76	1.12 / 63	1.25 / 53	1.41 / 45	1.60 / 39	1.80 / 34	2.02 / 30	2.24 / 27	2.46 / 24	2.69 / 22	2.93 / 20	3.16 / 18	3.40 / 17	3.64 / 16	3.88 / 15	4.12 / 14	4.37 / 13	4.61 / 13	4.85 / 12	5.10 / 11	5.34 / 11	5.59 / 10	5.84 / 10	6.08 / 9	6.33 / 9	6.58 / 9
1.25	1.27 / 79	1.35 / 68	1.46 / 59	1.60 / 51	1.77 / 45	1.95 / 40	2.15 / 36	2.36 / 32	2.57 / 29	2.80 / 27	3.02 / 24	3.25 / 23	3.48 / 21	3.72 / 20	3.95 / 18	4.19 / 17	4.43 / 16	4.67 / 16	4.91 / 15	5.15 / 14	5.40 / 13	5.64 / 13	5.88 / 12	6.13 / 12	6.37 / 11	6.62 / 11
1.50	1.52 / 81	1.58 / 72	1.68 / 63	1.80 / 56	1.95 / 50	2.12 / 45	2.30 / 41	2.50 / 37	2.70 / 34	2.92 / 31	3.13 / 29	3.35 / 27	3.58 / 25	3.81 / 23	4.04 / 22	4.27 / 21	4.51 / 19	4.74 / 18	4.98 / 18	5.22 / 17	5.46 / 16	5.70 / 15	5.94 / 15	6.18 / 14	6.43 / 13	6.67 / 13
1.75	1.77 / 82	1.82 / 74	1.90 / 67	2.02 / 60	2.15 / 54	2.30 / 49	2.47 / 45	2.66 / 41	2.85 / 38	3.05 / 35	3.26 / 32	3.47 / 30	3.69 / 28	3.91 / 27	4.14 / 25	4.37 / 24	4.60 / 22	4.83 / 21	5.06 / 20	5.30 / 19	5.53 / 18	5.77 / 18	6.01 / 17	6.25 / 16	6.49 / 16	6.73 / 15
2.00	2.02 / 83	2.06 / 76	2.14 / 69	2.24 / 63	2.36 / 58	2.50 / 53	2.66 / 49	2.83 / 45	3.01 / 42	3.20 / 39	3.40 / 36	3.61 / 34	3.82 / 32	4.03 / 30	4.25 / 28	4.47 / 27	4.70 / 25	4.92 / 24	5.15 / 23	5.39 / 22	5.62 / 21	5.85 / 20	6.09 / 19	6.32 / 18	6.56 / 18	6.80 / 17
2.25	2.26 / 84	2.30 / 77	2.37 / 72	2.46 / 66	2.57 / 61	2.70 / 56	2.85 / 52	3.01 / 48	3.18 / 45	3.36 / 42	3.55 / 39	3.75 / 37	3.95 / 35	4.16 / 33	4.37 / 31	4.59 / 29	4.81 / 28	5.03 / 27	5.26 / 25	5.48 / 24	5.71 / 23	5.94 / 22	6.17 / 21	6.41 / 21	6.64 / 20	6.88 / 19
2.50	2.51 / 84	2.55 / 79	2.61 / 73	2.69 / 68	2.80 / 63	2.92 / 59	3.05 / 55	3.20 / 51	3.36 / 48	3.54 / 45	3.72 / 42	3.91 / 40	4.10 / 38	4.30 / 36	4.51 / 34	4.72 / 32	4.93 / 30	5.15 / 29	5.37 / 28	5.59 / 27	5.81 / 25	6.04 / 24	6.27 / 23	6.50 / 23	6.73 / 22	6.96 / 21
2.75	2.76 / 85	2.80 / 80	2.85 / 75	2.93 / 70	3.02 / 66	3.13 / 61	3.26 / 58	3.40 / 54	3.55 / 51	3.72 / 47	3.89 / 45	4.07 / 43	4.26 / 40	4.45 / 38	4.65 / 36	4.85 / 35	5.06 / 33	5.27 / 31	5.49 / 30	5.71 / 29	5.93 / 28	6.15 / 27	6.37 / 26	6.60 / 25	6.83 / 24	7.06 / 23
3.00	3.01 / 85	3.04 / 81	3.09 / 76	3.16 / 72	3.25 / 67	3.35 / 63	3.47 / 60	3.61 / 56	3.75 / 53	3.91 / 50	4.07 / 47	4.24 / 45	4.42 / 43	4.61 / 41	4.80 / 39	5.00 / 37	5.20 / 35	5.41 / 34	5.62 / 32	5.83 / 31	6.05 / 30	6.26 / 29	6.49 / 28	6.71 / 27	6.93 / 26	7.16 / 25
3.25	3.26 / 86	3.29 / 81	3.34 / 77	3.40 / 73	3.48 / 69	3.58 / 65	3.69 / 62	3.82 / 58	3.95 / 55	4.10 / 52	4.26 / 50	4.42 / 47	4.60 / 45	4.78 / 43	4.96 / 41	5.15 / 39	5.35 / 37	5.55 / 36	5.76 / 34	5.96 / 33	6.17 / 32	6.39 / 31	6.60 / 29	6.82 / 28	7.04 / 27	7.27 / 27
3.50	3.51 / 86	3.54 / 82	3.58 / 78	3.64 / 74	3.72 / 70	3.81 / 67	3.91 / 63	4.03 / 60	4.16 / 57	4.30 / 54	4.45 / 52	4.61 / 49	4.78 / 47	4.95 / 45	5.13 / 43	5.32 / 41	5.51 / 39	5.70 / 38	5.90 / 36	6.10 / 35	6.31 / 34	6.52 / 32	6.73 / 31	6.95 / 30	7.16 / 29	7.38 / 28

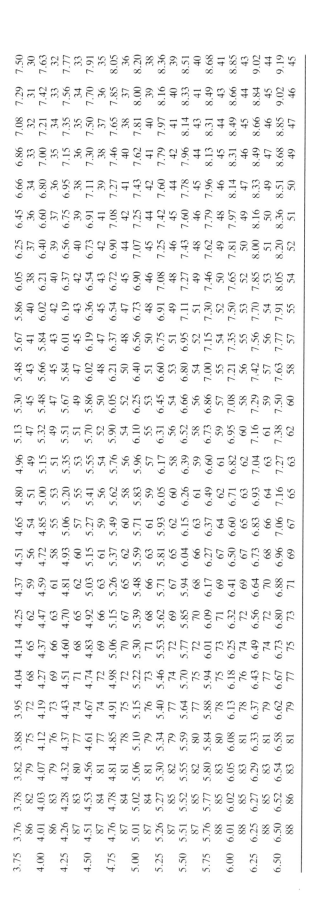

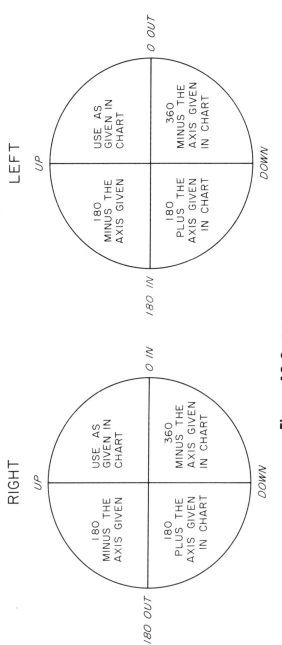

LEFT

RIGHT

Figure A2-2 Prism table conversion guide.

2-3 Prism Power Decentration Chart (Abridged)

Lens Power, D	Decentration, mm									
	0.5	1.0	1.5	2.0	2.5	3.0	3.5	4.0	4.5	5.0
0.125	0.01	0.01	0.02	0.03	0.03	0.04	0.04	0.05	0.06	0.06
0.250	0.01	0.03	0.04	0.05	0.06	0.08	0.09	0.10	0.11	0.13
0.375	0.02	0.04	0.06	0.08	0.09	0.11	0.13	0.15	0.17	0.19
0.500	0.03	0.05	0.08	0.10	0.13	0.15	0.18	0.20	0.23	0.25
0.625	0.03	0.06	0.09	0.13	0.16	0.19	0.22	0.25	0.28	0.31
0.750	0.04	0.08	0.11	0.15	0.19	0.23	0.26	0.30	0.34	0.38
0.875	0.04	0.09	0.13	0.18	0.22	0.26	0.31	0.35	0.39	0.44
1.000	0.05	0.10	0.15	0.20	0.25	0.30	0.35	0.40	0.45	0.50
1.125	0.06	0.11	0.17	0.23	0.28	0.34	0.39	0.45	0.51	0.56
1.250	0.06	0.13	0.19	0.25	0.31	0.38	0.44	0.50	0.56	0.63
1.375	0.07	0.14	0.21	0.28	0.34	0.41	0.48	0.55	0.62	0.69
1.500	0.08	0.15	0.23	0.30	0.38	0.45	0.53	0.60	0.68	0.75
1.625	0.08	0.16	0.24	0.33	0.41	0.49	0.57	0.65	0.73	0.81
1.750	0.09	0.18	0.26	0.35	0.44	0.53	0.61	0.70	0.79	0.88
1.875	0.09	0.19	0.28	0.38	0.47	0.56	0.66	0.75	0.84	0.94
2.000	0.10	0.20	0.30	0.40	0.50	0.60	0.70	0.80	0.90	1.00
2.125	0.11	0.21	0.32	0.43	0.53	0.64	0.74	0.85	0.96	1.06
2.250	0.11	0.23	0.34	0.45	0.56	0.68	0.79	0.90	1.01	1.13
2.375	0.12	0.24	0.36	0.48	0.59	0.71	0.83	0.95	1.07	1.19
2.500	0.13	0.25	0.38	0.50	0.63	0.75	0.88	1.00	1.13	1.25
2.625	0.13	0.26	0.39	0.53	0.66	0.79	0.92	1.05	1.18	1.31
2.750	0.14	0.28	0.41	0.55	0.69	0.83	0.96	1.10	1.24	1.38
2.875	0.14	0.29	0.43	0.58	0.72	0.86	1.01	1.15	1.29	1.44
3.000	0.15	0.30	0.45	0.60	0.75	0.90	1.05	1.20	1.35	1.50
3.125	0.16	0.31	0.47	0.63	0.78	0.94	1.09	1.25	1.41	1.56
3.250	0.16	0.33	0.49	0.65	0.81	0.98	1.14	1.30	1.46	1.63
3.375	0.17	0.34	0.51	0.68	0.84	1.01	1.18	1.35	1.52	1.69
3.500	0.18	0.35	0.53	0.70	0.88	1.05	1.23	1.40	1.58	1.75
3.625	0.18	0.36	0.54	0.73	0.91	1.09	1.27	1.45	1.63	1.81
3.750	0.19	0.38	0.56	0.75	0.94	1.13	1.31	1.50	1.69	1.88
3.875	0.19	0.39	0.58	0.78	0.97	1.16	1.36	1.55	1.74	1.94
4.000	0.20	0.40	0.60	0.80	1.00	1.20	1.40	1.60	1.80	2.00
4.125	0.21	0.41	0.62	0.83	1.03	1.24	1.44	1.65	1.86	2.06
4.250	0.21	0.43	0.64	0.85	1.06	1.28	1.49	1.70	1.91	2.13
4.375	0.22	0.44	0.66	0.88	1.09	1.31	1.53	1.75	1.97	2.19
4.500	0.23	0.45	0.68	0.90	1.13	1.35	1.58	1.80	2.03	2.25
4.625	0.23	0.46	0.69	0.93	1.16	1.39	1.62	1.85	2.08	2.31
4.750	0.24	0.48	0.71	0.95	1.19	1.43	1.66	1.90	2.14	2.38
4.875	0.24	0.49	0.73	0.98	1.22	1.46	1.71	1.95	2.19	2.44
5.000	0.25	0.50	0.75	1.00	1.25	1.50	1.75	2.00	2.25	2.50
5.250	0.26	0.53	0.79	1.05	1.31	1.58	1.84	2.10	2.36	2.63
5.500	0.28	0.55	0.83	1.10	1.38	1.65	1.93	2.20	2.48	2.75
5.750	0.29	0.58	0.86	1.15	1.44	1.73	2.01	2.30	2.59	2.88
6.000	0.30	0.60	0.90	1.20	1.50	1.80	2.10	2.40	2.70	3.00
6.250	0.31	0.63	0.94	1.25	1.56	1.88	2.19	2.50	2.81	3.13
6.500	0.33	0.65	0.98	1.30	1.63	1.95	2.28	2.60	2.93	3.25
6.750	0.34	0.68	1.01	1.35	1.69	2.03	2.36	2.70	3.04	3.38

2-3 *(Continued)*

Lens Power, D	Decentration, mm									
	0.5	*1.0*	*1.5*	*2.0*	*2.5*	*3.0*	*3.5*	*4.0*	*4.5*	*5.0*
7.000	0.35	0.70	1.05	1.40	1.75	2.10	2.45	2.80	3.15	3.50
7.500	0.38	0.75	1.13	1.50	1.88	2.25	2.63	3.00	3.38	3.75
8.000	0.40	0.80	1.20	1.60	2.00	2.40	2.80	3.20	3.60	4.00
8.500	0.43	0.85	1.28	1.70	2.13	2.55	2.98	3.40	3.83	4.25
9.000	0.45	0.90	1.35	1.80	2.25	2.70	3.15	3.60	4.05	4.50
9.500	0.48	0.95	1.43	1.90	2.38	2.85	3.33	3.80	4.28	4.75
10.000	0.50	1.00	1.50	2.00	2.50	3.00	3.50	4.00	4.50	5.00
11.000	0.55	1.10	1.65	2.20	2.75	3.30	3.85	4.40	4.95	5.50
12.000	0.60	1.20	1.80	2.40	3.00	3.60	4.20	4.80	5.40	6.00
13.000	0.65	1.30	1.95	2.60	3.25	3.90	4.55	5.20	5.85	6.50
14.000	0.70	1.40	2.10	2.80	3.50	4.20	4.90	5.60	6.30	7.00
15.000	0.75	1.50	2.25	3.00	3.75	4.50	5.25	6.00	6.75	7.50
16.000	0.80	1.60	2.40	3.20	4.00	4.80	5.60	6.40	7.20	8.00
17.000	0.85	1.70	2.55	3.40	4.25	5.10	5.95	6.80	7.65	8.50
18.000	0.90	1.80	2.70	3.60	4.50	5.40	6.30	7.20	8.10	9.00
19.000	0.95	1.90	2.85	3.80	4.75	5.70	6.65	7.60	8.55	9.50
20.000	1.00	2.00	3.00	4.00	5.00	6.00	7.00	8.00	9.00	10.00

2-4 Prism Power Decentration Chart (Unabridged)

Lens Power, D	Decentration, mm									
	0.5	1.0	1.5	2.0	2.5	3.0	3.5	4.0	4.5	5.0
0.125	0.01	0.01	0.02	0.03	0.03	0.04	0.04	0.05	0.06	0.06
0.250	0.01	0.03	0.04	0.05	0.06	0.08	0.09	0.10	0.11	0.13
0.375	0.02	0.04	0.06	0.08	0.09	0.11	0.13	0.15	0.17	0.19
0.500	0.03	0.05	0.08	0.10	0.13	0.15	0.18	0.20	0.23	0.25
0.625	0.03	0.06	0.09	0.13	0.16	0.19	0.22	0.25	0.28	0.31
0.750	0.04	0.08	0.11	0.15	0.19	0.23	0.26	0.30	0.34	0.38
0.875	0.04	0.09	0.13	0.18	0.22	0.26	0.31	0.35	0.39	0.44
1.000	0.05	0.10	0.15	0.20	0.25	0.30	0.35	0.40	0.45	0.50
1.125	0.06	0.11	0.17	0.23	0.28	0.34	0.39	0.45	0.51	0.56
1.250	0.06	0.13	0.19	0.25	0.31	0.38	0.44	0.50	0.56	0.63
1.375	0.07	0.14	0.21	0.28	0.34	0.41	0.48	0.55	0.62	0.69
1.500	0.08	0.15	0.23	0.30	0.38	0.45	0.53	0.60	0.68	0.75
1.625	0.08	0.16	0.24	0.33	0.41	0.49	0.57	0.65	0.73	0.81
1.750	0.09	0.18	0.26	0.35	0.44	0.53	0.61	0.70	0.79	0.88
1.875	0.09	0.19	0.28	0.38	0.47	0.56	0.66	0.75	0.84	0.94
2.000	0.10	0.20	0.30	0.40	0.50	0.60	0.70	0.80	0.90	1.00
2.125	0.11	0.21	0.32	0.43	0.53	0.64	0.74	0.85	0.96	1.06
2.250	0.11	0.23	0.34	0.45	0.56	0.68	0.79	0.90	1.01	1.13
2.375	0.12	0.24	0.36	0.48	0.59	0.71	0.83	0.95	1.07	1.19
2.500	0.13	0.25	0.38	0.50	0.63	0.75	0.88	1.00	1.13	1.25
2.625	0.13	0.26	0.39	0.53	0.66	0.79	0.92	1.05	1.18	1.31
2.750	0.14	0.28	0.41	0.55	0.69	0.83	0.96	1.10	1.24	1.38
2.875	0.14	0.29	0.43	0.58	0.72	0.86	1.01	1.15	1.29	1.44
3.000	0.15	0.30	0.45	0.60	0.75	0.90	1.05	1.20	1.35	1.50
3.125	0.16	0.31	0.47	0.63	0.78	0.94	1.09	1.25	1.41	1.56
3.250	0.16	0.33	0.49	0.65	0.81	0.98	1.14	1.30	1.46	1.63
3.375	0.17	0.34	0.51	0.68	0.84	1.01	1.18	1.35	1.52	1.69
3.500	0.18	0.35	0.53	0.70	0.88	1.05	1.23	1.40	1.58	1.75
3.625	0.18	0.36	0.54	0.73	0.91	1.09	1.27	1.45	1.63	1.81
3.750	0.19	0.38	0.56	0.75	0.94	1.13	1.31	1.50	1.69	1.88
3.875	0.19	0.39	0.58	0.78	0.97	1.16	1.36	1.55	1.74	1.94
4.000	0.20	0.40	0.60	0.80	1.00	1.20	1.40	1.60	1.80	2.00
4.125	0.21	0.41	0.62	0.83	1.03	1.24	1.44	1.65	1.86	2.06
4.250	0.21	0.43	0.64	0.85	1.06	1.28	1.49	1.70	1.91	2.13
4.375	0.22	0.44	0.66	0.88	1.09	1.31	1.53	1.75	1.97	2.19
4.500	0.23	0.45	0.68	0.90	1.13	1.35	1.58	1.80	2.03	2.25
4.625	0.23	0.46	0.69	0.93	1.16	1.39	1.62	1.85	2.08	2.31
4.750	0.24	0.48	0.71	0.95	1.19	1.43	1.66	1.90	2.14	2.38
4.875	0.24	0.49	0.73	0.98	1.22	1.46	1.71	1.95	2.19	2.44
5.000	0.25	0.50	0.75	1.00	1.25	1.50	1.75	2.00	2.25	2.50
5.125	0.26	0.51	0.77	1.03	1.28	1.54	1.79	2.05	2.31	2.56
5.250	0.26	0.53	0.79	1.05	1.31	1.58	1.84	2.10	2.36	2.63
5.375	0.27	0.54	0.81	1.08	1.34	1.61	1.88	2.15	2.42	2.69
5.500	0.28	0.55	0.83	1.10	1.38	1.65	1.93	2.20	2.48	2.75
5.625	0.28	0.56	0.84	1.13	1.41	1.69	1.97	2.25	2.53	2.81
5.750	0.29	0.58	0.86	1.15	1.44	1.73	2.01	2.30	2.59	2.88
5.875	0.29	0.59	0.88	1.18	1.47	1.76	2.06	2.35	2.64	2.94
6.000	0.30	0.60	0.90	1.20	1.50	1.80	2.10	2.40	2.70	3.00
6.125	0.31	0.61	0.92	1.23	1.53	1.84	2.14	2.45	2.76	3.06
6.250	0.31	0.63	0.94	1.25	1.56	1.88	2.19	2.50	2.81	3.13
6.375	0.32	0.64	0.96	1.28	1.59	1.91	2.23	2.55	2.87	3.19
6.500	0.33	0.65	0.98	1.30	1.63	1.95	2.28	2.60	2.93	3.25
6.625	0.33	0.66	0.99	1.33	1.66	1.99	2.32	2.65	2.98	3.31
6.750	0.34	0.68	1.01	1.35	1.69	2.03	2.36	2.70	3.04	3.38
6.875	0.34	0.69	1.03	1.38	1.72	2.06	2.41	2.75	3.09	3.44

| | | | | | Decentration, mm | | | | |
5.5	6.0	6.5	7.0	7.5	8.0	8.5	9.0	9.5	10.0
0.07	0.08	0.08	0.09	0.09	0.10	0.11	0.11	0.12	0.13
0.14	0.15	0.16	0.18	0.19	0.20	0.21	0.23	0.24	0.25
0.21	0.23	0.24	0.26	0.28	0.30	0.32	0.34	0.36	0.38
0.28	0.30	0.33	0.35	0.38	0.40	0.43	0.45	0.48	0.50
0.34	0.38	0.41	0.44	0.47	0.50	0.53	0.56	0.59	0.63
0.41	0.45	0.49	0.53	0.56	0.60	0.64	0.68	0.71	0.75
0.48	0.53	0.57	0.61	0.66	0.70	0.74	0.79	0.83	0.88
0.55	0.60	0.65	0.70	0.75	0.80	0.85	0.90	0.95	1.00
0.62	0.68	0.73	0.79	0.84	0.90	0.96	1.01	1.07	1.13
0.69	0.75	0.81	0.88	0.94	1.00	1.06	1.13	1.19	1.25
0.76	0.83	0.89	0.96	1.03	1.10	1.17	1.24	1.31	1.38
0.83	0.90	0.98	1.05	1.13	1.20	1.28	1.35	1.43	1.50
0.89	0.98	1.06	1.14	1.22	1.30	1.38	1.46	1.54	1.63
0.96	1.05	1.14	1.23	1.31	1.40	1.49	1.58	1.66	1.75
1.03	1.13	1.22	1.31	1.41	1.50	1.59	1.69	1.78	1.88
1.10	1.20	1.30	1.40	1.50	1.60	1.70	1.80	1.90	2.00
1.17	1.28	1.38	1.49	1.59	1.70	1.81	1.91	2.02	2.13
1.24	1.35	1.46	1.58	1.69	1.80	1.91	2.03	2.14	2.25
1.31	1.43	1.54	1.66	1.78	1.90	2.02	2.14	2.26	2.38
1.38	1.50	1.63	1.75	1.88	2.00	2.13	2.25	2.38	2.50
1.44	1.58	1.71	1.84	1.97	2.10	2.23	2.36	2.49	2.63
1.51	1.65	1.79	1.93	2.06	2.20	2.34	2.48	2.61	2.75
1.58	1.73	1.87	2.01	2.16	2.30	2.44	2.59	2.73	2.88
1.65	1.80	1.95	2.10	2.25	2.40	2.55	2.70	2.85	3.00
1.72	1.88	2.03	2.19	2.34	2.50	2.66	2.81	2.97	3.13
1.79	1.95	2.11	2.28	2.44	2.60	2.76	2.93	3.09	3.25
1.86	2.03	2.19	2.36	2.53	2.70	2.87	3.04	3.21	3.38
1.93	2.10	2.28	2.45	2.63	2.80	2.98	3.15	3.33	3.50
1.99	2.18	2.36	2.54	2.72	2.90	3.08	3.26	3.44	3.63
2.06	2.25	2.44	2.63	2.81	3.00	3.19	3.38	3.56	3.75
2.13	2.33	2.52	2.71	2.91	3.10	3.29	3.49	3.68	3.88
2.20	2.40	2.60	2.80	3.00	3.20	3.40	3.60	3.80	4.00
2.27	2.48	2.68	2.89	3.09	3.30	3.51	3.71	3.92	4.13
2.34	2.55	2.76	2.98	3.19	3.40	3.61	3.83	4.04	4.25
2.41	2.63	2.84	3.06	3.28	3.50	3.72	3.94	4.16	4.38
2.48	2.70	2.93	3.15	3.38	3.60	3.83	4.05	4.28	4.50
2.54	2.78	3.01	3.24	3.47	3.70	3.93	4.16	4.39	4.63
2.61	2.85	3.09	3.33	3.56	3.80	4.04	4.28	4.51	4.75
2.68	2.93	3.17	3.41	3.66	3.90	4.14	4.39	4.63	4.88
2.75	3.00	3.25	3.50	3.75	4.00	4.25	4.50	4.75	5.00
2.82	3.08	3.33	3.59	3.84	4.10	4.36	4.61	4.87	5.13
2.89	3.15	3.41	3.68	3.94	4.20	4.46	4.73	4.99	5.25
2.96	3.23	3.49	3.76	4.03	4.30	4.57	4.84	5.11	5.38
3.03	3.30	3.58	3.85	4.13	4.40	4.68	4.95	5.23	5.50
3.09	3.38	3.66	3.94	4.22	4.50	4.78	5.06	5.34	5.63
3.16	3.45	3.74	4.03	4.31	4.60	4.89	5.18	5.46	5.75
3.23	3.53	3.82	4.11	4.41	4.70	4.99	5.29	5.58	5.88
3.30	3.60	3.90	4.20	4.50	4.80	5.10	5.40	5.70	6.00
3.37	3.68	3.98	4.29	4.59	4.90	5.21	5.51	5.82	6.13
3.44	3.75	4.06	4.38	4.69	5.00	5.31	5.63	5.94	6.25
3.51	3.83	4.14	4.46	4.78	5.10	5.42	5.74	6.06	6.38
3.58	3.90	4.23	4.55	4.88	5.20	5.53	5.85	6.18	6.50
3.64	3.98	4.31	4.64	4.97	5.30	5.63	5.96	6.29	6.63
3.71	4.05	4.39	4.73	5.06	5.40	5.74	6.08	6.41	6.75
3.78	4.13	4.47	4.81	5.16	5.50	5.84	6.19	6.53	6.88

2-4 Prism Power Decentration Chart *(Continued)*

Lens Power, D	Decentration, mm									
	0.5	1.0	1.5	2.0	2.5	3.0	3.5	4.0	4.5	5.0
7.000	0.35	0.70	1.05	1.40	1.75	2.10	2.45	2.80	3.15	3.50
7.125	0.36	0.71	1.07	1.43	1.78	2.14	2.49	2.85	3.21	3.56
7.250	0.36	0.73	1.09	1.45	1.81	2.18	2.54	2.90	3.26	3.63
7.375	0.37	0.74	1.11	1.48	1.84	2.21	2.58	2.95	3.32	3.69
7.500	0.38	0.75	1.13	1.50	1.88	2.25	2.63	3.00	3.38	3.75
7.625	0.38	0.76	1.14	1.53	1.91	2.29	2.67	3.05	3.43	3.81
7.750	0.39	0.78	1.16	1.55	1.94	2.33	2.71	3.10	3.49	3.88
7.875	0.39	0.79	1.18	1.58	1.97	2.36	2.76	3.15	3.54	3.94
8.000	0.40	0.80	1.20	1.60	2.00	2.40	2.80	3.20	3.60	4.00
8.125	0.41	0.81	1.22	1.63	2.03	2.44	2.84	3.25	3.66	4.06
8.250	0.41	0.83	1.24	1.65	2.06	2.48	2.89	3.30	3.71	4.13
8.375	0.42	0.84	1.26	1.68	2.09	2.51	2.93	3.35	3.77	4.19
8.500	0.43	0.85	1.28	1.70	2.13	2.55	2.98	3.40	3.83	4.25
8.625	0.43	0.86	1.29	1.73	2.16	2.59	3.02	3.45	3.88	4.31
8.750	0.44	0.88	1.31	1.75	2.19	2.63	3.06	3.50	3.94	4.38
8.875	0.44	0.89	1.33	1.78	2.22	2.66	3.11	3.55	3.99	4.44
9.000	0.45	0.90	1.35	1.80	2.25	2.70	3.15	3.60	4.05	4.50
9.125	0.46	0.91	1.37	1.83	2.28	2.74	3.19	3.65	4.11	4.56
9.250	0.46	0.93	1.39	1.85	2.31	2.78	3.24	3.70	4.16	4.63
9.375	0.47	0.94	1.41	1.88	2.34	2.81	3.28	3.75	4.22	4.69
9.500	0.48	0.95	1.43	1.90	2.38	2.85	3.33	3.80	4.28	4.75
9.625	0.48	0.96	1.44	1.93	2.41	2.89	3.37	3.85	4.33	4.81
9.750	0.49	0.98	1.46	1.95	2.44	2.93	3.41	3.90	4.39	4.88
9.875	0.49	0.99	1.48	1.98	2.47	2.96	3.46	3.95	4.44	4.94
10.000	0.50	1.00	1.50	2.00	2.50	3.00	3.50	4.00	4.50	5.00
10.125	0.51	1.01	1.52	2.03	2.53	3.04	3.54	4.05	4.56	5.06
10.250	0.51	1.03	1.54	2.05	2.56	3.08	3.59	4.10	4.61	5.13
10.375	0.52	1.04	1.56	2.08	2.59	3.11	3.63	4.15	4.67	5.19
10.500	0.53	1.05	1.58	2.10	2.63	3.15	3.68	4.20	4.73	5.25
10.625	0.53	1.06	1.59	2.13	2.66	3.19	3.72	4.25	4.78	5.31
10.750	0.54	1.08	1.61	2.15	2.69	3.23	3.76	4.30	4.84	5.38
10.875	0.54	1.09	1.63	2.18	2.72	3.26	3.81	4.35	4.89	5.44
11.000	0.55	1.10	1.65	2.20	2.75	3.30	3.85	4.40	4.95	5.50
11.125	0.56	1.11	1.67	2.23	2.78	3.34	3.89	4.45	5.01	5.56
11.250	0.56	1.13	1.69	2.25	2.81	3.38	3.94	4.50	5.06	5.63
11.375	0.57	1.14	1.71	2.28	2.84	3.41	3.98	4.55	5.12	5.69
11.500	0.58	1.15	1.73	2.30	2.88	3.45	4.03	4.60	5.18	5.75
11.625	0.58	1.16	1.74	2.33	2.91	3.49	4.07	4.65	5.23	5.81
11.750	0.59	1.18	1.76	2.35	2.94	3.53	4.11	4.70	5.29	5.88
11.875	0.59	1.19	1.78	2.38	2.97	3.56	4.16	4.75	5.34	5.94
12.000	0.60	1.20	1.80	2.40	3.00	3.60	4.20	4.80	5.40	6.00
12.125	0.61	1.21	1.82	2.43	3.03	3.64	4.24	4.85	5.46	6.06
12.250	0.61	1.23	1.84	2.45	3.06	3.68	4.29	4.90	5.51	6.13
12.375	0.62	1.24	1.86	2.48	3.09	3.71	4.33	4.95	5.57	6.19
12.500	0.63	1.25	1.88	2.50	3.13	3.75	4.38	5.00	5.63	6.25
12.625	0.63	1.26	1.89	2.53	3.16	3.79	4.42	5.05	5.68	6.31
12.750	0.64	1.28	1.91	2.55	3.19	3.83	4.46	5.10	5.74	6.38
12.875	0.64	1.29	1.93	2.58	3.22	3.86	4.51	5.15	5.79	6.44
13.000	0.65	1.30	1.95	2.60	3.25	3.90	4.55	5.20	5.85	6.50
13.125	0.66	1.31	1.97	2.63	3.28	3.94	4.59	5.25	5.91	6.56
13.250	0.66	1.33	1.99	2.65	3.31	3.98	4.64	5.30	5.96	6.63
13.375	0.67	1.34	2.01	2.68	3.34	4.01	4.68	5.35	6.02	6.69
13.500	0.68	1.35	2.03	2.70	3.38	4.05	4.73	5.40	6.08	6.75
13.625	0.68	1.36	2.04	2.73	3.41	4.09	4.77	5.45	6.13	6.81
13.750	0.69	1.38	2.06	2.75	3.44	4.13	4.81	5.50	6.19	6.88

				Decentration, mm					
5.5	*6.0*	*6.5*	*7.0*	*7.5*	*8.0*	*8.5*	*9.0*	*9.5*	*10.0*
3.85	4.20	4.55	4.90	5.25	5.60	5.95	6.30	6.65	7.00
3.92	4.28	4.63	4.99	5.34	5.70	6.06	6.41	6.77	7.13
3.99	4.35	4.71	5.08	5.44	5.80	6.16	6.53	6.89	7.25
4.06	4.43	4.79	5.16	5.53	5.90	6.27	6.64	7.01	7.38
4.13	4.50	4.88	5.25	5.63	6.00	6.38	6.75	7.13	7.50
4.19	4.58	4.96	5.34	5.72	6.10	6.48	6.86	7.24	7.63
4.26	4.65	5.04	5.43	5.81	6.20	6.59	6.98	7.36	7.75
4.33	4.73	5.12	5.51	5.91	6.30	6.69	7.09	7.48	7.88
4.40	4.80	5.20	5.60	6.00	6.40	6.80	7.20	7.60	8.00
4.47	4.88	5.28	5.69	6.09	6.50	6.91	7.31	7.72	8.13
4.54	4.95	5.36	5.78	6.19	6.60	7.01	7.43	7.84	8.25
4.61	5.03	5.44	5.86	6.28	6.70	7.12	7.54	7.96	8.38
4.68	5.10	5.53	5.95	6.38	6.80	7.23	7.65	8.08	8.50
4.74	5.18	5.61	6.04	6.47	6.90	7.33	7.76	8.19	8.63
4.81	5.25	5.69	6.13	6.56	7.00	7.44	7.88	8.31	8.75
4.88	5.33	5.77	6.21	6.66	7.10	7.54	7.99	8.43	8.88
4.95	5.40	5.85	6.30	6.75	7.20	7.65	8.10	8.55	9.00
5.02	5.48	5.93	6.39	6.84	7.30	7.76	8.21	8.67	9.13
5.09	5.55	6.01	6.48	6.94	7.40	7.86	8.33	8.79	9.25
5.16	5.63	6.09	6.56	7.03	7.50	7.97	8.44	8.91	9.38
5.23	5.70	6.18	6.65	7.13	7.60	8.08	8.55	9.03	9.50
5.29	5.78	6.26	6.74	7.22	7.70	8.18	8.66	9.14	9.63
5.36	5.85	6.34	6.83	7.31	7.80	8.29	8.78	9.26	9.75
5.43	5.93	6.42	6.91	7.41	7.90	8.39	8.89	9.38	9.88
5.50	6.00	6.50	7.00	7.50	8.00	8.50	9.00	9.50	10.00
5.57	6.08	6.58	7.09	7.59	8.10	8.61	9.11	9.62	10.13
5.64	6.15	6.66	7.18	7.69	8.20	8.71	9.23	9.74	10.25
5.71	6.23	6.74	7.26	7.78	8.30	8.82	9.34	9.86	10.38
5.78	6.30	6.83	7.35	7.88	8.40	8.93	9.45	9.98	10.50
5.84	6.38	6.91	7.44	7.97	8.50	9.03	9.56	10.09	10.63
5.91	6.45	6.99	7.53	8.06	8.60	9.14	9.68	10.21	10.75
5.98	6.53	7.07	7.61	8.16	8.70	9.24	9.79	10.33	10.88
6.05	6.60	7.15	7.70	8.25	8.80	9.35	9.90	10.45	11.00
6.12	6.68	7.23	7.79	8.34	8.90	9.46	10.01	10.57	11.13
6.19	6.75	7.31	7.88	8.44	9.00	9.56	10.13	10.69	11.25
6.26	6.83	7.39	7.96	8.53	9.10	9.67	10.24	10.81	11.38
6.33	6.90	7.48	8.05	8.63	9.20	9.78	10.35	10.93	11.50
6.39	6.98	7.56	8.14	8.72	9.30	9.88	10.46	11.04	11.63
6.46	7.05	7.64	8.23	8.81	9.40	9.99	10.58	11.16	11.75
6.53	7.13	7.72	8.31	8.91	9.50	10.09	10.69	11.28	11.88
6.60	7.20	7.80	8.40	9.00	9.60	10.20	10.80	11.40	12.00
6.67	7.28	7.88	8.49	9.09	9.70	10.31	10.91	11.52	12.13
6.74	7.35	7.96	8.58	9.19	9.80	10.41	11.03	11.64	12.25
6.81	7.43	8.04	8.66	9.28	9.90	10.52	11.14	11.76	12.38
6.88	7.50	8.13	8.75	9.38	10.00	10.63	11.25	11.88	12.50
6.94	7.58	8.21	8.84	9.47	10.10	10.73	11.36	11.99	12.63
7.01	7.65	8.29	8.93	9.56	10.20	10.84	11.48	12.11	12.75
7.08	7.73	8.37	9.01	9.66	10.30	10.94	11.59	12.23	12.88
7.15	7.80	8.45	9.10	9.75	10.40	11.05	11.70	12.35	13.00
7.22	7.88	8.53	9.19	9.84	10.50	11.16	11.81	12.47	13.13
7.29	7.95	8.61	9.28	9.94	10.60	11.26	11.93	12.59	13.25
7.36	8.03	8.69	9.36	10.03	10.70	11.37	12.04	12.71	13.38
7.43	8.10	8.78	9.45	10.13	10.80	11.48	12.15	12.83	13.50
7.49	8.18	8.86	9.54	10.22	10.90	11.58	12.26	12.94	13.63
7.56	8.25	8.94	9.63	10.31	11.00	11.69	12.38	13.06	13.75

2-4 Prism Power Decentration Chart *(Continued)*

Lens Power, D	Decentration, mm									
	0.5	1.0	1.5	2.0	2.5	3.0	3.5	4.0	4.5	5.0
13.875	0.69	1.39	2.08	2.78	3.47	4.16	4.86	5.55	6.24	6.94
14.000	0.70	1.40	2.10	2.80	3.50	4.20	4.90	5.60	6.30	7.00
14.125	0.71	1.41	2.12	2.83	3.53	4.24	4.94	5.65	6.36	7.06
14.250	0.71	1.43	2.14	2.85	3.56	4.28	4.99	5.70	6.41	7.13
14.375	0.72	1.44	2.16	2.88	3.59	4.31	5.03	5.75	6.47	7.19
14.500	0.73	1.45	2.18	2.90	3.63	4.35	5.08	5.80	6.53	7.25
14.625	0.73	1.46	2.19	2.93	3.66	4.39	5.12	5.85	6.58	7.31
14.750	0.74	1.48	2.21	2.95	3.69	4.43	5.16	5.90	6.64	7.38
14.875	0.74	1.49	2.23	2.98	3.72	4.46	5.21	5.95	6.69	7.44
15.000	0.75	1.50	2.25	3.00	3.75	4.50	5.25	6.00	6.75	7.50
15.125	0.76	1.51	2.27	3.03	3.78	4.54	5.29	6.05	6.81	7.56
15.250	0.76	1.53	2.29	3.05	3.81	4.58	5.34	6.10	6.86	7.63
15.375	0.77	1.54	2.31	3.08	3.84	4.61	5.38	6.15	6.92	7.69
15.500	0.78	1.55	2.33	3.10	3.88	4.65	5.43	6.20	6.98	7.75
15.625	0.78	1.56	2.34	3.13	3.91	4.69	5.47	6.25	7.03	7.81
15.750	0.79	1.58	2.36	3.15	3.94	4.73	5.51	6.30	7.09	7.88
15.875	0.79	1.59	2.38	3.18	3.97	4.76	5.56	6.35	7.14	7.94
16.000	0.80	1.60	2.40	3.20	4.00	4.80	5.60	6.40	7.20	8.00
16.125	0.81	1.61	2.42	3.23	4.03	4.84	5.64	6.45	7.26	8.06
16.250	0.81	1.63	2.44	3.25	4.06	4.88	5.69	6.50	7.31	8.13
16.375	0.82	1.64	2.46	3.28	4.09	4.91	5.73	6.55	7.37	8.19
16.500	0.83	1.65	2.48	3.30	4.13	4.95	5.78	6.60	7.43	8.25
16.625	0.83	1.66	2.49	3.33	4.16	4.99	5.82	6.65	7.48	8.31
16.750	0.84	1.68	2.51	3.35	4.19	5.03	5.86	6.70	7.54	8.38
16.875	0.84	1.69	2.53	3.38	4.22	5.06	5.91	6.75	7.59	8.44
17.000	0.85	1.70	2.55	3.40	4.25	5.10	5.95	6.80	7.65	8.50
17.125	0.86	1.71	2.57	3.43	4.28	5.14	5.99	6.85	7.71	8.56
17.250	0.86	1.73	2.59	3.45	4.31	5.18	6.04	6.90	7.76	8.63
17.375	0.87	1.74	2.61	3.48	4.34	5.21	6.08	6.95	7.82	8.69
17.500	0.88	1.75	2.63	3.50	4.38	5.25	6.13	7.00	7.88	8.75
17.625	0.88	1.76	2.64	3.53	4.41	5.29	6.17	7.05	7.93	8.81
17.750	0.89	1.78	2.66	3.55	4.44	5.33	6.21	7.10	7.99	8.88
17.875	0.89	1.79	2.68	3.58	4.47	5.36	6.26	7.15	8.04	8.94
18.000	0.90	1.80	2.70	3.60	4.50	5.40	6.30	7.20	8.10	9.00
18.125	0.91	1.81	2.72	3.63	4.53	5.44	6.34	7.25	8.16	9.06
18.250	0.91	1.83	2.74	3.65	4.56	5.48	6.39	7.30	8.21	9.13
18.375	0.92	1.84	2.76	3.68	4.59	5.51	6.43	7.35	8.27	9.19
18.500	0.93	1.85	2.78	3.70	4.63	5.55	6.48	7.40	8.33	9.25
18.625	0.93	1.86	2.79	3.73	4.66	5.59	6.52	7.45	8.38	9.31
18.750	0.94	1.88	2.81	3.75	4.69	5.63	6.56	7.50	8.44	9.38
18.875	0.94	1.89	2.83	3.78	4.72	5.66	6.61	7.55	8.49	9.44
19.000	0.95	1.90	2.85	3.80	4.75	5.70	6.65	7.60	8.55	9.50
19.125	0.96	1.91	2.87	3.83	4.78	5.74	6.69	7.65	8.61	9.56
19.250	0.96	1.93	2.89	3.85	4.81	5.78	6.74	7.70	8.66	9.63
19.375	0.97	1.94	2.91	3.88	4.84	5.81	6.78	7.75	8.72	9.69
19.500	0.98	1.95	2.93	3.90	4.88	5.85	6.83	7.80	8.78	9.75
19.625	0.98	1.96	2.94	3.93	4.91	5.89	6.87	7.85	8.83	9.81
19.750	0.99	1.98	2.96	3.95	4.94	5.93	6.91	7.90	8.89	9.88
19.875	0.99	1.99	2.98	3.98	4.97	5.96	6.96	7.95	8.94	9.94
20.000	1.00	2.00	3.00	4.00	5.00	6.00	7.00	8.00	9.00	10.00

				Decentration, mm					
5.5	*6.0*	*6.5*	*7.0*	*7.5*	*8.0*	*8.5*	*9.0*	*9.5*	*10.0*
7.63	8.33	9.02	9.71	10.41	11.10	11.79	12.49	13.18	13.88
7.70	8.40	9.10	9.80	10.50	11.20	11.90	12.60	13.30	14.00
7.77	8.48	9.18	9.89	10.59	11.30	12.01	12.71	13.42	14.13
7.84	8.55	9.26	9.98	10.69	11.40	12.11	12.83	13.54	14.25
7.91	8.63	9.34	10.06	10.78	11.50	12.22	12.94	13.66	14.38
7.98	8.70	9.43	10.15	10.88	11.60	12.33	13.05	13.78	14.50
8.04	8.78	9.51	10.24	10.97	11.70	12.43	13.16	13.89	14.63
8.11	8.85	9.59	10.33	11.06	11.80	12.54	13.28	14.01	14.75
8.18	8.93	9.67	10.41	11.16	11.90	12.64	13.39	14.13	14.88
8.25	9.00	9.75	10.50	11.25	12.00	12.75	13.50	14.25	15.00
8.32	9.08	9.83	10.59	11.34	12.10	12.86	13.61	14.37	15.13
8.39	9.15	9.91	10.68	11.44	12.20	12.96	13.73	14.49	15.25
8.46	9.23	9.99	10.76	11.53	12.30	13.07	13.84	14.61	15.38
8.53	9.30	10.08	10.85	11.63	12.40	13.18	13.95	14.73	15.50
8.59	9.38	10.16	10.94	11.72	12.50	13.28	14.06	14.84	15.63
8.66	9.45	10.24	11.03	11.81	12.60	13.39	14.18	14.96	15.75
8.73	9.53	10.32	11.11	11.91	12.70	13.49	14.29	15.08	15.88
8.80	9.60	10.40	11.20	12.00	12.80	13.60	14.40	15.20	16.00
8.87	9.68	10.48	11.29	12.09	12.90	13.71	14.51	15.32	16.13
8.94	9.75	10.56	11.38	12.19	13.00	13.81	14.63	15.44	16.25
9.01	9.83	10.64	11.46	12.28	13.10	13.92	14.74	15.56	16.38
9.08	9.90	10.73	11.55	12.38	13.20	14.03	14.85	15.68	16.50
9.14	9.98	10.81	11.64	12.47	13.30	14.13	14.96	15.79	16.63
9.21	10.05	10.89	11.73	12.56	13.40	14.24	15.08	15.91	16.75
9.28	10.13	10.97	11.81	12.66	13.50	14.34	15.19	16.03	16.88
9.35	10.20	11.05	11.90	12.75	13.60	14.45	15.30	16.15	17.00
9.42	10.28	11.13	11.99	12.84	13.70	14.56	15.41	16.27	17.13
9.49	10.35	11.21	12.08	12.94	13.80	14.66	15.53	16.39	17.25
9.56	10.43	11.29	12.16	13.03	13.90	14.77	15.64	16.51	17.38
9.63	10.50	11.38	12.25	13.13	14.00	14.88	15.75	16.63	17.50
9.69	10.58	11.46	12.34	13.22	14.10	14.98	15.86	16.74	17.63
9.76	10.65	11.54	12.43	13.31	14.20	15.09	15.98	16.86	17.75
9.83	10.73	11.62	12.51	13.41	14.30	15.19	16.09	16.98	17.88
9.90	10.80	11.70	12.60	13.50	14.40	15.30	16.20	17.10	18.00
9.97	10.88	11.78	12.69	13.59	14.50	15.41	16.31	17.22	18.13
10.04	10.95	11.86	12.78	13.69	14.60	15.51	16.43	17.34	18.25
10.11	11.03	11.94	12.86	13.78	14.70	15.62	16.54	17.46	18.38
10.18	11.10	12.03	12.95	13.88	14.80	15.73	16.65	17.58	18.50
10.24	11.18	12.11	13.04	13.97	14.90	15.83	16.76	17.69	18.63
10.31	11.25	12.19	13.13	14.06	15.00	15.94	16.88	17.81	18.75
10.38	11.33	12.27	13.21	14.16	15.10	16.04	16.99	17.93	18.88
10.45	11.40	12.35	13.30	14.25	15.20	16.15	17.10	18.05	19.00
10.52	11.48	12.43	13.39	14.34	15.30	16.26	17.21	18.17	19.13
10.59	11.55	12.51	13.48	14.44	15.40	16.36	17.33	18.29	19.25
10.66	11.63	12.59	13.56	14.53	15.50	16.47	17.44	18.41	19.38
10.73	11.70	12.68	13.65	14.63	15.60	16.58	17.55	18.53	19.50
10.79	11.78	12.76	13.74	14.72	15.70	16.68	17.66	18.64	19.63
10.86	11.85	12.84	13.83	14.81	15.80	16.79	17.78	18.76	19.75
10.93	11.93	12.92	13.91	14.91	15.90	16.89	17.89	18.88	19.88
11.00	12.00	13.00	14.00	15.00	16.00	17.00	18.00	19.00	20.00

2-5 Vertical Imbalance Prism Compensation Tables (Prentice's Rule)

		Power Difference Between Left and Right 90-Degree Meridians										
		1.00	*1.25*	*1.50*	*1.75*	*2.00*	*2.25*	*2.50*	*2.75*	*3.00*	*3.25*	*3.50*
Difference from MRP to Reading Level	4	0.40	0.50	0.60	0.70	0.80	0.90	1.00	1.10	1.20	1.30	1.40
	5	0.50	0.63	0.75	0.88	1.00	1.13	1.25	1.38	1.50	1.63	1.75
	6	0.60	0.75	0.90	1.05	1.20	1.35	1.50	1.65	1.80	1.95	2.10
	7	0.70	0.88	1.05	1.23	1.40	1.58	1.75	1.93	2.10	2.28	2.45
	8	0.80	1.00	1.20	1.40	1.60	1.80	2.00	2.20	2.40	2.60	2.80
	9	0.90	1.13	1.35	1.58	1.80	2.03	2.25	2.48	2.70	2.93	3.15
	10	1.00	1.25	1.50	1.75	2.00	2.25	2.50	2.75	3.00	3.25	3.50
	11	1.10	1.38	1.65	1.93	2.20	2.48	2.75	3.03	3.30	3.58	3.85
	12	1.20	1.50	1.80	2.10	2.40	2.70	3.00	3.30	3.60	3.90	4.20

← Use FT-35 combination, dissimilar segs, or compensated segs →   ———————— Use slab-off ————————

3.75	4.00	4.25	4.50	4.75	5.00	5.25	5.50	5.75	6.00
1.50	1.60	1.70	1.80	1.90	2.00	2.10	2.20	2.30	2.40
1.88	2.00	2.13	2.25	2.38	2.50	2.63	2.75	2.88	3.00
2.25	2.40	2.55	2.70	2.85	3.00	3.15	3.30	3.45	3.60
2.63	2.80	2.98	3.15	3.33	3.50	3.68	3.85	4.03	4.20
3.00	3.20	3.40	3.60	3.80	4.00	4.20	4.40	4.60	4.80
3.38	3.60	3.83	4.05	4,28	4.50	4.73	4.95	5.18	5.40
3.75	4.00	4.25	4.50	4.75	5.00	5.25	5.50	5.75	6.00
4.13	4.40	4.68	4.95	5.23	5.50	5.78	6.05	6.33	6.60
4.50	4.80	5.10	5.40	5.70	6.00	6.30	6.60	6.90	7.20

Appendix

3   **Power**

3-1 "Power" of a Cylinder in the 180-Degree Meridian

Cyl Axis	Cyl Power													
	0.25	0.50	0.75	1.00	1.25	1.50	1.75	2.00	2.25	2.50	2.75	3.00	3.25	3.50
5 or 175	0.00	0.00	0.01	0.01	0.01	0.01	0.01	0.02	0.02	0.02	0.02	0.02	0.02	0.03
10 or 170	0.01	0.02	0.02	0.03	0.04	0.05	0.05	0.06	0.07	0.08	0.08	0.09	0.10	0.11
15 or 165	0.02	0.03	0.05	0.07	0.08	0.10	0.12	0.13	0.15	0.17	0.18	0.20	0.22	0.23
20 or 160	0.03	0.06	0.09	0.12	0.15	0.18	0.20	0.23	0.26	0.29	0.32	0.35	0.38	0.41
25 or 155	0.04	0.09	0.13	0.18	0.22	0.27	0.31	0.36	0.40	0.45	0.49	0.54	0.58	0.63
30 or 150	0.06	0.12	0.19	0.25	0.31	0.37	0.44	0.50	0.56	0.62	0.69	0.75	0.81	0.87
35 or 145	0.08	0.16	0.25	0.33	0.41	0.49	0.58	0.66	0.74	0.82	0.90	0.99	1.07	1.15
40 or 140	0.10	0.21	0.31	0.41	0.52	0.62	0.72	0.83	0.93	1.03	1.14	1.24	1.34	1.45
45 or 135	0.12	0.25	0.37	0.50	0.62	0.75	0.87	1.00	1.12	1.25	1.37	1.50	1.62	1.75
50 or 130	0.15	0.29	0.44	0.59	0.73	0.88	1.03	1.17	1.32	1.47	1.61	1.76	1.91	2.05
55 or 125	0.17	0.34	0.50	0.67	0.84	1.01	1.17	1.34	1.51	1.68	1.85	2.01	2.18	2.35
60 or 120	0.19	0.37	0.56	0.75	0.94	1.12	1.31	1.50	1.69	1.87	2.06	2.25	2.44	2.62
65 or 115	0.21	0.41	0.62	0.82	1.03	1.23	1.44	1.64	1.85	2.05	2.26	2.46	2.67	2.87
70 or 110	0.22	0.44	0.66	0.88	1.10	1.32	1.55	1.77	1.99	2.21	2.43	2.65	2.87	3.09
75 or 105	0.23	0.47	0.70	0.93	1.17	1.40	1.63	1.87	2.10	2.33	2.57	2.80	3.03	3.27
80 or 100	0.24	0.48	0.73	0.97	1.21	1.45	1.70	1.94	2.18	2.42	2.67	2.91	3.15	3.39
85 or 95	0.25	0.50	0.74	0.99	1.24	1.49	1.74	1.98	2.23	2.48	2.73	2.98	3.23	3.47
90 or 90	0.25	0.50	0.75	1.00	1.25	1.50	1.75	2.00	2.25	2.50	2.75	3.00	3.25	3.50

3-2 "Power" of a Cylinder in the 90-Degree Meridian

	Cyl Power													
Cyl Axis	*0.25*	*0.50*	*0.75*	*1.00*	*1.25*	*1.50*	*1.75*	*2.00*	*2.25*	*2.50*	*2.75*	*3.00*	*3.25*	*3.50*
5 or 175	0.25	0.50	0.75	1.00	1.25	1.49	1.74	1.99	2.24	2.49	2.74	2.99	3.24	3.49
10 or 170	0.25	0.49	0.74	0.98	1.23	1.48	1.72	1.97	2.22	2.46	2.71	2.95	3.20	3.45
15 or 165	0.24	0.48	0.72	0.97	1.21	1.45	1.69	1.93	2.17	2.41	2.66	2.90	3.14	3.38
20 or 160	0.23	0.47	0.70	0.94	1.17	1.41	1.64	1.88	2.11	2.35	2.58	2.82	3.05	3.29
25 or 155	0.23	0.45	0.68	0.91	1.13	1.36	1.59	1.81	2.04	2.27	2.49	2.72	2.95	3.17
30 or 150	0.22	0.43	0.65	0.87	1.08	1.30	1.52	1.73	1.95	2.17	2.38	2.60	2.81	3.03
35 or 145	0.20	0.41	0.61	0.82	1.02	1.23	1.43	1.64	1.84	2.05	2.25	2.46	2.66	2.87
40 or 140	0.19	0.38	0.57	0.77	0.96	1.15	1.34	1.53	1.72	1.92	2.11	2.30	2.49	2.68
45 or 135	0.18	0.35	0.53	0.71	0.88	1.06	1.24	1.41	1.59	1.77	1.94	2.12	2.30	2.47
50 or 130	0.16	0.32	0.48	0.64	0.80	0.96	1.12	1.29	1.45	1.61	1.77	1.93	2.09	2.25
55 or 125	0.14	0.29	0.43	0.57	0.72	0.86	1.00	1.15	1.29	1.43	1.58	1.72	1.86	2.01
60 or 120	0.13	0.25	0.38	0.50	0.63	0.75	0.88	1.00	1.13	1.25	1.38	1.50	1.63	1.75
65 or 115	0.11	0.21	0.32	0.42	0.53	0.63	0.74	0.85	0.95	1.06	1.16	1.27	1.37	1.48
70 or 110	0.09	0.17	0.26	0.34	0.43	0.51	0.60	0.68	0.77	0.86	0.94	1.03	1.11	1.20
75 or 105	0.06	0.13	0.19	0.26	0.32	0.39	0.45	0.52	0.58	0.65	0.71	0.78	0.84	0.91
80 or 100	0.04	0.09	0.13	0.17	0.22	0.26	0.30	0.35	0.39	0.43	0.48	0.52	0.56	0.61
85 or 95	0.02	0.04	0.07	0.09	0.11	0.13	0.15	0.17	0.20	0.22	0.24	0.26	0.28	0.31
90 or 90	0.00	0.00	0.00	0.00	0.00	0.00	0.00	0.00	0.00	0.00	0.00	0.00	0.00	0.00

these appear to be tables of Cos!
should be Cos² ??

3-3 Compensated Power Referenced to 1.53 Tool Index

Rx Power	CR-39 Plastic 1.498	Crown Glass 1.523	High-Index Plastic		Polycarb 1.586	High-Index		
			1.556	1.578		1.6	1.7	1.8
0.125	0.13	0.13	0.12	0.11	0.11	0.11	0.09	0.08
0.250	0.27	0.25	0.24	0.23	0.23	0.22	0.19	0.17
0.375	0.40	0.38	0.36	0.34	0.34	0.33	0.28	0.25
0.500	0.53	0.51	0.48	0.46	0.45	0.44	0.38	0.33
0.625	0.67	0.63	0.60	0.57	0.57	0.55	0.47	0.41
0.750	0.80	0.76	0.71	0.69	0.68	0.66	0.57	0.50
0.875	0.93	0.89	0.83	0.80	0.79	0.77	0.66	0.58
1.000	1.06	1.01	0.95	0.92	0.90	0.88	0.76	0.66
1.125	1.20	1.14	1.07	1.03	1.02	0.99	0.85	0.75
1.250	1.33	1.27	1.19	1.15	1.13	1.10	0.95	0.83
1.375	1.46	1.39	1.31	1.26	1.24	1.21	1.04	0.91
1.500	1.60	1.52	1.43	1.38	1.36	1.33	1.14	0.99
1.625	1.73	1.65	1.55	1.49	1.47	1.44	1.23	1.08
1.750	1.86	1.77	1.67	1.60	1.58	1.55	1.33	1.16
1.875	2.00	1.90	1.79	1.72	1.70	1.66	1.42	1.24
2.000	2.13	2.03	1.91	1.83	1.81	1.77	1.51	1.33
2.125	2.26	2.15	2.03	1.95	1.92	1.88	1.61	1.41
2.250	2.39	2.28	2.14	2.06	2.03	1.99	1.70	1.49
2.375	2.53	2.41	2.26	2.18	2.15	2.10	1.80	1.57
2.500	2.66	2.53	2.38	2.29	2.26	2.21	1.89	1.66
2.625	2.79	2.66	2.50	2.41	2.37	2.32	1.99	1.74
2.750	2.93	2.79	2.62	2.52	2.49	2.43	2.08	1.82
2.875	3.06	2.91	2.74	2.64	2.60	2.54	2.18	1.90
3.000	3.19	3.04	2.86	2.75	2.71	2.65	2.27	1.99
3.125	3.33	3.17	2.98	2.87	2.83	2.76	2.37	2.07
3.250	3.46	3.29	3.10	2.98	2.94	2.87	2.46	2.15
3.375	3.59	3.42	3.22	3.09	3.05	2.98	2.56	2.24
3.500	3.72	3.55	3.34	3.21	3.17	3.09	2.65	2.32
3.625	3.86	3.67	3.46	3.32	3.28	3.20	2.74	2.40
3.750	3.99	3.80	3.57	3.44	3.39	3.31	2.84	2.48
3.875	4.12	3.93	3.69	3.55	3.50	3.42	2.93	2.57
4.000	4.26	4.05	3.81	3.67	3.62	3.53	3.03	2.65
4.125	4.39	4.18	3.93	3.78	3.73	3.64	3.12	2.73
4.250	4.52	4.31	4.05	3.90	3.84	3.75	3.22	2.82
4.375	4.66	4.43	4.17	4.01	3.96	3.86	3.31	2.90
4.500	4.79	4.56	4.29	4.13	4.07	3.98	3.41	2.98
4.625	4.92	4.69	4.41	4.24	4.18	4.09	3.50	3.06
4.750	5.06	4.81	4.53	4.36	4.30	4.20	3.60	3.15
4.875	5.19	4.94	4.65	4.47	4.41	4.31	3.69	3.23
5.000	5.32	5.07	4.77	4.58	4.52	4.42	3.79	3.31
5.125	5.45	5.19	4.89	4.70	4.64	4.53	3.88	3.40
5.250	5.59	5.32	5.00	4.81	4.75	4.64	3.98	3.48
5.375	5.72	5.45	5.12	4.93	4.86	4.75	4.07	3.56
5.500	5.85	5.57	5.24	5.04	4.97	4.86	4.16	3.64
5.625	5.99	5.70	5.36	5.16	5.09	4.97	4.26	3.73
5.750	6.12	5.83	5.48	5.27	5.20	5.08	4.35	3.81
5.875	6.25	5.95	5.60	5.39	5.31	5.19	4.45	3.89

3-3 Compensated Power Referenced to 1.53 Tool Index *(Continued)*

Rx Power	CR-39 Plastic 1.498	Crown Glass 1.523	High-Index Plastic		Polycarb 1.586	High-Index		
			1.556	1.578		1.6	1.7	1.8
6.000	6.39	6.08	5.72	5.50	5.43	5.30	4.54	3.98
6.125	6.52	6.21	5.84	5.62	5.54	5.41	4.64	4.06
6.250	6.65	6.33	5.96	5.73	5.65	5.52	4.73	4.14
6.375	6.78	6.46	6.08	5.85	5.77	5.63	4.83	4.22
6.500	6.92	6.59	6.20	5.96	5.88	5.74	4.92	4.31
6.625	7.05	6.71	6.32	6.07	5.99	5.85	5.02	4.39
6.750	7.18	6.84	6.43	6.19	6.10	5.96	5.11	4.47
6.875	7.32	6.97	6.55	6.30	6.22	6.07	5.21	4.55
7.000	7.45	7.09	6.67	6.42	6.33	6.18	5.30	4.64
7.125	7.58	7.22	6.79	6.53	6.44	6.29	5.39	4.72
7.250	7.72	7.35	6.91	6.65	6.56	6.40	5.49	4.80
7.375	7.85	7.47	7.03	6.76	6.67	6.51	5.58	4.89
7.500	7.98	7.60	7.15	6.88	6.78	6.63	5.68	4.97
7.625	8.11	7.73	7.27	6.99	6.90	6.74	5.77	5.05
7.750	8.25	7.85	7.39	7.11	7.01	6.85	5.87	5.13
7.875	8.38	7.98	7.51	7.22	7.12	6.96	5.96	5.22
8.000	8.51	8.11	7.63	7.34	7.24	7.07	6.06	5.30
8.125	8.65	8.23	7.75	7.45	7.35	7.18	6.15	5.38
8.250	8.78	8.36	7.86	7.56	7.46	7.29	6.25	5.47
8.375	8.91	8.49	7.98	7.68	7.57	7.40	6.34	5.55
8.500	9.05	8.61	8.10	7.79	7.69	7.51	6.44	5.63
8.625	9.18	8.74	8.22	7.91	7.80	7.62	6.53	5.71
8.750	9.31	8.87	8.34	8.02	7.91	7.73	6.63	5.80
8.875	9.45	8.99	8.46	8.14	8.03	7.84	6.72	5.88
9.000	9.58	9.12	8.58	8.25	8.14	7.95	6.81	5.96
9.125	9.71	9.25	8.70	8.37	8.25	8.06	6.91	6.05
9.250	9.84	9.37	8.82	8.48	8.37	8.17	7.00	6.13
9.375	9.98	9.50	8.94	8.60	8.48	8.28	7.10	6.21
9.500	10.11	9.63	9.06	8.71	8.59	8.39	7.19	6.29
9.625	10.24	9.75	9.17	8.83	8.71	8.50	7.29	6.38
9.750	10.38	9.88	9.29	8.94	8.82	8.61	7.38	6.46
9.875	10.51	10.01	9.41	9.05	8.93	8.72	7.48	6.54
10.000	10.64	10.13	9.53	9.17	9.04	8.83	7.57	6.63
10.125	10.78	10.26	9.65	9.28	9.16	8.94	7.67	6.71
10.250	10.91	10.39	9.77	9.40	9.27	9.05	7.76	6.79
10.375	11.04	10.51	9.89	9.51	9.38	9.16	7.86	6.87
10.500	11.17	10.64	10.01	9.63	9.50	9.28	7.95	6.96
10.625	11.31	10.77	10.13	9.74	9.61	9.39	8.04	7.04
10.750	11.44	10.89	10.25	9.86	9.72	9.50	8.14	7.12
10.875	11.57	11.02	10.37	9.97	9.84	9.61	8.23	7.20
11.000	11.71	11.15	10.49	10.09	9.95	9.72	8.33	7.29
11.125	11.84	11.27	10.60	10.20	10.06	9.83	8.42	7.37
11.250	11.97	11.40	10.72	10.32	10.17	9.94	8.52	7.45
11.375	12.11	11.53	10.84	10.43	10.29	10.05	8.61	7.54
11.500	12.24	11.65	10.96	10.54	10.40	10.16	8.71	7.62
11.625	12.37	11.78	11.08	10.66	10.51	10.27	8.80	7.70
11.750	12.51	11.91	11.20	10.77	10.63	10.38	8.90	7.78
11.875	12.64	12.03	11.32	10.89	10.74	10.49	8.99	7.87

3-3 (Continued)

Rx Power	CR-39 Plastic 1.498	Crown Glass 1.523	High-Index Plastic		Polycarb 1.586	High-Index		
			1.556	1.578		1.6	1.7	1.8
12.000	12.77	12.16	11.44	11.00	10.85	10.60	9.09	7.95
12.125	12.90	12.29	11.56	11.12	10.97	10.71	9.18	8.03
12.250	13.04	12.41	11.68	11.23	11.08	10.82	9.28	8.12
12.375	13.17	12.54	11.80	11.35	11.19	10.93	9.37	8.20
12.500	13.30	12.67	11.92	11.46	11.31	11.04	9.46	8.28
12.625	13.44	12.79	12.03	11.58	11.42	11.15	9.56	8.36
12.750	13.57	12.92	12.15	11.69	11.53	11.26	9.65	8.45
12.875	13.70	13.05	12.27	11.81	11.64	11.37	9.75	8.53
13.000	13.84	13.17	12.39	11.92	11.76	11.48	9.84	8.61
13.125	13.97	13.30	12.51	12.04	11.87	11.59	9.94	8.70
13.250	14.10	13.43	12.63	12.15	11.98	11.70	10.03	8.78
13.375	14.23	13.55	12.75	12.26	12.10	11.81	10.13	8.86
13.500	14.37	13.68	12.87	12.38	12.21	11.93	10.22	8.94
13.625	14.50	13.81	12.99	12.49	12.32	12.04	10.32	9.03
13.750	14.63	13.93	13.11	12.61	12.44	12.15	10.41	9.11
13.875	14.77	14.06	13.23	12.72	12.55	12.26	10.51	9.19
14.000	14.90	14.19	13.35	12.84	12.66	12.37	10.60	9.28
14.125	15.03	14.31	13.46	12.95	12.78	12.48	10.69	9.36
14.250	15.17	14.44	13.58	13.07	12.89	12.59	10.79	9.44
14.375	15.30	14.57	13.70	13.18	13.00	12.70	10.88	9.52
14.500	15.43	14.69	13.82	13.30	13.11	12.81	10.98	9.61
14.625	15.56	14.82	13.94	13.41	13.23	12.92	11.07	9.69
14.750	15.70	14.95	14.06	13.53	13.34	13.03	11.17	9.77
14.875	15.83	15.07	14.18	13.64	13.45	13.14	11.26	9.85
15.000	15.96	15.20	14.30	13.75	13.57	13.25	11.36	9.94
15.125	16.10	15.33	14.42	13.87	13.68	13.36	11.45	10.02
15.250	16.23	15.45	14.54	13.98	13.79	13.47	11.55	10.10
15.375	16.36	15.58	14.66	14.10	13.91	13.58	11.64	10.19
15.500	16.50	15.71	14.78	14.21	14.02	13.69	11.74	10.27
15.625	16.63	15.83	14.89	14.33	14.13	13.80	11.83	10.35
15.750	16.76	15.96	15.01	14.44	14.24	13.91	11.93	10.43
15.875	16.90	16.09	15.13	14.56	14.36	14.02	12.02	10.52
16.000	17.03	16.21	15.25	14.67	14.47	14.13	12.11	10.60
16.125	17.16	16.34	15.37	14.79	14.58	14.24	12.21	10.68
16.250	17.29	16.47	15.49	14.90	14.70	14.35	12.30	10.77
16.375	17.43	16.59	15.61	15.02	14.81	14.46	12.40	10.85
16.500	17.56	16.72	15.73	15.13	14.92	14.58	12.49	10.93
16.625	17.69	16.85	15.85	15.24	15.04	14.69	12.59	11.01
16.750	17.83	16.97	15.97	15.36	15.15	14.80	12.68	11.10
16.875	17.96	17.10	16.09	15.47	15.26	14.91	12.78	11.18
17.000	18.09	17.23	16.21	15.59	15.38	15.02	12.87	11.26
17.125	18.23	17.35	16.32	15.70	15.49	15.13	12.97	11.35
17.250	18.36	17.48	16.44	15.82	15.60	15.24	13.06	11.43
17.375	18.49	17.61	16.56	15.93	15.71	15.35	13.16	11.51
17.500	18.62	17.73	16.68	16.05	15.83	15.46	13.25	11.59
17.625	18.76	17.86	16.80	16.16	15.94	15.57	13.34	11.68
17.750	18.89	17.99	16.92	16.28	16.05	15.68	13.44	11.76
17.875	19.02	18.11	17.04	16.39	16.17	15.79	13.53	11.84

3-3 Compensated Power Referenced to 1.53 Tool Index *(Continued)*

Rx Power	CR-39 Plastic 1.498	Crown Glass 1.523	High-Index Plastic		Polycarb 1.586	High-Index		
			1.556	1.578		1.6	1.7	1.8
18.000	19.16	18.24	17.16	16.51	16.28	15.90	13.63	11.93
18.125	19.29	18.37	17.28	16.62	16.39	16.01	13.72	12.01
18.250	19.42	18.49	17.40	16.73	16.51	16.12	13.82	12.09
18.375	19.56	18.62	17.52	16.85	16.62	16.23	13.91	12.17
18.500	19.69	18.75	17.63	16.96	16.73	16.34	14.01	12.26
18.625	19.82	18.87	17.75	17.08	16.85	16.45	14.10	12.34
18.750	19.95	19.00	17.87	17.19	16.96	16.56	14.20	12.42
18.875	20.09	19.13	17.99	17.31	17.07	16.67	14.29	12.50
19.000	20.22	19.25	18.11	17.42	17.18	16.78	14.39	12.59
19.125	20.35	19.38	18.23	17.54	17.30	16.89	14.48	12.67
19.250	20.49	19.51	18.35	17.65	17.41	17.00	14.58	12.75
19.375	20.62	19.63	18.47	17.77	17.52	17.11	14.67	12.84
19.500	20.75	19.76	18.59	17.88	17.64	17.23	14.76	12.92
19.625	20.89	19.89	18.71	18.00	17.75	17.34	14.86	13.00
19.750	21.02	20.01	18.83	18.11	17.86	17.45	14.95	13.08
19.875	21.15	20.14	18.95	18.22	17.98	17.56	15.05	13.17
20.000	21.29	20.27	19.06	18.34	18.09	17.67	15.14	13.25

3-4 Vertex Distance Compensation (plus lens moved toward the eye or minus lens moved away from the eye)

Change in Vertex Distance, mm

Rx Power	1	2	3	4	5	6	7	8	9	10	11	12	13	14	15
6.00	6.04	6.07	6.11	6.15	6.19	6.22	6.26	6.30	6.34	6.38	6.42	6.47	6.51	6.55	6.59
6.25	6.29	6.33	6.37	6.41	6.45	6.49	6.54	6.58	6.62	6.67	6.71	6.76	6.80	6.85	6.90
6.50	6.54	6.59	6.63	6.67	6.72	6.76	6.81	6.86	6.90	6.95	7.00	7.05	7.10	7.15	7.20
6.75	6.80	6.84	6.89	6.94	6.99	7.03	7.08	7.14	7.19	7.24	7.29	7.34	7.40	7.45	7.51
7.00	7.05	7.10	7.15	7.20	7.25	7.31	7.36	7.42	7.47	7.53	7.58	7.64	7.70	7.76	7.82
7.25	7.30	7.36	7.41	7.47	7.52	7.58	7.64	7.70	7.76	7.82	7.88	7.94	8.00	8.07	8.13
7.50	7.56	7.61	7.67	7.73	7.79	7.85	7.92	7.98	8.04	8.11	8.17	8.24	8.31	8.38	8.45
7.75	7.81	7.87	7.93	8.00	8.06	8.13	8.19	8.26	8.33	8.40	8.47	8.54	8.62	8.69	8.77
8.00	8.06	8.13	8.20	8.26	8.33	8.40	8.47	8.55	8.62	8.70	8.77	8.85	8.93	9.01	9.09
8.25	8.32	8.39	8.46	8.53	8.60	8.68	8.76	8.83	8.91	8.99	9.07	9.16	9.24	9.33	9.42
8.50	8.57	8.65	8.72	8.80	8.88	8.96	9.04	9.12	9.20	9.29	9.38	9.47	9.56	9.65	9.74
8.75	8.83	8.91	8.99	9.07	9.15	9.23	9.32	9.41	9.50	9.59	9.68	9.78	9.87	9.97	10.07
9.00	9.08	9.16	9.25	9.34	9.42	9.51	9.61	9.70	9.79	9.89	9.99	10.09	10.19	10.30	10.40
9.25	9.34	9.42	9.51	9.61	9.70	9.79	9.89	9.99	10.09	10.19	10.30	10.40	10.51	10.63	10.74
9.50	9.59	9.68	9.78	9.88	9.97	10.07	10.18	10.28	10.39	10.50	10.61	10.72	10.84	10.96	11.08
9.75	9.85	9.94	10.04	10.15	10.25	10.36	10.46	10.57	10.69	10.80	10.92	11.04	11.17	11.29	11.42
10.00	10.10	10.20	10.31	10.42	10.53	10.64	10.75	10.87	10.99	11.11	11.24	11.36	11.49	11.63	11.76
10.25	10.36	10.46	10.58	10.69	10.80	10.92	11.04	11.17	11.29	11.42	11.55	11.69	11.83	11.97	12.11
10.50	10.61	10.73	10.84	10.96	11.08	11.21	11.33	11.46	11.60	11.73	11.87	12.01	12.16	12.31	12.46
10.75	10.87	10.99	11.11	11.23	11.36	11.49	11.62	11.76	11.90	12.04	12.19	12.34	12.50	12.65	12.82
11.00	11.12	11.25	11.38	11.51	11.64	11.78	11.92	12.06	12.21	12.36	12.51	12.67	12.84	13.00	13.17
11.25	11.38	11.51	11.64	11.78	11.92	12.06	12.21	12.36	12.52	12.68	12.84	13.01	13.18	13.35	13.53
11.50	11.63	11.77	11.91	12.05	12.20	12.35	12.51	12.67	12.83	12.99	13.17	13.34	13.52	13.71	13.90
11.75	11.89	12.03	12.18	12.33	12.48	12.64	12.80	12.97	13.14	13.31	13.49	13.68	13.87	14.06	14.26
12.00	12.15	12.30	12.45	12.61	12.77	12.93	13.10	13.27	13.45	13.64	13.82	14.02	14.22	14.42	14.63
12.25	12.40	12.56	12.72	12.88	13.05	13.22	13.40	13.58	13.77	13.96	14.16	14.36	14.57	14.79	15.01
12.50	12.66	12.82	12.99	13.16	13.33	13.51	13.70	13.89	14.08	14.29	14.49	14.71	14.93	15.15	15.38
12.75	12.91	13.08	13.26	13.44	13.62	13.81	14.00	14.20	14.40	14.61	14.83	15.05	15.28	15.52	15.77
13.00	13.17	13.35	13.53	13.71	13.90	14.10	14.30	14.51	14.72	14.94	15.17	15.40	15.64	15.89	16.15
13.25	13.43	13.61	13.80	13.99	14.19	14.39	14.60	14.82	15.04	15.27	15.51	15.76	16.01	16.27	16.54
13.50	13.68	13.87	14.07	14.27	14.48	14.69	14.91	15.13	15.37	15.61	15.85	16.11	16.37	16.65	16.93
13.75	13.94	14.14	14.34	14.55	14.77	14.99	15.21	15.45	15.69	15.94	16.20	16.47	16.74	17.03	17.32
14.00	14.20	14.40	14.61	14.83	15.05	15.28	15.52	15.77	16.02	16.28	16.55	16.83	17.11	17.41	17.72
14.25	14.46	14.67	14.89	15.11	15.34	15.58	15.83	16.08	16.35	16.62	16.90	17.19	17.49	17.80	18.12
14.50	14.71	14.93	15.16	15.39	15.63	15.88	16.14	16.40	16.68	16.96	17.25	17.55	17.87	18.19	18.53
14.75	14.97	15.20	15.43	15.67	15.92	16.18	16.45	16.72	17.01	17.30	17.61	17.92	18.25	18.59	18.94

3-4 Vertex Distance Compensation (plus lens moved toward the eye or minus lens moved away from the eye) (Continued)

	Change in Vertex Distance, mm														
Rx Power	1	2	3	4	5	6	7	8	9	10	11	12	13	14	15
15.00	15.23	15.46	15.71	15.96	16.22	16.48	16.76	17.05	17.34	17.65	17.96	18.29	18.63	18.99	19.35
15.25	15.49	15.73	15.98	16.24	16.51	16.79	17.07	17.37	17.68	17.99	18.32	18.67	19.02	19.39	19.77
15.50	15.74	16.00	16.26	16.52	16.80	17.09	17.39	17.69	18.01	18.34	18.69	19.04	19.41	19.80	20.20
15.75	16.00	16.26	16.53	16.81	17.10	17.39	17.70	18.02	18.35	18.69	19.05	19.42	19.81	20.21	20.62
16.00	16.26	16.53	16.81	17.09	17.39	17.70	18.02	18.35	18.69	19.05	19.42	19.80	20.20	20.62	21.05
16.25	16.52	16.80	17.08	17.38	17.69	18.01	18.34	18.68	19.03	19.40	19.79	20.19	20.60	21.04	21.49
16.50	16.78	17.06	17.36	17.67	17.98	18.31	18.65	19.01	19.38	19.76	20.16	20.57	21.01	21.46	21.93
16.75	17.04	17.33	17.64	17.95	18.28	18.62	18.97	19.34	19.72	20.12	20.53	20.96	21.41	21.88	22.37
17.00	17.29	17.60	17.91	18.24	18.58	18.93	19.30	19.68	20.07	20.48	20.91	21.36	21.82	22.31	22.82
17.25	17.55	17.87	18.19	18.53	18.88	19.24	19.62	20.01	20.42	20.85	21.29	21.75	22.24	22.74	23.27
17.50	17.81	18.13	18.47	18.82	19.18	19.55	19.94	20.35	20.77	21.21	21.67	22.15	22.65	23.18	23.73
17.75	18.07	18.40	18.75	19.11	19.48	19.87	20.27	20.69	21.12	21.58	22.06	22.55	23.07	23.62	24.19
18.00	18.33	18.67	19.03	19.40	19.78	20.18	20.59	21.03	21.48	21.95	22.44	22.96	23.50	24.06	24.66
18.25	18.59	18.94	19.31	19.69	20.08	20.49	20.92	21.37	21.84	22.32	22.83	23.37	23.93	24.51	25.13
18.50	18.85	19.21	19.59	19.98	20.39	20.81	21.25	21.71	22.20	22.70	23.23	23.78	24.36	24.97	25.61
18.75	19.11	19.48	19.87	20.27	20.69	21.13	21.58	22.06	22.56	23.08	23.62	24.19	24.79	25.42	26.09
19.00	19.37	19.75	20.15	20.56	20.99	21.44	21.91	22.41	22.92	23.46	24.02	24.61	25.23	25.89	26.57
19.25	19.63	20.02	20.43	20.86	21.30	21.76	22.25	22.75	23.28	23.84	24.42	25.03	25.68	26.35	27.07
19.50	19.89	20.29	20.71	21.15	21.61	22.08	22.58	23.10	23.65	24.22	24.82	25.46	26.12	26.82	27.56
19.75	20.15	20.56	20.99	21.44	21.91	22.40	22.92	23.46	24.02	24.61	25.23	25.88	26.57	27.30	28.06
20.00	20.41	20.83	21.28	21.74	22.22	22.73	23.26	23.81	24.39	25.00	25.64	26.32	27.03	27.78	28.57
20.25	20.67	21.10	21.56	22.03	22.53	23.05	23.59	24.16	24.76	25.39	26.05	26.75	27.49	28.26	29.08
20.50	20.93	21.38	21.84	22.33	22.84	23.38	23.93	24.52	25.14	25.79	26.47	27.19	27.95	28.75	29.60
20.75	21.19	21.65	22.13	22.63	23.15	23.70	24.28	24.88	25.51	26.18	26.89	27.63	28.41	29.25	30.13
21.00	21.45	21.92	22.41	22.93	23.46	24.03	24.62	25.24	25.89	26.58	27.31	28.07	28.89	29.75	30.66
21.25	21.71	22.19	22.70	23.22	23.78	24.36	24.96	25.60	26.28	26.98	27.73	28.52	29.36	30.25	31.19
21.50	21.97	22.47	22.98	23.52	24.09	24.68	25.31	25.97	26.66	27.39	28.16	28.98	29.84	30.76	31.73
21.75	22.23	22.74	23.27	23.82	24.40	25.01	25.66	26.33	27.04	27.80	28.59	29.43	30.32	31.27	32.28
22.00	22.49	23.01	23.55	24.12	24.72	25.35	26.00	26.70	27.43	28.21	29.02	29.89	30.81	31.79	32.84
22.25	22.76	23.29	23.84	24.42	25.04	25.68	26.35	27.07	27.82	28.62	29.46	30.35	31.30	32.32	33.40
22.50	23.02	23.56	24.13	24.73	25.35	26.01	26.71	27.44	28.21	29.03	29.90	30.82	31.80	32.85	33.96
22.75	23.28	23.83	24.42	25.03	25.67	26.35	27.06	27.81	28.61	29.45	30.34	31.29	32.30	33.38	34.54
23.00	23.54	24.11	24.70	25.33	25.99	26.68	27.41	28.19	29.00	29.87	30.79	31.77	32.81	33.92	35.11

3-5 Vertex Distance Compensation (plus lens moved away from the eye or minus lens moved toward the eye)

Rx Power	Change in Vertex Distance, mm														
	1	2	3	4	5	6	7	8	9	10	11	12	13	14	15
6.00	5.96	5.93	5.89	5.86	5.83	5.79	5.76	5.73	5.69	5.66	5.63	5.60	5.57	5.54	5.50
6.25	6.21	6.17	6.13	6.10	6.06	6.02	5.99	5.95	5.92	5.88	5.85	5.81	5.78	5.75	5.71
6.50	6.46	6.42	6.38	6.34	6.30	6.26	6.22	6.18	6.14	6.10	6.07	6.03	5.99	5.96	5.92
6.75	6.70	6.66	6.62	6.57	6.53	6.49	6.45	6.40	6.36	6.32	6.28	6.24	6.21	6.17	6.13
7.00	6.95	6.90	6.86	6.81	6.76	6.72	6.67	6.63	6.59	6.54	6.50	6.46	6.42	6.38	6.33
7.25	7.20	7.15	7.10	7.05	7.00	6.95	6.90	6.85	6.81	6.76	6.71	6.67	6.63	6.58	6.54
7.50	7.44	7.39	7.33	7.28	7.23	7.18	7.13	7.08	7.03	6.98	6.93	6.88	6.83	6.79	6.74
7.75	7.69	7.63	7.57	7.52	7.46	7.41	7.35	7.30	7.24	7.19	7.14	7.09	7.04	6.99	6.94
8.00	7.94	7.87	7.81	7.75	7.69	7.63	7.58	7.52	7.46	7.41	7.35	7.30	7.25	7.19	7.14
8.25	8.18	8.12	8.05	7.99	7.92	7.86	7.80	7.74	7.68	7.62	7.56	7.51	7.45	7.40	7.34
8.50	8.43	8.36	8.29	8.22	8.15	8.09	8.02	7.96	7.90	7.83	7.77	7.71	7.65	7.60	7.54
8.75	8.67	8.60	8.53	8.45	8.38	8.31	8.24	8.18	8.11	8.05	7.98	7.92	7.86	7.80	7.73
9.00	8.92	8.84	8.76	8.69	8.61	8.54	8.47	8.40	8.33	8.26	8.19	8.12	8.06	7.99	7.93
9.25	9.17	9.08	9.00	8.92	8.84	8.76	8.69	8.61	8.54	8.47	8.40	8.33	8.26	8.19	8.12
9.50	9.41	9.32	9.24	9.15	9.07	8.99	8.91	8.83	8.75	8.68	8.60	8.53	8.46	8.38	8.32
9.75	9.66	9.56	9.47	9.38	9.30	9.21	9.13	9.04	8.96	8.88	8.81	8.73	8.65	8.58	8.51
10.00	9.90	9.80	9.71	9.62	9.52	9.43	9.35	9.26	9.17	9.09	9.01	8.93	8.85	8.77	8.70
10.25	10.15	10.04	9.94	9.85	9.75	9.66	9.56	9.47	9.38	9.30	9.21	9.13	9.04	8.96	8.88
10.50	10.39	10.28	10.18	10.08	9.98	9.88	9.78	9.69	9.59	9.50	9.41	9.33	9.24	9.15	9.07
10.75	10.64	10.52	10.41	10.31	10.20	10.10	10.00	9.90	9.80	9.71	9.61	9.52	9.43	9.34	9.26
11.00	10.88	10.76	10.65	10.54	10.43	10.32	10.21	10.11	10.01	9.91	9.81	9.72	9.62	9.53	9.44
11.25	11.12	11.00	10.88	10.77	10.65	10.54	10.43	10.32	10.22	10.11	10.01	9.91	9.81	9.72	9.63
11.50	11.37	11.24	11.12	10.99	10.87	10.76	10.64	10.53	10.42	10.31	10.21	10.11	10.00	9.91	9.81
11.75	11.61	11.48	11.35	11.22	11.10	10.98	10.86	10.74	10.63	10.51	10.41	10.30	10.19	10.09	9.99
12.00	11.86	11.72	11.58	11.45	11.32	11.19	11.07	10.95	10.83	10.71	10.60	10.49	10.38	10.27	10.17
12.25	12.10	11.96	11.82	11.68	11.54	11.41	11.28	11.16	11.03	10.91	10.80	10.68	10.57	10.46	10.35
12.50	12.35	12.20	12.05	11.90	11.76	11.63	11.49	11.36	11.24	11.11	10.99	10.87	10.75	10.64	10.53
12.75	12.59	12.43	12.28	12.13	11.99	11.84	11.71	11.57	11.44	11.31	11.18	11.06	10.94	10.82	10.70
13.00	12.83	12.67	12.51	12.36	12.21	12.06	11.92	11.78	11.64	11.50	11.37	11.25	11.12	11.00	10.88
13.25	13.08	12.91	12.74	12.58	12.43	12.27	12.13	11.98	11.84	11.70	11.56	11.43	11.30	11.18	11.05
13.50	13.32	13.15	12.97	12.81	12.65	12.49	12.33	12.18	12.04	11.89	11.75	11.62	11.48	11.35	11.23
13.75	13.56	13.38	13.21	13.03	12.87	12.70	12.54	12.39	12.24	12.09	11.94	11.80	11.66	11.53	11.40
14.00	13.81	13.62	13.44	13.26	13.08	12.92	12.75	12.59	12.43	12.28	12.13	11.99	11.84	11.71	11.57
14.25	14.05	13.86	13.67	13.48	13.30	13.13	12.96	12.79	12.63	12.47	12.32	12.17	12.02	11.88	11.74
14.50	14.29	14.09	13.90	13.71	13.52	13.34	13.16	12.99	12.83	12.66	12.51	12.35	12.20	12.05	11.91
14.75	14.54	14.33	14.12	13.93	13.74	13.55	13.37	13.19	13.02	12.85	12.69	12.53	12.38	12.23	12.08

3-5 Vertex Distance Compensation (plus lens moved away from the eye or minus lens moved toward the eye) (Continued)

	Change in Vertex Distance, mm														
Rx Power	1	2	3	4	5	6	7	8	9	10	11	12	13	14	15
15.00	14.78	14.56	14.35	14.15	13.95	13.76	13.57	13.39	13.22	13.04	12.88	12.71	12.55	12.40	12.24
15.25	15.02	14.80	14.58	14.37	14.17	13.97	13.78	13.59	13.41	13.23	13.06	12.89	12.73	12.57	12.41
15.50	15.26	15.03	14.81	14.60	14.39	14.18	13.98	13.79	13.60	13.42	13.24	13.07	12.90	12.74	12.58
15.75	15.51	15.27	15.04	14.82	14.60	14.39	14.19	13.99	13.79	13.61	13.42	13.25	13.07	12.90	12.74
16.00	15.75	15.50	15.27	15.04	14.81	14.60	14.39	14.18	13.99	13.79	13.61	13.42	13.25	13.07	12.90
16.25	15.99	15.74	15.49	15.26	15.03	14.81	14.59	14.38	14.18	13.98	13.79	13.60	13.42	13.24	13.07
16.50	16.23	15.97	15.72	15.48	15.24	15.01	14.79	14.58	14.37	14.16	13.97	13.77	13.59	13.40	13.23
16.75	16.47	16.21	15.95	15.70	15.46	15.22	14.99	14.77	14.56	14.35	14.14	13.95	13.75	13.57	13.39
17.00	16.72	16.44	16.18	15.92	15.67	15.43	15.19	14.96	14.74	14.53	14.32	14.12	13.92	13.73	13.55
17.25	16.96	16.67	16.40	16.14	15.88	15.63	15.39	15.16	14.93	14.71	14.50	14.29	14.09	13.89	13.70
17.50	17.20	16.91	16.63	16.36	16.09	15.84	15.59	15.35	15.12	14.89	14.68	14.46	14.26	14.06	13.86
17.75	17.44	17.14	16.85	16.57	16.30	16.04	15.79	15.54	15.31	15.07	14.85	14.63	14.42	14.22	14.02
18.00	17.68	17.37	17.08	16.79	16.51	16.25	15.99	15.73	15.49	15.25	15.03	14.80	14.59	14.38	14.17
18.25	17.92	17.61	17.30	17.01	16.72	16.45	16.18	15.92	15.68	15.43	15.20	14.97	14.75	14.54	14.33
18.50	18.16	17.84	17.53	17.23	16.93	16.65	16.38	16.11	15.86	15.61	15.37	15.14	14.91	14.69	14.48
18.75	18.40	18.07	17.75	17.44	17.14	16.85	16.57	16.30	16.04	15.79	15.54	15.31	15.08	14.85	14.63
19.00	18.65	18.30	17.98	17.66	17.35	17.06	16.77	16.49	16.23	15.97	15.72	15.47	15.24	15.01	14.79
19.25	18.89	18.54	18.20	17.87	17.56	17.26	16.96	16.68	16.41	16.14	15.89	15.64	15.40	15.16	14.94
19.50	19.13	18.77	18.42	18.09	17.77	17.46	17.16	16.87	16.59	16.32	16.06	15.80	15.56	15.32	15.09
19.75	19.37	19.00	18.65	18.30	17.97	17.66	17.35	17.06	16.77	16.49	16.23	15.97	15.72	15.47	15.24
20.00	19.61	19.23	18.87	18.52	18.18	17.86	17.54	17.24	16.95	16.67	16.39	16.13	15.87	15.63	15.38
20.25	19.85	19.46	19.09	18.73	18.39	18.06	17.74	17.43	17.13	16.84	16.56	16.29	16.03	15.78	15.53
20.50	20.09	19.69	19.31	18.95	18.59	18.25	17.93	17.61	17.31	17.01	16.73	16.45	16.19	15.93	15.68
20.75	20.33	19.92	19.53	19.16	18.80	18.45	18.12	17.80	17.48	17.18	16.89	16.61	16.34	16.08	15.82
21.00	20.57	20.15	19.76	19.37	19.00	18.65	18.31	17.98	17.66	17.36	17.06	16.77	16.50	16.23	15.97
21.25	20.81	20.38	19.98	19.59	19.21	18.85	18.50	18.16	17.84	17.53	17.22	16.93	16.65	16.38	16.11
21.50	21.05	20.61	20.20	19.80	19.41	19.04	18.69	18.34	18.01	17.70	17.39	17.09	16.80	16.53	16.26
21.75	21.29	20.84	20.42	20.01	19.62	19.24	18.88	18.53	18.19	17.86	17.55	17.25	16.96	16.67	16.40
22.00	21.53	21.07	20.64	20.22	19.82	19.43	19.06	18.71	18.36	18.03	17.71	17.41	17.11	16.82	16.54
22.25	21.77	21.30	20.86	20.43	20.02	19.63	19.25	18.89	18.54	18.20	17.88	17.56	17.26	16.97	16.68
22.50	22.00	21.53	21.08	20.64	20.22	19.82	19.44	19.07	18.71	18.37	18.04	17.72	17.41	17.11	16.82
22.75	22.24	21.76	21.30	20.85	20.43	20.02	19.62	19.25	18.88	18.53	18.20	17.87	17.56	17.25	16.96
23.00	22.48	21.99	21.52	21.06	20.63	20.21	19.81	19.43	19.06	18.70	18.36	18.03	17.71	17.40	17.10

Appendix

4

Lens Thickness

4-1 1.53 Tool Index Sag Chart for Various Chord Diameters

(D)	10	12	14	16	18	20	22	24	26	28	30	32	34	36	38	40	42	44	46
0.25	0.0	0.0	0.0	0.0	0.0	0.0	0.0	0.0	0.0	0.0	0.1	0.1	0.1	0.1	0.1	0.1	0.1	0.1	0.1
0.50	0.0	0.0	0.0	0.0	0.0	0.0	0.1	0.1	0.1	0.1	0.1	0.1	0.1	0.2	0.2	0.2	0.2	0.2	0.2
0.75	0.0	0.0	0.0	0.0	0.1	0.1	0.1	0.1	0.1	0.1	0.2	0.2	0.2	0.2	0.3	0.3	0.3	0.3	0.4
1.00	0.0	0.0	0.0	0.1	0.1	0.1	0.1	0.1	0.2	0.2	0.2	0.2	0.3	0.3	0.3	0.4	0.4	0.5	0.5
1.25	0.0	0.0	0.1	0.1	0.1	0.1	0.1	0.2	0.2	0.2	0.3	0.3	0.3	0.4	0.4	0.5	0.5	0.6	0.6
1.50	0.0	0.1	0.1	0.1	0.1	0.1	0.2	0.2	0.2	0.3	0.3	0.4	0.4	0.5	0.5	0.6	0.6	0.7	0.7
1.75	0.0	0.1	0.1	0.1	0.1	0.2	0.2	0.2	0.3	0.3	0.4	0.4	0.5	0.5	0.6	0.7	0.7	0.8	0.9
2.00	0.0	0.1	0.1	0.1	0.2	0.2	0.2	0.3	0.3	0.4	0.4	0.5	0.5	0.6	0.7	0.8	0.8	0.9	1.0
2.25	0.1	0.1	0.1	0.1	0.2	0.2	0.3	0.3	0.4	0.4	0.5	0.5	0.6	0.7	0.8	0.9	0.9	1.0	1.1
2.50	0.1	0.1	0.1	0.2	0.2	0.2	0.3	0.3	0.4	0.5	0.5	0.6	0.7	0.8	0.9	0.9	1.0	1.1	1.3
2.75	0.1	0.1	0.1	0.2	0.2	0.3	0.3	0.4	0.4	0.5	0.6	0.7	0.8	0.8	0.9	1.0	1.1	1.3	1.4
3.00	0.1	0.1	0.1	0.2	0.2	0.3	0.3	0.4	0.5	0.6	0.6	0.7	0.8	0.9	1.0	1.1	1.3	1.4	1.5
3.25	0.1	0.1	0.2	0.2	0.2	0.3	0.4	0.4	0.5	0.6	0.7	0.8	0.9	1.0	1.1	1.2	1.4	1.5	1.6
3.50	0.1	0.1	0.2	0.2	0.3	0.3	0.4	0.5	0.6	0.6	0.7	0.8	1.0	1.1	1.2	1.3	1.5	1.6	1.8
3.75	0.1	0.1	0.2	0.2	0.3	0.4	0.4	0.5	0.6	0.7	0.8	0.9	1.0	1.2	1.3	1.4	1.6	1.7	1.9
4.00	0.1	0.1	0.2	0.2	0.3	0.4	0.5	0.5	0.6	0.7	0.9	1.0	1.1	1.2	1.4	1.5	1.7	1.8	2.0
4.25	0.1	0.1	0.2	0.3	0.3	0.4	0.5	0.6	0.7	0.8	0.9	1.0	1.2	1.3	1.5	1.6	1.8	2.0	2.1
4.50	0.1	0.2	0.2	0.3	0.3	0.4	0.5	0.6	0.7	0.8	1.0	1.1	1.2	1.4	1.5	1.7	1.9	2.1	2.3
4.75	0.1	0.2	0.2	0.3	0.4	0.4	0.5	0.6	0.8	0.9	1.0	1.2	1.3	1.5	1.6	1.8	2.0	2.2	2.4
5.00	0.1	0.2	0.2	0.3	0.4	0.5	0.6	0.7	0.8	0.9	1.1	1.2	1.4	1.5	1.7	1.9	2.1	2.3	2.5
5.25	0.1	0.2	0.2	0.3	0.4	0.5	0.6	0.7	0.8	1.0	1.1	1.3	1.4	1.6	1.8	2.0	2.2	2.4	2.7
5.50	0.1	0.2	0.3	0.3	0.4	0.5	0.6	0.8	0.9	1.0	1.2	1.3	1.5	1.7	1.9	2.1	2.3	2.5	2.8
5.75	0.1	0.2	0.3	0.3	0.4	0.5	0.7	0.8	0.9	1.1	1.2	1.4	1.6	1.8	2.0	2.2	2.4	2.7	2.9
6.00	0.1	0.2	0.3	0.4	0.5	0.6	0.7	0.8	1.0	1.1	1.3	1.5	1.7	1.9	2.1	2.3	2.5	2.8	3.0
6.25	0.1	0.2	0.3	0.4	0.5	0.6	0.7	0.9	1.0	1.2	1.3	1.5	1.7	1.9	2.2	2.4	2.6	2.9	3.2
6.50	0.2	0.2	0.3	0.4	0.5	0.6	0.7	0.9	1.0	1.2	1.4	1.6	1.8	2.0	2.2	2.5	2.8	3.0	3.3
6.75	0.2	0.2	0.3	0.4	0.5	0.6	0.8	0.9	1.1	1.3	1.4	1.6	1.9	2.1	2.3	2.6	2.9	3.1	3.4
7.00	0.2	0.2	0.3	0.4	0.5	0.7	0.8	1.0	1.1	1.3	1.5	1.7	1.9	2.2	2.4	2.7	3.0	3.3	3.6
7.25	0.2	0.2	0.3	0.4	0.6	0.7	0.8	1.0	1.2	1.4	1.6	1.8	2.0	2.3	2.5	2.8	3.1	3.4	3.7
7.75	0.2	0.3	0.4	0.5	0.6	0.7	0.9	1.1	1.2	1.4	1.7	1.9	2.1	2.4	2.7	3.0	3.3	3.6	4.0
8.00	0.2	0.3	0.4	0.5	0.6	0.8	0.9	1.1	1.3	1.5	1.7	2.0	2.2	2.5	2.8	3.1	3.4	3.8	4.1
8.25	0.2	0.3	0.4	0.5	0.6	0.8	0.9	1.1	1.3	1.5	1.8	2.0	2.3	2.6	2.9	3.2	3.5	3.9	4.3
8.50	0.2	0.3	0.4	0.5	0.7	0.8	1.0	1.2	1.4	1.6	1.8	2.1	2.4	2.7	3.0	3.3	3.6	4.0	4.4
8.75	0.2	0.3	0.4	0.5	0.7	0.8	1.0	1.2	1.4	1.6	1.9	2.2	2.4	2.7	3.1	3.4	3.8	4.1	4.5
9.00	0.2	0.3	0.4	0.5	0.7	0.9	1.0	1.2	1.5	1.7	1.9	2.2	2.5	2.8	3.1	3.5	3.9	4.3	4.7
9.25	0.2	0.3	0.4	0.6	0.7	0.9	1.1	1.3	1.5	1.7	2.0	2.3	2.6	2.9	3.2	3.6	4.0	4.4	4.8
9.50	0.2	0.3	0.4	0.6	0.7	0.9	1.1	1.3	1.5	1.8	2.1	2.3	2.7	3.0	3.3	3.7	4.1	4.5	5.0
9.75	0.2	0.3	0.5	0.6	0.8	0.9	1.1	1.3	1.6	1.8	2.1	2.4	2.7	3.1	3.4	3.8	4.2	4.7	5.1
10.00	0.2	0.3	0.5	0.6	0.8	1.0	1.2	1.4	1.6	1.9	2.2	2.5	2.8	3.2	3.5	3.9	4.3	4.8	5.3
10.25	0.2	0.3	0.5	0.6	0.8	1.0	1.2	1.4	1.7	1.9	2.2	2.5	2.9	3.2	3.6	4.0	4.5	4.9	5.4
10.50	0.2	0.4	0.5	0.6	0.8	1.0	1.2	1.4	1.7	2.0	2.3	2.6	2.9	3.3	3.7	4.1	4.6	5.0	5.5
11.00	0.3	0.4	0.5	0.7	0.8	1.0	1.3	1.5	1.8	2.1	2.4	2.7	3.1	3.5	3.9	4.3	4.8	5.3	5.8
11.50	0.3	0.4	0.5	0.7	0.9	1.1	1.3	1.6	1.9	2.2	2.5	2.9	3.2	3.7	4.1	4.6	5.1	5.6	6.1
12.00	0.3	0.4	0.6	0.7	0.9	1.1	1.4	1.7	2.0	2.3	2.6	3.0	3.4	3.8	4.3	4.8	5.3	5.9	6.5
12.50	0.3	0.4	0.6	0.8	1.0	1.2	1.5	1.7	2.0	2.4	2.7	3.1	3.6	4.0	4.5	5.0	5.6	6.2	6.8

48	50	52	54	56	58	60	62	64	66	68	70	72	74	76	78	80	82	84	86
0.1	0.1	0.2	0.2	0.2	0.2	0.2	0.2	0.2	0.3	0.3	0.3	0.3	0.3	0.3	0.4	0.4	0.4	0.4	0.4
0.3	0.3	0.3	0.3	0.4	0.4	0.4	0.5	0.5	0.5	0.5	0.6	0.6	0.6	0.7	0.7	0.8	0.8	0.8	0.9
0.4	0.4	0.5	0.5	0.6	0.6	0.6	0.7	0.7	0.8	0.8	0.9	0.9	1.0	1.0	1.1	1.1	1.2	1.2	1.3
0.5	0.6	0.6	0.7	0.7	0.8	0.8	0.9	1.0	1.0	1.1	1.2	1.2	1.3	1.4	1.4	1.5	1.6	1.7	1.7
0.7	0.7	0.8	0.9	0.9	1.0	1.1	1.1	1.2	1.3	1.4	1.4	1.5	1.6	1.7	1.8	1.9	2.0	2.1	2.2
0.8	0.9	1.0	1.0	1.1	1.2	1.3	1.4	1.5	1.5	1.6	1.7	1.8	1.9	2.0	2.2	2.3	2.4	2.5	2.6
1.0	1.0	1.1	1.2	1.3	1.4	1.5	1.6	1.7	1.8	1.9	2.0	2.1	2.3	2.4	2.5	2.7	2.8	2.9	3.1
1.1	1.2	1.3	1.4	1.5	1.6	1.7	1.8	1.9	2.1	2.2	2.3	2.5	2.6	2.7	2.9	3.0	3.2	3.3	3.5
1.2	1.3	1.4	1.6	1.7	1.8	1.9	2.0	2.2	2.3	2.5	2.6	2.8	2.9	3.1	3.3	3.4	3.6	3.8	4.0
1.4	1.5	1.6	1.7	1.9	2.0	2.1	2.3	2.4	2.6	2.7	2.9	3.1	3.3	3.4	3.6	3.8	4.0	4.2	4.4
1.5	1.6	1.8	1.9	2.0	2.2	2.3	2.5	2.7	2.8	3.0	3.2	3.4	3.6	3.8	4.0	4.2	4.4	4.6	4.9
1.6	1.8	1.9	2.1	2.2	2.4	2.6	2.7	2.9	3.1	3.3	3.5	3.7	3.9	4.1	4.4	4.6	4.8	5.1	5.3
1.8	1.9	2.1	2.3	2.4	2.6	2.8	3.0	3.2	3.4	3.6	3.8	4.0	4.3	4.5	4.7	5.0	5.2	5.5	5.8
1.9	2.1	2.2	2.4	2.6	2.8	3.0	3.2	3.4	3.6	3.9	4.1	4.3	4.6	4.8	5.1	5.4	5.7	5.9	6.2
2.1	2.2	2.4	2.6	2.8	3.0	3.2	3.4	3.7	3.9	4.2	4.4	4.7	4.9	5.2	5.5	5.8	6.1	6.4	6.7
2.2	2.4	2.6	2.8	3.0	3.2	3.4	3.7	3.9	4.2	4.4	4.7	5.0	5.3	5.6	5.9	6.2	6.5	6.8	7.2
2.3	2.5	2.7	3.0	3.2	3.4	3.7	3.9	4.2	4.4	4.7	5.0	5.3	5.6	5.9	6.3	6.6	6.9	7.3	7.6
2.5	2.7	2.9	3.1	3.4	3.6	3.9	4.2	4.4	4.7	5.0	5.3	5.6	6.0	6.3	6.6	7.0	7.4	7.7	8.1
2.6	2.8	3.1	3.3	3.6	3.8	4.1	4.4	4.7	5.0	5.3	5.6	6.0	6.3	6.7	7.0	7.4	7.8	8.2	8.6
2.8	3.0	3.2	3.5	3.8	4.0	4.3	4.6	4.9	5.3	5.6	5.9	6.3	6.7	7.0	7.4	7.8	8.3	8.7	9.1
2.9	3.1	3.4	3.7	4.0	4.3	4.6	4.9	5.2	5.5	5.9	6.3	6.6	7.0	7.4	7.8	8.3	8.7	9.2	9.6
3.0	3.3	3.6	3.9	4.2	4.5	4.8	5.1	5.5	5.8	6.2	6.6	7.0	7.4	7.8	8.2	8.7	9.2	9.6	10.1
3.2	3.5	3.7	4.0	4.4	4.7	5.0	5.4	5.7	6.1	6.5	6.9	7.3	7.8	8.2	8.7	9.1	9.6	10.1	10.6
3.3	3.6	3.9	4.2	4.6	4.9	5.3	5.6	6.0	6.4	6.8	7.2	7.7	8.1	8.6	9.1	9.6	10.1	10.6	11.2
3.5	3.8	4.1	4.4	4.8	5.1	5.5	5.9	6.3	6.7	7.1	7.6	8.0	8.5	9.0	9.5	10.0	10.6	11.1	11.7
3.6	3.9	4.3	4.6	5.0	5.3	5.7	6.1	6.5	7.0	7.4	7.9	8.4	8.9	9.4	9.9	10.5	11.1	11.6	12.3
3.8	4.1	4.4	4.8	5.2	5.6	6.0	6.4	6.8	7.3	7.7	8.2	8.7	9.3	9.8	10.4	11.0	11.6	12.2	12.8
3.9	4.2	4.6	5.0	5.4	5.8	6.2	6.6	7.1	7.6	8.1	8.6	9.1	9.7	10.2	10.8	11.4	12.1	12.7	13.4
4.1	4.4	4.8	5.2	5.6	6.0	6.4	6.9	7.4	7.9	8.4	8.9	9.5	10.1	10.7	11.3	11.9	12.6	13.3	14.0
4.3	4.7	5.1	5.6	6.0	6.5	6.9	7.4	7.9	8.5	9.1	9.6	10.2	10.9	11.5	12.2	12.9	13.7	14.4	15.2
4.5	4.9	5.3	5.8	6.2	6.7	7.2	7.7	8.2	8.8	9.4	10.0	10.6	11.3	12.0	12.7	13.4	14.2	15.0	15.9
4.7	5.1	5.5	5.9	6.4	6.9	7.4	8.0	8.5	9.1	9.7	10.4	11.0	11.7	12.4	13.2	14.0	14.8	15.6	16.5
4.8	5.2	5.7	6.1	6.6	7.2	7.7	8.3	8.8	9.4	10.1	10.7	11.4	12.2	12.9	13.7	14.5	15.4	16.3	17.2
5.0	5.4	5.9	6.4	6.9	7.4	8.0	8.5	9.1	9.8	10.4	11.1	11.9	12.6	13.4	14.2	15.1	16.0	16.9	17.9
5.1	5.6	6.1	6.6	7.1	7.6	8.2	8.8	9.5	10.1	10.8	11.5	12.3	13.1	13.9	14.8	15.7	16.6	17.6	18.7
5.3	5.7	6.2	6.8	7.3	7.9	8.5	9.1	9.8	10.5	11.2	11.9	12.7	13.5	14.4	15.3	16.3	17.3	18.3	19.4
5.4	5.9	6.4	7.0	7.5	8.1	8.8	9.4	10.1	10.8	11.6	12.3	13.2	14.0	14.9	15.9	16.9	18.0	19.1	20.2
5.6	6.1	6.6	7.2	7.8	8.4	9.0	9.7	10.4	11.2	11.9	12.8	13.6	14.5	15.5	16.5	17.6	18.7	19.8	21.1
5.7	6.3	6.8	7.4	8.0	8.6	9.3	10.0	10.8	11.5	12.3	13.2	14.1	15.1	16.1	17.1	18.2	19.4	20.7	22.0
5.9	6.4	7.0	7.6	8.2	8.9	9.6	10.3	11.1	11.9	12.8	13.6	14.6	15.6	16.6	17.8	18.9	20.2	21.5	23.0
6.1	6.6	7.2	7.8	8.5	9.2	9.9	10.6	11.4	12.3	13.2	14.1	15.1	16.1	17.3	18.4	19.7	21.0	22.5	24.0
6.4	7.0	7.6	8.3	9.0	9.7	10.5	11.3	12.2	13.1	14.0	15.1	16.2	17.3	18.6	19.9	21.3	22.9	24.6	26.4
6.7	7.4	8.0	8.7	9.5	10.3	11.1	12.0	12.9	13.9	15.0	16.1	17.3	18.6	20.0	21.5	23.2	25.0	27.1	29.5
7.1	7.8	8.5	9.2	10.0	10.9	11.8	12.7	13.7	14.8	16.0	17.2	18.6	20.0	21.7	23.4	25.4	27.7	30.5	34.1
7.4	8.2	8.9	9.7	10.6	11.5	12.4	13.5	14.6	15.8	17.1	18.5	20.0	21.7	23.6	25.8	28.3	31.6	36.6	

4-1 1.53 Tool Index Sag Chart for Various Chord Diameters *(Continued)*

(D)	10	12	14	16	18	20	22	24	26	28	30	32	34	36	38	40	42	44	46
13.00	0.3	0.4	0.6	0.8	1.0	1.2	1.5	1.8	2.1	2.5	2.9	3.3	3.7	4.2	4.7	5.2	5.8	6.4	7.1
13.50	0.3	0.5	0.6	0.8	1.0	1.3	1.6	1.9	2.2	2.6	3.0	3.4	3.9	4.4	4.9	5.5	6.1	6.7	7.4
14.00	0.3	0.5	0.7	0.9	1.1	1.3	1.6	2.0	2.3	2.7	3.1	3.5	4.0	4.6	5.1	5.7	6.4	7.0	7.8
14.50	0.3	0.5	0.7	0.9	1.1	1.4	1.7	2.0	2.4	2.8	3.2	3.7	4.2	4.7	5.3	6.0	6.6	7.4	8.1
15.00	0.4	0.5	0.7	0.9	1.2	1.4	1.8	2.1	2.5	2.9	3.3	3.8	4.4	4.9	5.5	6.2	6.9	7.7	8.5
15.50	0.4	0.5	0.7	0.9	1.2	1.5	1.8	2.2	2.6	3.0	3.5	4.0	4.5	5.1	5.8	6.5	7.2	8.0	8.9
16.00	0.4	0.5	0.7	1.0	1.2	1.5	1.9	2.3	2.7	3.1	3.6	4.1	4.7	5.3	6.0	6.7	7.5	8.4	9.3
16.50	0.4	0.6	0.8	1.0	1.3	1.6	1.9	2.3	2.7	3.2	3.7	4.3	4.9	5.5	6.2	7.0	7.8	8.7	9.7
17.00	0.4	0.6	0.8	1.0	1.3	1.6	2.0	2.4	2.8	3.3	3.8	4.4	5.0	5.7	6.5	7.3	8.1	9.1	10.1
17.50	0.4	0.6	0.8	1.1	1.4	1.7	2.1	2.5	2.9	3.4	4.0	4.6	5.2	5.9	6.7	7.5	8.5	9.5	10.6
18.00	0.4	0.6	0.8	1.1	1.4	1.8	2.1	2.6	3.0	3.5	4.1	4.7	5.4	6.1	7.0	7.8	8.8	9.9	11.1
18.50	0.4	0.6	0.9	1.1	1.5	1.8	2.2	2.6	3.1	3.7	4.2	4.9	5.6	6.4	7.2	8.1	9.2	10.3	11.6
19.00	0.5	0.7	0.9	1.2	1.5	1.9	2.3	2.7	3.2	3.8	4.4	5.0	5.8	6.6	7.5	8.4	9.5	10.7	12.1
19.50	0.5	0.7	0.9	1.2	1.5	1.9	2.3	2.8	3.3	3.9	4.5	5.2	6.0	6.8	7.7	8.8	9.9	11.2	12.7
20.00	0.5	0.7	0.9	1.2	1.6	2.0	2.4	2.9	3.4	4.0	4.7	5.4	6.2	7.1	8.0	9.1	10.3	11.7	13.3

4-2 Vision-Ease Diopteric Compensation for Changes in Center Thickness

Index	Plano	2	4	6	8	10	12	14	16	18	20	22	24
1.498	0	0	0.010	0.026	0.047	0.070	0.100	0.140	0.163	0.247	0.313	0.390	0.487
1.523	0	0	0.011	0.027	0.049	0.071	0.103	0.143	0.166	0.250			
1.586	0	0	0.012	0.028	0.050	0.073							
1.601	0	0	0.012	0.029	0.052	0.076							
1.701	0	0	0.012										
1.805	0	0.003	0.013	0.033	0.063	0.093							

To use chart, locate index of material in the left margin and read over to the base curve being used. Multiply the actual change in center thickness by the multiplier listed under the base curve and round to the nearest 0.01 diopter.
Source: Vision-Ease Laboratory Processing Data, Vision-Ease Corporation, St. Cloud, Minn., revised May 18, 1988, p. 96, used by permission.

48	50	52	54	56	58	60	62	64	66	68	70	72	74	76	78	80	82	84	86
7.8	8.6	9.4	10.2	11.1	12.1	13.2	14.3	15.5	16.8	18.3	19.9	21.6	23.6	26.0	28.9	32.9			
8.2	9.0	9.8	10.8	11.7	12.8	13.9	15.2	16.5	18.0	19.6	21.5	23.6	26.1	29.4	34.8				
8.6	9.4	10.3	11.3	12.4	13.5	14.8	16.1	17.6	19.3	21.2	23.4	26.1	29.8						
9.0	9.9	10.9	11.9	13.1	14.3	15.7	17.2	18.9	20.8	23.1	26.0	30.2							
9.4	10.4	11.4	12.5	13.8	15.1	16.7	18.4	20.4	22.7	25.7	30.5								
9.8	10.9	12.0	13.2	14.6	16.1	17.8	19.8	22.1	25.2	30.6									
10.3	11.4	12.6	13.9	15.4	17.1	19.1	21.5	24.6	30.3										
10.8	12.0	13.3	14.7	16.4	18.3	20.6	23.7	29.3											
11.3	12.5	14.0	15.6	17.5	19.7	22.7	27.9												
11.8	13.2	14.8	16.6	18.7	21.8	26.1													
12.4	13.9	15.6	17.7	20.3	24.3														
13.0	14.7	16.6	19.1	22.6															
13.7	15.5	17.8	20.9																
14.4	16.5	19.3	24.1																
15.3	17.7	21.4																	

4-3 Segment Thickness Chart for Bifocals and Trifocals

Add Power	22 mm		25 mm		28 mm		35 mm	
	All Bases	Except	All Bases	Except	All Bases	Except	All Bases	Except
0.50	0.5	10 0.8	0.7	10 1.0	0.8	10 1.2	1.3	PL-2 1.4
0.75	0.8		1.0		1.2		2.0	
1.00	1.0	PL 0.5	1.3	PL 0.7	1.6	PL 0.8	1.4	10 2.5
1.25	0.7	8-10 1.3	0.8	8-10 1.6	1.0	8-10 2.0	1.7	3.3
1.50	0.8	10 1.5	1.0	10 1.9	1.2	10 2.4	2.0	
1.75	0.9	PL 0.7	1.1	PL 0.9	1.4	PL 1.1	1.8	10 2.2
2.00	1.0	PL 0.8	1.3	PL 1.1	1.6	PL 1.3	2.0	
2.25	1.1	PL-2 0.9	1.5	PL-2 1.2	1.8	PL-2 1.5	2.2	PL-2 2.3
2.50	1.3	1.0	1.6	PL-2 1.3	2.0	1.6	2.4	PL-2-4 2.5
2.75	1.4	PL-2-4 1.1	1.8	PL-2-4 1.4	2.2	PL-2-4 1.8	2.7	PL-2 2.8
3.00	1.5	1.2	1.9	1.5	2.4	1.9	2.8	PL-2-4 3.0
3.25	1.3	7-8-10 1.6	1.7	7-8-10 2.1	2.1	7-8-10 2.6	3.1	PL-2 3.3

4-3 Segment Thickness Chart for Bifocals and Trifocals *(Continued)*

Add Power	22 mm All Bases	Except	25 mm All Bases	Except	28 mm All Bases	Except	35 mm All Bases	Except
3.50	1.4		1.8		2.2	PL 2.3	3.4	PL 3.6
3.75	1.5		1.9		2.3	PL-2 2.4	3.6	PL-2 3.8
4.00	1.6		2.0	PL 2.1	2.5	PL 2.6	3.9	PL 4.2
4.25	1.7		2.1	PL-2 2.2	2.6	PL-2 2.7	4.1	PL-2 4.3
4.50	1.8		2.3		2.8	2.9	4.4	4.7
4.75	1.9		2.4		3.0		4.5	PL-2-4 4.8
5.00	2.0		2.6		3.1	PL-2 3.3	4.8	5.2
5.25	2.1		2.7		3.2	3.4		
5.50	2.2		2.9		3.4	3.6		
5.75	2.3		3.0		3.7	7-8-10 3.5		
6.00	2.4		3.1		3.7	PL-2 4.0		
6.25	2.5		3.3		4.0	PL 4.3		
6.50	2.5		3.4		4.1	2 4.3		
6.75	2.6		3.5		4.3	4.4 / 2-4		
7.00	2.7		3.6		4.4	4.6 / 4		
7.25	2.8		3.7		4.6	4.7		
7.50	2.9		3.9		4.7	4.9		
7.75	3.0		4.0		5.0			
8.00	3.1		4.0		5.1			

For glass polarized segment thickness, add 1.4 mm for cover plate.
Source: Vision-Ease Laboratory Processing Data, Vision-Ease Corporation, St. Cloud, Minn., revised May 18, 1988, p. 7, used by permission.

4-4 Crown-Glass Thickness Difference of Sharp-Edged Prisms (refractive index 1.523)

Prism	Diameter, mm 50	54	58	62	66	70	74	78
0.5	0.5	0.5	0.6	0.6	0.6	0.7	0.7	0.8
1.0	1.0	1.0	1.1	1.2	1.3	1.3	1.4	1.5
1.5	1.4	1.6	1.7	1.8	1.9	2.0	2.1	2.2
2.0	1.9	2.1	2.2	2.4	2.5	2.7	2.8	3.0
2.5	2.4	2.6	2.8	3.0	3.2	3.3	3.5	3.7
3.0	2.9	3.1	3.3	3.6	3.8	4.0	4.2	4.5

4-4   Crown-Glass Thickness Difference of Sharp-Edged Prisms (refractive index 1.523) *(Continued)*

				Diameter, mm				
Prism	50	54	58	62	66	70	74	78
3.5	3.3	3.6	3.9	4.1	4.4	4.7	4.9	5.2
4.0	3.8	4.1	4.4	4.7	5.0	5.3	5.7	6.0
4.5	4.3	4.6	5.0	5.3	5.7	6.0	6.4	6.7
5.0	4.8	5.1	5.5	5.9	6.3	6.7	7.1	7.4
5.5	5.2	5.7	6.1	6.5	6.9	7.3	7.8	8.2
6.0	5.7	6.2	6.6	7.1	7.5	8.0	8.5	8.9
6.5	6.2	6.7	7.2	7.7	8.2	8.7	9.1	9.6
7.0	6.6	7.2	7.7	8.2	8.8	9.3	9.8	10.4
7.5	7.1	7.7	8.3	8.8	9.4	10.0	10.5	11.1
8.0	7.6	8.2	8.8	9.4	10.0	10.6	11.2	11.8
8.5	8.0	8.7	9.3	10.0	10.6	11.3	11.9	12.6
9.0	8.5	9.2	9.9	10.6	11.2	11.9	12.6	13.3
9.5	9.0	9.7	10.4	11.1	11.8	12.6	13.3	14.0
10.0	9.4	10.2	10.9	11.7	12.4	13.2	14.0	14.7
10.5	9.9	10.7	11.5	12.3	13.0	13.8	14.6	15.4
11.0	10.3	11.2	12.0	12.8	13.6	14.5	15.3	16.1
11.5	10.8	11.7	12.5	13.4	14.2	15.1	16.0	16.8
12.0	11.2	12.1	13.0	13.9	14.8	15.7	16.6	17.5

Source: Vision-Ease Laboratory Processing Data, Vision-Ease Corporation, St. Cloud, Minn., revised May 18, 1988, p. 101, used by permission.

4-5   Thickness Difference of Sharp-Edged Prisms (refractive index 1.498)

				Diameter, mm				
Prism	50	54	58	62	66	70	74	78
0.5	0.5	0.5	0.6	0.6	0.7	0.7	0.7	0.8
1.0	1.0	1.1	1.2	1.2	1.3	1.4	1.5	1.6
1.5	1.5	1.6	1.8	1.9	2.0	2.1	2.2	2.4
2.0	2.0	2.2	2.3	2.5	2.7	2.8	3.0	3.1
2.5	2.5	2.7	2.9	3.1	3.3	3.5	3.7	3.9
3.0	3.0	3.3	3.5	3.7	4.0	4.2	4.5	4.7
3.5	3.5	3.8	4.1	4.4	4.6	4.9	5.2	5.5
4.0	4.0	4.3	4.7	5.0	5.3	5.6	5.9	6.3
4.5	4.5	4.9	5.2	5.6	6.0	6.3	6.7	7.0
5.0	5.0	5.4	5.8	6.2	6.6	7.0	7.4	7.8
5.5	5.5	5.9	6.4	6.8	7.3	7.7	8.1	8.6
6.0	6.0	6.5	7.0	7.4	7.9	8.4	8.9	9.4
6.5	6.5	7.0	7.5	8.0	8.6	9.1	9.6	10.1
7.0	7.0	7.5	8.1	8.7	9.2	9.8	10.3	10.9
7.5	7.5	8.1	8.7	9.3	9.9	10.5	11.1	11.7
8.0	8.0	8.6	9.2	9.9	10.5	11.1	11.8	12.4
8.5	8.4	9.1	9.8	10.5	11.1	11.8	12.5	13.2
9.0	8.9	9.6	10.4	11.1	11.8	12.5	13.2	13.9
9.5	9.4	10.2	10.9	11.7	12.4	13.2	13.9	14.7
10.0	9.9	10.7	11.5	12.3	13.1	13.9	14.6	15.4
10.5	10.4	11.2	12.0	12.9	13.7	14.5	15.4	16.2
11.0	10.9	11.7	12.6	13.5	14.3	15.2	16.1	16.9
11.5	11.3	12.2	13.1	14.0	14.9	15.9	16.8	17.7
12.0	11.8	12.7	13.7	14.6	15.6	16.5	17.5	18.4

Source: Vision-Ease Laboratory Processing Data, Vision-Ease Corporation, St. Cloud, Minn., revised May 18, 1988, p. 100, used by permission.

Appendix
5

Lap Tool Charts

5-1 Pad Thickness Compensation Values

To cut compensated tools: Cut the tool steeper by the amount shown in the column corresponding to the pad thickness being used. For glass lenses this is the total pad thickness at fining. For plastic lenses this is the total pad thickness at second fining.

To find the best tool when using uncompensated tools: Find what the compensated tool curve ought to have been. Use the uncompensated tool that is closest to this value.

	Pad Flattens Actual Curve on Lap by					
	Pad Thickness Options					
For Curve	*0.008 inch*	*0.012 inch*	*0.016 inch*	*0.018 inch*	*0.022 inch*	*0.025 inch*
0–2.00	0.00	0.00	0.00	0.00	0.00	0.00
2.50	0.00	0.00	0.00	0.00	0.00	0.01
3.00	0.00	0.01	0.01	0.01	0.01	0.01
3.50	0.00	0.01	0.01	0.01	0.01	0.01
4.00	0.01	0.01	0.01	0.01	0.02	0.02
4.50	0.01	0.01	0.02	0.02	0.02	0.02
5.00	0.01	0.01	0.02	0.02	0.03	0.03
5.50	0.01	0.02	0.02	0.03	0.03	0.04
6.00	0.01	0.02	0.03	0.03	0.04	0.04
6.50	0.02	0.02	0.03	0.04	0.04	0.05
7.00	0.02	0.03	0.04	0.04	0.05	0.06
7.50	0.02	0.03	0.04	0.05	0.06	0.07
8.00	0.02	0.04	0.05	0.05	0.07	0.08
8.50	0.03	0.04	0.06	0.06	0.08	0.09
9.00	0.03	0.05	0.06	0.07	0.08	0.10
9.50	0.03	0.05	0.07	0.08	0.09	0.11
10.00	0.04	0.06	0.08	0.09	0.10	0.12
10.50	0.04	0.06	0.08	0.09	0.11	0.13
11.00	0.05	0.07	0.09	0.10	0.13	0.14
11.50	0.05	0.08	0.10	0.11	0.14	0.16
12.00	0.05	0.08	0.11	0.12	0.15	0.17
12.50	0.06	0.09	0.12	0.13	0.16	0.18

For Curve	Pad Flattens Actual Curve on Lap by					
	Pad Thickness Options					
	0.008 inch	*0.012 inch*	*0.016 inch*	*0.018 inch*	*0.022 inch*	*0.025 inch*
13.00	0.06	0.10	0.13	0.14	0.18	0.20
13.50	0.07	0.10	0.14	0.16	0.19	0.21
14.00	0.07	0.11	0.15	0.17	0.20	0.23
14.50	0.08	0.12	0.16	0.18	0.22	0.25
15.00	0.09	0.13	0.17	0.19	0.23	0.26
15.50	0.09	0.14	0.18	0.20	0.25	0.28
16.00	0.10	0.15	0.19	0.22	0.27	0.30
16.50	0.10	0.16	0.21	0.23	0.28	0.32
17.00	0.11	0.16	0.22	0.25	0.30	0.34
17.50	0.12	0.17	0.23	0.26	0.32	0.36
18.00	0.12	0.18	0.25	0.28	0.34	0.38
18.50	0.13	0.19	0.26	0.29	0.35	0.40
19.00	0.14	0.21	0.27	0.31	0.37	0.42
19.50	0.14	0.22	0.29	0.32	0.39	0.45
20.00	0.15	0.23	0.30	0.34	0.41	0.47
20.50	0.16	0.24	0.32	0.36	0.43	0.49
21.00	0.17	0.25	0.33	0.37	0.45	0.52
21.50	0.18	0.26	0.35	0.39	0.48	0.54
22.00	0.18	0.27	0.36	0.41	0.50	0.56
22.50	0.19	0.29	0.38	0.43	0.52	0.59
23.00	0.20	0.30	0.40	0.45	0.54	0.62
23.50	0.21	0.31	0.42	0.47	0.57	0.64
24.00	0.22	0.33	0.43	0.49	0.59	0.67
24.50	0.23	0.34	0.45	0.51	0.62	0.70
25.00	0.24	0.35	0.47	0.53	0.64	0.73

Source: Vision-Ease Laboratory Processing Data, Vision-Ease Corporation, St. Cloud, Minn., revised May 18, 1988, p. 95, used by permission.

5-2   Uncompensated Sag Charts for Convex Surfaces Using a Bar Gauge, 5/32-inch Ball

These charts are accurate when a bar gauge with 5/32-inch ball tips are used on a convex surface. If this bar gauge is used on concave surfaces, the charts are not valid. Neither are they valid when using a bell gauge.

1.530 index   50-mm convex cylinder   0.000 pad compensation

Diopter	Sag	Diopter	Sag	Diopter	Sag	Diopter	Sag
0.062	0.04	3.125	1.83	6.187	3.64	9.250	5.53
0.125	0.07	3.187	1.87	6.250	3.68	9.312	5.57
0.187	0.11	3.250	1.90	6.312	3.72	9.375	5.61
0.250	0.15	3.312	1.94	6.375	3.75	9.437	5.65
0.312	0.18	3.375	1.98	6.437	3.79	9.500	5.69
0.375	0.22	3.437	2.01	6.500	3.83	9.562	5.73
0.437	0.26	3.500	2.05	6.562	3.87	9.625	5.77
0.500	0.29	3.562	2.09	6.625	3.90	9.687	5.81
0.562	0.33	3.625	2.12	6.687	3.94	9.750	5.85
0.625	0.37	3.687	2.16	6.750	3.98	9.812	5.89
0.687	0.40	3.750	2.20	6.812	4.02	9.875	5.93
0.750	0.44	3.812	2.23	6.875	4.06	9.937	5.97
0.812	0.48	3.875	2.27	6.937	4.09	10.000	6.01
0.875	0.51	3.937	2.31	7.000	4.13	10.062	6.05
0.937	0.55	4.000	2.34	7.062	4.17	10.125	6.09
1.000	0.59	4.062	2.38	7.125	4.21	10.187	6.13
1.062	0.62	4.125	2.42	7.187	4.25	10.250	6.18
1.125	0.66	4.187	2.45	7.250	4.28	10.312	6.22
1.187	0.70	4.250	2.49	7.312	4.32	10.375	6.26
1.250	0.73	4.312	2.53	7.375	4.36	10.437	6.30
1.312	0.77	4.375	2.56	7.437	4.40	10.500	6.34
1.375	0.81	4.437	2.60	7.500	4.44	10.562	6.38
1.437	0.84	4.500	2.64	7.562	4.48	10.625	6.42
1.500	0.88	4.562	2.68	7.625	4.51	10.687	6.46
1.562	0.92	4.625	2.71	7.687	4.55	10.750	6.51
1.625	0.95	4.687	2.75	7.750	4.59	10.812	6.55
1.687	0.99	4.750	2.79	7.812	4.63	10.875	6.59
1.750	1.03	4.812	2.82	7.875	4.67	10.937	6.63
1.812	1.06	4.875	2.86	7.937	4.71	11.000	6.67
1.875	1.10	4.937	2.90	8.000	4.74	11.062	6.72
1.937	1.14	5.000	2.93	8.062	4.78	11.125	6.76
2.000	1.17	5.062	2.97	8.125	4.82	11.187	6.80
2.062	1.21	5.125	3.01	8.187	4.86	11.250	6.84
2.125	1.25	5.187	3.04	8.250	4.90	11.312	6.88
2.187	1.28	5.250	3.08	8.312	4.94	11.375	6.93
2.250	1.32	5.312	3.12	8.375	4.98	11.437	6.97
2.312	1.36	5.375	3.16	8.437	5.02	11.500	7.01
2.375	1.39	5.437	3.19	8.500	5.06	11.562	7.06
2.437	1.43	5.500	3.23	8.562	5.09	11.625	7.10
2.500	1.47	5.562	3.27	8.625	5.13	11.687	7.14
2.562	1.50	5.625	3.30	8.687	5.17	11.750	7.18
2.625	1.54	5.687	3.34	8.750	5.21	11.812	7.23
2.687	1.58	5.750	3.38	8.812	5.25	11.875	7.27
2.750	1.61	5.812	3.42	8.875	5.29	11.937	7.31
2.812	1.65	5.875	3.45	8.937	5.33	12.000	7.36
2.875	1.68	5.937	3.49	9.000	5.37	12.062	7.40
2.937	1.72	6.000	3.53	9.062	5.41	12.125	7.45
3.000	1.76	6.062	3.57	9.125	5.45	12.187	7.49
3.062	1.79	6.125	3.60	9.187	5.49	12.250	7.53

5-2 *(Continued)*

Diopter	Sag	Diopter	Sag	Diopter	Sag	Diopter	Sag
12.312	7.58	15.000	9.61	17.687	12.06	20.375	15.39
12.375	7.62	15.062	9.66	17.750	12.12	20.437	15.49
12.437	7.67	15.125	9.71	17.812	12.19	20.500	15.59
12.500	7.71	15.187	9.77	17.875	12.25	20.562	15.69
12.562	7.76	15.250	9.82	17.937	12.32	20.625	15.80
12.625	7.80	15.312	9.87	18.000	12.38	20.687	15.90
12.687	7.84	15.375	9.92	18.062	12.45	20.750	16.01
12.750	7.89	15.437	9.97	18.125	12.52	20.812	16.11
12.812	7.93	15.500	10.03	18.187	12.58	20.875	16.22
12.875	7.98	15.562	10.08	18.250	12.65	20.937	16.34
12.937	8.03	15.625	10.13	18.312	12.72	21.000	16.45
13.000	8.07	15.687	10.19	18.375	12.79	21.062	16.56
13.062	8.12	15.750	10.24	18.437	12.86	21.125	16.68
13.125	8.16	15.812	10.29	18.500	12.93	21.187	16.80
13.187	8.21	15.875	10.35	18.562	13.00	21.250	16.93
13.250	8.25	15.937	10.40	18.625	13.07	21.312	17.05
13.312	8.30	16.000	10.46	18.687	13.15	21.375	17.18
13.375	8.35	16.062	10.51	18.750	13.22	21.437	17.31
13.437	8.39	16.125	10.57	18.812	13.29	21.500	17.45
13.500	8.44	16.187	10.62	18.875	13.37	21.562	17.58
13.562	8.49	16.250	10.68	18.937	13.44	21.625	17.72
13.625	8.53	16.312	10.74	19.000	13.52	21.687	17.87
13.687	8.58	16.375	10.79	19.062	13.59	21.750	18.02
13.750	8.63	16.437	10.85	19.125	13.67	21.812	18.17
13.812	8.68	16.500	10.91	19.187	13.75	21.875	18.33
13.875	8.72	16.562	10.96	19.250	13.82	21.937	18.50
13.937	8.77	16.625	11.02	19.312	13.90	22.000	18.66
14.000	8.82	16.687	11.08	19.375	13.98	22.062	18.84
14.062	8.87	16.750	11.14	19.437	14.06	22.125	19.02
14.125	8.92	16.812	11.20	19.500	14.15	22.187	19.21
14.187	8.96	16.875	11.26	19.562	14.23	22.250	19.41
14.250	9.01	16.937	11.31	19.625	14.31	22.312	19.62
14.312	9.06	17.000	11.37	19.687	14.40	22.375	19.84
14.375	9.11	17.062	11.43	19.750	14.48	22.437	20.07
14.437	9.16	17.125	11.49	19.812	14.57	22.500	20.32
14.500	9.21	17.187	11.56	19.875	14.66	22.562	20.58
14.562	9.26	17.250	11.62	19.937	14.74	22.625	20.86
14.625	9.31	17.312	11.68	20.000	14.83	22.687	21.18
14.687	9.36	17.375	11.74	20.062	14.92	22.750	21.52
14.750	9.41	17.437	11.80	20.125	15.02	22.812	21.91
14.812	9.46	17.500	11.87	20.187	15.11	22.875	22.38
14.875	9.51	17.562	11.93	20.250	15.20	22.937	22.96
14.937	9.56	17.625	11.99	20.312	15.30		

Source: Coburn Optical Industries, Muskogee, Okla., used by permission.

5-3 0.018-inch Tool Compensation

1.530 index	50-mm convex cylinder		0.018-inch tool compensation				
Diopter	Sag	Diopter	Sag	Diopter	Sag	Diopter	Sag
0.062	0.04	3.125	1.84	6.187	3.66	9.250	5.58
0.125	0.07	3.187	1.87	6.250	3.70	8.312	5.62
0.187	0.11	3.250	1.91	6.312	3.74	9.375	5.66
0.250	0.15	3.312	1.95	6.375	3.78	9.437	5.70
0.312	0.18	3.375	1.98	6.437	3.81	9.500	5.74
0.375	0.22	3.437	2.02	6.500	3.85	9.562	5.78
0.437	0.26	3.500	2.06	6.562	3.89	9.625	5.82
0.500	0.29	3.562	2.09	6.625	3.93	9.687	5.86
0.562	0.33	3.625	2.13	6.687	3.97	9.750	5.90
0.625	0.37	3.687	2.17	6.750	4.00	9.812	5.94
0.687	0.40	3.750	2.20	6.812	4.04	9.875	5.99
0.750	0.44	3.812	2.24	6.875	4.08	9.937	6.03
0.812	0.48	3.875	2.28	6.937	4.12	10.000	6.07
0.875	0.51	3.937	2.32	7.000	4.16	10.062	6.11
0.937	0.55	4.000	2.35	7.062	4.20	10.125	6.15
1.000	0.59	4.062	2.39	7.125	4.23	10.187	6.19
1.062	0.62	4.125	2.43	7.187	4.27	10.250	6.24
1.125	0.66	4.187	2.46	7.250	4.31	10.312	6.28
1.187	0.70	4.250	2.50	7.312	4.35	10.375	6.32
1.250	0.74	4.312	2.54	7.375	4.39	10.437	6.36
1.312	0.77	4.375	2.57	7.437	4.43	10.500	6.40
1.375	0.81	4.437	2.61	7.500	4.47	10.562	6.45
1.437	0.85	4.500	2.65	7.562	4.51	10.625	6.49
1.500	0.88	4.562	2.69	7.625	4.54	10.687	6.53
1.562	0.92	4.625	2.72	7.687	4.58	10.750	6.57
1.625	0.96	4.687	2.76	7.750	4.62	10.812	6.62
1.687	0.99	4.750	2.80	7.812	4.66	10.875	6.66
1.750	1.03	4.812	2.83	7.875	4.70	10.937	6.70
1.812	1.07	4.875	2.87	7.937	4.74	11.000	6.74
1.875	1.10	4.937	2.91	8.000	4.78	11.062	6.79
1.937	1.14	5.000	2.95	8.062	4.82	11.125	6.83
2.000	1.18	5.062	2.98	8.125	4.86	11.187	6.87
2.062	1.21	5.125	3.02	8.187	4.90	11.250	6.92
2.125	1.25	5.187	3.06	8.250	4.94	11.312	6.96
2.187	1.29	5.250	3.10	9.312	4.98	11.375	7.00
2.250	1.32	5.312	3.13	8.375	5.02	11.437	7.05
2.312	1.36	5.375	3.17	8.437	5.06	11.500	7.09
2.375	1.40	5.437	3.21	8.500	5.10	11.562	7.14
2.437	1.43	5.500	3.25	8.562	5.13	11.625	7.18
2.500	1.47	5.562	3.28	8.625	5.17	11.687	7.22
2.562	1.51	5.625	3.32	8.687	5.21	11.750	7.27
2.625	1.54	5.687	3.36	8.750	5.25	11.812	7.31
2.687	1.58	5.750	3.40	8.812	5.29	11.875	7.36
2.750	1.62	5.812	3.43	8.875	5.33	11.937	7.40
2.812	1.65	5.875	3.47	8.937	5.37	12.000	7.45
2.875	1.69	5.937	3.51	9.000	5.42	12.062	7.49
2.937	1.73	6.000	3.55	9.062	5.46	12.125	7.54
3.000	1.76	6.062	3.59	9.125	5.50	12.187	7.58
3.062	1.80	6.125	3.62	9.187	5.54	12.250	7.63

5-3 *(Continued)*

Diopter	Sag	Diopter	Sag	Diopter	Sag	Diopter	Sag
12.312	7.67	14.875	9.67	17.437	12.07	19.937	15.26
12.375	7.72	14.937	9.72	17.500	12.14	20.000	15.36
12.437	7.76	15.000	9.77	17.562	12.21	20.062	15.46
12.500	7.81	15.062	9.83	17.625	12.27	20.125	15.56
12.562	7.85	15.125	9.88	17.687	12.34	20.187	15.67
12.625	7.90	15.187	9.93	17.750	12.41	20.250	15.77
12.687	7.95	15.250	9.99	17.812	12.48	20.312	15.88
12.750	7.99	15.312	10.04	17.875	12.55	20.375	15.99
12.812	8.04	15.375	10.10	17.937	12.62	20.437	16.10
12.875	8.09	15.437	10.15	18.000	12.69	20.500	16.21
12.937	8.13	15.500	10.21	18.062	12.76	20.562	16.33
13.000	8.18	15.562	10.26	18.125	12.83	20.625	16.45
13.062	8.23	15.625	10.32	18.187	12.90	20.687	16.57
13.125	8.27	15.687	10.37	18.250	12.98	20.750	16.69
13.187	8.32	15.750	10.43	18.312	13.05	20.812	16.81
13.250	8.37	15.812	10.49	18.375	13.13	20.875	16.94
13.312	8.42	15.875	10.54	18.437	13.20	20.937	17.07
13.375	8.46	15.937	10.60	18.500	13.28	21.000	17.21
13.467	8.51	16.000	10.66	18.562	13.35	21.062	17.34
13.500	8.56	16.062	10.71	18.625	13.43	21.125	17.48
13.562	8.61	16.125	10.77	18.687	13.51	21.187	17.63
13.625	8.66	16.187	10.83	18.750	13.59	21.250	17.78
13.687	8.71	16.250	10.89	18.812	13.67	21.312	17.93
13.750	8.75	16.312	10.95	18.875	13.75	21.375	18.08
13.812	8.80	16.375	11.01	18.937	13.83	21.437	18.25
13.875	8.85	16.437	11.07	19.000	13.91	21.500	18.41
13.937	8.90	16.500	11.13	19.062	13.99	21.562	18.59
14.000	8.95	16.562	11.19	19.125	14.08	21.625	18.76
14.062	9.00	16.625	11.25	19.187	14.16	21.687	18.95
14.125	9.05	16.687	11.31	19.250	14.25	21.750	19.15
14.817	9.10	16.750	11.37	19.312	14.33	21.812	19.35
14.250	9.15	16.812	11.43	19.375	14.42	21.875	19.56
14.312	9.20	16.875	11.49	19.437	14.51	21.937	19.79
14.375	9.25	16.937	11.56	19.500	14.60	22.000	20.02
14.437	9.30	17.000	11.62	19.562	14.69	22.062	20.28
14.500	9.36	17.062	11.68	19.625	14.78	22.125	20.55
14.562	9.41	17.125	11.75	19.687	14.87	22.187	20.84
14.625	9.46	17.817	11.81	19.750	14.97	22.250	21.17
14.687	9.51	17.250	11.88	19.812	15.06	22.312	21.52
14.750	9.56	17.312	11.94	19.875	15.16	22.375	21.93
14.812	9.62	17.375	12.01				

Source: Coburn Optical Industries, Muskogee, Okla., used by permission.

5-4 0.022-inch Tool Compensation

1.530 index		50-mm convex cylinder		0.022-inch tool compensation			
Diopter	Sag	Diopter	Sag	Diopter	Sag	Diopter	Sag
0.062	0.04	3.125	1.84	6.187	3.67	9.250	5.59
0.125	0.07	3.187	1.87	6.250	3.70	9.312	5.63
0.187	0.11	3.250	1.91	6.312	3.74	9.375	5.67
0.250	0.15	3.312	1.95	6.375	3.78	9.437	5.71
0.312	0.18	3.375	1.98	6.437	3.82	9.500	5.75
0.375	0.22	3.437	2.02	6.500	3.86	9.562	5.79
0.437	0.26	3.500	2.06	6.562	3.89	9.625	5.83
0.500	0.29	3.562	2.10	6.625	3.93	9.687	5.87
0.562	0.33	3.625	2.13	6.687	3.97	9.750	5.92
0.625	0.37	3.687	2.17	6.750	4.01	9.812	5.96
0.687	0.40	3.750	2.21	6.812	4.05	9.875	6.00
0.750	0.44	3.812	2.24	6.875	4.09	9.937	6.04
0.812	0.48	3.875	2.28	6.937	4.12	10.000	6.08
0.875	0.51	3.937	2.32	7.000	4.16	10.062	6.12
0.937	0.55	4.000	2.35	7.062	4.20	10.125	6.17
1.000	0.59	4.062	2.39	7.125	4.24	10.187	6.21
1.062	0.63	4.125	2.43	7.187	4.28	10.250	6.25
1.125	0.66	4.187	2.47	7.250	4.32	10.312	6.29
1.187	0.70	4.250	2.50	7.312	4.36	10.375	6.33
1.250	0.74	4.312	2.54	7.375	4.40	10.437	6.38
1.312	0.77	4.375	2.58	7.437	4.43	10.500	6.42
1.375	0.81	4.437	2.61	7.500	4.47	10.562	6.46
1.437	0.85	4.500	2.65	7.562	4.51	10.625	6.50
1.500	0.88	4.562	2.69	7.625	4.55	10.687	6.55
1.562	0.92	4.625	2.73	7.687	4.59	10.750	6.59
1.625	0.96	4.687	2.76	7.750	4.63	10.812	6.63
1.687	0.99	4.750	2.80	7.812	4.67	10.875	6.67
1.750	1.03	4.812	2.84	7.875	4.71	10.937	6.72
1.812	1.07	4.875	2.87	7.937	4.75	11.000	6.76
1.875	1.10	4.937	2.91	8.000	4.79	11.062	6.80
1.937	1.14	5.000	2.95	8.062	4.83	11.125	6.85
2.000	1.18	5.062	2.99	8.125	4.87	11.187	6.89
2.062	1.21	5.125	3.02	8.187	4.91	11.250	6.93
2.125	1.25	5.187	3.06	8.250	4.94	11.312	6.98
2.187	1.29	5.250	3.10	8.312	4.98	11.375	7.02
2.250	1.32	5.312	3.14	8.375	5.02	11.437	7.07
2.312	1.36	5.375	3.17	8.437	5.06	11.500	7.11
2.375	1.40	5.437	3.21	8.500	5.10	11.562	7.15
2.437	1.43	5.500	3.25	8.562	5.14	11.625	7.20
2.500	1.47	5.562	3.29	8.625	5.18	11.687	7.24
2.562	1.51	5.625	3.32	8.687	5.22	11.750	7.29
2.625	1.54	5.687	3.36	8.750	5.26	11.812	7.33
2.687	1.58	5.750	3.40	8.812	5.30	11.875	7.38
2.750	1.62	5.812	3.44	8.875	5.34	11.937	7.42
2.812	1.65	5.875	3.48	8.937	5.38	12.000	7.47
2.875	1.69	5.937	3.51	9.000	5.43	12.062	7.51
2.937	1.73	6.000	3.55	9.062	5.47	12.125	7.56
3.000	1.76	6.062	3.59	9.125	5.51	12.187	7.60
3.062	1.80	6.125	3.63	9.187	5.55	12.250	7.65

5-4 *(Continued)*

Diopter	Sag	Diopter	Sag	Diopter	Sag	Diopter	Sag
12.312	7.69	13.250	8.39	14.187	9.13	15.125	9.92
12.375	7.74	13.312	8.44	14.250	9.18	15.187	9.97
12.437	7.78	13.375	8.49	14.312	9.24	15.250	10.03
12.500	7.83	13.437	8.54	14.375	9.29	15.312	10.08
12.562	7.88	13.500	8.59	14.437	9.34	15.375	10.14
12.625	7.92	13.562	8.64	14.500	9.39	15.437	10.19
12.687	7.97	13.625	8.68	14.562	9.44	15.500	10.25
12.750	8.02	13.687	8.73	14.625	9.49	15.562	10.30
12.812	8.06	13.750	8.78	14.687	9.55	15.625	10.36
12.875	8.11	13.812	8.83	14.750	9.60	15.687	10.42
12.937	8.16	13.875	8.88	14.812	9.65	15.750	10.47
13.000	8.20	13.937	8.93	14.875	9.70	15.812	10.53
13.062	8.25	14.000	8.98	14.937	9.76	15.875	10.59
13.125	8.30	14.062	9.03	15.000	9.81	15.937	10.64
13.187	8.35	14.125	9.08	15.062	9.86	16.000	10.70

Source: Coburn Optical Industries, Muskogee, Okla., used by permission.

5-5 0.030-inch Tool Compensation

1.530 index		50-mm convex cylinder		0.030-inch tool compensation			
Diopter	Sag	Diopter	Sag	Diopter	Sag	Diopter	Sag
0.062	0.04	3.125	1.84	6.187	3.67	9.250	5.61
0.125	0.07	3.187	1.88	6.250	3.71	9.312	5.65
0.187	0.11	3.250	1.91	6.312	3.75	9.375	5.69
0.250	0.15	3.312	1.95	6.375	3.79	9.437	5.73
0.312	0.18	3.375	1.99	6.437	3.83	9.500	5.77
0.375	0.22	3.437	2.02	6.500	3.87	9.562	5.82
0.437	0.26	3.500	2.06	6.562	3.90	9.625	5.86
0.500	0.29	3.562	2.10	6.625	3.94	9.687	5.90
0.562	0.33	3.625	2.14	6.687	3.98	9.750	5.94
0.625	0.37	3.687	2.17	6.750	4.02	9.812	5.98
0.687	0.40	3.750	2.21	6.812	4.06	9.875	6.02
0.750	0.44	3.812	2.25	6.875	4.10	9.937	6.07
0.812	0.48	3.875	2.28	6.937	4.14	10.000	6.11
0.875	0.52	3.937	2.32	7.000	4.18	10.062	6.15
0.937	0.55	4.000	2.36	7.062	4.21	10.125	6.19
1.000	0.59	4.062	2.39	7.125	4.25	10.187	6.23
1.062	0.63	4.125	2.43	7.187	4.29	10.250	6.28
1.125	0.66	4.187	2.47	7.250	4.33	10.312	6.32
1.187	0.70	4.250	2.51	7.312	4.37	10.375	6.36
1.250	0.74	4.312	2.54	7.375	4.41	10.437	6.40
1.312	0.77	4.375	2.58	7.437	4.45	10.500	6.45
1.375	0.81	4.437	2.62	7.500	4.49	10.562	6.49
1.437	0.85	4.500	2.66	7.562	4.53	10.625	6.53
1.500	0.88	4.562	2.69	7.625	4.57	10.687	6.58
1.562	0.92	4.625	2.73	7.687	4.60	10.750	6.62
1.625	0.96	4.687	2.77	7.750	4.64	10.812	6.66
1.687	0.99	4.750	2.81	7.812	4.68	10.875	6.71
1.750	1.03	4.812	2.84	7.875	4.72	10.937	6.75
1.812	1.07	4.875	2.88	7.937	4.76	11.000	6.79
1.875	1.10	4.937	2.92	8.000	4.80	11.062	6.84
1.937	1.14	5.000	2.96	8.062	4.84	11.125	6.88
2.000	1.18	5.062	2.99	8.125	4.88	11.187	6.92
2.062	1.21	5.125	3.03	8.187	4.92	11.250	6.97
2.125	1.25	5.187	3.07	8.250	4.96	11.312	7.01
2.187	1.29	5.250	3.11	8.312	5.00	11.375	7.06
2.250	1.32	5.312	3.14	8.375	5.04	11.437	7.10
2.312	1.36	5.375	3.18	8.437	5.08	11.500	7.15
2.375	1.40	5.437	3.22	8.500	5.12	11.562	7.19
2.437	1.43	5.500	3.26	8.562	5.16	11.625	7.23
2.500	1.47	5.562	3.29	8.625	5.20	11.687	7.28
2.562	1.51	5.625	3.33	8.687	5.24	11.750	7.32
2.625	1.54	5.687	3.37	8.750	5.28	11.812	7.37
2.687	1.58	5.750	3.41	8.812	5.32	11.875	7.41
2.750	1.62	5.812	3.45	8.875	5.36	11.937	7.46
2.812	1.65	5.875	3.48	8.937	5.40	12.000	7.51
2.875	1.69	5.937	3.52	9.000	5.45	12.062	7.55
2.937	1.73	6.000	3.56	9.062	5.49	12.125	7.60
3.000	1.77	6.062	3.60	9.125	5.53	12.187	7.64
3.062	1.80	6.125	3.64	9.187	5.57	12.250	7.69

5-5 *(Continued)*

Diopter	Sag	Diopter	Sag	Diopter	Sag	Diopter	Sag
12.312	7.74	14.812	9.72	17.312	12.12	19.812	15.42
12.375	7.78	14.875	9.78	17.375	12.19	19.875	15.53
12.437	7.83	14.937	9.83	17.437	12.26	19.937	15.63
12.500	7.87	15.000	9.89	17.500	12.33	20.000	15.74
12.562	7.92	15.062	9.94	17.562	12.40	20.062	15.85
12.625	7.97	15.125	9.99	17.625	12.47	20.125	15.96
12.687	8.02	15.187	10.05	17.687	12.54	20.187	16.08
12.750	8.06	15.250	10.11	17.750	12.61	20.250	16.19
12.812	8.11	15.312	10.16	17.812	12.69	20.312	16.31
12.875	8.16	15.375	10.22	17.875	12.76	20.375	16.43
12.937	8.21	15.437	10.27	17.937	12.83	20.437	16.55
13.000	8.25	15.500	10.33	18.000	12.91	20.500	16.68
13.062	8.30	15.562	10.39	18.062	12.98	20.562	16.81
13.125	8.35	15.625	10.44	18.125	13.06	20.625	16.94
13.187	8.40	15.687	10.50	18.187	13.13	20.687	17.07
13.250	8.45	15.750	10.56	18.250	13.21	20.750	17.21
13.312	8.49	15.812	10.62	18.312	13.29	20.812	17.35
13.375	8.54	15.875	10.68	18.375	13.36	20.875	17.49
13.437	8.59	15.937	10.74	18.437	13.44	20.937	17.64
13.500	8.64	16.000	10.79	18.500	13.52	21.000	17.79
13.562	8.69	16.062	10.85	18.562	13.60	21.062	17.95
13.625	8.74	16.125	10.91	18.625	13.68	21.125	18.11
13.687	8.79	16.187	10.97	18.687	13.77	21.187	18.28
13.750	8.84	16.250	11.03	18.750	13.85	21.250	18.45
13.812	8.89	16.312	11.10	18.812	13.93	21.312	18.63
13.875	8.94	16.375	11.16	18.875	14.02	21.375	18.81
13.937	8.99	16.437	11.22	18.937	14.10	21.437	19.01
14.000	9.04	16.500	11.28	19.000	14.19	21.500	19.21
14.062	9.09	16.562	11.34	19.062	14.28	21.562	19.42
14.125	9.14	16.625	11.41	19.125	14.37	21.625	19.64
14.187	9.20	16.687	11.47	19.187	14.46	21.687	19.88
14.250	9.25	16.750	11.53	19.250	14.55	21.750	20.13
14.312	9.30	16.812	11.60	19.312	14.64	21.812	20.39
14.375	9.35	16.875	11.66	19.375	14.73	21.875	20.68
14.437	9.40	16.937	11.73	19.437	14.83	21.937	21.00
14.500	9.46	17.000	11.79	19.500	14.92	22.000	21.34
14.562	9.51	17.062	11.86	19.562	15.02	22.062	21.74
14.625	9.56	17.125	11.92	19.625	15.12	22.125	22.20
14.687	9.62	17.187	11.99	19.687	15.22	22.187	22.77
14.750	9.67	17.250	12.06	19.750	15.32	22.250	23.58

Source: Coburn Optical Industries, Muskogee, Okla., used by permission.

5-6 0.040-inch Tool Compensation

1.530 index		50-mm convex cylinder		0.040-inch tool compensation			
Diopter	Sag	Diopter	Sag	Diopter	Sag	Diopter	Sag
0.062	0.04	3.125	1.84	6.187	3.69	9.250	5.64
0.125	0.07	3.187	1.88	6.250	3.72	9.312	5.68
0.187	0.11	3.250	1.92	6.312	3.76	9.375	5.72
0.250	0.15	3.312	1.95	6.375	3.80	9.437	5.76
0.312	0.18	3.375	1.99	6.437	3.84	9.500	5.80
0.375	0.22	3.437	2.03	6.500	3.88	9.562	5.84
0.437	0.26	3.500	2.06	6.562	3.92	9.625	5.89
0.500	0.29	3.562	2.10	6.625	3.96	9.687	5.93
0.562	0.33	3.625	2.14	6.687	3.99	9.750	5.97
0.625	0.37	3.687	2.18	6.750	4.03	9.812	6.01
0.687	0.40	3.750	2.21	6.812	4.07	9.875	6.05
0.750	0.44	3.812	2.25	6.875	4.11	9.937	6.10
0.812	0.48	3.875	2.29	6.937	4.15	10.000	6.14
0.875	0.52	3.937	2.32	7.000	4.19	10.062	6.18
0.937	0.55	4.000	2.36	7.062	4.23	10.125	6.22
1.000	0.59	4.062	2.40	7.125	4.27	10.187	6.27
1.062	0.63	4.125	2.44	7.187	4.31	10.250	6.31
1.125	0.66	4.187	2.47	7.250	4.35	10.312	6.35
1.187	0.70	4.250	2.51	7.312	4.39	10.375	6.40
1.250	0.74	4.312	2.55	7.375	4.43	10.437	6.44
1.312	0.77	4.375	2.59	7.437	4.46	10.500	6.48
1.375	0.81	4.437	2.62	7.500	4.50	10.562	6.53
1.437	0.85	4.500	2.66	7.562	4.54	10.625	6.57
1.500	0.88	4.562	2.70	7.625	4.58	10.687	6.61
1.562	0.92	4.625	2.74	7.687	4.62	10.750	6.66
1.625	0.96	4.687	2.77	7.750	4.66	10.812	6.70
1.687	0.99	4.750	2.81	7.812	4.70	10.875	6.74
1.750	1.03	4.812	2.85	7.875	4.74	10.937	6.79
1.812	1.07	4.875	2.89	7.937	4.78	11.000	6.83
1.875	1.10	4.937	2.92	8.000	4.82	11.062	6.88
1.937	1.14	5.000	2.96	8.062	4.86	11.125	6.92
2.000	1.18	5.062	3.00	8.125	4.90	11.187	6.97
2.062	1.21	5.125	3.04	8.187	4.94	11.250	7.01
2.125	1.25	5.187	3.08	8.250	4.98	11.312	7.06
2.187	1.29	5.250	3.11	8.312	5.02	11.375	7.10
2.250	1.32	5.312	3.15	8.375	5.06	11.437	7.15
2.312	1.36	5.375	3.19	8.437	5.10	11.500	7.19
2.375	1.40	5.437	3.23	8.500	5.14	11.562	7.24
2.437	1.44	5.500	3.27	8.562	5.18	11.625	7.28
2.500	1.47	5.562	3.30	8.625	5.23	11.687	7.33
2.562	1.51	5.625	3.34	8.687	5.27	11.750	7.37
2.625	1.55	5.687	3.38	8.750	5.31	11.812	7.42
2.687	1.58	5.750	3.42	8.812	5.35	11.875	7.46
2.750	1.62	5.812	3.46	8.875	5.39	11.937	7.51
2.812	1.66	5.875	3.49	8.937	5.43	12.000	7.56
2.875	1.69	5.937	3.53	9.000	5.47	12.062	7.60
2.937	1.73	6.000	3.57	9.062	5.51	12.125	7.65
3.000	1.77	6.062	3.61	9.125	5.55	12.187	7.70
3.062	1.81	6.125	3.65	9.187	5.59	12.250	7.74

5-6 *(Continued)*

Diopter	Sag	Diopter	Sag	Diopter	Sag	Diopter	Sag
12.312	7.79	14.750	9.76	17.187	12.14	19.625	15.42
12.375	7.84	14.812	9.81	17.250	12.21	19.687	15.53
12.437	7.88	14.875	9.87	17.312	12.28	19.750	15.64
12.500	7.93	14.937	9.92	17.375	12.35	19.812	15.75
12.562	7.98	15.000	9.98	17.437	12.43	19.875	15.86
12.625	8.03	15.062	10.04	17.500	12.50	19.937	15.97
12.687	8.07	15.125	10.09	17.562	12.57	20.000	16.09
12.750	8.12	15.187	10.15	17.625	12.64	20.062	16.21
12.812	8.17	15.250	10.21	17.687	12.72	20.125	16.33
12.875	8.22	15.312	10.26	17.750	12.79	20.187	16.45
12.937	8.27	15.375	10.32	17.812	12.87	20.250	16.57
13.000	8.32	15.437	10.38	17.875	12.94	20.312	16.70
13.062	8.36	15.500	10.44	17.937	13.02	20.375	16.83
13.125	8.41	15.562	10.49	18.000	13.09	20.437	16.97
13.187	8.46	15.625	10.55	18.062	13.17	20.500	17.10
13.250	8.51	15.687	10.61	18.125	13.25	20.562	17.25
13.312	8.56	15.750	10.67	18.187	13.33	20.625	17.39
13.375	8.61	15.812	10.73	18.250	13.41	20.687	17.54
13.437	8.66	15.875	10.79	18.312	13.49	20.750	17.69
13.500	8.71	15.937	10.85	18.375	13.57	20.812	17.85
13.562	8.76	16.000	10.91	18.437	13.65	20.875	18.01
13.625	8.81	16.062	10.97	18.500	13.74	20.937	18.17
13.687	8.86	16.125	11.03	18.562	13.82	21.000	18.35
13.750	8.91	16.187	11.10	18.625	13.91	21.062	18.53
13.812	8.97	16.250	11.16	18.687	13.99	21.125	18.71
13.875	9.02	16.312	11.22	18.750	14.08	21.187	18.90
13.937	9.07	16.375	11.28	18.812	14.17	21.250	19.10
14.000	9.12	16.437	11.35	18.875	14.26	21.312	19.32
14.062	9.17	16.500	11.41	18.937	14.35	21.375	19.54
14.125	9.22	16.562	11.48	19.000	14.44	21.437	19.77
14.187	9.28	16.625	11.54	19.062	14.53	21.500	20.02
14.250	9.33	16.687	11.61	19.125	14.62	21.562	20.28
14.312	9.38	16.750	11.67	19.187	14.72	21.625	20.57
14.375	9.44	16.812	11.74	19.250	14.82	21.687	20.88
14.437	9.49	16.875	11.80	19.312	14.91	21.750	21.22
14.500	9.54	16.937	11.87	19.375	15.01	21.812	21.61
14.562	9.60	17.000	11.94	19.437	15.11	21.875	22.05
14.625	9.65	17.062	12.01	19.500	15.21	21.937	22.60
14.687	9.70	17.125	12.08	19.562	15.32	22.000	23.34

Source: Coburn Optical Industries, Muskogee, Okla., used by permission.

5-7 0.050-inch Tool Compensation

1.530 index	50-mm convex cylinder		0.050-inch tool compensation				
Diopter	*Sag*	*Diopter*	*Sag*	*Diopter*	*Sag*	*Diopter*	*Sag*
0.062	0.04	3.125	1.84	6.187	3.70	9.250	5.66
0.125	0.07	3.187	1.88	6.250	3.74	9.312	5.71
0.187	0.11	3.250	1.92	6.312	3.77	9.375	5.75
0.250	0.15	3.312	1.96	6.375	3.81	9.437	5.79
0.312	0.18	3.375	1.99	6.437	3.85	9.500	5.83
0.375	0.22	3.437	2.03	6.500	3.89	9.562	5.87
0.437	0.26	3.500	2.07	6.562	3.93	9.625	5.92
0.500	0.29	3.562	2.11	6.625	3.97	9.687	5.96
0.562	0.33	3.625	2.14	6.687	4.01	9.750	6.00
0.625	0.37	3.687	2.18	6.750	4.05	9.812	6.04
0.687	0.41	3.750	2.22	6.812	4.09	9.875	6.09
0.750	0.44	3.812	2.25	6.875	4.13	9.937	6.13
0.812	0.48	3.875	2.29	6.937	4.17	10.000	6.17
0.875	0.52	3.937	2.33	7.000	4.20	10.062	6.22
0.937	0.55	4.000	2.37	7.062	4.24	10.125	6.26
1.000	0.59	4.062	2.40	7.125	4.28	10.187	6.30
1.062	0.63	4.125	2.44	7.187	4.32	10.250	6.35
1.125	0.66	4.187	2.48	7.250	4.36	10.312	6.39
1.187	0.70	4.250	2.52	7.312	4.40	10.375	6.43
1.250	0.74	4.312	2.55	7.375	4.44	10.437	6.48
1.312	0.77	4.375	2.59	7.437	4.48	10.500	6.52
1.375	0.81	4.437	2.63	7.500	4.52	10.562	6.56
1.437	0.85	4.500	2.67	7.562	4.56	10.625	6.61
1.500	0.88	4.562	2.71	7.625	4.60	10.687	6.65
1.562	0.92	4.625	2.74	7.687	4.64	10.750	6.70
1.625	0.96	4.687	2.78	7.750	4.68	10.812	6.74
1.687	0.99	4.750	2.82	7.812	4.72	10.875	6.78
1.750	1.03	4.812	2.86	7.875	4.76	10.937	6.83
1.812	1.07	4.875	2.89	7.937	4.80	11.000	6.87
1.875	1.10	4.937	2.93	8.000	4.84	11.062	6.92
1.937	1.14	5.000	2.97	8.062	4.88	11.125	6.96
2.000	1.18	5.062	3.01	8.125	4.92	11.187	7.01
2.062	1.22	5.125	3.05	8.187	4.96	11.250	7.05
2.125	1.25	5.187	3.08	8.250	5.00	11.312	7.10
2.187	1.29	5.250	3.12	8.312	5.04	11.375	7.15
2.250	1.33	5.312	3.16	8.375	5.08	11.437	7.19
2.312	1.36	5.375	3.20	8.437	5.13	11.500	7.24
2.375	1.40	5.437	3.24	8.500	5.17	11.562	7.28
2.437	1.44	5.500	3.27	8.562	5.21	11.625	7.33
2.500	1.47	5.562	3.31	8.625	5.25	11.687	7.37
2.562	1.51	5.625	3.35	8.687	5.29	11.750	7.42
2.625	1.55	5.687	3.39	8.750	5.33	11.812	7.47
2.687	1.59	5.750	3.43	8.812	5.37	11.875	7.51
2.750	1.62	5.812	3.47	8.875	5.41	11.937	7.56
2.812	1.66	5.875	3.50	8.937	5.45	12.000	7.61
2.875	1.70	5.937	3.54	9.000	5.50	12.062	7.65
2.937	1.73	6.000	3.58	9.062	5.54	12.125	7.70
3.000	1.77	6.062	3.62	9.125	5.58	12.187	7.75
3.062	1.81	6.125	3.66	9.187	5.62	12.250	7.80

5-7 *(Continued)*

Diopter	Sag	Diopter	Sag	Diopter	Sag	Diopter	Sag
12.312	7.84	14.750	9.85	17.125	12.23	19.500	15.52
12.375	7.89	14.812	9.91	17.187	12.30	19.562	15.63
12.437	7.94	14.875	9.96	17.250	12.38	19.625	15.74
12.500	7.99	14.937	10.02	17.312	12.45	19.687	15.86
12.562	8.04	15.000	10.08	17.375	12.52	19.750	15.97
12.625	8.08	15.062	10.14	17.437	12.60	19.812	16.09
12.687	8.13	15.125	10.19	17.500	12.67	19.875	16.21
12.750	8.18	15.187	10.25	17.562	12.74	19.937	16.34
12.812	8.23	15.250	10.31	17.625	12.82	20.000	16.46
12.875	8.28	15.312	10.37	17.687	12.90	20.062	16.59
12.937	8.33	15.375	10.43	17.750	12.97	20.125	16.72
13.000	8.38	15.437	10.49	17.812	13.05	20.187	16.85
13.062	8.43	15.500	10.54	17.875	13.13	20.250	16.99
13.125	8.48	15.562	10.60	17.937	13.21	20.312	17.13
13.187	8.53	15.625	10.66	18.000	13.29	20.375	17.28
13.250	8.58	15.687	10.73	18.062	13.37	20.437	17.42
13.312	8.63	15.750	10.79	18.125	13.45	20.500	17.58
13.375	8.68	15.812	10.85	18.187	13.54	20.562	17.73
13.437	8.73	15.875	10.91	18.250	13.62	20.625	17.89
13.500	8.78	15.937	10.97	18.312	13.70	20.687	18.06
13.562	8.83	16.000	11.03	18.375	13.79	20.750	18.23
13.625	8.89	16.062	11.10	18.437	13.87	20.812	18.41
13.687	8.94	16.125	11.16	18.500	13.96	20.875	18.59
13.750	8.99	16.187	11.22	18.562	14.05	20.937	18.79
13.812	9.04	16.250	11.29	18.625	14.14	21.000	18.99
13.875	9.09	16.312	11.35	18.687	14.23	21.062	19.20
13.937	9.15	16.375	11.42	18.750	14.32	21.125	19.42
14.000	9.20	16.437	11.48	18.812	14.41	21.187	19.65
14.062	9.25	16.500	11.55	18.875	14.51	21.250	19.89
14.125	9.31	16.562	11.61	18.937	14.60	21.312	20.15
14.187	9.36	16.625	11.68	19.000	14.70	21.375	20.44
14.250	9.41	16.687	11.75	19.062	14.80	21.437	20.74
14.312	9.47	16.750	11.82	19.125	14.90	21.500	21.07
14.375	9.52	16.812	11.88	19.187	15.00	21.562	21.45
14.437	9.58	16.875	11.95	19.250	15.10	21.625	21.88
14.500	9.63	16.937	12.02	19.312	15.20	21.687	22.39
14.562	9.68	17.000	12.09	19.375	15.31	21.750	23.05
14.625	9.74	17.062	12.16	19.437	15.41	21.812	24.23
14.687	9.80						

Source: Coburn Optical Industries, Muskogee, Okla., used by permission.

5-8 Tool Curves for Minus Cylinders
(1.498-index CR 39)

Desired Cylinder Power	Additional Cross Curve Required	Desired Cylinder Power	Additional Cross Curve Required
0.12	0.13	3.75	3.99
0.25	0.26	4.00	4.25
0.37	0.40	4.25	4.52
0.50	0.53	4.50	4.78
0.62	0.66	4.75	5.05
0.75	0.80	5.00	5.32
0.87	0.93	5.25	5.58
1.00	1.07	5.50	5.85
1.25	1.33	5.75	6.11
1.50	1.60	6.00	6.38
1.75	1.86	6.25	6.65
2.00	2.13	6.50	6.91
2.25	2.23	6.75	7.18
2.50	2.66	7.00	7.44
2.75	2.93	7.25	7.71
3.00	3.19	7.50	7.98
3.25	3.46	7.75	8.24
3.50	3.72	8.00	8.51

Source: Vision-Ease Laboratory Processing Data, Vision-Ease Corporation, St. Cloud, Minn., revised May 18, 1988, p. 50, used by permission.

Appendix 6

Lens and Frame Measurement Standards*

How much lenses are decentered for edging depends entirely on the method by which lenses and frames are measured. Two main systems are used throughout the English-speaking world, one based on a "boxed" lens size and another on a mid-lens width measurement. The *boxing system* is pictured in Figure A6-1 and is used in the United States and Canada. The *datum system*, as further defined in the *British Standards*, is used in England and many of the British Commonwealth nations. It is imperative that one standard or the other be used consistently, since the pattern is made for either one standard or the other and cannot be used interchangeably.

In the boxing system the *eye* or *lens* size is determined by the horizontal distance between two vertical tangents enclosing the lens on the left and right. The point halfway between these vertical tangents and also halfway between horizontal tangents enclosing the lens in a box is the primary reference point. This is known as the *boxing center*, since it is the center of the box enclosing the lens. It is alternately referred to as the *geometric center*, because *after* the lens is edged, it is the geometric center point. (The term "geometric center" must usually be qualified, since the geometric center of an uncut lens blank will not be at the geometric center of the lens once it has been edged.)

The *British Standards* define the lens or eyesize as being the width of the lens along the datum line.

See Figure A6-2. The *datum line* is a horizontal line halfway between the two horizontal tangents that border the top and bottom of the lens. This measure corresponds to the so-called *C* dimension of the boxing system and is known as the *datum length*, or simply the *eyesize*. The central reference point in the datum system is halfway across the lens as measured along the datum line and is called the *datum center*.

The distance between lenses (DBL) is measured differently between the two standards as well. The British Standard measures this along the datum line. As can be seen from Figure A6-2, this distance between lenses may not necessarily be the *smallest* distance between lenses. Therefore, the British Standards define the smallest measurable distance between the two lenses (regardless of the level where this minimum occurs) as the *minimum between lenses* (MBL). The datum MBL is the same as the boxing system's DBL.

When patterns are being manufactured, the center of rotation is drilled to correspond to the central reference point of the standard being used. And because the boxing center is not located at the same point for a given shape as the datum center, a pattern drilled for the boxing system will not work if the British Standard is being used to calculate lens decentration and vice versa.

Fortunately, decentration calculations are made in exactly the same manner, regardless of the system being used. However, the results must not be interchanged.

---

*From C. W. Brooks, *Essentials for Ophthalmic Lens Work*, Butterworth-Heinemann, Boston, 1983, pp. 224–229.

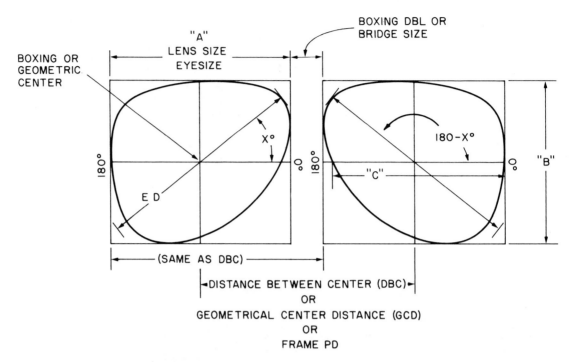

Figure A6-1 In the boxing system, *ED* is the abbreviation for effective diameter, which is twice the longest radius of the shape as measured from the boxing (geometric) center. The angle from the zero-degree side of the 180-degree line to the effective diameter axis is *X* for the right lens. The measure is used in accurate calculation of the minimum lens blank size and blank thickness required to fabricate the prescription.

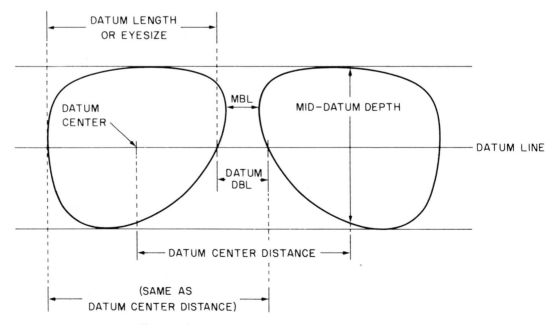

Figure A6-2 The datum system.

For example, suppose a frame has the following dimensions:

Boxing eyesize (A) = 52
Boxing DBL = 15
Datum length = 49
Datum DBL = 19
Wearer's PD = 63

Decentration for the boxing system is

$$\frac{(\text{Eyesize} + \text{DBL}) - \text{PD}}{2} = \frac{(52 + 15) - 63}{2}$$

so

$$\text{Decentration} = 2 \text{ mm per lens}$$

Decentration for British Standards is

$$\frac{(\text{Eyesize} + \text{DBL}) - \text{PD}}{2} = \frac{(49 + 19) - 63}{2}$$

so

Decentration = 2.5 mm per lens

Now if a pattern intended for the boxing standard is used when British Standard calculations have been made, the distance between the two lens optical centers will be 1 mm smaller than ordered.

A third system was established by a group representing the European Economic Community and referred to as the Groupement des Opticiens du Marché Commun (GOMAC). As Figure A6-3 shows, the attempt was to reach a compromise between boxing and datum systems. The results have not been universally accepted, even among Common Market countries.

Differences and similarities in systems are summarized in Figure A6-4, while corresponding terms are listed in Appendix 6-1. Similarities and differences between U.S. and British multifocal placement terminology are summarized in Figures A6-5 and A6-6.

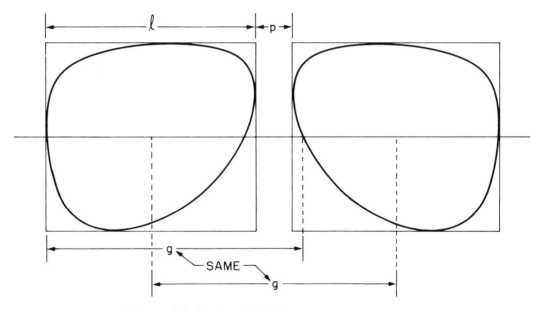

Figure A6-3 The GOMAC system.
l = boxed length of lens ("largeur totale du verre")
p = boxing DBL ("distance minima entre verres," or "pont")
g = datum center distance ("grandeur, ou taille de la monture")
Not pictured:
n = base of the frame bridge on the datum line, a type of anatomical inside bridge measure ("largeur nasale anatomique")
t = width of a rimless mounting front measured from barrel center to barrel center ["largeur temporale de la face, mesurée entre les axes d'articulation (seulement pour les monture glaces)"]
[From L.S. Sasieni, Optical Standards, *Manufacturing Optics International,* 25 (10): 395–398 (May 1972).]

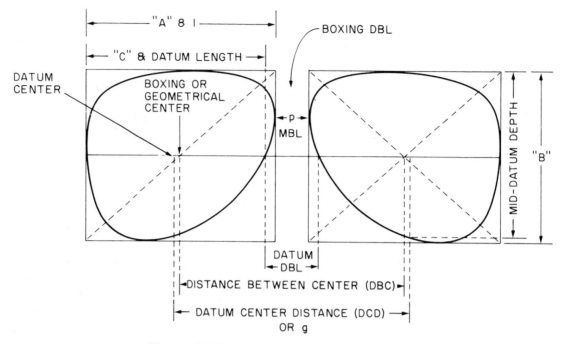

Figure A6-4 Diagrammatic comparison of boxing, datum, and GOMAC systems. Note that the datum center will not always be outset with respect to the boxing center. For an upswept harlequin shape, the datum center will be inset as compared to the boxing center.

6-1 Comparison of Standard Terms

Boxing	Datum or British Standards	GOMAC
Mechanical center		R
A	—	ℓ
B	—	—
C	Datum length	—
Boxing DBL	MBL	p
—	Datum DBL	—
—	Datum center distance (DCD)	g
Distance between centers (DBC) (Geometric center distance) (GCD) ("Frame PD") (Boxing center distance)	—	—
—	Mid-datum depth	—
Major reference point (MRP)	Distance centration point (DCP) (or simply centration point)	

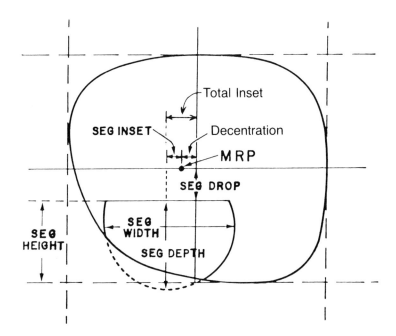

Figure A6-5 Accepted U.S. multifocal placement terminology. Decentration is sometimes referred to as *inset*. This must not be confused with *seg inset* or *total inset*.

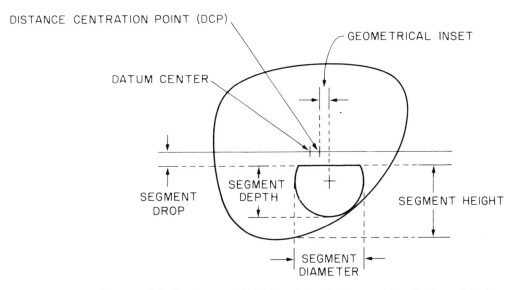

Figure A6-6 Accepted British multifocal placement terminology. (It will be noted that a right lens is shown in this diagram, whereas a left lens was shown in Figure A6-5.) Because the datum center and boxing center do not necessarily correspond, the decentration required for the MRP (DCP) will not likely be the same.

ANSI Z80 Standards

Standards established by the American National Standards Institute (ANSI) are summarized here in tabular form. The tables are not meant to be all-inclusive. For complete information consult *American National Standard Recommendations for Prescription Ophthalmic Lenses, Z80.1* It may be obtained from:

American National Standards
1430 Broadway
New York, New York 10018

7-1 ANSI Refractive Power Tolerances*

Refractive Power	Tolerance
For the sphere component:	
From 0.00 to ±6.50 D	±0.13 D
Above ± 6.50 D	2% of the sphere power
For the cylinder component:	
From 0.00 to 2.00 D cyl	±0.13 D
From 2.12 to 4.50 D cyl	±0.15 D
Above 4.50 D cyl	4% of the cylinder power
For the near addition:	
For multifocals whose *distance* powers are 8.00 D and below, the add power tolerance is	±0.13 D
For multifocals whose *distance* powers are above 8.00 D, the add power tolerance is	±0.18 D

*Based on *American Standard Recommendations for Prescription Ophthalmic Lenses*, Z80.1-1987, American National Standards Institute, Inc., New York, 1987, p. 11.

---

*All tables from C. W. Brooks, *Essentials for Ophthalmic Lens Work*, Butterworth-Heinemann, Boston, 1983, pp. 230–231.

7-2 Tolerance for Cylinder Axis*

Cylinder Power	Tolerance
0.125 D to 0.375 D	±7 degrees
0.500 D to 0.750 D	±5 degrees
0.875 D to 1.50 D	±3 degrees
1.625 D and above	±2 degrees

*Tolerances are based on *American National Standard Recommendations for Prescription Ophthalmic Lenses*, Z80.1-1987, p. 12.

7-3 ANSI Prism Power and Major Reference Point Location*

	Tolerance
For lenses in the frame:	
Vertical prism or MRP placement	⅓ prism diopter *or* 1.0-mm difference between left and right MRP heights in high-power Rx with no prism ordered
Horizontal prism or MRP placement	⅔ prism diopter (total from both lenses combined) *or* ±2.5-mm variation from the specified distance PD for high-powered Rxs
For "lenses only" (not yet mounted) *and* uncut multifocals:	
Prism power	± ⅓ prism diopter in any direction on the lens
MRP position placement	±1.0 mm in any direction for high-powered lenses

*Based on *American National Standard Recommendations for Precription Ophthalmic Lenses*, Z80.1-1987, pp. 12–13.

7-4 ANSI Segment Location Tolerances*

	Tolerance
Vertical (segment height):	
Unmounted single lens	±1.0 mm
Lens pair: mounted or unmounted	+1.0 mm (but both lenses in pair should be at matching heights)
Horizontal (segment inset):	
Unmounted single lenses	±1.0 mm
Mounted lens pair	±2.5 mm
	Inset should appear symmetrical and balanced

*Based on *American National Standard Recommendations for Prescription Ophthalmic Lenses*, Z80.1-1987, p. 13.

7-5 ANSI Miscellaneous Tolerances*

	Tolerance
Thickness	±0.3 mm (when specified on order)
Warpage	1.00 D (does not apply within 6 mm of eyewire)
Base curve	±0.75 D (when specified on order)

*Based on *American National Standard Recommendations for Prescription Ophthalmic Lenses*, Z80.1-1987, pp. 13–14.

Comparison of Surfacing Techniques

	GLASS	*CR-39 PLASTIC*
CENTER THICKNESS: Minimum Recommended	2.2 mm	2.2 mm
BLOCKING Block Size	43 mm or larger	Large blocks advised
Alloy Type	158 degrees	117 degrees
Alloy Temperature	165 to 170 degrees	125 degrees or less
Special comments		
Minimum Recommended Cooling Time Before Generating	Opinion varies	Opinion varies, but cooling time needed. Solid alloy blocks need additional cooling time.
GENERATING Wet or Dry	Wet: oil or water based	Wet or dry
Maximum Recommended Cut	One cut with oil coolant if photochromic generator wheel is used. 1 mm with water based coolant	3 to 4 mm with correct generator wheel and chilled coolant. 0.3 to 0.8 mm per pass if a multipurpose (glass and plastic) wheel is used, or if coolant is not refrigerated.
Final Cut	0.2 to 0.3 mm	Wet: 0.2 mm Two cuts of 0.2 mm each if coolant is not refrigerated or if a multipurpose wheel is used. Dry: 0.5 to 1.0 mm

POLYCARBONATE	*POLYURETHANE* *Thin & Lite 1.6 and Varilux 1.6* *Recommendations*	*PHOTOCHROMIC PLASTIC* *Transitions Recommendations*
1.5 mm (2.4 mm for low-powered lenses)	1.5 mm	2.0 mm (2.4 mm for low-powered lenses)
Slightly less than lens blank diameter to make shock deblocking easier	Largest block available (such as 68-mm block)	Largest block possible. Use 68-mm block for best results
117 degree	117 degree	117 degree
Not more than 125 at stem of blocker	122 to 125 degrees	120 to 122 degrees
Do not use a varnish coating. Use blocking tape.	Keep the alloy flowing smoothly. This will prevent voids in the alloy. Voids cause waves in the surface. The blocking coolant ring should be 60 to 65 degrees F.	Keep the alloy flowing smoothly. This will prevent voids in the alloy. Voids cause waves in the surface.
15 minutes Solid alloy blocks need additional cooling time.	20 to 30 minutes Solid alloy blocks need additional cooling time.	15 minutes Solid alloy blocks need additional cooling time.
Wet or dry, but wet recommended. Coolant temperature 65–75 degrees.	Wet—with a plated generator wheel recommended. Use fly cutter generator wheel if dry used.	Wet or dry
2 to 3 mm per pass. Some advise limiting first cuts to between 0.5 and 1.0 mm.	1.0 mm or 2.0 mm. Use manual sweep on slow speed. Or if normal speed is 7 to 8, turn speed down to 5.	2 mm
Remove 0.5 mm with a 15-second final sweep, or do two final sweeps of 0.5 and 0.2 mm each. For plus power lenses some advise taking a heavy (2 to 3 mm) cut on the final pass.	0.2-mm final cut if wet (0.7 mm if using dry fly cutter wheel). Final cut should be as slow as possible. When using automatic thickness, a zero cut final cut is recommended.	0.5 mm at slow speed

	GLASS	CR-39 PLASTIC
Thickness Allowance for Fining	0.3 mm	0.3 mm
FINING Pressure	20 psi	One-step process: 20 psi Two-step process: 15 to 20 psi
One-step pads	Aluminum oxide slurry on metal pads	Option 1: 15-micron aluminum oxide Option 2: 4-micron pad
One-step time		Option 1: 1 minute Option 2: 1 to 3 minutes
Two-step pads	Does not apply	15-micron silicon carbide first fine (black or gray) 12-micron aluminum oxide second fine
Two-step time	Does not apply	1 to 1½ minutes first fine 2 minutes second fine

Comments	Stroke:
	  Upper use long stroke
	  Lower use medium stroke
		Stroke:
		  Upper use long stroke
		  Lower use medium stroke

POLISHING Pressure	mid 30's	20 psi
Time	Varies; 4 to 5 minutes average	5 to 6 minutes
Polish Temperature		55 to 60 degrees

Comments	Stroke:
	  Upper use long stroke
	  Lower use long stroke
		Stroke:
		  Upper use long stroke
		  Lower use long stroke

DEBLOCKING	Hot water	Hot water or shock
CLEANING	Most anything works	Mild detergent or normal solvents such as alcohol or acetone

POLYCARBONATE	POLYURETHANE *Thin & Lite 1.6 and Varilux 1.6* *Recommendations*	PHOTOCHROMIC PLASTIC *Transitions Recommendations*
0.35 mm	0.2 to 2.5 mm (MAXIMUM) for one-step fining. If take-off exceeds 2.5 mm during fining, reduce cylinder machine head pressure 2–3 lbs at a time until the correct amount of stock removal is achieved. 0.4 mm for two-step fining	0.3 to 0.4 mm
18 to 20 psi	15 to 17 psi (Varilux recommends) 18 to 20 psi (Thin & Lite recommends)	15 psi (at the pins)
	1200 grit (seven leaf pad recommended)	1200 grit
	1½ minutes	1 minute
280 grit (40 micron) first fine 1200 (13 to 15 micron) grit second fine	40-micron aluminum oxide first fine. Yellow 12-micron aluminum oxide second fine or 600 grit first fine, 1200 grit second fine	600 grit first fine 12-micron second fine
2 minutes first fine 2 minutes second fine	1 minute first fine 1½ to 2 minutes second fine	½ minute first fine 1 minute second fine
Bevel the backside of the generated lens to remove sharp edges and allow for better coolant flow during fining and polishing.	1. Fining at high speed is recommended. 2. Adjust the stroke to maximum. 3. Use a 5-second fine to check correctness of curve. There should be a 30-mm size hole if curve is correct. If hole is larger, the curve is coming off the generator too steep. 4. Use fresh water. If recirculated water must be used, filter the water or change it frequently. 5. Dip in alcohol bath immediately after fining to prevent oxidation. (Do not spray.) Air dry.	
20 psi	15 to 17 psi (Varilux recommends) 18 to 20 psi (Thin & Lite recommends)	15 psi
4 to 6 minutes	6 minutes (Flood the pad with polish during polishing process.)	4 minutes
65 to 70 degrees	Cooled	50 to 60 degrees
	1. Rinse in warm water immediately after polish cycle. Use natural sponges. 2. Handle lens by edges. Never touch surface.	
Shock	Shock	Shock only
Wash with diluted mild detergent. Rinse with fresh running water. Dry with HyperClean™ tissue or equivalent. Do not use air dryer. Never let water or polish dry on the lens.	See "Comments" in the Fining and Polishing portions of this table.	Use mild detergent or normal solvents as with CR-39.

Bibliography

American National Standards Recommendations for Occupational and Educational Eye and Face Protection, Z87.1-1989. American National Standards Institute, New York, 1989.

American National Standard Recommendations for Prescription Ophthalmic Lenses, ANSI Z80.1-1987. American National Standards Institute, New York, 1987.

Back-side Coating Technical Information. Essilor of America, Inc., 1991.

Brooks, C.W. *Essentials for Ophthalmic Lens Work.* Butterworth-Heinemann, Boston, 1983.

Brooks, C.W., and Borish, I.M. *System for Ophthalmic Dispensing.* Butterworth-Heinemann, Boston, 1979.

Check, W. Slab-off Grinding. *Optical Index,* 56 (3):54–56 (March 1981).

Cline, D., Hofstetter, H.W., and Griffin, J.R. *The Dictionary of Visual Science,* 4th ed. Chilton Trade Book Publishing, Radmor, Pa., 1989, p. 573.

Coating Manual. Gentex Corporation, Dudley, Mass., 1988.

Coburn/LTI Coating System Owner's Manual. Coburn Optical Industries, Muskogee, Okla., August, 1990.

Coburn Optical Industries. *Operation and Maintenance Manual, Manual and Semi-Automatic Generators, Series 108.* Coburn Optical Industries, Muskogee, Okla., n.d.

Coburnsystem Bulletin No. 4. Coburn Optical Industries, Muskogee, Okla., n.d.

Coburnsystem Bulletin No. 7. Coburn Optical Industries, Muskogee, Okla., n.d.

Coburnsystem Bulletin No. 9. Coburn Optical Industries, Muskogee, Okla., n.d.

Coburnsystem Bulletin No. 11. Coburn Optical Industries, Muskogee, Okla., n.d.

Coburnsystem Bulletin, Standard Glass Procedure. Coburn Optical Industries, Muskogee, Okla., revised 10/80.

A Coburnsystem™ Procedure for Processing Polycarbonate Lenses. Coburn Optical Industries, Muskogee, Okla., Copyright 1989, February 1990 edition.

Coburnsystem Procedure for Surfacing Polycarbonate Lenses. Coburn Optical Industries, Inc., Muskogee. Okla., n.d.

Coburnsystem Program Outline, Coburn Optical Industries, Muskogee, Okla., n.d.

Denison, J. Surfacing Optical Plastic Lenses Made from CR-39® Monomer—Part 1. *Optical Index,* 55 (8):61 (August 1980).

Drew, R. CR-39 Slab-off Lenses: Now Ready Cast. *Optical Management,* 13:21–29 (January 1980).

Drew, R. In-Office Lens Casting Can Offer a Marketing Edge. *Optometric Management,* 23 (11):40–46 (November 1987).

Fry, G.A. The Optometrist's New Role in the Use of Corrected Curve Lenses. *Journal of the American Optometric Association,* 50 (5):561–562 (May 1970).

Gentex Corporation Surfacing Manual. Gentex Corporation, Dudley, Mass., 1988.

Hirschhorn, H. Lens-Blocking Materials. *Optical Index,* 55 (3):95–98 (March 1980).

Horne, D.F. *Spectacle Lens Technology.* Adam Hilger, Bristol, England, 1978.

How to Cut Aluma-Laps. PSI Technical Bulletin. Practical Systems, Inc., Tarpon Springs, Fla., n.d.

Introducing One Step Plastic Lens Polishing. FB Optical Manufacturing, Inc., Saint Cloud, Minn., n.d.

Jalie, M. *Tables for Surfacing Instruction; Spectacle Crown Glass and CR-39.* ICP Science and Technology Press, Guildford, England, 1972.

Job Coach for Prescription Laboratory Operations. Bausch and Lomb, Rochester, NY, 1946 (reprinted 1970).

Kors, Kermit. Part 1—Seg Inset for the "Executive" Multifocal. *Journal of the American Optometric Association,* 52 (6):513–517 (June 1981).

Kors, Kermit. Part II—Seg Inset for the "Executive" Multifocal. *Journal of the American Optometric Association,* 52 (7):575–577 (July 1981).

Laboratory Manual for Processing Varilux Lenses. Varilux Corporation, Foster City, Calif., n.d.

Lens Learning System. Nova Communications, for Titmus Optical, Petersburg, Va., 1976.

Mancusi, R.L. *Ophthalmic Surfacing for Plastic and Glass Lenses.* Butterworth-Heinemann, Boston, 1982.

Mullins, P. Accurately Measuring Lens Surfaces During Manufacturing. *Optical Index,* 56 (2):39–40 (February 1981).

Optical Laboratory Marketing Plan. Gentex, Dudley Mass., 1980.

Polycarbonate Lens Processing Guide. Sola Optical, Inc., Petaluma, Calif., undated.

Polycarbonate Processing Guide, Poly T × 3. Orcolite, Azusa, Calif., January 1991.

Rosen, K. Premolded Slab-offs Bring Results. *Optical Management,* 13:27–32 (September 1984).

Seamless Plus Layout for Surfacing (Publication 104 TF). Younger Optics, Los Angeles, Calif., n.d.

Sheedy, J.E., and Parson, S.D. Vertical Yoked Prism—Patient Acceptance and Postural Adjustment. *Ophthalamic and Physiological Opt.,* 7(3):225–257 (1987).

Silvernail, W.L. *Reopol Technical Bulletin Series.* Shieldalloy Corporation, Newfield, N.J.

Stone, G. Varilux Labs Helpful Hints. *Progressive Addition,* V (3):(August 15, 1985).

Titmus Polycristyl™ Comprehensive Processing Guide for Polycarbonate Lenses. Titmus Optical, Petersburg, Va., n.d.

Thin & Lite™ 1.6 High Index Lenses Technical Guide. Silor Optical, Pinellas Park, Fla., 1990.

Transitions Comfort Lenses Technical Guide. Silor Optical, Pinellas Park, Fla., January 1991.

Varilux Infinity 1.6 (High Index Plastic) Lab Manual. Varilux Corporation, Foster City, Calif., undated.

Vision-Ease Laboratory Processing Data. Vision-Ease, St. Cloud, Minn., January 1985, revised May 18, 1988.

Whitman, P.C. Fundamentals of Glass Polishing for the Prescription Laboratory—Part 2: Polishing Theory and Cerium Oxide. *Optical Index,* 54 (17):58–60 (December 1979).

Woodcock, F.R. Prescription Shop Machinery, Part 3: Automatic Cylinder Surfacing Machines. *Manufacturing Optics International,* 27 (3):105–116 (March 1974).

Woodcock, F.R. Prescription Shop Machinery, Part 6: Lap Cutting Machines. *Manufacturing Optics International,* 27 (6):296–301 (June 1974).

Glossary

Δ Symbol for prism. When following a number, it denotes the units known as prism diopters.

A Horizontal dimension of the boxing system rectangle that encloses a lens or lens opening.

Accelerator An additive to a polishing slurry that is used to increase the efficiency of the slurry.

Accurate sag formula *See* Formula, accurate sag.

Actual power *See* Power, actual.

Adapter, offset block A small metal device used on a lens that has been blocked off center. It is used for the purpose of transferring pressure back to the center of the lens so that unwanted prism may be avoided.

Add *See* Addition, near.

Addition, near The power that a lens segment has in addition to that power already present in the main portion of the lens.

Alignment, standard An impersonal standard, independent of facial shape, for the alignment of spectacle frames.

Allowance, vertex power The amount by which the front surface curvature of a lens must be flattened in order to compensate for a thickness-related gain in power.

Angle, apical The angle formed by the junction of two nonparallel prism surfaces.

Angle, effective diameter The angle from the zero-degree side of the 180-degree line to the axis of the effective diameter. The angle is referred to by the letter X and is measured using the right lens.

Angle of deviation The difference between the angle of incidence and the angle of refraction.

Angle, pantoscopic 1. In standard alignment, that angle by which the frame front deviates from the vertical (lower rims farther inward than upper rims) when the spectacles are held with the temples horizontal. 2. In fitting, that angle which the frame front makes with the frontal plane of the wearer's face when the lower rims are closer to the face than the upper rims (opposite-retroscopic angle). (Synonym: Pantoscopic tilt.)

Angle, retroscopic That angle which the frame front makes with the frontal plane of the wearer's face when the lower rims are farther from the face than the upper rims (opposite-pantoscopic angle). (Synonym: Retroscopic tilt.)

Anisometropia A condition in which one eye differs significantly in refractive power from the other.

Antireflection coating *See* Coating, antireflection.

Antiscratch coating *See* Coating, antiscratch.

Aperture An opening or hole that admits only a portion of light from a given source or sources.

Aperture, lens The portion of the spectacle frame that accepts the lens. (Synonym: Lens opening.)

Apex The junction point at which the two nonparallel surfaces of a prism meet.

Aphakic A person whose crystalline lens has been removed.

Aspheric A nonspherical surface. An aspheric lens surface generally decreases in power peripherally in order to correct for aberrations found in the periphery of a lens.

Aspheric, full-field An aspheric lens that begins its asphericity where the small central spheric region leaves off. It continues in its asphericity all the way to the edge of the lens blank.

Aspheric lenticular *See* Lenticular, aspheric.

Astigmatism The presence of two different curves on a single refracting surface on or within the eye. This causes light to focus as two line images instead of a single point.

Axis, of a cylinder An imaginary reference line used to specify cylinder or spherocylinder lens orientation and corresponding to the meridian perpendicular to that of maximum cylinder power.

Axis, prism The base direction of an ophthalmic prism, expressed in degrees.

Axis, optical That line which passes through the center of a lens on which the radii of curvature of the front and back surfaces fall.

B The vertical dimension of the boxing system rectangle that encloses a lens or lens opening.

Back base curve *See* Curve, back base.

Back cut *See* Cut, back.

Back vertex power *See* Power, back vertex.

Ball gauge *See* Gauge, ball.

Bar gauge *See* Gauge, bar.

Base In a prism, the edge of maximum surface separation opposite the apex.

Base curve *See* Curve, base.

Base down Vertical placement of prism such that the base is at 270 degrees on a degree scale.

Base in Horizontal placement of prism such that the base is toward the nose.

Base out Horizontal placement of prism such that the base is toward the side of the head.

Base up Vertical placement of prism such that the base is at 90 degrees on a degree scale.

Baumé degrees A system used to quantify the concentration of a slurry based on the specific gravity of the slurry; $°Bé = 145 - 145/SG$, where SG = specific gravity.

BCD Boxing center distance. *See* Distance, boxing center.

°Bé An abbreviation for degrees Baumé.

Bell gauge *See* Gauge, bell.

Bevel The angled edge of the spectacle lens.

Bevel, pin Synonym for safety bevel.

Bevel, safety 1. To remove the sharp interface between lens surface and bevel surface and the sharp point at the bevel apex. 2. The smoothed interface between lens surface and bevel surface and the smoothed lens bevel apex.

Bevel, V A lens edge configuration having the form of a V across the whole breadth of the lens edge.

Bicentric grind Synonym for slab-off.

Bifocals Lenses having two areas for viewing, each with its own focal power. Usually the upper portion of the lens is for distance vision, the lower for near vision.

Bifocal, blended A bifocal lens constructed from one piece of lens material and having the demarcation line smoothed out so as not to be visible to an observer.

Bifocal, curved-top A bifocal lens having a segment that is round in the lower portion and gently curved on the top of the segment.

Bifocal, Executive American Optical's trade name for the Franklin-style bifocal.

Bifocal, flat-top A bifocal with a segment that is round in the lower half but flat on the top.

Bifocal, Franklin A bifocal having a segment that extends the entire width of the lens blank.

Bifocals, round seg A bifocal with a segment that is perfectly round. The width of the segment is usually 22 mm, but may be larger (usually 38 mm).

Blank, finished lens A lens having both front and back surfaces ground to the desired powers, but not yet edged to the shape of the frame.

Blank geometric center *See* Center, blank geometric.

Blank, rough A lens-shaped piece of glass with neither side having the finished curvature. Both sides must yet be surfaced in order to bring the lens to its desired power and thickness.

Blank seg drop *See* Drop, blank seg.

Blank seg inset *See* Inset, blank seg.

Blank, semifinished lens A lens with only one side having the desired curvature. The second side must yet be surfaced in order to bring the lens to its desired power and thickness.

Blended myodisc *See* Lens, blended myodisc.

Block That which is attached to the surface of a lens in order to hold it in place during the surfacing or edging process.

Block decentration *See* Decentration, block.

Block mark *See* Mark, block.

Blocker The device used to place a block on the lens in order to hold the lens in place during the surfacing or edging process.

Blocking bodies Surfacing blocks used in conjunction with pitch.

Blocking, finish The application of a holding block to an ophthalmic lens so that it may be edged to fit a frame.

Blocking, off-center The practice of placing the surfacing lens block at the desired location for the major reference point of the lens. Off-center blocking does not grind prism for decentration.

Blocking, on-center The practice of placing the surfacing block at the blank geometric center of the lens and moving the major reference point of the lens to its desired location by grinding prism for decentration.

Blocking, simplified on-center The practice of using sine-squared methods to move the optical center horizontally. The surfacing block is centered horizontally but positioned vertically above the seg top by an amount equal to the seg drop.

Blocking, surface The application of a holding block to an ophthalmic lens so that one side may be ground to the correct curvature and polished.

Blocks, glass A small, thick disk used to hold a glass lens in place during the surfacing process. These are generally 43 mm in diameter and may be adapted for use in blocking plastic lenses.

Blocks, plastic A curved disk used to hold a plastic lens in place during the surfacing process. These blocks vary in diameter, but are normally larger than glass blocks to prevent lens flex during processing.

Box-o-Graph A flat device containing grids and slides, used in the measurement of pattern and edged lens size.

Boxing center *See* Center, boxing.

Boxing center distance *See* Distance, boxing center.

Boxing system *See* System, boxing.

Bridge The area of the frame front between the lenses.

Burn, polishing A lens surface defect that looks like a blister or a small group of blisters on the lens surface. Polishing burn may be the result of a polishing pad that has not been sufficiently wetted with polish.

C The horizontal width of a lens at a level halfway between the two horizontal tangents of the top and bottom of the lens shape. (Synonym: Datum length.)

Carrier The optically unusable outer portion of a lenticular lens that "carries" the optically usable central portion.

Cataract A loss in clarity of the crystalline lens of the eye, which results in reduced vision or loss of vision.

Center, boxing The midpoint of the rectangle that encloses a lens in the boxing system.

Center, blank geometric The physical center of a semifinished lens blank or an uncut finished lens blank. The blank geometric center is the center of the smallest square or rectangle that completely encloses the lens blank.

Center, datum The midpoint of the datum length (C dimension) of a lens along the datum line.

Center, geometric 1. The boxing center. 2. The middle point on an uncut lens blank.

Center, optical That point on an ophthalmic prescription lens through which no prismatic effect is manifested.

Center, reading That point on a lens at the reading level that corresponds to the near PD.

Center, seg optical That location on the segment of a bifocal lens that shows zero prismatic effect when there is no refractive power in the distance portion of the lens.

Centers Three short, replaceable, cylinder-shaped pieces that fit into a surfacing block and serve as pivot points during fining and polishing.

Centrad (∇) A unit of measurement of the displacement of light by a prism. One centrad is the prism power required to displace a ray of light 1 cm from the position it would otherwise strike on the arc of a circle having a 1-m radius.

Centration The act of positioning a lens for edging such that it will conform optically to prescription specifications.

Chart, prism A circular chart used to find the sum of two prismatic effects graphically. This sum is expressed with the amount given in prism diopters and the base direction given in degrees.

Charts, surfacing Synonym for surfacing tables.

Chiller A refrigeration unit used for cooling generator coolant, fining or polishing slurry, or blocking alloy in the ophthalmic surfacing laboratory.

Chord A straight line intersecting two points of an arc.

Chord diameter *See* Diameter, chord.

Clock, seg Designed like a conventional lens measure except that the three points of contact are closely spaced.

Coating, antiscratch A thin, hard coating applied to plastic lens surfaces in order to make them more resistant to scratching.

Coating, antireflection A thin layer or series of layers of material applied to the surface of a lens for the purpose of reducing unwanted reflections from the lens surface and thus increasing the amount of light that passes through to the eye.

Collector, mist A vacuum system installed above the generator grinding chamber, which removes droplets of generator coolant caused by the rapidly spinning grinding wheel that would otherwise form a mist.

Colmascope An instrument that utilizes polarized light to show strain patterns in glass or plastic.

Compensated lap tool *See* Tool, compensated lap.

Compensating pad *See* Pad, tool compensating.

Compensated power *See* Power, compensated.

Compounding (of prism) The process of combining two or more prisms to obtain the equivalent prismatic effect expressed as a single prism.

Concave An inward-curved surface.

Convergence 1. An inward turning of the eyes, as when looking at a near object. 2. The action of light rays traveling toward a specific real image point.

Convex An outward-curved surface.

Coolant A recirculating liquid used to cool and lubricate the lens/grinding wheel interface during the grinding process.

Coolant manifold *See* Manifold, coolant.

Countersink curve *See* Curve, countersink.

Cover lens *See* Lens, cover.

CR-39 A registered trademark of Pittsburgh Plate Glass Co. for an optical plastic known as Columbia Resin 39. It is the standard material from which conventional plastic lenses are made.

Cribbing The process of reducing a semifinished lens blank to a smaller size in order to speed the surfacing process or reduce the probability of difficulty in surfacing.

Cross curve *See* Curve, cross.

Cross, fitting A reference point 2 to 4 mm above the major reference point on progressive-addition lenses. The fitting cross is positioned in front of the pupil.

Cross, power A schematic representation on which the two major meridians of a lens or lens surface are depicted.

Curvature The reciprocal of the radius of curvature of a curved surface, quantified in m^{-1}, abbreviated by R.

Curve, back base The weaker back-surface curve of a minus cylinder-form lens. When the lens is a minus cylinder-form lens, the back base curve and the toric base curve are the same.

Curve, base The surface curve of a lens that becomes the basis from which the other remaining curves are calculated.

Curve, cross The stronger curve of a toric lens surface.

Curve, countersink For the manufacture of semifinished bi- and trifocal lenses, the countersink curve is that curve which is ground into the main lens in the area where the segment is to be placed. The countersink curve matches the back curve of the bi- or trifocal segment. When the segment is placed on the countersink curve of the main lens, the two may then be fused together.

Curve, nominal base A 1.53-index-referenced number assigned to the base curve of a semifinished lens. For moderately powered crown-glass lenses the needed back-surface tool curve may be found by subtracting the nominal base curve from the prescribed back vertex power.

Curve, tool The 1.53-index-referenced surface power of a lap tool used in the fining and polishing of ophthalmic lenses.

Curve, true base Synonym for true power.

Cut, back In generating, the practice of beginning with the back edge of the lens and making only a partial grinding cut across the surface. This prepares the lens for a deep, full sweep across the surface of the lens from the front edge and avoids tearing a chunk off the back edge of the lens.

Cutter, lap A machine used to cut a lap tool to its correct curvature.

Cutter, template A lap cutter that uses individual templates to guide the accurate cutting of the lap tool. Template cutters will cut laps with especially low base curves and saddleback tools, which many standard lap cutters are not able to do.

Cylinder A lens having a refractive power in one meridian only and used in the correction of astigmatism.

D An abbreviation for diopter of refractive power. *See also* Diopter, lens.

Datum center *See* Center, datum.

Datum center distance *See* Distance, datum center.

Datum line *See* Line, datum.

Datum system *See* System, datum.

DBC Distance between centers.

DBL Distance between lenses.

DCD Datum center distance.

Decentration 1. The displacement of the lens optical center or major reference point away from the boxing or datum center of the frame's lens aperture. 2. The displacement of a lens optical center away from the wearer's line of sight for the purpose of creating a prismatic effect.

Decentration, block The distance a lens surfacing block is moved from the blank geometric center of a lens.

Degrees Baumé *See* Baumé degrees.

Depth, mid-datum The depth of the lens measured through the datum center.

Depth, reading The vertical position in the lens through which the wearer's line of sight passes when reading.

Depth, seg The longest vertical dimension of the lens segment.

Depth, sagittal (sag) The height or depth of a given segment of a circle.

Diamater, chord The diameter of a lens used for calculating lens thickness. Chord diameter = ED + (*A* + DBL − PD).

Diameter, effective Twice the longest radius of a frame's lens aperture as measured from the boxing center. Abbreviated ED.

Difference, frame In the boxing system, the difference between frame *A* and frame *B* dimensions, expressed in millimeters.

Diopter, lens (D) Unit of lens refractive power, equal to the reciprocal of the lens focal length in meters.

Diopter, prism (Δ) The unit of measurement that quantifies prism deviating power; one prism diopter (1 Δ) is the power required to deviate a ray of light 1 cm from the position it would otherwise strike at a point 1 m away from the prism.

Disk, trueing An abrasive disk that may be selectively spun across certain areas of a spinning spherical lap tool for the purpose of bringing that tool back to its proper curvature.

Dissimilar segs *See* Segs, dissimilar.

Distance between centers In a frame or finished pair of glasses, the distance between the boxing (geometric) centers.

Distance between lenses 1. In the boxing system, the distance between the two boxed lenses as positioned in the frame. [Synonym: datum minimum between lenses (MBL)]. 2. In the datum system, the distance between lenses in the frame as measured at the level of the datum line.

Distance, boxing center Synonym for distance between centers.

Distance, datum center The distance between the datum centers in a frame or pair of glasses.

Distance, frame center Synonym for distance between centers.

Distance, geometric center The distance between the boxing (geometric) centers of a frame.

Distance, interpupillary (PD) The distance from the center of one pupil to the center of the other when either an infinitely distant object is being viewed (distance PD) or a near object is being viewed (near PD).

Distance, near centration The distance between the geometric centers of the near segments.

Distance, vertex The distance from the back surface of the lens to the front of the eye.

Divergence The action of light rays going out from a point source.

Dress To resharpen the cutting surface of a grinding wheel.

Drop, blank seg The vertical distance from the blank geometric center to the top of the multifocal segment.

Drop, seg 1. The vertical distance from the major reference point (MRP) to the top of the seg when the seg top is lower than the MRP. 2. The vertical distance from the datum line to the top of the seg when the seg top is lower than the datum line (laboratory usage). (Antonym: seg raise.)

ED Effective diameter.

Edger The piece of machinery used to physically grind the uncut lens blank to fit the shape of the frame.

Edger, hand A grinding wheel made especially for grinding lenses by hand.

Effective diameter *See* Diameter, effective.

Effective diameter angle *See* Angle, effective diameter.

Effective power *See* Power, effective.

Elliptical error *See* Error, elliptical.

Emery An impure form of aluminum oxide containing certain iron oxides.

Emery, rough A commonly used term for a coarse abrasive used to obtain a curve on a glass lens that is beyond the range of the generator. The term is a misnomer, because the abrasive is really carborundum, not emery.

Equithin A term used by the Varilux Corporation when referring to the use of yoked prism for thickness reduction on a pair of Varilux progressive-addition lenses. *See also* Prism, yoked.

Equivalent, spherical The sum of the spherical component and one-half of the cylinder component of an ophthalmic lens prescription.

Error, elliptical The slight deviation of a lens surface away from a sphere and toward an ellipse that occurs during lens generating when using a cup-shaped generator wheel.

Executive bifocal *See* Bifocal, Executive.

Executive water ring *See* Ring, Executive water.

Extender An additive to a polishing slurry, used to reduce the amount of cerium needed in the slurry.

Eyesize 1. In the boxing system, the *A* dimension. 2. In the datum system, the datum length.

Eyewire The rim of the frame that goes around the lenses.

F Often used in equations to denote lens refractive power in diopters. Alternate symbol for F is D.

Fiber ring *See* Ring, fiber.

Fining In surfacing, the process of bringing a generated lens surface to the smoothness needed so that it will be capable of being polished.

Finishing The process in the production of spectacles that begins with a pair of uncut lenses of the correct refractive power and ends with a completed pair of spectacles.

Finished lap tool *See* Tool, finished lap.

Finished lens *See* Lens, finished.

Fitting cross *See* Cross, fitting.

Flat-top bifocal *See* Bifocal, flat-top.

Focal point *See* Point, focal.

Focal power *See* Power, focal.

Form, minus cylinder The form a prescription takes when the value of the cylinder is expressed as a negative number.

Form, plus cylinder The form a prescription takes when the value of the cylinder is expressed as a positive number.

Formula, accurate sag The formula used to find sagittal depth, which states that $s = r - \sqrt{(r^2 - y^2)}$, where r is the radius of curvature of the surface and y is the semidiameter of the chord.

Formula, lensmaker's A formula used to find the dioptric power of a surface from radius of curvature or vice versa, which states that $D = (n' - n)/r$, where $D =$ lens refractive power in diopters, n' is the refractive index of the lens, and n is the refractive index of the media surrounding the lens. Now, since there is only one letter n in the equation, n is used to denote the refractive index of the lens instead of n'. For a lens surface in air this becomes $D = \dfrac{(n - 1)}{r}$.

Formula, sine-squared A formula used to obtain the "power" of an oblique cylinder in the 180-degree meridian.

Frame center distance *See* Distance, frame center.

Frame difference *See* Difference, frame

Frame, combination 1. A frame having a metal chassis with plastic top rims and temples. 2. A frame having some major parts of plastic construction and some of metal.

Frame PD *See* PD, frame.

Franklin bifocal *See* Bifocal, Franklin.

Front vertex power *See* Power, front vertex.

Full-field aspheric *See* Aspheric, full-field.

Gauge, ball A zero-in gauge consisting of a small metal ball of known diameter, mounted on a handle.

Gauge, bar A type of sag gauge that has three contact points on the end of three "legs," which pass through a bar and contact the lap or lens surface.

Gauge, bell A type of sag gauge used to measure spherical surfaces and having a domelike outer rim and a movable center pin. The circular rim contacts the spherical surface and the pin measures how steep or flat that surface is.

Gauge, center thickness A device used to measure the thickness of a semifinished lens while it is mounted on a lens surfacing block.

Gauge, lap One of a set of flat pieces of metal, usually brass, having one edge that is precision-cut to a known radius of curvature. The lap gauge is used as a standard and is placed against a surface in order to determine whether or not the surface in question is true to the standard.

Gauge, prism A device used to measure thickness differences at two opposite points on a lens blocked for surfacing. Using thickness differences, the amount of prism present in the lens is determined.

Gauge, saddle A type of zero-in gauge that uses a cylindrical pin of known length and is steadied on the generator ram with a saddlelike mounting.

Gauge, zero-in An object of known thickness, such as a ball or pin, which is used to assure an exact distance between generator wheel and lens center. The zero-in gauge is needed when using a manual or semi-automatic lens generator. Common types are a saddle gauge and a ball gauge.

Geometric center *See* Center, geometric

GCD Geometric center distance.

Generating The process of rapidly cutting the desired surface curvature onto a semifinished lens blank.

Generator marks *See* Marks, generator.

Generator ring *See* Ring, generator.

Generator wheel *See* Wheel, generator.

Geometric center distance *See* Distance, geometric center.

Glazing 1. The insertion of lenses into a spectacle frame. 2. The clogging of empty spaces between the exposed abrasive particles of an abrasive wheel, resulting in reduced grinding ability.

Grayness A lens surface defect caused by incomplete polishing.

Grind, bicentric Synonym for slab-off.

Gripper pad *See* Pad, gripper.

Hand edger *See* Edger, hand.

Hand stone *See* Stone, hand.

Height, seg The vertically measured distance from the lowest point on the lens or lens opening to the level of the top of the seg.

Hide-a-Bevel Tradename for an edge-grinding system that produces a shelf effect behind the bevel on thick-edged lenses.

Hollow tool *See* Tool, hollow.

Hydrometer An instrument used to measure the specific gravity of a liquid. In surfacing, the specific gravity of an abrasive slurry is measured in degrees Baumé.

Hyperopia Farsightedness.

Imbalance, vertical A differential vertical prismatic effect between the two eyes. At near this can be induced by right and left lenses of unequal powers when the wearer drops his or her eyes below the optical centers of the lenses.

Implant, intraocular lens A plastic lens placed inside the eye as a replacement for a crystalline lens that has lost its clarity.

Index, refractive The ratio of the speed of light in a medium (such as air) to the speed of light in another medium (such as glass).

Inset The amount of lens decentration nasally from the boxing (or datum) center of the frame's lens aperture. (Antonym: outset.)

Inset, blank seg The horizontal distance from the blank geometric center to the center of the multifocal segment.

Inset, net seg The amount of additional seg inset (or outset) required to produce a desired amount of horizontal prismatic effect at near, added to the normal seg inset required by the near PD.

Inset, seg The lateral distance from the major reference point to the geometric center of the segment.

Inset, total The amount the near segment must move from the boxing (or datum) center to place it at the near PD (near centration distance).

Intermediate The area of a trifocal lens between the distance viewing portion and the near portion.

Interpupillary distance *See* Distance, interpupillary.

Intraocular lens implant *See* Implant, intraocular lens.

Iseikonic lenses *See* Lenses, iseikonic.

Knife-edge A plus lens ground to an absolute minimum thickness such that the edge of the lens is so thin that it has a knifelike sharpness to it, i.e., an edge thickness of zero.

Laminated lens *See* Lens, laminated.

Lap A tool having a curvature matching that of the curvature desired for a lens surface. The lens surface is rubbed across the face of the tool and, with the aid of pads, abrasives, and polishes, the lens surface is brought to optical quality.

Lap cutter *See* Cutter, lap.

Lap gauge *See* Gauge, lap.

Lap tool *See* Tool, lap.

Layout The process of preparing a lens for blocking and edging or surfacing.

Layout marker *See* Marker.

Length, datum The horizontal width of a lens or lens opening as measured along the datum line.

Lens, blended myodisc A minus lens, lenticular in design, with the edges of the bowl blended so as to improve the cosmetic aspects of the lens.

Lens center locator *See* Locator, lens center.

Lens, cover A thin lens that is temporarily glued to the surface of a semifinished blank in order to protect the surface of the lens and facilitate accurate grinding, as in the case of a slab-off grind on a glass lens.

Lens, finished A spectacle lens that has been surfaced on both front and back to the needed power and thickness. A finished lens has not been edged for a spectacle frame, but is still in uncut form.

Lens, laminated An ophthalmic lens that is made up of more than one layer. Examples include polarized lenses, lenses that have a glass front and a polyurethane back surface, and plastic bifocal lenses made from front and back sections in order to bypass conventional surfacing procedures.

Lens measure *See* Measure, lens.

Lens, meniscus A lens having a convex front surface and a concave back surface.

Lens, mineral Synonym for glass lens.

Lens, minus cylinder form A lens ground such that it obtains its cylinder power from a difference in surface curvature between two back surface meridians.

Lens, minus lenticular A high-minus lens that is lenticular in design, having a central area containing the prescribed refractive power and a peripheral carrier that is plus in power for maximum edge thinning.

Lens, multidrop A high-plus, full-field aspheric lens in which the surface power drops rapidly as the edge of the lens is approached.

Lens, myodisc 1. Traditional definition: a high-minus lens that is lenticular in design, having a central area containing the prescribed refractive power and a peripheral carrier that is plano in power. The front curve is either plano in power or very close to plano. 2. General usage: any high-minus lens that is lenticular in design.

Lens, photochromic A lens that changes its transmission characteristics when exposed to light.

Lens, plus cylinder form A lens ground so that it obtains its cylinder power from a difference in surface curvature between two front surface meridians.

Lens, progressive-addition A lens having optics that vary in power gradually from the distance to near zones.

Lens, reverse-slab A slab-off lens that has base-down prism below the slab line, instead of base-up. Reverse-slab lenses are usually precast plastic.

Lens, single-vision A lens with the same sphere and/or cylinder power throughout the whole lens, as distinguished from a multifocal lens.

Lens size *See* Size, lens.

Lensmaker's formula *See* Formula, lensmaker's.

Lenses, iseikonic A lens pair with their curvatures and thicknesses specially chosen in order to produce a difference in image magnification between the left and right eyes. Also known as size lenses.

Lensmeter The instrument used for finding power and prism in spectacle lenses.

Lenticular A high-powered lens with the desired prescription power found only in the central portion. The outer carrier portion is ground so as to reduce edge thickness and weight in minus prescriptions and center thickness and weight in plus prescriptions.

Lenticular, aspheric A lenticular lens whose optically usable central portion has a front surface with a changing radius of curvature. The farther from the center of the lens, the longer the front surface radius of curvature becomes.

Lenticular, negative A high-minus lens that has had the peripheral portion flattened for the purpose of reducing weight and edge thickness. (Synonym: myodisc.)

Lenticular, spheric A lenticular lens whose optically usable central portion has a front surface that does not vary in curvature, but is entirely spherical.

Level, reading A synonym for reading depth. *See* Depth, reading.

Line, datum A line drawn parallel to and halfway between horizontal lines tangent to the lowest and highest edges of the lens.

Loading Occurs when plastic lens material gets in be-

tween the diamond grit of a generator or edger wheel, causing a glazing effect and decreased cutting ability.

Locator, lens center A device that finds and spots the blank geometric center of a round lens.

Major reference point *See* Point, major reference.

Manifold, coolant The part of the lens generator that divides the incoming coolant into separate streams of fluid, which are directed onto the grinding wheel for purposes of cooling, cleaning, and lubrication.

Marker A centering device used to position a lens accurately and stamp it with reference lines for use in lens blocking.

Mark, block A surface defect on a plastic lens caused by pressure from the block or heat from the blocking alloy.

Marks, generator A surface defect on a lens that consists of parallel, curved marks across the surface of the lens caused by the generator wheel.

Marks, swirl A lens surface defect that indicates that a larger grain of abrasive material was trapped in the pad and scratched the surface in a swirl pattern.

MBL Minimum between lenses.

MBS Minimum blank size. *See* Size, minimum blank.

Measure, lens A small, pocket-watch-sized instrument for measuring the surface curve of a lens. (Also called lens clock, lens gauge.)

Meniscus A lens form having one concave and one convex surface.

Meniscus lens *See* Lens, meniscus.

Meridian, axis The meridian of least power of a cylinder or spherocylinder lens; for a minus cylinder the least minus meridian, for a plus cylinder the least plus meridian.

Meridian, major One of two meridians in a cylinder or spherocylinder lens. These meridians are 90 degrees apart and correspond to the maximum and minimum powers in the lens.

Meridian, power The meridian of maximum power of a cylinder or spherocylinder lens; for a minus cylinder the most minus meridian, for a plus cylinder the most plus meridian.

Method, monocentric A surfacing technique for Franklin-style (Executive) lenses that grinds the lens with no seg inset and no seg drop.

Method, near-prism reduction A surfacing technique for Franklin-style (Executive) lenses that grinds the lens in such a way as to reduce the horizontal prismatic effect at the reading center caused by the distance lens.

Method, optically poor A surfacing technique for Franklin-style (Executive) lenses that grinds the lens with a seg drop, but in grinding for decentration completely ignores the location of the seg optical center.

Method, preferred (flat-top style) inset A surfacing technique for Franklin-style (Executive) lenses that grinds the lens with the customary seg inset and seg drop characteristic of flat-top bifocal lenses.

Method, zero inset A surfacing technique for Franklin-style (Executive) lenses that grinds the lens with no seg inset, but with the customary seg drop.

Mid-datum depth *See* Depth, mid-datum.

Minimum between lenses The datum system equivalent of the boxing distance between lenses.

Minus cylinder form *See* Form, minus cylinder.

Minus cylinder-form lens *See* Lens, minus cylinder form.

Minus lenticular lens *See* Lens, minus lenticular.

Mist collector *See* Collector, mist.

Monocentric method *See* Method, monocentric.

MRP Major reference point.

Multidrop lens *See* Lens, multidrop.

Multifocal A lens having a sector or sectors where the refractive power is different from the rest of the lens, such as bifocals or trifocals.

Mushroom tool *See* Tool, mushroom.

Myodisc *See* Lens, myodisc.

Myopia Nearsightedness.

Nasal The side of a lens or frame that is toward the nose (inner edge).

NBC Nominal base curve.

Near power *See* Power, near.

Near prism reduction method *See* Method, near prism reduction.

Near Rx The net power resulting from the combination of the add power and the distance power.

Net seg inset *See* Inset, net seg.

Neutralize To determine the refractive power of a lens.

Nominal base curve *See* Curve, nominal base.

OC Optical center.

OD Latin, *oculus dexter* (right eye).

Off-center blocking *See* Blocking, off-center.

Offset block adapter *See* Adapter, offset block.

On-center blocking *See* Blocking, on-center.

Opening, lens The portion of the spectacle frame that accepts the spectacle lens. (Synonym: lens aperture.)

Optical axis *See* Axis, optical.

Optical center *See* Center, optical.

Optically poor method *See* Method, optically poor.

Orange peel A surface defect on a lens that looks like the peel of an orange and is caused by watery polishing compound.

OS Latin, *oculus sinister* (left eye).

Outset The amount of lens decentration temporally from the boxing (or datum) center of the frame's lens aperture. (Antonym: inset.)

Overhang The portion of an off-center-blocked semifinished lens that is farthest away from the lens block and may prove to be problematic during the surfacing process.

Pad, gripper A friction-grip fining/polishing pad system that eliminates difficulty in stripping the pad from the tool. By using a special backing on the tool, the pad sticks to the backing.

Pad press *See* Press, pad.

Pad, tool-compensating A pad that lengthens the radius of curvature of a convex tool, flattening the tool and causing it to grind a slightly weaker minus curve.

Pan, hand A large, round metal tub containing a rotating spindle that spins concave or convex lap tools. Used to hand-work a lens surface.

Pantoscopic angle or tilt *See* Angle, pantoscopic.

PD Interpupillary distance; the distance from the center of one pupil to the center of the other.

PD, binocular The interpupillary distance specified as a single number, without reference to the center of the frame.

PD, distance The wearer's interpupillary distance specified for a situation equivalent to when the wearer is viewing a distant object.

PD, frame Synonym for distance between centers.

PD, monocular Half the interpupillary distance as specified for each eye individually with the center of the frame's bridge as a reference point.

PD, near The interpupillary distance as specified for a near viewing situation.

Pellon A brand of material used for polishing pads reputed to hold polish within the pad microstructure while still allowing the individual polishing particles to roll and polish.

Phoria The direction of the line of sight of one eye with reference to that of the partner eye when fusion is interrupted, as when one eye is covered.

Photochromic lens *See* Lens, photochromic.

Plano A term referring to a lens or lens surface having zero refracting power.

Pliers, chipping Pliers used to chip or break away the outer portions of an uncut or semifinished lens in order either to reduce its size or bring it into the rough shape needed to approximate the finished shape.

Plus cylinder form *See* Form, plus cylinder.

Plus-cylinder-form lens *See* Lens, plus cylinder form.

Point One-tenth of a millimeter of lens thickness.

Point, distance centration The British equivalent of the major reference point.

Point, focal A point to or from which light rays converge or diverge.

Point, major reference The point on a lens where the prism equals that called for by the prescription.

Polishing The last step in bringing a lens surface to its needed state of optical clarity.

Polishing rouge *See* Rouge, polishing.

Polish, water Synonym for an orange-peel lens surface defect.

Polycarbonate A strong, plastic lens material often used for safety eyewear.

Power cross *See* Cross, power

Power, actual   Synonym for true power.

Power, back vertex   The reciprocal of the distance in air from the rear surface of the lens to the second principal focus, which serves as a specific measure of the power of a lens.

Power, compensated   Back vertex power that has been converted to a 1.53-index frame of reference. Used for the purpose of finding a 1.53-index-referenced tool curve for a lens with a different index of refraction.

Power, effective   1. The vergence power of a lens at a designated position other than that occupied by the principal point of the lens itself. 2. That power lens required for a new position which will replace the original reference lens and yet maintain the same focal point.

Power, focal   A measure of the ability of a lens or lens surface to change the vergence of entering light rays.

Power, front vertex   The reciprocal of the distance in air from the front surface of a lens to the first principal focus.

Power, near   The sum of the distance power and the near add. (Synonym: near Rx.)

Power, nominal   1. An estimate of total lens power, calculated as the sum of front and back surface powers. (Not to be confused with nominal base curve.)

Power, refractive   The dioptric value that accurately describes the ability of a lens or lens surface to converge or diverge light. For a lens surface in air the refractive power is expressed as $D = \dfrac{(n - 1)}{r}$, where n is the refractive index of the lens material and r is the radius of the surface expressed in meters.

Power, true   The 1.53-index-referenced curvature of the base curve of a lens. True power is found by using a lens clock or sagometer (sag gauge) that is 1.53-index-referenced.

Precoat   A spray or brush-on liquid that, when applied to a lens, protects the surface during processing and/or makes the adhesion of a block to the lens possible.

Preferred (flat-top style) inset method   *See* Method, preferred (flat-top style) inset.

Prentice's rule   *See* Rule, Prentice's.

Press, pad   A machine used to press a pad onto a lap tool. There are two types of pad presses. One type presses a fining or polishing pad onto the lap tool with moderately heavy pressure. The second type uses extremely high pressure to press a metal pad onto a lap tool.

Prism   That part of an optical lens or system that deviates the path of light.

Prism axis   *See* Axis, prism.

Prism chart   *See* Chart, prism.

Prism gauge   *See* Gauge, prism.

Prism ring   *See* Ring, prism.

Prism, Rx   Prism in an ophthalmic lens prescription that has been called for by the prescribing doctor.

Prism table   *See* Table, prism.

Prism wedge   *See* Wedge, prism.

Prism, yoked   Base-down prism of equal value ground on both right and left lenses of a progressive or Franklin-style lens for the purpose of reducing lens thickness.

Progressive-addition lens   *See* Lens, progressive-addition.

Protractor, lens   A millimeter grid on a 360-degree protractor used in the lens centration process for both surfacing and finishing.

R-compensated segs   *See* Segs, R-compensated.

Raise, seg   1. The vertical distance from the major reference point to the top of the seg when the seg top is higher than the MRP. 2. The vertical distance from the datum line to the top of the seg when the seg top is higher than the datum line (laboratory usage). (Antonym: seg drop.)

Reading center   *See* Center, reading.

Reading depth   *See* Depth, reading.

Reading level   *See* Level, reading.

Reduced thickness   Thickness of a medium divided by its refractive index.

Refraction   1. The bending of light by a lens or optical system. 2. The process of determining the needed power of a prescription lens for an individual.

Refractive index   *See* Index, refractive.

Refractive power   *See* Power, refractive.

Removal, stock   The thickness of semifinished lens material that must be removed to bring the lens to its desired thickness.

Resolving (of prism)   The process of expressing a single prism as two prisms whose base directions are perpendicular to each other but whose combined effect equals that of the original prism.

Retroscopic angle or tilt   *See* Angle, retroscopic.

Reverse-slab lens   *See* Lens, reverse-slab.

Rim   *See* Eyewire.

Rimless   Having to do with frames (mountings) that hold lenses in place by some method other than eyewires. Most rimless mountings have two points of attachment per lens.

Ring, Executive water   A hollow, coolant-cooled mold, which casts blocking alloy into the shape of a fiber ring so that the glass Franklin-style (Executive) lens can be generated successfully.

Ring, fiber   A ring that fits around the glass block and against the lens during the generating process. Its purpose is to level the lens, assuring that no unwanted prism is ground in during generating.

Ring, generator   Synonym for fiber ring.

Ring, prism   A ring that fits around a surfacing block and is thick on one side and thin on the other. The ring causes the blocked lens to tilt by a known amount during the generating process in order to create a specific amount of prismatic effect. *See also* Wedge, prism.

Rings, prism blocking   Rings used in conjunction with 43-mm glass blocks for the purpose of molding prism into the block, eliminating the need for prism rings or prism wedges during generating.

Ring, Ultex A special fiber ring with a section cut out. This ring allows Ultex multifocal lenses to be generated even though the front surface of the lens segment "humps up."

Ring, water A hollow device that fits around the lens block on the surface blocker. It is connected to circulating coolant or cold running water and causes the lens block and alloy to chill, "freezing" the alloy.

Rouge, polishing Iron oxide used in the polishing of ophthalmic glass surfaces.

Rough-in An extra step in the fining of some lenses to remove roughness present after generating.

Roughing Using a lap tool and rough abrasive to generate a curve on a lens blank.

Round-seg bifocal *See* Bifocal, round-seg.

Rule, Prentice's A rule which states that the decentration of a lens in centimeters times the power of the lens is equal to the prismatic effect ($\Delta = cD$).

Rx prism *See* Prism, Rx.

Saddle gauge *See* Gauge, saddle.

Safety bevel *See* Bevel, safety.

Sag A synonym or abbreviation for sagittal depth. *See also* Depth, sagittal.

Sagittal depth *See* Depth, sagittal.

Sag tables *See* Tables, sag.

Score To cut parallel grooves into the surface of a lap tool at regular intervals for the purpose of allowing slurry to flow under a lens more easily when fining on the bare surface of the lap tool.

Scratch A furrowed-out line that has jagged edges.

Seg *See* Segment.

Seg clock *See* Clock, seg.

Seg depth *See* Depth, seg.

Seg drop *See* Drop, seg.

Seg height *See* Height, seg.

Seg inset *See* Inset, seg.

Seg optical center *See* Center, seg optical.

Seg width *See* Width, seg.

Segment (seg) An area of a spectacle lens with power differing from that of the main portion.

Segs, dissimilar A method of correcting vertical imbalance at near that uses different bifocal segment styles for the right and left eyes.

Segs, R-compensated A method for correcting vertical imbalance at near that uses ribbon-style bifocal segments which have been modified so that the segment optical center for one lens is high in one segment, and low in the other.

Semidiameter Diameter divided by 2. In ophthalmic optics, semidiameter refers to half of the chord for the arc of a given surface and is used in calculating the sagittal depth of the surface.

Semifinished blank *See* Blank, semifinished.

Semifinished lap tool *See* Tool, semifinished lap.

Shop, back Synonym for surfacing laboratory.

Shop, front Synonym for finishing laboratory.

Simplified on-center blocking *See* Blocking, simplified on-center.

Sine-squared formula *See* Formula, sine-squared.

Single-vision lens *See* Lens, single-vision.

Size, lens 1. In the boxing system, the *A* dimension of a lens or lens opening. 2. In the datum system, the datum length of a lens.

Size lenses *See* Lenses, iseikonic.

Size, minimum blank The smallest lens blank that can be used for a given prescription lens and frame combination.

Slab-off Grinding a portion of a lens so as to add a second optical center. Often used to create vertical prism in the lower portion of one lens for the purpose of alleviating vertical imbalance at near.

Sleek A furrowed-out line on a lens, which resembles a scratch but whose edges are smooth instead of jagged.

Slurry Particles suspended in a liquid. In surfacing, abrasive particles are suspended in the fining and polishing slurries.

Sphere A lens having a single refractive power in all meridians.

Spherical equivalent *See* Equivalent, spherical.

Spheric lenticular *See* Lenticular, spheric.

Spherocylinder The combination of sphere and cylinder powers into a single lens.

Spotting The placing of spots on a lens with a lensmeter in such a manner that the lens will be oriented correctly for axis and positioned for major reference point and horizontal meridian locations.

Standard alignment *See* Alignment, standard.

Stick, trueing A long, rectangular abrasive stick that can be (1) held against certain areas of a spinning spherical lap tool for the purpose of bringing that tool back to its proper curvature, or (2) held against an edger or generator wheel to expose more of the diamond-cutting surface and "sharpen" the wheel. There are different types of abrasive sticks for different purposes.

Stock, lens 1. An inventory of lenses. 2. The material from which a semifinished blank is made, as in the amount of stock removal required to bring the blank to its needed thickness.

Stock removal *See* Removal, stock.

Stone 1. An abrasive grinding wheel. 2. To sharpen the cutting ability of a grinding wheel by honing it with an abrasive stick.

Stone, hand Synonym for hand edger.

Surfacing The process of creating the prescribed refractive power, prism, and major reference point location on a lens by generating the required curves and bringing the surface to a polished state.

Surfacing charts *See* Tables, surfacing.

Surfacing tables *See* Tables, surfacing.

Swarf Accumulated waste material present as a result of the grinding process.

Swirl marks *See* Marks, swirl.

System, boxing A system of lens measurement based on the enclosure of a lens by horizontal and vertical tangents to form a box or rectangle.

System, datum A system of lens measurement that defines the lens or eyesize as being the width of the lens along the datum line.

System, GOMAC A European Economic Community standard incorporating portions of both the boxing and datum systems.

Table, Fry's A table developed by Glenn Fry to determine the appropriate base curve for a lens of any given refractive power.

Table, prism A table used to convert combined horizontal and vertical prismatic effects into a single, new prism. Amount is expressed in prism diopters and base direction in degrees.

Tables, sag A set of tables used for finding sagittal depth when surface power and lens diameter are known.

Tables, surfacing Tables supplied by a lens manufacturer for the purpose of helping the surfacing laboratory accurately determine the tool curves and lens thicknesses needed in order to grind lenses to the specified back vertex power.

Take-off Synonym for stock removal.

Tangent For a right triangle, the ratio of the side opposite the angle considered to the side adjacent:

$$\tan = \frac{\text{opp}}{\text{adj}}.$$

Template cutter *See* Cutter, template.

Temporal The area of a lens or frame that is toward the temples (outer edge).

Tool, compensated lap A surfacing lap tool that has been cut with a radius of curvature so as to allow for a correctly curved surface after the lap pad has been applied to the lap.

Tool curve *See* Curve, tool.

Tool, finished lap A lap tool that has been purchased from the supplier after having already been cut to the correct curvature.

Tool, hollow A spherical concave tool used to fine and polish spherical convex lens surfaces. It is called a hollow tool because the concave surface on the top of the tool appears to be hollowed out. This type of tool is used on sphere machines only.

Tool, lap A tool used for fining and polishing lens surfaces. The tool used must have a surface identical in curvature to that of the lens for which it is to be used; that is, if the lens surface is convex, the tool must be concave.

Tool, mushroom A spherical convex lap tool used to fine and polish spherical concave lens surfaces. This type of tool is shaped like a mushroom and is used on sphere machines only.

Tool, semifinished lap A lap tool with an approximate base and cross curve molded onto the tool. A semifinished tool with rough curves close to the needed finished curves is chosen and then the tool is cut to the desired curvature.

Tool, uncompensated lap A surfacing lap tool that has been cut without taking lap pad thickness into consideration. It is of the correct curvature without a pad, but will be slightly off with fining or polishing pads in place.

Toric A surface having separate curves at right angles to one another.

Toric base curve *See* Curve, toric base.

Toric transposition *See* Transposition, toric.

Total inset *See* Inset, total.

Transposition, toric The process of transposing a prescription from the form in which it is written to another form, such as from a plus to a minus cylinder form.

Trifocals Lenses having three areas of viewing, each with its own focal power. Usually the upper portion is for distance viewing, the lower for near, and the middle or intermediate portion for distance in between.

True 1. To reshape the cutting surface of a worn grinding wheel so that it cuts at the angles and in the manner originally intended. 2. To bring a pair of glasses into a position of correct alignment. 3. In surfacing, when using a hand pan, a step following roughing and smoothing, using a somewhat finer grade of abrasive in order to bring the lens to an exact curve.

True base curve *See* Curve, true base.

Trueing *See* True.

True power *See* Power, true.

Trueing disk *See* Disk, trueing.

Trueing stick *See* Stick, trueing.

Ultex ring *See* Ring, Ultex.

Ultraviolet Rays having a wavelength somewhat shorter than those at the violet end of the visible spectrum.

Uncompensated lap tool *See* Tool, uncompensated.

Uncut A lens that has been surfaced on both sides but not yet edged for a frame.

V-bevel *See* Bevel, V.

Vertex distance *See* Distance, vertex.

Vertex power allowance *See* Allowance, vertex power.

Vertical imbalance *See* Imbalance, vertical.

Water polish *See* Polish, water.

Water ring *See* Ring, water.

Wave A defect in lens surface curvature, which causes a slight, irregular variation in the surface power.

Wedge, prism A wedge of known thickness and angle placed at one side of a chucked lens for the purpose of causing the lens to tilt, resulting in a specific amount of prismatic effect. *See also* Ring, prism.

Wheel, electroplated An abrasive wheel made by electrolytically depositing metal on the wheel in such a manner as to encompass diamond particles. This type of wheel is often used to grind plastic lenses.

Wheel, generator A cup-shaped wheel with a diamond impregnated rim, small cutter blades, or both, that is used to rapidly cut or grind a specifically curved surface onto a lens.

Wheel, roughing An edger or cribber wheel that rapidly cuts a lens to near its finished size.

Width, seg The size of a bi- or trifocal segment measured horizontally across its widest section.

Yoked prism *See* Prism, yoked.

Younger blended myodisc *See* Lens, blended myodisc.

Younger Seamless Trade name for a blended bifocal made by Younger Optics.

Zero-cut A generator sweep across a lens surface with the generator set for zero stock removal. The purpose of a zero-cut is to smooth out the lens surface, or to remove unwanted prism. Unwanted prism will show up as a partial cut across the lens surface.

Zero-in gauge *See* Gauge, zero-in.

Zero inset method *See* Method, zero inset.

Zone, blended The blurred area between distance and near areas on an "invisible" bifocal. (Not to be confused with the progressive zone of a progressive-add lens.)

Zone, progressive That portion of a progressive-addition lens between the distance and near portions where lens power is gradually increasing.

Answers to Questions and Problems

Chapter 1

1. +2.50 D
2. −10.00 D
3. d
4. b
5. 2.8 prism diopters
6. 5 mm
7. c
   d
8. a
9. 4.5 Base 207
   4.5 Base 27 DN
10. 3.25 Base 107 DN
11. 1.50 Base 181
12. Induce Rx prism by moving the optical center of the uncut lens into the prism position. Otherwise, grind prism onto a semifinished blank during the surfacing process.
13. 5.38 Base 158
14. 3.35 Base 153
15. **a.** 4 Base at 150 Down
       2 Base Down and 3.5 Base In
    b. 4 Base at 150 Down
       2 Base Down and 3.5 Base Out
16. 3.90 Base 140
    3.90 Base 140 Up
    3.90 Base 40
    3.90 Base 40 Up
17. 2.50 Base 233
    2.50 Base 53 Down
    2.50 Base 307
    2.50 Base 127 Down
18. 7.81 Base 140
    7.81 Base 140 Up
    7.81 Base 320
    7.81 Base 140 Down
19. 5.00 Base 127
    5.00 Base 127 Up
    5.00 Base 307
    5.00 Base 127 Down
20. 5.4 Base 146 Down
    5.4 Base 326
    4.1 Base 101 Down
    4.1 Base 281
21. 5.6 Base 10 Down
    5.6 Base 190
    4.6 Base 60 Down
    4.6 Base 240
22. 4.24 Base 45 DN
    4.24 Base 225
    4.24 Base 45 UP
    4.24 Base 45
23. 2.61 Base 107 DN
    2.61 Base 287
    2.61 Base 107 UP
    2.61 Base 107
24. 4.93 Base 60 DN
    4.93 Base 240
    4.70 Base 115 UP
    4.70 Base 115
25. 1.82 Base 74 UP
    1.82 Base 74
    1.82 Base 74 DN
    1.82 Base 254
26. 4.07 Base 11 UP
    4.07 Base 11
    4.32 Base 10 DN
    4.32 Base 190
27. 4.70 Base 25 UP
    4.70 Base 25
    4.25 Base 28 DN
    4.25 Base 208
28. 5.25 Base 31 UP
    5.25 Base 31
    5.25 Base 49 DN
    5.25 Base 229
29. 1.25 Base 53 DN
    1.25 Base 233
    1.25 Base 101 DN
    1.25 Base 281

30. 1.50 Base 149 DN
 1.50 Base 329
 1.50 Base 135 UP
 1.50 Base 135
31. 3.25 Base 171 UP
 3.25 Base 171
 3.37 Base 153 DN
 3.37 Base 333

Chapter 2

1. a. 67 mm
 b. 59 mm
2. a
3. 54 mm
4. 50 mm
5. 60 mm
6. 54 mm
7. b. plano
8. b
9. c
10. +9.00 D
11. +9.75 D
12. +7.75 D
13. +4.00 D
14. +5.25 D
15. +4.43 D
16. +3.94 D
17. +3.00 D
18. 6.50 D
19. R +8.50 D
 L +4.50 D
20. R +10.50 D
 L +10.50 D
21. R +2.50 D
 L +2.50 D
22. R +6.50 D
 L +6.50 D
23. 72 mm
24. 63 mm
25. a. 72 or 74 mm
 b. 61 mm
26. See Chapter 2 text and Figures 2-2 and 2-3.
27. Raise the seg and increase the near PD.
28. No. Both will give identical results, because the lens is a minus lens.
29. No

Chapter 3

1. The prescription could contain prescribed prism.
2. 1.0 Base 180
3. 1.8 Base 0
4. a. R: 4.50 Base 180
 L: 3.90 Base 0
 b. 67 mm
5. a. 2.8 Base 154
 2.37 Base 162 DN
 b. MBS = 63 mm

6. R: 1.095 Base 0
 L: 1.575 Base 180

Questions 7–14 assume that the lens is marked with the convex side up.

7. The marked cross is 2.5 mm to the right of the blank geometric center.
8. The marked cross is 3 mm to the left of the blank geometric center.
9. The marked cross is 4 mm to the right of the blank geometric center.
10. The marked cross is 3.5 mm to the left of the blank geometric center.
11. The marked cross is 3.5 mm to the right of the blank geometric center.
12. The marked cross is 3.5 mm to the left of the blank geometric center.
13. The marked cross is 2 mm to the right of the blank geometric center.
14. The marked cross is 5.5 mm to the left of the blank geometric center.
15. Prism amount 0.62
 Prism base direction
 R: 180
 L: 0
16. Prism amount 0.45
 Prism base direction
 R: 0
 L: 180
17. Prism amount 0.3
 Prism base direction
 R: 180
 L: 0
18. Prism amount 0.7
 Prism base direction
 R: 0
 L: 180
19. Prism amount 0.34
 Prism base direction
 R: 180
 L: 0
20. Prism amount 0.53
 Prism base direction
 R: 180
 L: 0
21. Prism amount 0.50
 Prism base direction
 R: 0
 L: 180
22. Prism amount 0.14
 Prism base direction
 R: 180
 L: 0
23. a. 0 mm
 b. R: 1.2 Base 0
 L: 1.0 Base 180

   c. 63 mm
   d. 55 mm
24. a. 0 mm
   b. R: 1.0 Base 0
      L: 0.875 Base 180
   c. 67 mm
   d. 57 mm
25. a. 0 mm
   b. R: 1.87 Base 0
      L: 1.75 Base 180
   c. 63 mm
   d. 55 mm
26. a. 0 mm
   b. R: 2.25 Base 180
      L: 2.50 Base 0
   c. 73.5 mm
   d. 67 mm
27. a. 0 mm
   b. R: 1.75 Base 180
      L: 1.40 Base 0
   c. 72 mm
   d. 61 mm
28. a. R: 4.5 mm
      L: 4.5 mm
   b. R: 3.35 Base 0
      L: 2.4 Base 180
   c. 64 mm
   d. 55 mm
29. a. R: 5 mm
      L: 5 mm
   b. R: 2.125 Base 152
      L: 2.46 Base 156 DN
   c. 72 mm
   d. 62 mm
30. a. R: 4.5 mm
      L: 4.5 mm
   b. R: 4.15 Base 166
      L: 4.85 Base 168 DN
   c. 70 mm
   d. 61 mm
31. a. R: 4 mm
      L: 5.6 mm
   b. R: 1.00 Base 180
      L: 0.15 Base 0
   c. 79 mm
   d. 67 mm

Chapter 4
1. Seg drop = 1 mm
Seg inset = 2 mm
Cylinder axis = 35
Prism = none
With the lens convex side up, the marked cross is centered 1 mm above and 2 mm to the left of the center of the seg top.
2. Seg inset = 3 mm
Seg drop = 2 mm

Cylinder axis = 65
Prism = none
With the lens convex side up, the marked cross is centered 3 mm above and 2 mm to the right of the center of the seg top.
3. Seg drop = 0 mm
Seg inset = 1.5 mm
Cylinder axis = 110
Prism = none
With the lens convex side up, the marked cross is centered 0 mm above and 1.5 mm to the left of the center of the seg top.
4. Seg drop = 4 mm
Seg inset = 1 mm
Cylinder axis = 15
Prism = none
With the lens convex side up, the marked cross is centered 4 mm above and 1 mm to the left of the center of the seg top.
5. Seg drop = 4.5 mm
Seg inset = 1.5 mm
Cylinder axis = 120
Prism = 1 Base 0
With the lens convex side up, the marked cross is centered 4.5 mm above and 1.5 mm to the right of the center of the seg top.
6. Seg drop = 4 mm
Seg inset = 1 mm
Cylinder axis = 175
Prism = 2.24 Base 297 or 117 DN
With the lens convex side up, the marked cross is centered 4 mm above and 1 mm to the left of the center of the seg top.
7. Seg drop = 1 mm
Seg inset = 1.5 mm
Cylinder axis = 167
Prism = 3.58 Base 335 or 155 DN
With the lens convex side up, the marked cross is centered 1 mm above and 1.5 mm to the left of the center of the seg top.
8. With the lens convex side up, the marked crosses are centered 4 mm above and 1.5 mm to the left of the center of the seg top.
Cylinder axis = 17
Prism axis = Base 0
9. With the lens convex side up, the marked crosses are centered 4 mm above and 1.5 to the left of the center of the seg top.
Cylinder axis = 75
Prism axis = Base 117
10. With the lens convex side up, the marked crosses are centered 4.5 mm above and 2 mm to the left of the center of the seg top.
Cylinder axis = 35
Prism axis = Base 153
11. With the lens convex side up, the MRP is 1.75 mm

(really 2 mm) and 1.5 mm to the right of the center of the seg top.

12. With the lens convex side up, the MRP is 0.5 mm above and 1.5 mm to the left of the center of the seg top.
13. With the lens convex side up, the MRP is 4 mm above and 1.5 mm to the right of the center of the seg top.
14. With the lens convex side up, the MRP is .5 mm above and 1.5 mm to the right of the center of the seg top.
15. With the lens convex side up, the MRP is 2 mm above and 2.5 mm to the right of the center of the seg top.
16. With the lens convex side up, the MRP is 2 mm above and 2.5 mm to the left of the center of the seg top.
17. With the lens convex side up, the MRP is 1.25 mm (really 1 mm) above and 2 mm to the right of the center of the seg top.
18. With the lens convex side up, the MRP is 1.25 mm (really 1 mm) above and 2 mm to the left of the center of the seg top.
19. With the lens convex side up, the marked cross is centered 6 mm above and 7 mm to the left of the center of the seg top.
Cylinder axis = none
Prism = 1.5 Base 0
20. With the lens convex side up, the marked crosses are centered 5 mm above and 6 mm to the right of the center of the seg top.
Cylinder axis = 90
Prism = 1.6 Base 180
21. With the lens convex side up, the marked crosses are centered 3 mm above and 6 mm to the left of the center of the seg top.
Cylinder axis = 60
Prism = 2.1 Base 0
22. With the lens convex side up, the marked crosses are centered 2 mm above and 7 mm to the right of the center of the seg top.
Cylinder axis = 30
Prism = 3.5 Base 0
23. With the lens convex side up, the marked crosses are centered 3 mm above and 6 mm to the left of the center of the seg top.
Cylinder axis = 90
Prism = 0.3 Base 180
24. With the lens convex side up, the marked crosses are centered 4.5 mm above and 7 mm to the right of the center of the seg top.
Cylinder axis = 80
Prism = 0.8 Base 0
25. With the lens convex side up, the marked crosses are centered 5 mm above and 6 mm to the left of the center of the seg top.

Cylinder axis = 20
Prism = 1.3 Base 146 DN

Chapter 5
1. False
2. d
3. a
4. b
5. d
6. True
7. b
8. Seg drop = 4
Seg inset = 1.5
9. Seg drop = 1
Scg inset = 2
10. Seg drop = 0
Seg inset = 1.5
11. Seg drop = 6.5
Seg inset = 1.5
12. Seg drop = 0.5
Seg inset = 2
13. Seg drop = 3
Seg inset = 1.5
14. Seg drop = 3.5
Seg inset = 1.5
15. Seg drop = 4.5
Seg inset = 1.5
16. Seg drop = 1.75
Seg inset = 1.5
17. Seg drop = 0.5
Seg inset = 1.5
18. Seg drop = 4
Seg inset = 1.5
19. Seg drop = 1.75
Seg inset = 1.5
20. Seg drop = 2
Seg inset = 2.5
21. Seg drop = 2
Seg inset = 2.5
22. Seg drop = 1.25
Seg inset = 2
23. Seg drop = 1.25
Seg inset = 2

Chapter 6
1. c
2. a
3. a
4. d
5. a and b
6. d and e
7. d
8. a
9. False
10. d
11. a and b
12. d

13. To determine the horizontal location of the near optical center
14. It is possible to view the reflected image of a straight fluorescent bulb in the front surface of the Franklin-style lens. The seg optical center is located at the place where the two halves of the reflected image form one straight line.
15. **a.** The distance and seg optical centers are at the same place. Both are located on the seg line and in the middle of the line.
    b. The seg optical center is on the line and in the middle of the line. The distance optical center is 4 mm above the seg optical center.
    c. The seg optical center is on the line and in the middle of the line. The distance optical center is 4 mm above the seg optical center and 2 mm outward (temporally).
16. The optically questionable method is to treat the lens almost like a single-vision lens that has been blocked on center. The location of the seg optical center is ignored and decentration prism is ground. This causes the distance PD to come out as ordered, but the near PD may end up being considerably larger than the distance PD.
17. Mark the lens for cylinder axis at the center of the seg line.
18. Seg drop = 6.5 mm
    Seg inset = zero
19. Seg drop = 5.5 mm
    Seg inset = zero
20. Seg drop = 6.5 mm
    Seg inset = zero
    Right lens prism Base 0
    Left lens prism Base 180
21. Seg drop = 5.5 mm
    Seg inset = zero
    Right lens prism 2.36 Base 32
    Left lens prism 1.95 Base 40 DN
22. Seg drop = 5 mm
    Seg inset = 1 mm
23. Seg drop = 1.5 mm raise
    Seg inset = 1.5 mm
24. Seg drop = 3 mm
    Seg inset = 2.5 mm
    R: prism 5.38 Base 158
    L: prism 5.75 Base 162
25. Seg drop = 7.5 mm
    Seg inset = 2 mm
    R: prism 3.00 Base 24
    L: prism 2.69 Base 22 DN
26. R: 1.3   L: 1.3
    R: Base 0 L: Base 180
    Resulting near PD = 77
27. R: 3.08   L: 3.41
    R: Base 180   L: Base 0
    Resulting near PD = 74

28. R: 0.825   L: 1.65
    R: Base 0   L: Base 180
    Resulting near PD = 75
29. R: 3.25   L: 3.25
    R: 161   L: 163 DN
    Resulting near PD = 75

Chapter 7
1. **a.** +8.062 D
   b. −6.00 D
   c. +8.17 D
2. Nominal power = +8.25 D
   True power = +8.17 D
   Refractive power = +10.79 D
3. Nominal power = +6.25 D
   True power = +6.18 D
   Refractive power = +5.81 D
4. True power = +10.17 D
   Anticipated nominal power = +10.25 D
5. **a.** −6.63 D
   b. a −8.62 D tool
6. **a.** −4.35 D
   b. a 6.37 D tool
7. 7.50 D tool
8. $K = 1.062$
9. 4.90 mm
10. 3.20 mm
11. Chord diameter = 60 mm
    Tool curve = 5.75
    Center thickness = 9.3 − 5.0 + 1.5 = 5.8 mm
12. Chord diameter = 58 mm
    Tool curve = 5.00
    Center thickness = 7.2 − 4.0 + 2.3 = 5.5 mm
13. Chord diameter = 41 mm
    Tool curve = 4.50/5.00
    Center thickness = 5.05 − 1.8 + 1.6 = 4.85 mm
14. $r = (n − 1)/D$

    $= (1.53 − 1)/4.25$

    $= 0.1247$ m or 124.7 mm

    $s = r − \sqrt{r^2 − y^2}$

    $= 124.7 − \sqrt{124.7^2 − 25^2}$

    $= 124.7 − 122.2$

    $= 2.5$ mm

15. **a.** Compensated power = −4.75 D
        Tool curve = 6.75
    b. 6.25 mm
16. 0.828

Chapter 8
1. **a.** Thickness = $K(D)$ + (edge or center thickness), where K is a constant that depends on lens size

   b. An increase in center thickness of 0.5 mm for each prism diopter
2. 8.7 mm
3. **a.** $(1.0 \times 5) + 2 = 7$ mm
   b. $7 + (4/2) = 9$ mm
4. 5.9 mm
5. 0.26 Base 180
6. 2.4 mm
7. 4.05 mm difference
8. 1.8 Base In
9. a
10. The lens will be thicker temporally by 4 mm.
11. The lens will be thickened temporally by 2 mm, which means that since the temporal edge limits how thin the lens can be ground, the lens can be thinned in the center (overall, really) by 2 mm.
12. c
13. c
14. c
15. a
16. c
17. b
18. b

Chapter 9
1. False
2. b
3. c
4. a
5. b
6. True
7. a
8. c
9. False (Too much pressure will distort plastic lenses.)
10. True
11. a and d
12. True
13. b
14. a
15. a and d
16. False
17. b and c
18. Extra long centers are sometimes used in the center hole only. This allows the lens to be held in place by the center pin alone, permitting the lens to rotate freely during fining and polishing. Some operators maintain that this rotation produces a sphere that is better optically.
19. **a.** True
   b. True
20. 58 mm
21. False
22. The lens segment stands away from the lens (or is cut into the lens, in the case of Franklin-style lenses). Therefore the segment can cause the lens

to tilt in the blocking process if it contacts the block surface, resulting in prism in the lens.
23. When the lens has already been surfaced once and one wants to resurface the lens. This would be done basically to protect the lens from heat and stress, which might result in a wavy lens.
24. d

Chapter 10
1. d
2. b
3. d
4. a
5. d
6. b
7. b
8. d
9. b
10. False
11. b and d
12. d
13. d
14. a
15. b
16. e
17. a
18. False
19. a and b
20. b and c
21. False
22. True
23. It is necessary to make an individualized chart in order to use the 3-inch wheel. Lenses must be ground for every power and the curves recorded. One starts, for example, from $+11.00$ D and goes in 0.25 D steps up to -11.00 D. Thus a homemade chart is created that can be trusted as being accurate.
24. True
25. False
26. False
27. True
28. a
29. b
30. a
31. False
32. False
33. True

Chapter 11
1. 3.00 mm
2. $r = 47.72$ mm; 11.11 D compensated
3. mushroom and hollow
4. b
5. **a.** 7.04 D
   b. 4.27 mm

6. **a.** 75.26 mm

   b. $D = \dfrac{1.53 - 1}{0.07526} = 7.04 \text{ D}$

7. **a.** cast iron
   b. plastic
   c. aluminum
8. a
9. False
10. False
11. b
12. False
13. b
14. False
15. 81.5 mm
16. c
17. 60.1 mm
18. 8.82 D
19. True
20. 8.19 D

Chapter 12

1. False
2. a
3. d
4. a
5. b
6. b
7. b
8. c
9. False
10. a
11. a
12. b
13. d
14. b
15. e
16. True
17. d
18. c
19. d
20. e
21. False
22. b
23. c
24. c
25. d
26. True
27. False
28. c
29. b
30. True
31. e
32. c
33. b
34. a
35. e
36. True
37. d
38. b
39. False
40. **a.** crib
    b. off-set block
    c. off-set holes on regular block
41. b
42. To extend the generator range for CR-39 lenses
43. Pellon
44. iron oxide
45. False
46. chemical action
    mechanical abrasion
    thermal flow
47. diamond-impregnated pads
    diamond-impregnated lap tool facings
    scoring of cast iron lap tools
48. rouge, iron oxide
49. Extend slurry life.
    Decrease polishing time.
    Allow for less slurry concentration.
    Reduce foaming (somewhat).
50. A pad on a tool, on which nonadhesive pads can be placed.
51. No, because the curve must be exceptionally accurate. Normally, fining is done on diamond tools if polyurethane polishing pads are used.

Chapter 13

1. True
2. False
3. True
4. True
5. c
6. d
7. d
8. a
9. a
10. e

Chapter 14

1. d
2. chord diameter = $49 + [0.75(47 + 19 - 62)]$ = 52 mm
3. **a.** $+6.50 - 0.62 = +5.88 \text{ D}$
   b. $+6.50 - 1.32 = +5.13 \text{ D}$
4. d
5. c
6. False
7. False
8. c
9. R: $+10.80$ D (or $+10.75$ D)
   L: $+10.25$ D
10. R: $+12.35 \ -2.28 \times 75$
    L: $+12.93 \ -2.93 \times 105$

11. b and c
12. a
13. c
14. 56.25 mm
15. 5.42 D
16. **a.** 66 mm
    b. 58 mm
    c. 64 mm
    d. 62 mm
17. $+13.51 -2.30 \times 015$ or $+13.50 -2.25 \times 015$ rounded off

Chapter 15

1. False
2. c
3. False
4. c
5. d
6. c
7. a
8. b
9. c
10. a
11. a
12. c
13. 1.50 Base Down on both right and left lenses

Chapter 16

1. **a.** (2)
   b. (2)
2. d
3. **a.** $1.5 \times c = 3.00$
   $c = 0.5$ cm $= 5$ mm
   Direction is nasal
   b. Net seg inset $= 7$ mm per lens
   c. 50 mm
4. A flat-top 35
5. b
6. **a.** (4)
   b. (1)
7. 1.8 prism diopters Base In
8. 1.2 Base Out
9. 1.4 Base In
10. 1.2 Base In
11. **a.** 4.5 mm of net seg inset per lens.
    b. Right eye: 0.2 mm of net seg outset
    Left eye: 0.2 mm of net seg inset
    (Rounded, both amount to zero net seg inset.)
    c. Right eye: 4.5 mm of net seg inset
    Left eye: 4 mm of net seg inset
12. **a.** Right lens: The net seg inset is 7 mm. The blank geometric center is decentered 2 mm inward.
    Left lens: The net seg inset is 6.5 mm. The blank geometric center is decentered 1.5 mm inward.
    b. Right lens: The net seg inset is 13 mm outward. The left blank is used. This gives a 5-mm seg outset to start with. The blank geometric center is decentered 8 mm more outward.
    Left lens: The net seg inset is 14 mm outward. The right blank is used. This also gives a 5-mm seg outset to start with. The blank geometric center is decentered 9 mm more outward. Cut out will depend upon frame size and blank size.

Chapter 17

1. The reading depth is 5 below the seg line. Since the seg drop is 4 mm, the reading depth is 9 mm below the MRP.
2. **a.** $+4.00$ D
   b. $+3.00$ D
   c. -6.50 D
   d. -3.50 D
   e. -2.75 D
   f. -1.75 D
   g. -1.27 D
   h. -7.08 D
   i. -3.75 D
   j. -4.25 D
   k. $+0.08$ D
   l. -0.88 D
3. **a.** 3.2 Base Up
   b. 2.4 Base Up
   c. 5.2 Base Down
   d. 2.8 Base Down
   e. 2.2 Base Down
   f. 1.4 Base Down
   g. 1.02 Base Down
   h. 5.66 Base Down
   i. 3 Base Down
   j. 3.4 Base Down
   k. 0.06 Base Up
   l. 0.70 Base Down
4. d
5. a
6. b
7. **a.** (2)
   b. (2)
   c. (1)
8. Find the reading depth by adding the seg drop to 5 mm.
   Drop $= 48/2 - 20 = 4$ mm
   Reading depth $= 9$ mm
   Multiply 0.9 by the dioptric imbalance of 3.00 D, which is 2.7 prism diopters. Use a slab-off prescription. In a Younger precast lens this would be placed on the left eye. In a fused-glass or regular plastic lens this would be on the right eye.
9. 3.04 prism diopters
10. Needed seg separation is 6 mm. The higher seg must be on the left eye. The wearer should not be overcorrected, but can be undercorrected. Two flat-top 35s are the most logical, one with the seg OC

on the line (on the left eye), the other with the seg OC 5 mm below the seg line.

11. the right eye
12. There is 2.4 prism diopters Base Up before the left eye (or Base Down before the right) of vertical imbalance.
13. $7.5 \times 0.9 = 6.75$ prism diopters. Reverse slab is on the left lens.
14. The seg centers must be $c = \Delta/\text{add power} = 1.50/2 = 0.75$ cm or approximately 8 mm apart. Two segs whose centers are 8 mm apart are the 22 round and the 38 round. The 38 round would go on the right eye.
15. The imbalance is 8.28 Base Down right eye, or 8.28 Base Up left eye.
16. The imbalance is 3.38 Base Up right eye, or 3.38 Base Down left eye.
17. The imbalance is 5.83 Base Down right eye, or 5.83 Base Up left eye.

Chapter 18
1. a, b, c, d, e
2. False
3. c
4. b
5. False

Chapter 19
1. b
2. b, c, d, g, h, i
3. d
4. e
5. a
6. False
7. A 1-inch steel ball is dropped from 50 inches onto the front surface of the lens.

Index